MOLECULAR PATHOLOGY: ADVANCES AND TECHNIQUES

Levan Maglakelidze

ALLIED
HEALTH
PRESS

Molecular Pathology: Advances and Techniques

Author: **Levan Maglakelidze**

Allied Health Press
4164 Lakeshore Road
Burlington ON L7L 1A4
Canada
www.alliedhealthpress.com
Email: orders@arclereducation.com

ISBN: 978-1-77956-839-7

ABOUT THE AUTHOR

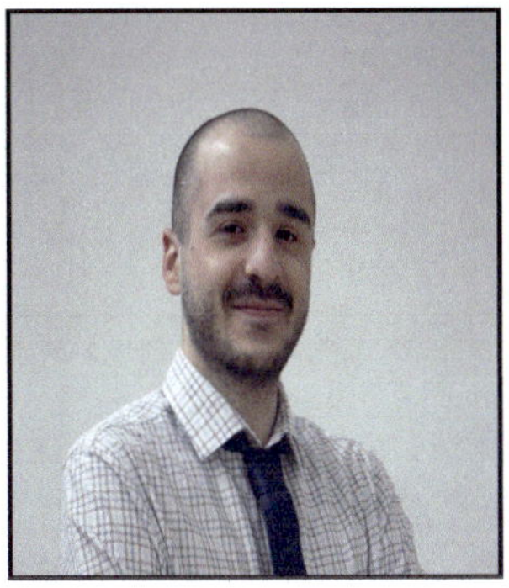

Levan Maglakelidze holds an M.D. from David Tvildiani Medical University, Tbilisi, with a clinical background in intensive care, cardiac and neurosurgical assistance, and psychiatry. He is currently working as a Research Study Coordinator at Evexi Clinic, Tbilisi, contributing to international clinical trials with organizations including ICON, Merck, and PPD. He also serves as an invited lecturer in American medical programs at the University of Georgia. His research interests include psychiatry, precision medicine, and medical data analysis. He holds a Good Clinical Practice (GCP) certificate obtained through his research work, and has previous experience as an ICU junior doctor, surgical assistant, and junior psychiatrist.

Brief Table of Contents

Detailed Table of Contents

CHAPTER 12

Molecular Cytogenetics 411

CHAPTER 13

Quality Assurance and Laboratory Management 449

CHAPTER 14

Ethical, Legal, and Social Implications (ELSI) 483

CHAPTER 15

Emerging Technologies and Future Directions 517

LIST OF FIGURES

PREFACE

The field of molecular pathology has transformed our understanding of disease mechanisms by uncovering the genetic and biochemical substrates of health and disease. No longer limited to simple microscopic observations, pathology laboratories are now going out into the field of translating the language of nucleic acids and proteins to detect minute changes that happen before actual clinical manifestations. This molecular insight has not just enhanced diagnostic precision but also allowed personalized treatment strategies, meaning interventions that can be tailored to an individual's own genetic blueprint. With advances in technology, our ability to identify biomarkers for early diagnosis, monitor minimal residual disease, and predict therapeutic outcomes in various diseases has similarly advanced.

These advances have echoed through almost every specialty in medicine, ranging from oncology and infectious disease to genetic conditions and autoimmune diseases. Previously reliant solely on histology and immunohistochemistry, the laboratory now includes high-throughput sequencing, gene expression arrays, and sophisticated bioinformatic pipelines to generate high-resolution molecular portraits of patient samples. The result is a rapidly evolving, data-driven field in which cross-disciplinary groups of clinicians, laboratory scientists, and computer biologists work together to convert discoveries at the molecular level into better outcomes for patients. As we push back the boundaries of technology, concern for careful quality control, ethical oversight, and wise utilization cannot be too strongly stressed.

Molecular Pathology: Advances and Techniques addresses both fundamental concepts and newer methodological developments. The book is organized to take the reader through a rational progression: from foundational laboratory techniques to more advanced applications in disease conditions, to a consideration of new tools in development and more general implications for molecular diagnosis. Each chapter offers easy-to-read exposition, easy-to-follow guidelines, and example case studies to illustrate the issues, making this book not just a handy reference for senior practitioners but also a learning tool for trainees.

Chapter 1 presents the historical evolution and conceptual basis of molecular pathology, explaining how molecular assays complement standard histopathology. It explains the principles of assay selection, sampling requirements, and integration of molecular information into the diagnosis.

Chapter 2 covers nucleic acid extraction and quantification from different types of samples , including fresh tissue, formalin-fixed paraffin-embedded blocks, and liquid biopsies. The chapter compares manual and automated extraction platforms and factors influencing yield and purity.

Chapter 3 delves into the polymerase chain reaction and its many derivatives—real-time PCR, digital PCR, and multiplex assays, among others. Primer design considerations, primer verification, and data analysis are combined with troubleshooting recommendations to ensure successful amplification.

Chapter 4 explores next-generation sequencing technologies in depth, from short-read platforms to emerging long-read strategies. It addresses library preparation pipelines, sequencing chemistry, and targeted panel, whole-exome, and whole-genome analysis methodologies.

Chapter 5 covers microarrays for gene expression profiling, DNA copy-number analysis, and methylation analysis. Experimental design, normalization strategies, and data mining statistical methods for research and clinical applications are accorded great importance.

Chapter 6 covers molecular oncology, the way in which the somatic mutation profiling, gene fusions, and the measurement of tumor mutational burden drive diagnostic classification and treatment choice. The chapter also mentions minimal residual disease assessment and liquid biopsy use.

Chapter 7 addresses the molecular diagnosis of infectious diseases, detailing pathogen detection technologies from multiplex PCR panels to metagenomic sequencing. It notes applications in outbreak investigation, antimicrobial resistance surveillance, and transplant infectious diseases management.

Chapter 8 covers the molecular pathogenesis of inherited genetic disease, with a focus on variant detection approaches, such as targeted gene panels, exome sequencing, and copy-number variation analysis. Genetic counseling and guidelines for variant classification are also discussed.

Chapter 9 outlines epigenetic mechanisms—DNA methylation, histone marks, and non-coding RNAs—and disease involvement. Hands-on protocols for bisulfite sequencing and chromatin immunoprecipitation assays are included, as well as clinical examples of utility.

Chapter 10 deals with the integration of bioinformatics into molecular pathology, presenting workflows for sequence alignment, variant calling, annotation, and visualization. Strong pipelines, quality metrics, and data security are emphasized as the most important considerations in the chapter.

Chapter 11 depicts CRISPR-mediated genome editing technologies, including functional genomics, disease modeling, and novel diagnostic assays applications. Ethical considerations and off-target effect identification are addressed in the context of clinical translation.

Chapter 12 condenses molecular cytogenetics techniques, including fluorescent *in situ* hybridization (FISH) and comparative genomic hybridization (CGH), detailing how chromosomal abnormalities are detected and interpreted within neoplastic and constitutional disorders.

Chapter 13 deals with the practice of quality assurance and laboratory management, which involves accreditation requirements, proficiency testing, and method validation. It describes the setting up of standard operating procedures, staff training, and continuous improvement indicators.

Chapter 14 presents the ethical, legal, and social consequences of molecular pathology, from patient consent to data privacy, incidental findings, and equitable access to high-tech diagnostics. Case studies illustrate policy challenges and stakeholder issues.

Chapter 15 looks toward the future of emerging technologies—single-cell sequencing, spatial transcriptomics, nanopore-based assays—and their potential effects on diagnostic paradigms. It also considers the role of artificial intelligence in decision support and pattern recognition.

This publication is addressed to a general readership of practicing pathologists, molecular laboratory staff, clinical fellows, and graduate students in pathology and biomedical sciences. It will also be of use for clinicians who rely on molecular diagnostic information—e.g., oncologists, infectious disease physicians, and geneticists—bioinformaticians, and quality managers who would like to gain more insight into laboratory practice and regulatory requirements.

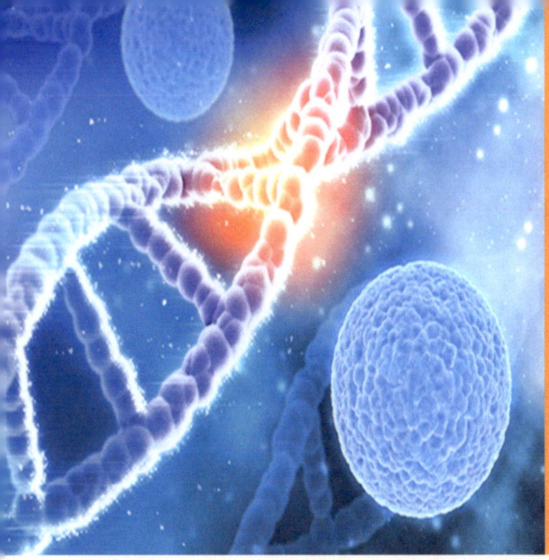

Chapter 1

FOUNDATIONS OF MOLECULAR PATHOLOGY

Contents

Introduction

The field of molecular pathology is being viewed more and more as a bridge science that integrates traditional pathology and molecular diagnostics. The field is better at explaining the molecular mechanisms of disease, and this is what translates into diagnosis and therapy planning. The new technologies in molecular sciences, such as next-generation sequencing and polymerase chain reaction (PCR), have played a major role in changing the field and allowing a better understanding of disease at the genetic level. For instance, the ability to identify specific mutations associated with cancers has transformed therapeutic approaches from a one-size-fits-all model to more tailored paradigms for medicine. Such gains not only enhance the accuracy of diagnosis but also offer chances at targeted therapy that profoundly change patient outcomes, emphasizing the relevance of molecular pathology to modern health and requiring intensive education and training in the discipline (Virginia Commonwealth University, 2018). Besides, with emerging human-animal-environment health complexities, the role of molecular pathology is on the rise. Emerging diseases are a result of intricate human-animal-environment interactions, and the stakes are greater for mechanisms of pathogens and transmission pathways. Molecular pathology provides significant insights into such complexities so that healthcare professionals may have a better understanding of the etiology and potential impacts of infectious disease. As it is becoming easier with globalization for diseases to travel across the world, it is crucial that education in the domain shifts to encompass a broader ecological perspective. In the fast-paced transformation of laboratory tools and their applications, it is now a pressing need to accelerate the process of developing a workforce with skills to employ these devices in the fight against emerging health challenges. In response, the building of stronger educational structures that include molecular pathology and conservation and ecology principles is important for guaranteeing an efficient response to future health crises (Kaufman et al., 2008). Moreover, the integration of molecular pathology into medical and veterinary education curricula is needed to properly prepare future professionals. Well-balanced education encompassing theoretical knowledge as well as practical skills in molecular diagnostics will be capable of providing graduates with the skills they need to counter the challenge from emerging health hazards. Educational institutions should consider expanding their curricula to provide multidisciplinary study options that incorporate molecular biology, genomics, and epidemiology. Such an educational configuration will enable students to realize the relevance of molecular pathology within the framework of health. Moreover, the amalgamation of instructional objectives with real research and case studies will consolidate the pragmatic application of knowledge, hence enhancing the overall performance of prospective health practitioners. Ultimately, a firm foundation in molecular pathology will not only improve individual professions but also make substantial contributions to the formulation of global health programs (Virginia Commonwealth University, 2018) (Figure 1.1).

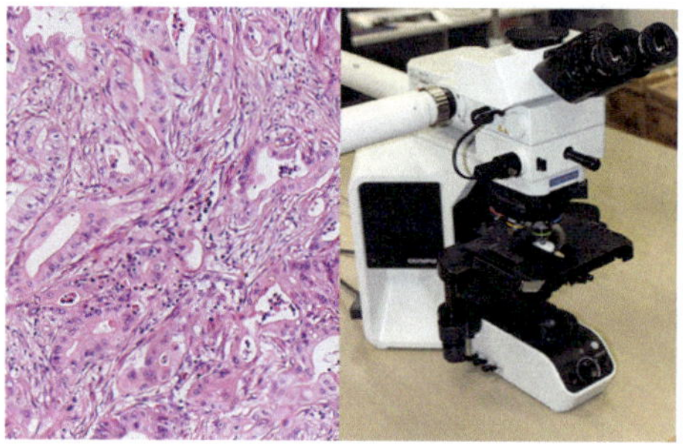

Figure 1.1. Molecular pathology.

Source: https://pod.ncc.go.jp/jp/ri/division/molecular_pathology/sub.png.

Definition and Scope of Molecular Pathology

Molecular pathology refers to the integration of traditional pathology along with molecular biology techniques to define disease mechanisms at the molecular level. Emphasizing genetic, biochemical, and molecular alterations that control various diseases, molecular pathology is a significant component of contemporary medicine due to the generation of knowledge beyond histopathological examination. This discipline has gained a greater understanding of the etiology of diseases, particularly in cancer and genetic disorders, where specific alterations in mutations or molecular pathways can significantly influence the disease course as well as responsiveness to therapy. Molecular pathologists utilize an assortment of methods, including genomic sequencing and proteomics, to identify biomarkers that can lead to improved diagnostic specificity and accuracy and targeted therapies, thus enhancing the strategy of personalized medicine immensely. The field of molecular pathology is not only limited to cancer diagnosis but extends to an enormous spectrum of diseases, such as infectious and autoimmune diseases. Molecular pathologists can further differentiate among disease subtypes using high-throughput technologies , such as next-generation sequencing, thereby aiding in the creation of personalized treatment protocols. For instance, in CRC, molecular subtyping has been seen to be key to the stratification of patients and treatment optimization. The integration of molecular data not only allows for improved prognostic estimation but also helps identify possible therapeutic targets that can lower off-target activity in therapy. This union of molecular insight and practice heralds a new age of precision medicine, where drugs can be customized to a patient's genetic and molecular profile. Furthermore, the significance of molecular pathologies is also highlighted by the continuous evolution of diagnostic tools and treatment approaches.

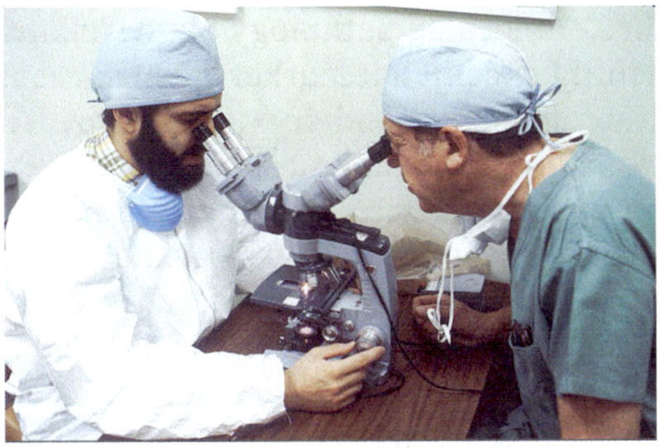

Figure 1.2. Pathology – definition.

Source: https://biologydictionary.net/wp-content/uploads/2017/04/Pathologists-looking-into-microscopes.jpg.

With burgeoning knowledge in glycoproteomics, the potential for novel biomarker discovery increases—for example, the exploration of glycan biomarkers , such as sialyl-Tn (STn) and sialyl-Lewis A (SLeA), which have the potential to enhance non-invasive cancer prognosis. These developments testify to the dual focus of the discipline towards finding markers for disease and developing novel treatment modalities. With the evolution of therapeutic modalities, for example, with targeted drugs and immunotherapy, the role of molecular pathology progressively becomes crucial in bridging gaps between basic science and clinical application. By advocating for improved approaches to study molecular alterations, molecular pathology is well-poised for improving healthcare outcomes and its place in modern medical practice and research, as evidenced in recent publications on disease burdens and research spending efficiency to improve patient care (Kaufman et al., 2008; Fernandes et al., 2020) (Figure 1.2).

Historical Development of the Field

Historically, the evolution of molecular pathology is marked by critical breakthroughs in comprehending genetic mutations and their consequences for disease. Based initially on classical pathology, the discipline came to take great leaps forward in the latter part of the 20th century with the emergence of molecular biology methods. This revolution enabled scientists to explore mechanisms of disease at the genetic level, gaining a deeper appreciation for the subtleties of cell function and dysfunction. Of special interest is the identification of specific mutations that lead to diseases , such as fibrous dysplasia (FD) as a landmark, where the discovery helped emphasize the significance of the genetic basis in pathology. The recent reviews affirm the manner in which mutations within genes , such as GNAS lead to bone growth regulation disorders, pushing the field to move towards an integrated field that captures both molecular genetics and clinical practice (Zyma et al., 2025). This early change paved the way for ground-breaking diagnostic and treatment protocols that are now standard in clinical practice. Parallel with molecular advancement, the emergence of sophisticated diagnostic technology has also played an important role in shaping the course of molecular pathology. The introduction of methods , such as polymerase chain reaction (PCR), next-generation sequencing, and bioinformatics has revolutionized the identification and diagnosis of diseases. This progression has enabled us to identify genetic faults in numerous illnesses, including glioblastoma, which outlines the complexity of tumor biology. With researchers studying the tumor microenvironment and immune marker-glioblastoma cell communication, the study is extending its scope further. These discoveries not only augment our understanding of oncogenesis but also form the foundation of the creation of targeted therapy to overcome resistance to treatment and improve patient benefit. This synergistic advancement of molecular techniques and diagnostic innovation has therefore strengthened the foundation of current molecular pathology (Świątek et al., 2024).

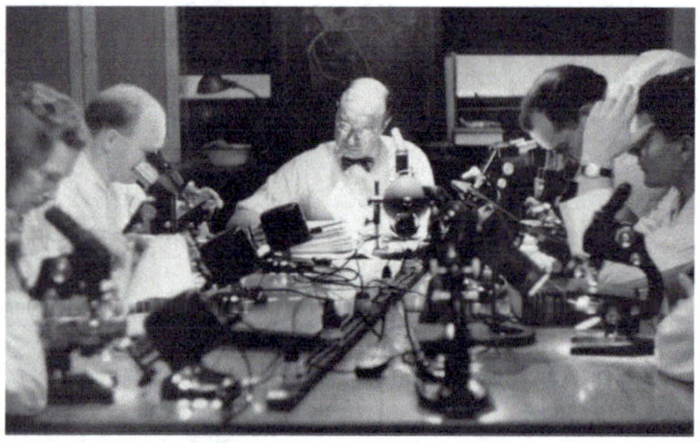

Figure 1.3. History of pathology.

Source: https://www.massgeneral.org/assets/mgh/images/pathology/history-scope.jpg.

Furthermore, milestones of molecular pathology are marked by a continued commitment to translational research that bridges the divide between laboratory findings and clinical medicine. The transition from basic science to the application of stem cell therapy is a case in point. For instance, the recognition of fibrous dysplasia as a disease of stem cells has yielded possibilities for new therapeutic modalities that leverage mesenchymal stem cells (MSCs) to restore bone integrity. Similarly, glioblastoma research has illuminated potential avenues for immunotherapy and individualized medicine and underscored the value of further research into genetic variables influencing responsiveness to treatment. As molecular pathology's historical contexts remain to be uncovered, these further reinforce calls for interdisciplinary strategies to addressing complex pathologies. As the future unfolds, coordination of historical knowledge with cutting-edge research will be needed to steer the field toward innovative solutions that enhance patient care and therapeutic options (Figure 1.3).

Importance in Modern Medicine

The progress of molecular pathology has ushered in a new era in modern medicine that revolutionizes the diagnosis and treatment of diseases. This is most clearly seen in the area of personalized medicine, where patients are treated based on their individual genetic profiles. Molecular pathology allows clinicians to identify specific biomarkers, which result in accurate diagnoses and specific therapy. These developments have made a significant difference in improving results in patients with complicated disease, such as cancer, where knowledge of the molecular basis is the difference between a strategy treating the disease on a one-size-fits-all basis to one that addresses variations of response to treatment in individuals. The role of educational forums, like the Golden Helix Pharmacogenomics Days, is to put emphasis on the importance of shared endeavors and knowledge sharing in promoting individualized medicine with the tool of molecular pathology (Squassina et al., 2012). Molecular pathology not only enriched diagnostic potential but also served a large role in preventive medicine. The discovery of genetic risk factors for specific diseases makes it possible for clinicians to provide preventive interventions that can truncate risk factors years before disease onset. This proactive approach not only places patient autonomy first by empowering individuals with the ability to make informed decisions concerning their health, but it also pressures healthcare systems economically by being capable of reducing the incidence of severe illness. For instance, patients with a family history of breast cancer can be subjected to screening tests through genetic testing, thus facilitating early detection and treatment. The growing attention given to such preventive care reflects the pivotal role of molecular pathology in guiding clinical decisions and the formulation of public health policies favoring improved population health outcomes (Camilleri et al., 2004). Furthermore, the collaboration of molecular pathology with new technology widens its contribution to modern medicine. Next-generation sequencing and CRISPR gene editing are some of those technologies that have advanced medical research and clinical practice to a new era, making molecular pathology a pioneer field of medicine. Apart from raising the ability to diagnose genetic disorders associated with diseases, such technologies provide avenues for new therapeutic approaches. With continuing growth in clinical uses of these technologies, molecular pathology will increasingly play a central role in optimizing therapy regimens and developing new therapies. Thus, the intersection of molecular pathology and new technology constitutes a paradigm shift in the practice of healthcare, again justifying a firm comprehension of molecular mechanisms to continue driving modern medical practice forward (Figure 1.4).

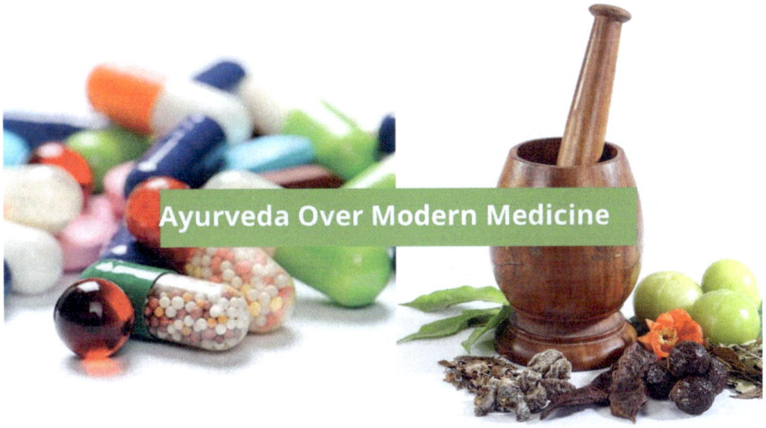

Figure 1.4. Health benefits of Ayurveda over modern medicine.

Source: https://www.ayurvedacollege.net/images/blogs/blog40.jpg.

1.1. Key Concepts in Molecular Biology

The intertwined interaction between pathology and molecular biology is nicely explained by the study of macrophages, the primary immune protectors of the body. In terms of molecular biology, macrophage polarization is described as a key process through which macrophages adapt to various physiological statuses. Macrophages are classified into M1 and M2 phenotypes, each with dissimilar functions in immunological responses and cancerous microenvironments. M1 macrophages are typically pro-inflammatory and are actively engaged in the destruction of pathogens, while M2 macrophages favor tissue repair and the control of inflammation. Polarization is not only a main element of immune homeostasis but also significantly influences tumorigenesis and cancer development. As highlighted by emerging research, the signaling mechanisms regulating such processes are one focus of ongoing research, with implications for therapeutic approaches in cancer treatment and immune regulation (Chen et al., 2023). Another key term in molecular biology is the basis for understanding tumor microenvironments, particularly in highly aggressive cancers , such as pancreatic ductal adenocarcinoma (PDAC). PDAC is characterized by a dynamic interaction between tumor cells and the stroma that influences tumor behavior and patient prognosis. The tumor microenvironment is composed of heterogeneous cell types, including fibroblasts, immune cells, and extracellular matrix elements, all of which contribute to metabolic alterations maintaining tumor growth. Emerging evidence identifies the importance of these cellular interactions in defining the pathophysiology of PDAC because they create a favorable environment for tumorigenesis. Investigation of these interactions is the foundation of building new therapeutic strategies aimed at interfering with the supportive framework of the tumor microenvironment, which can result in improved survival rates for patients suffering from this devastating disease (Collyar et al., 2024). Furthermore, integration with leading-edge technologies has additionally unraveled the molecular processes that propagate disease. High-throughput sequencing, proteomics, and advanced imaging techniques are revolutionizing the discipline of molecular biology and pathology. These technologies enable scientists to dissect the molecular intricacies of disease, establishing novel biomarkers and therapeutic targets. For example, the elucidation of metabolic pathways with macrophages unveiled their dual role in stimulating and inhibiting cancer, informing potential therapy. Aside from that, their use can lead to practices in personalized medicine, as treatments are tailored from individual to individual based on their unique molecular profiles. The advances hold much potential in revolutionizing the face of cancer treatment and patient outcomes, with a direct application of molecular biology to practical use in pathology (Chen et al., 2023; Collyar et al., 2024) (Figure 1.5).

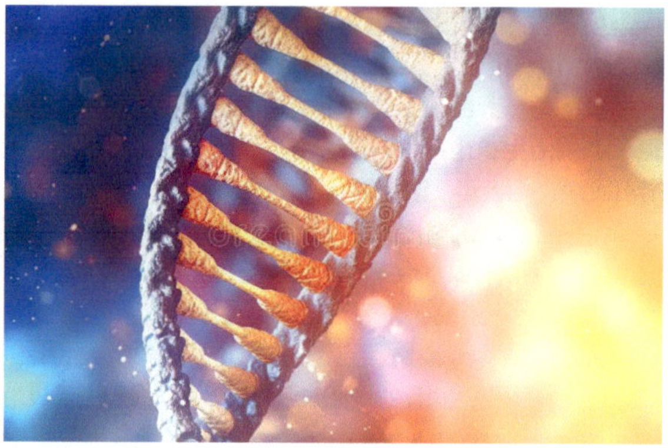

Figure 1.5. Molecular biology.

Source: https://thumbs.dreamstime.com/b/dna-strain-molecular-biology-scientific-concept-generative-ai-illustration-282218055.jpg.

1.1.1. DNA Structure and Function

It is its intricate DNA structure that is the basis for its role in carrying genetic information. Deoxyribonucleic acid, or DNA, is a double helix molecule proposed by James Watson and Francis Crick in 1953. The helix structure is made up of two strands that are oriented in opposite directions, with a backbone composed of sugar and phosphate groups. Every strand is also characterized by nucleotide sequences made up of four bases: thymine, adenine, cytosine, and guanine. The specific pairing of the bases—adenine with thymine and cytosine with guanine—is the basis of accurate replication and transmission of genetic information upon cell division. Stability provided by hydrogen bonds between pairs of bases is critical in maintaining the integrity of genetic information and therefore, signifies the structural significance of DNA in biological processes. The biological role of DNA extends far beyond the preservation of genetic information; DNA also plays a key role in the regulation and expression of genes. Central to this process is the transcription of DNA to messenger RNA (mRNA), and subsequent translation into polypeptide chains that fold into proteins. Proteins, in turn, are engaged in virtually all cellular activities, ranging from catalyzing metabolic reactions to providing structural support and facilitating communication between cells. Interestingly, gene expression can be influenced by numerous intrinsic and extrinsic factors, leading to changes in gene expression. Understanding such dynamics comes under the principles of molecular pathology since aberrations in DNA structure or function may give rise to disease states, including cancers and genetic disorders. For instance, tumorigenesis can be promoted by mutations of tumor suppressor genes or oncogenes, disrupting normal cellular functions. Also, the recent advances in molecular biology have shown how epigenetic modifications could influence DNA function without modifying its sequence. Such modifications, DNA methylation and histone modification, are chemical labels that regulate gene expression and can be heritable from cell division to cell division.

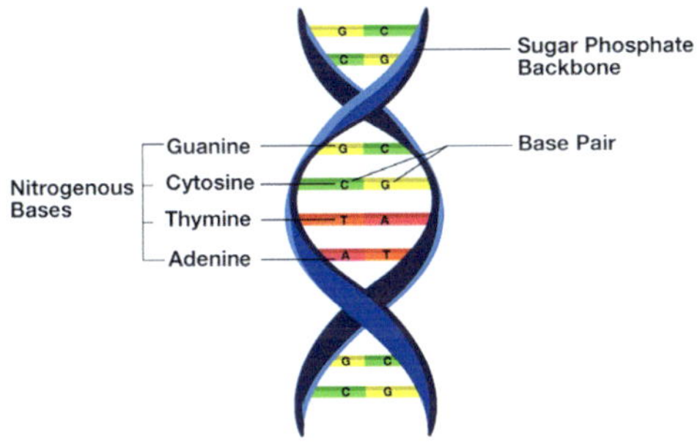

Figure 1.6. DNA structure.

Source: https://cdn1.byjus.com/wp-content/uploads/2018/12/DNA-Structure1.png.

As evidenced by studies in cancer biology, such as the role of the mTORC1 pathway and TP53 mutations in type II endometrial carcinomas, understanding these molecular mechanisms is imperative to create biotherapies. Such new therapies aim to repair or regulate the expression of disease-altered genes, underscoring the integrity of DNA structure and its functional consequence in health and disease settings (Gallucci et al., 1995; Wild et al., 2012). With research ongoing to reveal more of these mechanisms, the foundation of molecular pathology becomes progressively important to clinical application and treatment (Figure 1.6).

1.1.2. RNA and Protein Synthesis

The intricate processes of RNA and protein synthesis are the hallmark of cellular life and ultimately play a role in the pathology of the majority of diseases. Transcription and translation are at the heart of these functions, in which genetic information contained in DNA is transcribed into messenger RNA (mRNA) before being translated into proteins. When the transcription is done, RNA polymerase binds to a specific location on the DNA, unzipping its double helix and synthesizing a complementary strand of RNA. The mRNA strand then undergoes certain modifications, including capping, polyadenylation, and splicing, which are required for its stability as well as for the efficiency of translation. By such modifications, the cell can ensure that the mRNA is already processed and in readiness to be used by the ribosomal apparatus, hence playing a fundamental role in ensuring cellular homeostasis and responding to pathological signals emanating from the extracellular environment. Protein synthesis, or translation, occurs in the ribosome, where the sequence of the mRNA dictates the order of the arrangement of amino acids in a polypeptide chain. Transfer RNA (tRNA) molecules play a role in this sense in that they bring the correct amino acids to the ribosome according to the sequence of the codon on the mRNA. Each tRNA molecule has an anticodon that is complementary to the same codon on the mRNA, meaning the appropriate amino acid is added. This stringently controlled step directly impacts protein function. Proteins, once synthesized, can also undergo post-translational modification, which affects their stability and activity further. The information on protein synthesis, therefore, sheds light on how deficiencies in such processes can lead to states of disease, particularly those that entail dysfunction of regulatory proteins. Advances in molecular biology techniques have led to a greater understanding of RNA and protein synthesis, shedding light on their role in disease conditions.

Techniques , such as Western blotting and confocal microscopy allow scientists to analyze patterns of protein expression and their localization in tissues, and this represents a snapshot of the molecular response to myocardial infarction-type diseases. Identification of inflammatory mediators , such as cytokines and chemokines, by such techniques dictates how protein synthesis is intricately interwoven with inflammation and tissue repair. In addition, studies on molecules like Galectin-1 illustrate the bipartite role of proteins in immune regulation and tissue repair, underlining the equilibrium utilized in pathological events (Riezzo et al., 2015; Potikha et al., 2016). Therefore, more understanding of the pathways that control RNA and protein synthesis will be required for the development of targeted therapies to establish normal cellular function and alleviate disease symptoms (Figure 1.7).

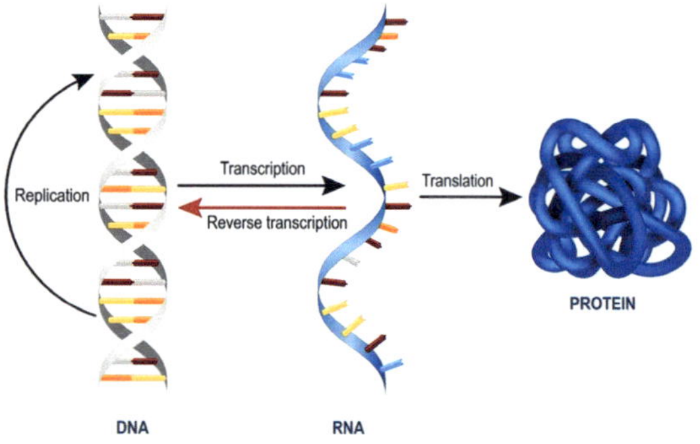

Figure 1.7. RNA and protein synthesis.

Source: https://cdn4.vectorstock.com/i/1000x1000/13/93/dna-replication-protein-synthesis-transcription-vector-21211393.jpg.

1.1.3. Genetic Mutations and Their Implications

Genetic mutational understanding has transformed molecular pathology because such alterations form the core of the etiology of numerous diseases , such as congenital spinal deformity and cancer. For instance, research indicates that congenital spinal deformity (CSD) is linked with genetic disorder in vertebral development during embryogenesis. Mutations in essential genes , such as TBX6 and PAX1, could lead to diseases , such as scoliosis and kyphosis that strongly impair patients' quality of life. Identifying the genetic mechanisms for such diseases reveals potential pathways , such as Wnt and Hedgehog, that are pivotal for normal skeletal development. Thus, the role of genetic mutations is not limited by the fact that they are employed to identify the presence of specific defects; they can predetermine directed therapeutic strategies and enhance the accuracy of diagnosis, ultimately revolutionizing patient care in molecular pathology (Samarkhanova et al., 2025). In addition to bone disease, genetic mutations play a significant role in the field of oncology as well, particularly in ovarian cancer. Identification of the precancerous cells and early tumors in the fallopian tubes reflects the importance of understanding genetic alterations in cancer progression. For individuals with BRCA1/2 gene mutations, risk-reducing salpingo-oophorectomy is typically recommended to prevent the occurrence of ovarian cancer. The practice highlights anticipatory management on the basis of the identification of genetic predisposition and its influence on clinical practice. Moreover, the discovery of serous tubal intraepithelial carcinomas (STIC) as a precursor to high-grade serous ovarian cancer has rocked traditional beliefs regarding tumor origin, revealing the complex interplay between genetic mutation and cancer initiation. Such insights underscore the critical importance of molecular pathology in prevention and clinical decision-making in oncology (Pölcher et al., 2025). Genetic mutation in molecular pathology also extends beyond an examination of mutations themselves to examine the impact of environmental and epigenetic factors on gene expression. While some mutations may put individuals at risk for certain diseases, environmental stimuli, combined with these mutations, can create additional phenotypic effects. Lifestyle, exposure to toxins, and other extrinsic factors, for example, can influence expression of mutant genes and result in disease presentation.

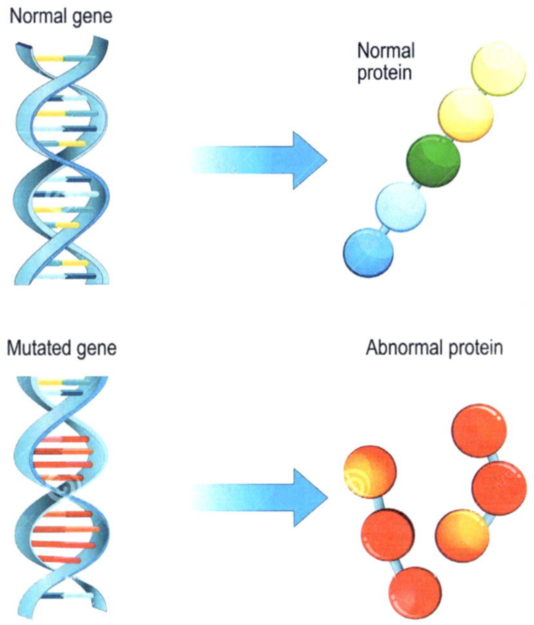

Figure 1.8. Genetic mutation.

Source: https://thumbs.dreamstime.com/z/genetic-mutation-normal-mutated-genes-synthesis-abnormal-proteins-vector-poster-education-science-257038816.jpg.

In addition, technological advances , such as CRISPR-Cas9 provide promising avenues for future therapeutic interventions through the ability to make precise edits in mutant genes. With continuing advancement in these technologies, there is a critical need for continued research that gives us insight into the intricate dynamics of genetic mutations, environmental factors, and outcomes among patients. Lastly, a complete comprehension of these dynamics is poised to advance personalized medicine and improved preventive measures in molecular pathology considerably (Figure 1.8).

1.2. Techniques in Molecular Pathology

The evolving landscape in molecular pathology is well-funded by a variety of sophisticated techniques that enable diseases to be diagnosed and described at the molecular level. They include highly sensitive techniques , such as polymerase chain reaction (PCR), which can amplify traces of DNA as small as a few molecules to enable comprehensive examination of genetic material. PCR's versatility allows for the detection of some mutations within various malignancies that enhance diagnostic accuracy immensely. Finally, next-generation sequencing has revolutionized the practice with the ability to perform wide genomic profiling and offer insight into tumor heterogeneity and targeted therapy potential. This not only enhances diagnosis but also allows for informing treatment protocols and makes molecular pathologies an outstanding contribution to modern medicine. One of the most important uses of molecular pathology is genetic algorithms utilized to decode complex structure-activity relationships. Maximizing the identification of important genetic markers of some diseases by utilizing these algorithms leads to targeted therapeutic interventions. As illustrated in more recent studies, the application of genetic algorithms makes possible a new exploration of gene interaction and its resultant phenotypic expressions within various farming and gardening situations (Lorentz et al., 2010). This combination of molecular pathology and genetics is a prime indicator of the consequential potentiality of interdisciplinary collaboration that promises much in our education regarding the mechanisms of disease as well as the provision of treatment protocols. Ongoing study of such cutting-edge methodologies is imperative to overcome the challenge presented by conditions , such as cancer, in which intervention can only be effectively initiated through an all-around approach. Furthermore, improvements in imaging technology have contributed significantly to molecular pathology. Techniques , such as fluorescence *in situ* hybridization (FISH) allow for focused targeting of individual DNA sequences within cells, which is of tremendous utility in detecting genetic aberrations.

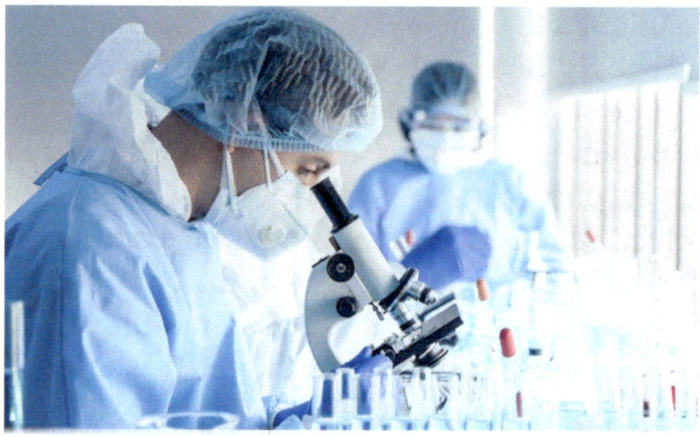

Figure 1.9. Molecular pathology lab techniques.

Source: https://i.ytimg.com/vi/xIzV94bIerQ/maxresdefault.jpg.

While traditional histopathology is founded on tissue morphology, the integration with molecular techniques enhances disease diagnosis at a minute level. As evident in institutional curricula, such as those of Virginia Commonwealth University, the curriculum shines a light on the importance of such methods in the education of prospective pathologists (Virginia Commonwealth University, 2018). Through bridging the divide between diagnostic pathology and molecular biology, these educational systems are developing a new generation of practitioners who can proficiently use molecular techniques, ultimately leading to the enhancement of patient outcome in clinical practice (Figure 1.9).

1.2.1. Polymerase Chain Reaction (PCR)

The Polymerase Chain Reaction (PCR) technique was a milestone in molecular pathology, allowing the amplification of single DNA sequences to an unprecedented degree of accuracy and speed. The innovative technique was discovered by Kary Mullis in 1983, relying on denaturation, annealing, and extension cycles to duplicate target DNA. The ability to generate millions of copies from a single small sample of DNA has not just facilitated genetic analysis but has also transformed diagnostic approaches to infectious diseases and genetic diseases. PCR facilitates quick detection of infectious disease agents, and it's worth is invaluable during public health crises, such as the recent pandemic, where quick identification of viral genetic material is important for containment activities and studies (Ulrich et al., 2023). PCR is, therefore, a leading tool in the modern era of molecular pathology, facilitating improved research and clinical applications. Besides, the universality of PCR has rendered it widely used in most fields, with significant impacts on cancer studies and disease diagnosis. One such fascinating application is CTC analysis, which, based on recent studies, is a critical marker of cancer initiation and metastasis (Yang et al., 2019). With the use of PCR techniques, researchers are able to concentrate CTC DNA to reveal essential genetic alterations that inform therapy and predictive results. The use of PCR in this capacity not only enhances sensitivity in detecting trace CTCs in blood but also provides an understanding of tumor kinetics. As our knowledge of CTCs expands, the combination of PCR with ancillary techniques has the potential to advance cancer biology knowledge and improve therapeutic intervention, a bright prospect in molecular pathology. While PCR has indeed revolutionized molecular diagnosis, its application is also fraught with difficulties that need to be carefully balanced. One of the better-known issues is the risk of contamination that will lead to false-positive findings, thereby leading to misdiagnosis and mismanagement of patients. Furthermore, PCR assay specificity and sensitivity are also influenced by primer and reagent design, involving optimal adjustment and verification to ensure the reliability of test outcomes. Furthermore, with the advancement in technology, efforts are being made to take into account the evolution of PCR technology, e.g., multiplex PCR, which allows for amplifying more than a single target at once. These developments will further strengthen its position in molecular pathology, particularly in understanding complicated disorders and refining personalized medicine approaches (Ulrich et al., 2023). Therefore, continuous research and discussion by scientists are still of utmost importance in overcoming these challenges while tapping PCR's potential in demystifying molecular intricacies (Figure 1.10).

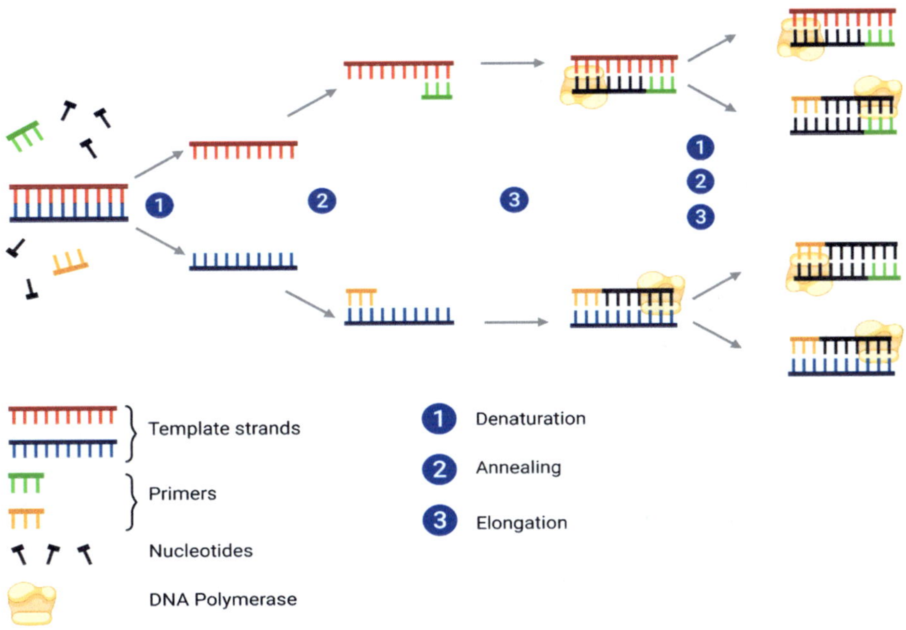

Figure 1.10. Polymerase chain reaction (PCR).

Source: https://www.researchgate.net/profile/Olivier-Tytgat/publication/362991666/figure/fig4/AS:11431281081198081@1661584823008/Polymerase-Chain-Reaction-A-PCR-reaction-consists-of-three-phases-1-denaturation.png.

1.2.2. Next-Generation Sequencing (NGS)

The advent of next-generation sequencing (NGS) has transformed the world of molecular pathology beyond recognition, with unmatched entry into the genetic etiology of diseases. Unlike traditional sequencing methods, NGS allows for the sequencing of vast amounts of DNA simultaneously and at very low cost, making global genomic profiling feasible. This aspect has been more beneficial in oncology, where NGS has made the detection of somatic mutations in neoplastic cells a reality, thereby guiding personalized therapy decisions. These tailored therapies not only enhance the outcomes of the patients but also provide a clearer perspective of disease mechanisms at the molecular level. As NGS continues to advance, its incorporation into clinical practice becomes inevitable for driving innovations in diagnosis, therapy, and overall disease management in molecular pathology. Moreover, utilization of NGS has, to a large extent, facilitated the work related to pathogen genomic surveillance, especially infectious disease outbreaks. By means of high-throughput genomics of pathogens, NGS has played a major role in the monitoring of new emerging variants and epidemiological patterns. An example in this regard is the large-scale sequencing of SARS-CoV-2, which has played a significant role in the public health response to the COVID-19 pandemic. Through the delivery of real-time whole genome sequence (WGS) data, NGS enables clinical decision-making and infection control, highlighting the requirement for highly efficient surveillance systems that integrate diagnostics and genomic data. Transition to integrated, One Health approaches highlight the importance of intersectoral collaboration to deal with global health issues, as laid out by Struelens et al. (2024). The nexus of next-generation sequencing with bioinformatics further underscores the transformative potential of such technologies for individualized molecular pathology. The coming together of advanced bioinformatics tools further simplifies the application of NGS data, allowing for rigorous analysis and interpretation of genomic information. This association ensures the transition from traditional diagnostic approaches to more individualized methods aimed at predicting disease susceptibility and treatment response. Along with the escalation of healthcare systems to integrate these developments, ethical issues regarding information protection and security gain increased significance. Besides, building collaborations between researchers, clinicians, and technology developers will be key to overcoming challenges towards integrating into clinics and unlocking the maximum benefits of NGS within personalized medicine, as emphasized by Struelens et al. (2024). This interdisciplinarity-oriented movement can take the form of a new paradigm for healthcare where patient-centered practices are put at the center of disease prediction and treatment (Figure 1.11).

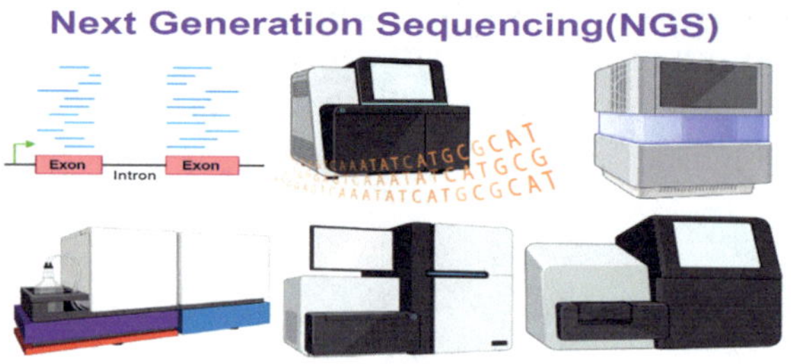

Figure 1.11. Next-generation sequencing (NGS).

Source: https://sciencevivid.com/wp-content/uploads/2022/12/Untitled-2-3.png.

1.2.3. In Situ Hybridization

In situ hybridization (ISH) is an important technique used in molecular pathology to detect specific nucleic acid sequences in fixed tissue sections. By the use of nucleic acid probes labeled with fluorescent or enzymatic labels and tissue preparations, ISH provides a spatial basis for the study of gene expression. This is particularly pertinent in the explanation of the molecular etiology of disease, in which the intracellular localization of RNA may reveal information regarding pathophysiological processes. Progress in ISH techniques has paralleled developments in molecular genetics, borrowing from methodologies like Southern blotting, an innovation required in the 1970s for the investigation of genetic disease. Specific attention was attracted to hemoglobinopathies at breakthrough meetings like the one organized in Crete in 1978, where the need for gene probing was emphasized, as well as for interfacing opportunities that it allowed to molecular geneticists in the new field of molecular genetics (Jones & Tansey, 2014). *In situ* hybridization techniques extend beyond detection; they allow the study of patterns of gene expression in various tissues and conditions. In cardiovascular disease, for example, ISH may be used to assess the expression of inflammatory genes in the events that take place following myocardial infarction. The cascade of inflammation with its interactive phases of tissue response can be defined by the application of ISH in conjunction with other modalities. This becomes essential for the comprehension of how some of the gene expressions are associated with clinical endpoints and therefore become part of the knowledge of myocardial healing and scar formation. Techniques , such as confocal microscopy and Western blotting complement ISH by offering quantitative and qualitative descriptions of patterns of protein expression in the setting of cardiac tissue remodeling, thereby providing an in-depth representation of the molecular dynamics of infarction (Riezzo et al., 2015). Furthermore, integrating *in situ* hybridization with high-resolution imaging technologies has revolutionized molecular pathology through enhanced visualization qualities. Confocal laser scanning microscopy (CLSM), for instance, gives three-dimensional reconstructions of tissues through which the detailed assessment of the spatial organization of gene expression is enabled. The technology is a precious tool in both research and diagnostics, with the capability to give the accurate localization of RNA transcripts in a given cell type. The merging of ISH with advanced imaging modalities underpins a more advanced understanding of gene regulation within disease processes, from the molecular fundamentals through to clinical practice. With ongoing research and advancements in molecular pathology, the use of ISH alongside ancillary methodologies has the ability to provide an understanding of disease initiation and therapeutic targeting of specific molecular pathways (Figure 1.12).

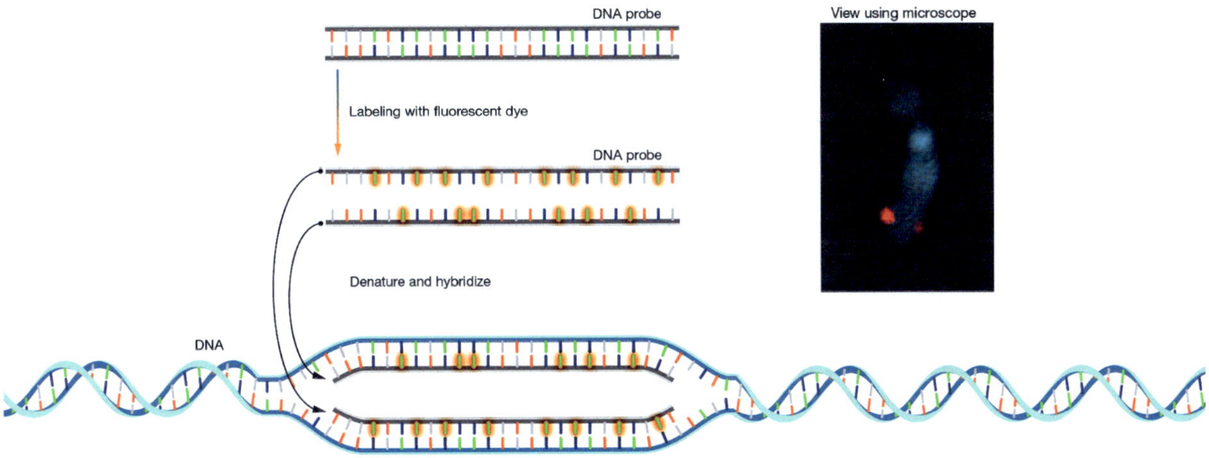

Figure 1.12. Fluorescent *in situ* hybridization (FISH).

Source: https://www.genome.gov/sites/default/files/media/images/tg/FISH.jpg.

1.3. Role of Molecular Pathology in Disease Diagnosis

The integration of molecular pathology into the realm of disease diagnosis is transforming the process of diagnosing various medical conditions. The discipline utilizes genetic, genomic, and proteomic data to shed light on the molecular etiology of diseases, which may enable healthcare professionals to provide more precise diagnoses than the traditional methods offer. By analyzing alterations at the molecular level—e.g., specific mutations, gene expression changes, and protein post-translational modifications—molecular pathology enhances the diagnostic accuracy for complicated diseases, e.g., cancers and genetic diseases. For instance, molecular tests can detect the occurrence of oncogenic mutations that determine the prognosis and treatment selection of cancer patients. With this paradigm shift to molecular pathology, thus, not only are diagnostic processes more sophisticated, but also new avenues are provided for personalized medicine, pointing out the central role that molecular understanding plays in determining therapeutic interventions and fine-tuning patient outcomes. Beyond cancer, molecular pathology is used to diagnose diseases, spanning an extensive list of ailments , such as infectious diseases and genetic disorders. The ability to identify specific pathogens at the genetic level, for instance, by polymerase chain reaction (PCR) techniques, allows rapid and accurate detection of infection that may be overlooked by standard culture. Furthermore, in the framework of genetic investigation, molecular pathology allows for the early recognition of inherited disorders, thus increasing the possibility of interventions whose impact will alter disease direction. As part of precision medicine, the contribution of molecular pathology in deciphering complex disease mechanisms enhances the diagnostic capabilities of modern healthcare systems, highlighting its fundamental role in improving overall patient care and management for all categories of medical specialties. Moreover, constant advances in molecular pathology technologies also prove its central contribution to the diagnosis of diseases. Technologies , such as next-generation sequencing (NGS) make it possible to conduct comprehensive genomic profiling, something that can uncover new mutations and variations implicated in disease pathology. This high-throughput capability cuts the process of diagnosis drastically short while concurrently increasing molecular-level insight into disease mechanisms. As the discipline continues to advance, there is not only an expansion of the arsenal available to clinicians but also an increasing demand for advanced bioinformatics platforms that can make sense of complex collections of data. Hence, according to the Virginia Commonwealth University professional programs bulletin for 2018–2019, the field has to alter its educational systems so that it can prepare the next generation of pathologists with the competencies required by them to utilize these advances meaningfully. These preparations will ensure the therapeutic potential of molecular pathology is actualized to the maximum level in clinical practice, ultimately increasing the quality of care for the patients afflicted by diseases with varying characters (Camilleri et al., 2004; Virginia Commonwealth University, 2018).

1.3.1. Cancer Diagnostics and Personalized Medicine

Advances in the diagnosis of cancer have transformed the practice of personalized medicine, allowing physicians to pair treatments with an individual molecular signature. Standard diagnostic methods are generally not able to expose the intricate heterogeneity of tumors, but molecular pathology supplies the data on the genetic and epigenetic alterations underlying cancer progression. The paradigm shift recognizes the move toward precision medicine, whereby treatments are paired against the specific biomolecular characteristics of a patient's cancer. Accordingly, the integration of molecular diagnostic testing into the clinical environment has a greater significance in that it makes possible earlier detection and more accurate prognostic evaluation. The knowledge of tumor dynamics in terms of molecules has made it possible to obtain information that ensures a good outcome of treatments, which eventually leads to better control of various forms of cancer. One of the significant developments in cancer diagnosis is the development of liquid biopsy, offering a less invasive procedure than traditional tissue biopsies. Liquid biopsy allows real-time monitoring of tumor dynamics through the measurement of circulating tumor cells, cell-free DNA, and extracellular vesicles. The new technology provides significant information on the tumor mutational profile and treatment response with the absence of invasive surgery. The Liquid Biopsy Consortium, which is part of the National Cancer Institute, describes both the technical and clinical challenges for liquid biopsies, which promote the development of validated assays capable of identifying tumor-derived material (Batool et al., 2023). Hence, liquid biopsy serves not only as a diagnosis but also as a means to ongoing patient management and monitoring treatment response throughout the course of therapy. Central to the success of personalized medicine is biomarker discovery and application to guide therapy decisions. Biomarkers are quantitative indicators of normal or disease pathology, and their relevance has increased with advances in omics technologies. These technologies allow for the discovery of new biomarkers through genomic, proteomic, and metabolomic profiling with results that are essential for disease diagnosis, prognosis, and therapeutic selection (Ahmad et al., 2023). For instance, specific biomarkers have been associated with specific cancer subtypes and treatment results, making it increasingly probable for the health providers to select the optimal drugs for their patients. As our understanding of the role of various biomarkers in cancer continues to advance, the integration of this knowledge into clinical practice holds the potential to transform patient outcomes through increasingly tailored patterns of therapy (Figure 1.13).

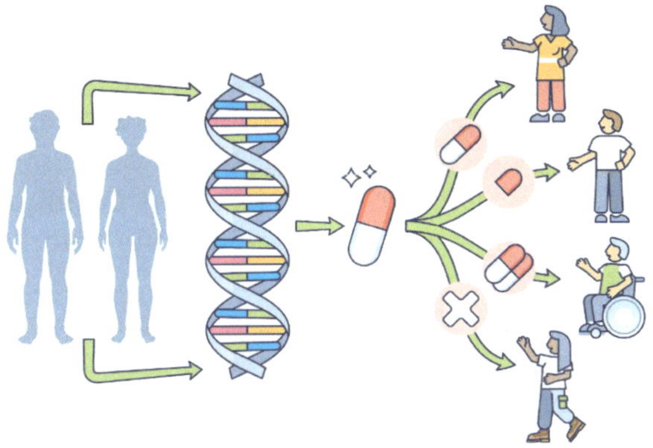

Figure 1.13. Precision and personalized medicine in healthcare.

Source: https://www.medznat.ru/uploads/images/post_content/7182/image_3/1690458980image_3.webp.

1.3.2. Infectious Disease Identification

Infectious disease identification is critical in molecular pathology because it is the foundation of disease mechanisms, transmission dynamics, and treatment principles. With increasing complexities of interactions between humans and the environment, new pathogens are being discovered and evolving, so new means of identification and control must be devised to combat the threats. Molecular techniques , such as polymerase chain reaction (PCR) and next-generation sequencing (NGS) have revolutionized the practice by allowing for rapid detection and identification of etiological infectious agents at the genomic level. These procedures are far better compared to traditional culture-based techniques, which are slow and insensitive. In accordance with

Kaufman et al. (2008), training programs ought to be improved to equip professionals with the capability of managing such dynamic challenges, with particular emphasis on the integration of molecular diagnostics into public health facilities. Detection of infectious diseases also involves the understanding of the dynamic interplay of pathogens and host factors that result in disease phenotypes. Single-cell analysis technologies offer unprecedented insight into heterogeneous cell populations' reactions to infection, which is pivotal for the establishment of accurate diagnostic criteria. Using techniques like flow cytometry and machine learning classification, researchers can separate distinct disease states and monitor treatment responses more aptly. For instance, the technique outlined by Candia et al. (2013) illustrates how unique phenotypic markers can identify diseases that may have clinically indistinguishable presentations. Single-cell-level classification enhances diagnostic precision and allows for the administration of targeted therapy to patients with improved outcomes. The landscape of infectious disease identification is also altered by the impact of global health programs and the interconnectedness of populations worldwide. The etiology of zoonotic origin diseases and the globalization of trade and travel accelerate the imperative for robust identification practices. The contribution of molecular pathology toward the use of genetic and environmental data in tracking outbreaks and predicting potential pandemics is paramount. Interdisciplinary collaborations are essential to formulate integrated surveillance systems that can respond in real time to health hazards. As Kaufman et al. (2008) identify, it is essential to have innovative models of training and research collaborations to formulate effective counter-strategies against the evolving dynamics of infectious diseases. This transdisciplinary approach will ultimately improve our capacity for timely identification and action, laying the groundwork of molecular pathology to meet impending health crises (Figure 1.14).

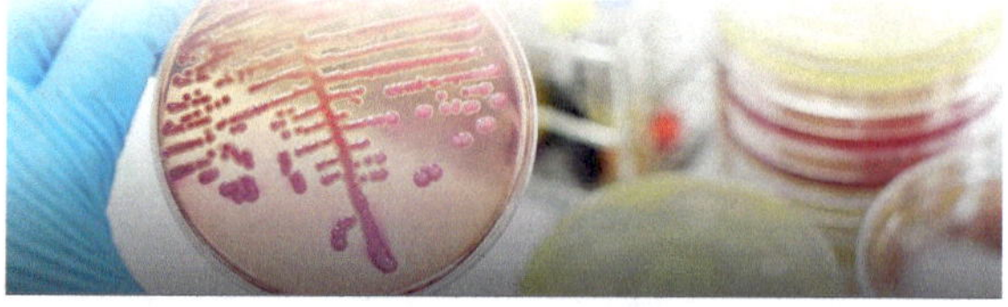

Figure 1.14. Infectious diseases.

Source: https://healthcare.utah.edu/sites/g/files/zrelqx136/files/styles/billboard_tablet/public/media/images/2021/infectious-disease.jpg?itok=nKOJvm2C.

1.3.3. Genetic Disorder Screening

The history of screening for genetic disorders has been radically impacted by developments in molecular pathology. Over the past decades, techniques have progressed from rudimentary approaches to sophisticated genomic screening, which has led to the diagnosis of a wide range of genetic disorders. One of the major highlights of this development was the identification of techniques , such as Southern blotting in the 1970s, which facilitated the exploration of complex genetic disorders. This technology not only allowed researchers to identify specific DNA sequences but also opened up studies into inherited diseases like thalassemia, which was aided through specific investigations and molecular techniques. As was the subject of recent seminars, critical networking meetings , such as the Crete conference of 1978 had a pivotal effect in ensuring scientific exchange and collaboration between geneticists globally, ultimately making screening methods more efficient and securing genetic research as an integral part of modern medicine (Jones & Tansey, 2014). Moreover, ethical issues with respect to screening for genetic conditions emphasize the importance of informed consent and the autonomy of the patient. With the expansion of genetic screening comes the amplification of the effects of the resultant information. The 2003 ALRC Report analyzes the ethical, legal, and social effects of genetic technologies and how genetic information affects individual and collective decision-making. The paper presents 144 recommendations for managing the niceties of the New Genetics, and expresses concerns about privacy, discrimination, and the potential psychological impact on families and patients. Such ethical issues are important in that they promote conducting the methodology of genetic screening in a responsible way so as to balance the advances in molecular pathology with the inherent dignity of individuals undergoing such screening tests (Otlowski, 2006). Introduction of screening for genetic disorders into general medical practice has also caused controversy regarding accessibility and equity in health care systems. As there becomes more widespread availability of screening technologies, unequal access can start to emerge, particularly among disadvantaged groups. This understandably raises significant questions regarding how equitable such developments are. For instance, whereas some patients may benefit from early detection and targeted interventions through state-of-the-art screening techniques, there are others who may be disadvantaged by socioeconomic factors or because they are unaware of the value of genetic screening. The issue is to bridge these disparities to ensure that genetic screening is not merely an elite luxury, but a fair service that ensures public health benefits. This balance can be achieved only through continued discussion among healthcare providers, policymakers, and advocacy groups, supporting the necessity for health-inclusive strategies as we move forward in the area of molecular pathology (Figure 1.15).

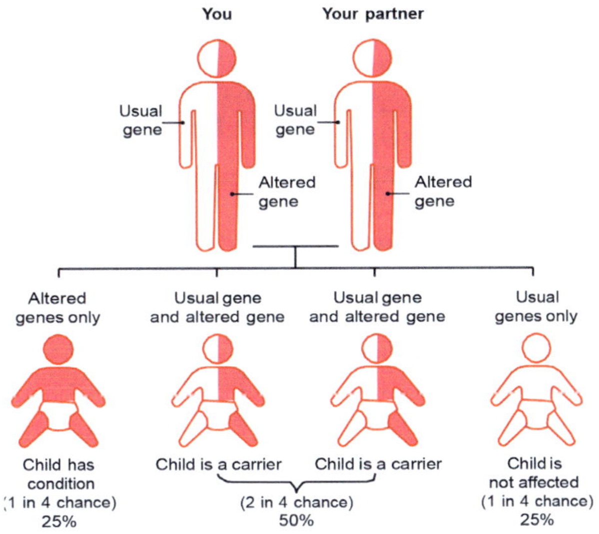

Figure 1.15. Genetic disorders chart.

Source: https://phescreening.blog.gov.uk/wp-content/uploads/sites/152/2015/09/inheritance-diagram-620x544.jpg.

1.4. Molecular Pathology in Cancer Research

Molecular pathology is a cornerstone of cancer research, where the intricately related fields of molecular biology, genetics, and pathology are brought together to enhance understanding of tumor behavior and response to treatment. Methods , such as genomic sequencing can be utilized to identify mutations and alterations that cause oncogenesis and progression. Not only does this platform facilitate characterization of specific tumor entities, but also the development of targeted treatments aimed at individual molecularly defined subgroups of patients. Integration of molecular diagnostics into daily pathology practice has transformed cancer treatment, from the old one-size-fits-all approach to personalized medicine based on individual genomic profiles. This change underscores the pivotal role of molecular pathology in optimizing treatment methods and improving patient care for numerous forms of cancer. Additionally, the setting of molecular pathology is regularly being revolutionized, particularly through programs concentrating on collaborative research as well as information sharing among institutions. An example of this is the Children's Brain Tumor Network (CBTN), which operates under an open science model to accelerate pediatric brain tumor research. Through the concerted effort of the Open Pediatric Brain Tumor Atlas (OpenPBTA), large-scale molecular characterization of pediatric brain tumor specimens has been achieved, including multimodal data types like genomic, transcriptomic, and proteomic data. These efforts are reliant on systematic procurement and analysis of biospecimens with the ability to deliver comprehensive characterization of tumor heterogeneity and actionable biomarkers. Such projects illustrate how collaborative models can enhance molecular pathology research, thereby informing new directions of therapy and clinical trial design for the greater good of patient care, specifically that of vulnerable populations like children with cancer. Finally, the role of patient advocates within translational research models, including the COMET study, helps to illustrate the imperatives of stakeholder participation in molecular pathology research. By locating patient advocates in the Translational Working Group (TWG), the research community is more likely to address the complexities of biospecimen management, data sharing, and patient-centered policy making. Advocates create an arena for debate regarding the ethical concerns of research, so as to have equitable access to trials and use of data. Their involvement not only makes the scientific process more robust but also fosters public confidence and openness, critical for the success of molecular pathology initiatives. With the science continuing to develop, the integration of molecular findings with patient experience is set to remain vital in dictating the direction of cancer therapy's future face, projecting a trend of increasingly personalized and effective treatment modes as attested by continued endeavors as seen through studies like COMET and CBTN (Figure 1.16).

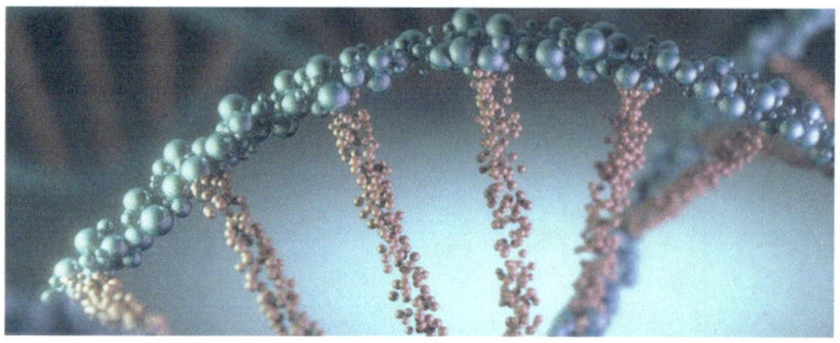

Figure 1.16. Translational molecular pathology.

Source: https://www.mdanderson.org/research/departments-labs-institutes/departments-divisions/translational-molecular-pathology/jcr:content/heroparsys/herodescription/lvpimage.resize.high.dir.jpg/1599680873246.jpg.

1.4.1. Tumor Markers and Their Significance

The role of tumor markers in oncological clinics extends beyond mere diagnostic significance, with significant roles in illuminating cancer biology as well as patient management. Tumor markers are substances produced by cancer cells or by the body of an individual in response to cancer and are generally detectable in blood, urine, or tissue. Their significance is not just in malignancy detection but also in monitoring disease course, treatment, and recurrence. For example, tumor markers , such as prostate-specific antigen (PSA) are a key component of prostate cancer management, where alterations in levels correlate with response to therapy or disease progression. Hence, the addition of tumor markers enhances the clinician's capabilities to tailor treatment strategies for individual patients and hence, enhance precision medicine treatment paradigms. The landscape of tumor marker research is a multi-system paradigm for cancer care using both established and emerging markers. Established markers like carcinoembryonic antigen (CEA) and alpha-fetoprotein (AFP) have been utilized for decades in many malignancies, such as gastrointestinal and liver neoplasms. But with the advent of high-level molecular techniques, there has arisen a new generation of biomarkers that reach deeper into the molecular pathology of the tumor. Circulating tumor cells (CTCs), for instance, are now known to be significant biomarkers since they have been discovered to be valuable in prognosis, treatment selection, and monitoring response to therapy (Che et al., 2016). Research has determined that CTCs can offer insights into tumor heterogeneity and metastasis and document evidence for their value in longitudinal patient analysis and treatment selection. Furthermore, fluidic processes of tumor markers also highlight the power of utilizing them to define disease mechanisms and develop new therapies. Recent research has proven that biomarkers like Galectin-1 (Gal1) have functions in important biological functions, which are involved in inflammation and liver regeneration, and thus must have an extremely important function in tumor biology outside the classical boundaries (Potikha et al., 2016). The above observations vindicate the potential of novel therapeutic targets and the need for continued investigation into tumor marker development. The evolution of biomarker science in molecular pathology not only enhances diagnosis but also the door to tailored therapies, ultimately leading to better survival and patient outcomes. Continued research into these markers is important as cancer therapy becomes increasingly more personalized, taking advantage of the molecular heterogeneity of tumorigenesis.

1.4.2. Genomic Profiling of Tumors

Tumor genomic profiling has transformed the science of molecular pathology to its very essence, whereby critical information regarding the genetic etiology of malignancies is revealed. Through the examination of tumor cell DNA sequence, researchers can establish specific mutations, copy number alterations, and chromosomal rearrangements on which cancer growth is initiated. This precision medicine approach facilitates a more targeted therapeutic approach as opposed to the traditional one-size-fits-all method. Improved understanding of genomic alterations not only directs therapeutic approaches but also allows for the prediction of disease prognosis. Greater utilization of more comprehensive genomic evaluation will likely enhance the identification of characteristic tumor features to further the development of individualized therapies, particularly for the use of targeted agents against specific genetic drivers. Importantly, dynamic tumor heterogeneity complicates the genomic profiling process. Tumors are not homogeneous populations; they are subclonal, having distinct genetic mutations that may vary with time depending on factors , such as therapy and the tumor microenvironment. New evidence has illustrated that even between synchronous tumors developing from an identical tissue, a broad genomic diversity can be present which determines the responsiveness of treatment regimens. Specifically, it has been proven that oncogenic mutations may vary, but some conserved pathways are necessarily involved in tumorigenesis (Ma et al., 2017). Realization of such enhances the need for continuous monitoring of tumor genomic characterization to steer treatment in accordance with changing tumor biology. In addition to genetic mutations, epigenetic changes , such as DNA methylation are also critical components in tumor initiation and drug resistance. The discovery of 5-hydroxymethylcytosine has added complexity to the field, since it is now suggested that the epigenetic landscape of cancer is not fixed but dynamic and may be a novel field of therapeutic intervention. By profiling the changes of 5-hydroxymethylcytosine, scientists are able to gain better insight into tumor behavior regulation mechanisms and can suggest potential biomarkers for diagnosis and prognosis (Laird et al., 2013). Furthermore, a better comprehension of the interaction between genetic and epigenetic factors can better account for carcinogenesis and direct therapeutic interventions that exploit such knowledge. Genomic profiling thus not only delineates the molecular features of tumors but also provides the basis for new cancer treatment strategies (Figure 1.17).

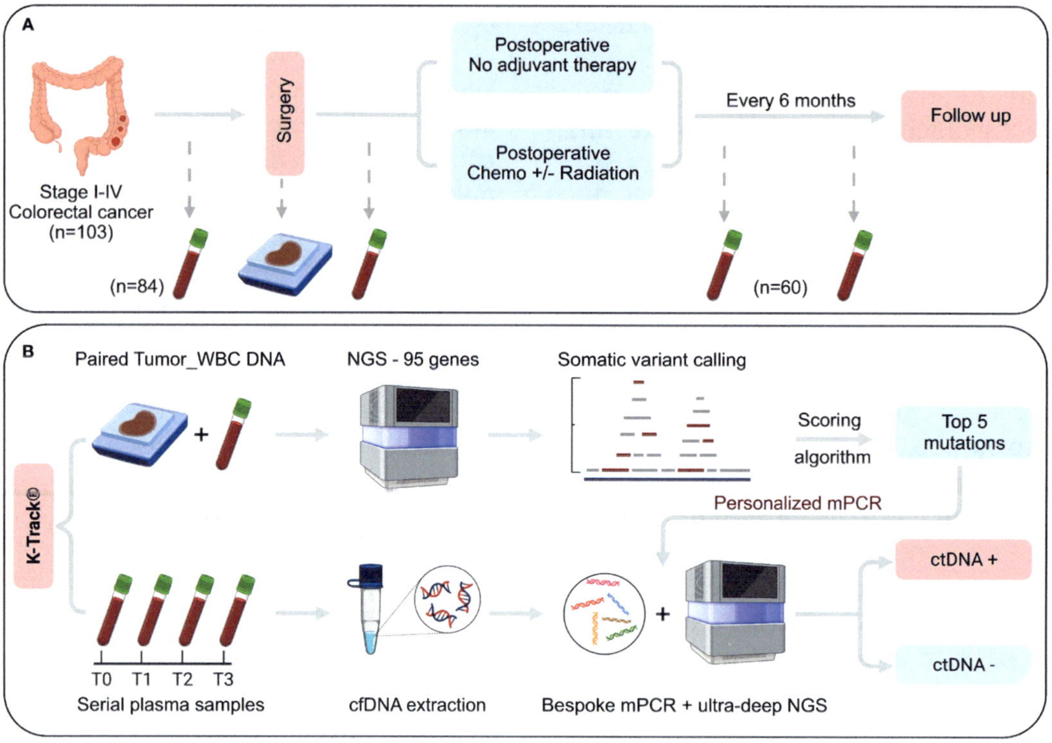

Figure 1.17. Tumor genomic profiling.

Source: https://www.frontiersin.org/files/Articles/1069296/fonc-12-1069296-HTML/image_m/fonc-12-1069296-g001.jpg.

1.4.3. Targeted Therapies and Their Development

The establishment of targeted therapies is a significant step in the field of molecular pathology, signaling the necessity for the elucidation of the genetic and molecular foundations of diseases. This allows for the development of interventions that are tailored to specific patient populations, namely patients with complicated illnesses , such as cancer and autoimmune diseases. Through the use of holistic genomic investigations, researchers are able to discover new mutations and biomarkers that induce susceptibility to personalized agents. Through this, not just is the therapeutic effect enhanced, but also unwanted toxicity that tends to result from standard therapies is minimized. Furthermore, this revolution rests on the integration of network pharmacology concepts, which provide platforms for the discovery of possible drug targets in biological networks. Therefore, targeted therapies are an encouraging avenue for the improvement of clinical results as they hold the promise of delivering safer and more effective treatment to patients in need (Watkins et al., 2010). Development of targeted therapies demands a team effort beyond basic research to include clinical use and patient involvement. The iterative treatment development process involves extremely large clinical trials that yield efficacy and safety data gathered carefully. Real-world evidence is required to define the heterogeneity of patient response and therefore, guide the iterations of treatment strategy in the future. In addition, because therapies are tailored based on molecular profiles, the requirement for efficient screening methods becomes increasingly relevant. Biomarker assays, such as liquid biopsies, can potentially facilitate monitoring of how the patient responds to therapy and mechanisms of resistance, to keep treatment protocols up to date with the evolving character of a patient's disease. Such an adaptive and dynamic approach is vital in maximizing the benefits of targeted therapies (Guido et al., 2019). Despite the promise of targeted therapies, there are several challenges that persist, which can preclude their widespread use. Such issues as the availability of high-end genomic diagnostics and the price of precision medicine can bring about disparities in treatment among vulnerable groups. Further, the complexity of biological networks is also a challenge to identifying productive therapeutic targets, as isolated mutations cannot account for drug response or resistance very well. Further investigation is required to overcome such obstacles, testifying to the value of multidisciplinary research between genetics, pharmacology, and healthcare policy disciplines. Overcoming such challenges, the field of molecular pathology can evolve, rendering development and application of targeted therapy available to a larger pool of patients and fostering innovation in individualized medicine (Watkins et al., 2010).

1.5. Ethical Considerations in Molecular Pathology

The evolution of molecular pathology holds huge potential for diagnostic medicine but also raises serious ethical questions that must be examined very rigorously. Among the concerns is the one of informed consent, particularly as increased genetic testing is undertaken in clinical medicine. Patients may have trouble comprehending intricate genetics, and this may lead to misconceptions about the meaning of their results. This complexity is further amplified when test results can impact members of the family, requiring careful communication processes that leave patients well aware of the implications of their choices. Additionally, since most molecular tests are linked to genetic disorders, the ethical context of privacy and information sharing comes to the forefront, where protecting individuals' genetic information becomes critical in the face of rising data breaches and abuse in the healthcare sector. Furthermore, the integration of machine learning and artificial intelligence into molecular pathology holds revolutionary possibilities but poses a range of ethical questions. The employment of AI technologies in decision-making for diagnosis poses challenges regarding accountability and transparency, especially because algorithms can function as so-called black boxes, which hide the reason for their recommendations. This lack of transparency can lead to distrust in healthcare professionals as well as patients, spurring fears of algorithmic bias that may disproportionately affect marginalized groups. Ethical standards must therefore be developed that will ensure that AI technologies are created and deployed ethically to enhance, not undermine, clinical judgment. Continuous assessment of these technologies from an ethical perspective will be instrumental in unlocking their potential while preventing inherent risks to their application (Najjar, 2023). Ultimately, as molecular pathology becomes increasingly integrated into digital health, ethical concerns regarding data ownership and control come into play. The analysis, compilation, and storage of vast quantities of genomic and health information need comprehensive policies that promote the integrity and confidentiality of patient information. Ethical issues also arise regarding the ownership of this information and its uses, particularly in light of the potential threat that commercial interests will be able to utilize personal health information for profit. Regulatory bodies must navigate this complex landscape by fostering stringent ethical standards that serve patients, not just by protecting patient rights, but also by enabling effective innovations in the field. Facilitating cooperative action between industry, academia, and regulatory bodies, the ethical paradigms that shape molecular pathology can be made to evolve with technology, always striving for a patient-centered approach respecting individual autonomy and public trust (Shah et al., 2019) (Figure 1.18).

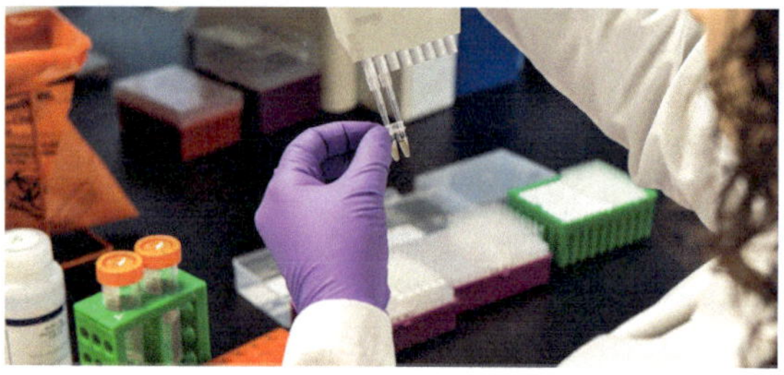

Figure 1.18. Molecular pathology division.

Source: https://pathology.jhu.edu/build/assets/department/_image1200/molecular-pathology-research.jpg.

1.5.1. Patient Consent and Privacy Issues

In molecular pathology, patient consent and patient privacy are major ethical as well as legal issues. These arise particularly with regard to the handling of genetic information that not only reveals the health status of a person but also offers information about the susceptibility of relatives to disease. The privacy surrounding genetic data demands rigorous controls for verifying that patients are actually informed before samples are taken from them and used for research or diagnostic testing. Physicians must work within a challenging tightrope of advancing scientific knowledge and upholding individual rights. Without open and transparent consent protocols, patients will become disenfranchised and lose faith in healthcare systems that utilize molecular pathology. Besides, the job of maintaining patient confidentiality is complicated by the rise of digital health technology that functions on enormous amounts of genetic information. The storing and transmission of such information exposes it to various threats of unauthorized breach that can leak confidential personal health data. Institutions handling molecular pathology, thus, must implement strong data governance systems for protection against illicit use. Steering from the ALRC Report 96, which enumerated concerns of ethical and legal character attached to genetic information, underscores the necessity of visionary policies directing practitioners on best practices in data privacy and consent. The report endorses the acknowledgment that patients' rights should always be at the center of all progress in molecular diagnosis and therapy. As molecular pathology progresses, discussion of patient privacy and consent remains vital. This discussion has to involve actively involving patients, clinicians, and ethicists to come to terms with the problems presented by varying technology and methods for the field. Involvement of stakeholders facilitates guidelines that are attuned to both scientific advancement and patient rights. Efforts must work towards harmonization of research needs and moral concerns, such that consent becomes not just a process but an affirmation of patient autonomy. These discourses can lead to broader practice in consent that incorporates patients' opinions and enhances greater confidence in the utilization of molecular pathology in clinical practice, ultimately resulting in better-quality patient care while safeguarding individual rights.

1.5.2. Implications of Genetic Testing

The implications of genetic testing are profoundly revolutionizing the world of molecular pathology, offering unprecedented information on the prevention, diagnosis, and treatment of disease. Genetic testing enables clinicians to detect genetic mutations and predispositions, thereby making it possible for them to tailor prevention strategies and therapeutic interventions for patients. For instance, individuals who have a genetic susceptibility to breast or ovarian cancer can actively take steps , such as enhanced monitoring and prophylactic surgery. This specific approach not only has better outcomes for the patient but also shifts the model from reactive to proactive medicine, ultimately leading to reduced morbidity and mortality rates. Nevertheless, growing utilization of genetic testing necessitates consideration of ethical concerns, data privacy issues, and emotional influence on patients and their families. In addition, integrating genetic testing into clinical practice also generates serious issues about accessibility and equity within healthcare systems. While genetic testing holds promise, disparity in access to these technologies has the potential to maintain existing health inequities. The vulnerable populations of individuals might not receive the correct genetic counseling and testing services, negating the opportunities for early detection and intervention. Additionally, the interpretation and comprehension of genetic tests are based on the degree of health literacy that is not possessed by all patients. This inequality raises an ethical concern because it can lead to the underutilization of genetic testing among those individuals who stand to gain most from it. It is thus necessary that healthcare professionals not only offer genetic test services but also that they be accompanied by proper education and support to foster an open environment for all patients. With molecular pathology development, the effect of genetic testing will likely extend beyond the treatment of individual patients to influence models of public health. Detection of genetic risk factors will inform population-level preventive strategies for disease, targeting screening recommendations and policy to health. As an example, genetic susceptibility studies of diseases like PDAC do not just necessitate targeted screening programs but also more research budgets (Collyar et al., 2024). In addition, what is learned through genetic testing can give us a clearer understanding of disease mechanisms, creating the possibility for new therapies with targeted solutions from individualized genetic profiles. But everything , such as that must be pursued with caution, with ethical guidelines keeping pace with technological innovation, with faith being maintained and the public interest in genetic technology (Najjar, 2023) (Figure 1.19).

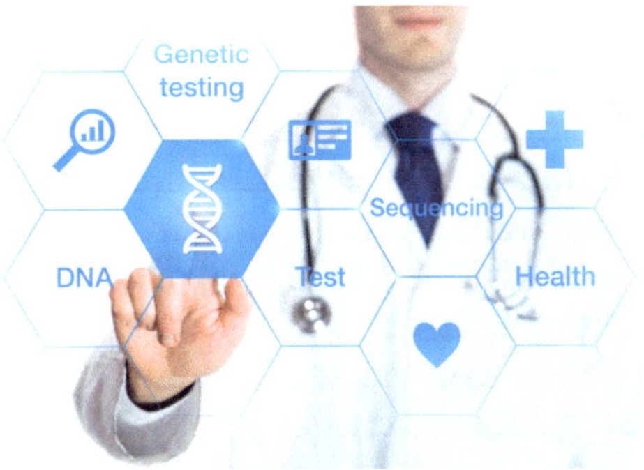

Figure 1.19. Genetic testing.

Source: https://www.coriell.com/wp-content/uploads/AdobeStock_132367929-scaled.jpeg.

1.5.3. Equity in Access to Molecular Diagnostics

Equity of access to molecular diagnostics is a central challenge in the field of molecular pathology when contrasts are considered within healthcare systems. The invention of new diagnostic procedures has the potential for more accurate detection of disease and more personalized treatment. Socioeconomic inequalities, however, usually decide who has access to these advantages. For instance, low-income patients may not reach the basic healthcare centers, let alone more advanced molecular diagnostic procedures that require specialized infrastructure and human capacity. As a result, disparities in disease control are aggravated, with significant effects on patient outcomes. Correcting these imbalances necessitates a multi-faceted approach that involves policy reform, restructuring of healthcare systems, and public education to bridge the gap between what is technologically achievable and what can realistically be implemented in the real world, and to ensure that innovations are accessible for all sections of society, particularly the underprivileged. For equity in molecular diagnostics, policy change advocacy needs to intersect with clinical practice and education. This can be facilitated by programs that provide more health literacy to underprivileged populations, which have the potential to enhance the understanding and utilization of available diagnostic options. Further, utilization of telemedicine and mobile health platforms can facilitate access to molecular diagnostics in remote or underserved areas. These sites not only democratize health access but also make possible real-time data generation, increasing the capability of offering successful interventions in diverse populations. By leveraging technology, actors within the healthcare system can drive the adoption of molecular diagnostics into standard practice, ultimately getting these advances to become the standard in various populations and closing the general health disparities. In addition to the educational and infrastructural components, public-private partnerships are of utmost significance in providing equal access to molecular diagnostics. Public health programs must partner with industry innovation to create merged avenues of implementation. Incidents like the meeting hosted by the Eunice Kennedy Shriver National Institute of Child Health and Human Development emphasize the necessity of bringing together stakeholders with similar interests to deliberate on knowledge gaps and opportunities in translational research. These partnerships can lead to breakthroughs that directly address health disparities, particularly reproductive health, where disparities are particularly important. As seen with the heightened emphasis on menstrual health, there's tremendous potential for molecular diagnostics to inform tailored care strategies that not only improve individual health but also have broader societal benefits as these innovations spread to other cultural and economic environments (Critchley et al., 2020). Ultimately, resolving the inequities in access to molecular diagnostics is key to realizing the full potential of molecular pathology in improving population health.

1.6. Future Directions in Molecular Pathology

While molecular pathology continues to grow, its future will be shaped immensely by the coupling of new technologies with the demand for personalized medicine. One underlying direction is the integration of high-throughput genomic sequencing technologies, which promise to revolutionize the diagnosis and treatment of cancer. By enabling in-depth analysis of genetic mutations and molecular alterations, these technologies will enable individualized treatments to focus on specific pathways in an individual's tumor. This shift towards precision medicine is necessitated by the collaborative input of multi-disciplinary teams of bioinformaticians, geneticists, and pathologists to make sure that the large volumes of data generated are effectively interpreted and translated to the clinic. These advancements contribute not just to better diagnostic precision but also to the ability to identify novel targets for therapy, thus positioning molecular pathology at the focal point of personalized healthcare strategies, eventually leading to improved patient outcomes and transforming paradigms of disease management. Another hopeful region of inquiry for the molecular pathology of the future is the application of new imaging technologies. The ever-more-advanced state-of-the-art medical imaging instruments have the potential to provide unprecedented images of tissue morphology and cell-to-cell molecular interactions at the tissue level. High-image-quality-improving techniques have to be used to accurately image the complex structural and functional characteristics of numerous disparate diseases. For instance, the use of artificial intelligence in image evaluation can significantly improve diagnostic interpretation with minimal chances for human error. Through the use of such technologies, molecular pathologists will be suitably placed to diagnose disease sooner and monitor response to treatment more accurately. Consequently, these developments not only add support to rising interest in accurate diagnostic agents but also allow for more personalized treatment protocols, further underlining the significance of advanced imaging to molecular pathology's future (Sohail et al., 2018). Another field of future use includes the exploration of liquid biopsies, a non-invasive method for cancer diagnosis and surveillance. Unlike traditional tissue biopsies, liquid biopsies analyze circulating tumor DNA (ctDNA) in blood samples carrying essential information about tumor heterogeneity and evolution. This technique holds the major advantage of allowing for real-time monitoring of treatment responses and the detection of emerging resistance mutations. Moreover, ongoing advances in technologies , such as microfluidics and nanopore sequencing will likely enhance the sensitivity and specificity of liquid biopsy tests. With the progress of the method, liquid biopsies can easily become an integral component of clinical practice, offer a more dynamic cancer profile of patients and significantly contribute to individualized therapy. Integrating such advanced diagnostic methods into molecular pathology can revolutionize patient management strategies and results (Winkleman, 1986).

1.6.1. Advances in Technology and Methodology

The rapid technological and methodological advancements have significantly influenced the terrain of molecular pathology, particularly with the integration of artificial intelligence (AI). The groundbreaking technology has permeated every facet of its subfields, one of which is radiology. AI facilitates enhanced imaging evaluation through the use of machine learning and deep learning algorithms, which increase diagnostic accuracy and efficiency. As mentioned in recent literature, these innovations have propelled changes in clinical workflows and precision medicine to facilitate more precise diagnoses of patient conditions. However, as the potential benefits of AI in molecular pathology are broad, challenges exist, including data quality issues and concerns of ethical transparency in algorithmic decision-making. These complexities must be addressed to ensure that AI is a responsible agent for change that, ultimately, benefits patient care in diagnostic practices (Najjar, 2023). As parallel to the developments in AI, biomarker research has emerged as a hallmark feature of molecular pathology. Biomarkers are quantifiable indications of physiological phenomena, and they can warn clinicians about the presence and progression of disease. Emergent advances in omics technologies have made major contributions to the identification and confirmation of new biomarkers in a range of pathological conditions. These emerging methods include genomic, proteomic, and metabolomic approaches that unveil extensive knowledge about the molecular basis of the disease. Clinicians become increasingly able to navigate therapeutic options through elevated awareness of the role of biomarkers, and personalized treatment regimens can be implemented with greater fidelity according to the needs of individual patients. The continuous development of detection methods and analytical tools ensures that the clinical application of biomarkers will remain a cornerstone of modern molecular pathology (Ahmad et al., 2023). The correspondence between technology and methodological advancements proves the dynamic nature of molecular pathology as a discipline. The accuracy and efficacy of diagnostic processes are constantly improved by integrating sophisticated tools, whether through computational processes like AI or through the use of biomarkers in real clinical practice. There has to be an effort to ensure that research activity goes on, not just to enhance technology but also to highlight cooperation among laboratory scientists, clinicians, and technology developers. These multidisciplinary approaches will foster the ethical application of revolutionary technologies, balancing a moral compass with the betterment of molecular pathology practice. Ultimately, all these advances cumulatively usher in the efficiency of health care delivery, highlighting the significant role of technology in disease diagnosis and management in the future (Ahmad et al., 2023; Najjar, 2023).

1.6.2. Integration with Other Medical Disciplines

The unification of molecular pathology with other medical fields is increasingly regarded as important in enhancing patient care and the outcome of health. Interdisciplinary practice, through the integration of information from biochemistry, genetics, and pathology into clinical decision-making, improves the diagnostic process. By combining the molecular pathogenesis of disease with mainstream clinical practices, health practitioners can envision a more holistic approach to diagnosis and treatment. For example, molecular techniques enable the identification of specific genetic mutations causing various cancers, leading to more specific treatments. The synergy is also enhanced by the emergence of artificial intelligence techniques in radiology, which is revolutionizing imaging analysis and allowing accurate interpretations based on results of molecular pathology (Najjar, 2023). With collaborative efforts, different fields not only get to share information but can also advance their approaches and technologies that will result in comprehensive patient management processes. Apart from enhancing the diagnostic systems, integration of molecular pathology with other sciences also results in innovation in personalized medicine. Personalized medicine itself greatly relies on accurate molecular profiles that may direct treatment therapies that are tailored to the unique needs of individual patients. Through collaboration with specialists in genomics, pharmacogenomics, and indeed psychiatry, molecular pathologists can contribute to the knowledge of genetic variation and how it influences drug response and disease state. For instance, in psychiatric illnesses, the application of techniques like genomics can explain the biological mechanisms of mental diseases, ultimately modifying diagnosis criteria and treatment based on the Hierarchical Taxonomy of Psychopathology (HiTOP) model (Kotov et al., 2021). Thus, the integration of molecular pathology with other medical specialties not only enhances the specificity of diagnoses but also gets the treatment protocols attuned to the individual profile of the patient so that overall treatment efficacy is increased. In addition, interdisciplinary communication in molecular pathology assists in addressing daunting challenges in health care, such as integrating data and ethical concerns. As healthcare organizations become increasingly reliant on huge volumes of data, bringing in input from other specialties is essential in meeting the challenges of patient privacy and interoperability of data. In radiology, for instance, implementation of AI-based solutions is hindered by problems in the black box complexity of these systems, with quite a lot of debate needed among radiologists, pathologists, and ethicists (Najjar, 2023). This uniting of knowledge allows for the development of integrated frameworks that not only prioritize technological advancement but also consider ethical precepts, so that innovations are respectful to patient autonomy and improve data integrity. Convergence between molecular pathology and other specialty medical sciences is therefore significant, not just for scientific advancement but for being able to keep pace with the subtleties of the ethical healthcare environment of today.

1.6.3. Potential for New Therapeutic Approaches

The identification of new potential therapeutic approaches in the field of molecular pathology is a necessity since it offers a platform to challenge unmet medical requirements in various conditions. Progress in molecular diagnostics over the past several years has identified previously enigmatic disease pathways, paving the way for targeted therapies with the potential to alter disease progression at the molecular level. There continues to be a significant challenge in translating preclinical findings into successful therapies, particularly in diseases like progressive MS, whose existing treatments have not yielded satisfying results.

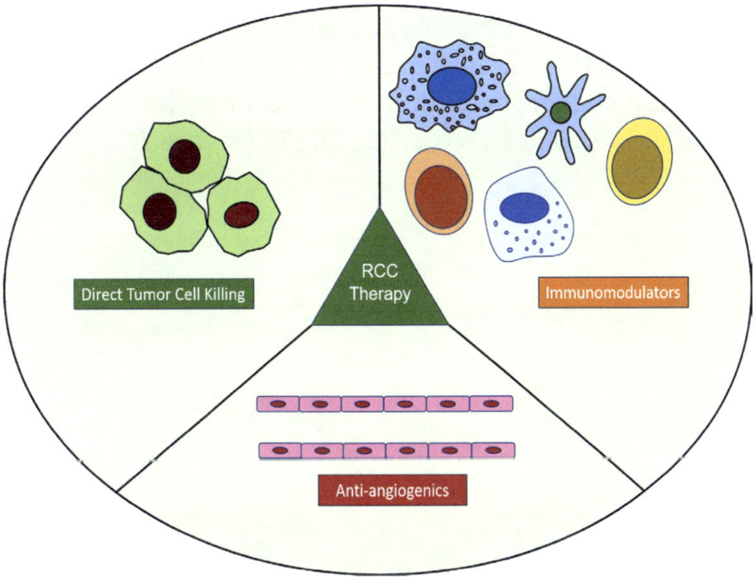

Figure 1.20. Potential for new therapeutic approaches.

Source: https://www.seminarsinnephrology.org/cms/attachment/a57e2908-cb99-4e08-b1d7-fcb3c2488a75/gr1_lrg.jpg.

To overcome such limitations, scientists are calling for an integrated, multi-disciplinary approach that brings together resources and expertise from diverse disciplines, thereby enhancing successful disease-modifying therapy development. Such collaborative effort is important to accelerate progress in therapeutic methods that can restrict the impact of disease with complex molecular etiology, like progressive MS. New therapeutic paradigms should be discussed in the future to evolve patient management (Fox et al., 2012). Yet another exciting avenue in molecular pathology is the emergence of personalized medicine, intending to optimize therapeutic strategies using individualized genetic and molecular profiles and disease specifics. Leveraging the platform of network pharmacology, researchers are beginning to engineer therapies based on the complex interactions between multiple biological molecules and pathways. This shift to thinking about disease and health in a networked framework can lead to the development of new drugs that work on numerous pathways at once, thus providing a more integrated system for treatment. Not only does this represent a breakthrough in treatment efficiency, but it also has the promise of reducing undesirable side effects by tailoring therapy to the metabolic niche of an individual patient. As this paradigm develops, a symbiotic interaction between pharmacology and personalized medicine will be ready to redefine therapeutic approaches and facilitate new drug discovery strategies (Watkins et al., 2010). The search for new therapeutic approaches in molecular pathology also raises the need for continued research in experimental models and biomarker identification. With the help of cutting-edge technologies , such as CRISPR gene editing, researchers are now more able than ever before to investigate the roles of individual genes and how they contribute to disease processes, simplifying the design of targeted treatments. Furthermore, the addition of new trial designs, such as adaptive trials that allow for real-time modification based on trial results, can significantly optimize the efficiency of science to actionable treatments. Identification of precise biomarkers will also enable more precise patient stratification, as long as treatments are administered only to patients who are most likely to derive benefit. This robust system for setting and implementing new therapies is a central shift in surmounting long-standing challenges within the field of molecular pathology and ultimately resulting in improved patient outcomes (Fox et al., 2012) (Figure 1.20).

SUMMARY

In summarizing a study of molecular pathology, it is evident that the integration of advanced technologies significantly supports our understanding and management of diseases, particularly cancers , such as prostate cancer. The application of next-generation sequencing (NGS) has achieved great strides into the genetics of cancers. As mentioned in some research, e.g., the study that established the correlation of pathogenic mutations of the androgen receptor with tumor volume, these molecular changes are highly useful for both treatment planning and prognosis. This highlights the function of molecular pathology as a cornerstone of the new wave of personalized medicine, whereby plans of treatment are made based on personal genetic configuration (Balta et al., 2024). Furthermore, the role of artificial intelligence (AI) in molecular pathology cannot be overemphasized. New advances in image recognition technology have presented new avenues for pathology diagnosis. Bibliometric analyses have shown that there is a rising trend in research on deep learning applications to pathological image analysis, evidence of rising consciousness of the potential of AI to improve diagnostic performance and automate procedures. By incorporating algorithms that effectively identify features , such as microsatellite instability, AI is going to transform the efficiency and impact of molecular pathology assessments (Yu et al., 2024). Consequently, the union of computational techniques and molecular expertise is a milestone in disease diagnosis and therapy. In essence, the foundations of molecular pathology are being strengthened by emerging technological advancements and research achievements. The significance of identifying molecular changes cannot be overstated, as it not only aids in prognosis and general therapy but also supports targeted therapeutic strategies and facilitates a deeper understanding of disease pathomechanisms. The demands like quality, standardization, and infrastructure need to be met on an ongoing basis as research progresses. Equivalence of these demands with the promise held by new technologies will be crucial to maximize the therapeutic potential of molecular pathology in influencing outcomes. Generally, establishing cooperation in multidisciplinary fields will be essential to make full use of molecular pathology for better healthcare (Balta et al., 2024; Yu et al., 2024).

The foundations of molecular pathology are centuries-old in the study of various omics technologies, as a collective that enhances our understanding of disease pathogenesis. Among the significant progresses in molecular pathology is metabolomics, a study of metabolites that is vital biomarkers of biological processes and disease states. Such an analysis facilitates the development of novel biomarkers that not only supplement diagnostic requirements but also the construction of targeted therapies. The metabolomic uses for oral and maxillofacial pathology illustrate this potential, particularly with regard to common diseases. Studies of diseases , such as oral cancer and ameloblastomas reflect a variety of metabolic changes that can guide clinicians both in diagnosis and treatment, highlighting the necessity for integrating metabolomic analysis into the greater scheme of molecular pathology (Hu et al., 2025). Another essential area of research within molecular pathology is the role of epigenetics in multi-factorial disease , such as depression. Epigenetic modifications, which determine gene expression without altering sequences in DNA, are central to the deciphering of the biological mechanisms controlling mood regulation and mental health. Current research points to how environmental influences have the potential to cause such changes with significant effects on neuroplasticity and synaptic function. The identification of novel epigenetic targets not only holds the potential for new antidepressant treatments but also advances the use of personalized medicine approaches that target distinct epigenetic patterns. This offers a greater understanding of the molecular mechanisms of depression and can lead to improved treatment, thus highlighting the revolutionary potential of epigenetic discovery in molecular pathology (Batool et al., 2023). In summary, the integration of metabolomics and epigenetics in molecular pathology offers a complete stage for improving the understanding of disease and designing efficient treatments. Based on these advanced analytic techniques, researchers can identify important metabolic changes and identify epigenetic alterations that explain the pathophysiology of diseases. This comprehensive understanding is essential in not just diagnosing and treating disease more ideally, but also developing specific therapeutic strategies that account for variation in the individual. Further research on these issues will undoubtedly bring about fantastic breakthroughs, forming the basis of fantastic advances in clinical practice and eventually improving patient care across a broad spectrum of health disciplines. Thus, the molecular pathology roots form a basis for impending practice and research in clinical disease warfare for difficult diseases (Batool et al., 2023; Hu et al., 2025).

A LOOK TO THE FUTURE

SEROUS TUBAL INTRAEPITHELIAL CARCINOMA (STIC):

Serous Tubal Intraepithelial Carcinoma (STIC) has emerged over the past two decades as a pivotal lesion in gynecologic oncology, fundamentally reshaping our understanding of the origin and early pathogenesis of the most lethal form of pelvic serous carcinoma. Historically, high-grade serous carcinomas involving the ovary, fallopian tube, or peritoneum were classified primarily as ovarian cancers; however, detailed morphologic and molecular investigations have revealed that a substantial proportion of these malignancies originate not in the ovary itself but in the epithelium of the distal fallopian tube, most often at the fimbrial end. This paradigm shift owes much to rigorous pathological protocols such as the Sectioning and Extensively Examining the FIMbria (SEE-FIM) technique, which has dramatically increased the detection of microscopic precursor lesions in fallopian tubes removed from women at high risk for ovarian carcinoma.

STIC is defined by a population of cytologically malignant epithelial cells confined to the tubal mucosa without evidence of stromal invasion. These cells exhibit characteristic morphological features—including increased nuclear-to-cytoplasmic ratios, marked nuclear atypia, and epithelial stratification—and distinct immunohistochemical profiles such as aberrant p53 expression and elevated Ki-67 proliferative indices. Molecularly, STIC lesions almost universally harbor TP53 mutations, which are also a hallmark of high-grade serous carcinomas, providing strong evidence of a clonal relationship and supporting the role of STIC as a precursor lesion.

The clinical significance of STIC extends beyond its pathological definition. It is frequently detected incidentally during risk-reducing bilateral salpingo-oophorectomy in women carrying pathogenic BRCA1 or BRCA2 mutations, in whom the estimated incidence ranges from approximately 0.6% to 7%. However, STIC can also be found in women without known hereditary cancer syndromes, underscoring its relevance to both high-risk and average-risk populations. Despite this, the natural history and optimal management of isolated STIC remain areas of ongoing investigation, particularly because reliable early detection strategies for progression to invasive carcinoma are lacking.

STIC represents the earliest morphologically identifiable step in the carcinogenic sequence leading to many high-grade serous carcinomas of the pelvis. Its recognition as a lesion of critical clinical importance has profound implications for cancer prevention, surgical management, and the conceptual framework of ovarian and tubal carcinogenesis. Future research aimed at refining diagnostic criteria, clarifying progression risk, and tailoring management strategies promises to further improve outcomes and deepen insight into this early and enigmatic lesion.

REFERENCES

1. Ahmad, A., Imran, M., & Ahsan, H. (2023). Biomarkers as biomedical bioindicators: Approaches and techniques for the detection, analysis, and validation of novel biomarkers of diseases. *Pharmaceutics, 15*, 1630–1630. https://doi.org/10.3390/pharmaceutics15061630 (accessed on 17th July 2025).
2. Ayaz, H., Baker, W. B., Blaney, G., Boas, D. A., Bortfeld, H., Brady, K. M., Brake, J., et al. (2022). Optical imaging and spectroscopy for the study of the human brain: Status report. *Neurophotonics, 9*. https://doi.org/10.1117/1.nph.9.s2.s24001 (accessed on 17th July 2025).
3. Fox RJ, Thompson A, Baker D, et al. Setting a research agenda for progressive multiple sclerosis: the International Collaborative on Progressive MS. *Mult Scler*. 2012;18(11):1534-1540. doi:10.1177/1352458512458169(accessed on 17th July 2025).
4. Balta, M. Ç., Erdogdu, I., Oktay, E., & Çulhac, N. (2024). Comparison of molecular analysis results determined by next-generation sequencing to immunohistochemical indicators and clinicopathological parameters in prostate adenocarcinomas. *Indian Journal of Pathology & Microbiology, 4*. https://www.semanticscholar.org/paper/4994cbdcc9d0284b8923026903d0cc2418aecd69 (accessed on 17th July 2025).
5. Candia, J., Maunu, R., Driscoll, M., Biancotto, A., Dagur, P., McCoy, J. P., Jr, Sen, H. N., Wei, L., Maritan, A., Cao, K., Nussenblatt, R. B., Banavar, J. R., & Losert, W. (2013). From cellular characteristics to disease diagnosis: uncovering phenotypes with supercells. *PLoS computational biology, 9*(9), e1003215. https://doi.org/10.1371/journal.pcbi.1003215(accessed on 17th July 2025).
6. Batool, S. M., Yekula, A., Khanna, P., Hsia, T., Gamblin, A. S., Ekanayake, E., Escobedo, A., et al. (2023). The Liquid Biopsy Consortium: Challenges and opportunities for early cancer detection and monitoring. *Cell Reports Medicine, 4*, 101198–101198. https://doi.org/10.1016/j.xcrm.2023.101198 (accessed on 17th July 2025).
7. Sohail, A., Bég, O. A., Li, Z., & Celik, S. (2018). Physics of fractional imaging in biomedicine. *Progress in biophysics and molecular biology, 140*, 13–20. https://doi.org/10.1016/j.pbiomolbio.2018.03.002(accessed on 17th July 2025).
8. Betz, U. A. K., Arora, L., Assal, R. A., Azevedo, H., Baldwin, J., Becker, M., Bostock, S., et al. (2023). Game changers in science and technology–now and beyond. *Technological Forecasting and Social Change, 193*, 122588–122588. https://doi.org/10.1016/j.techfore.2023.122588 (accessed on 17th July 2025).
9. Ma, Peng-Fei & Fu, Yujie & Cai, Meichun & Yan, Ying & Jing, Ying & Zhang, Shengzhe & Chen, Minjiang & Wu, Jie & Shen, Ying & Zhu, Liang & Chen, Hong-Zhuan & Gao, Wei-Qiang & Wang, Mengzhao & Gu, Zhenyu & Bivona, Trever & Zhao, Xiaojing & Zhuang, Guanglei. (2017). Simultaneous evolutionary expansion and constraint of genomic heterogeneity in multifocal lung cancer. Nature Communications. 8. 10.1038/s41467-017-00963-0. (accessed on 17th July 2025).
10. Squassina, A., Severino, G., Grech, G., Fenech, A., Borg, J., & Patrinos, G. P. (2012). Conference Scene: Golden Helix Pharmacogenomics Days: Educational Activities on Pharmacogenomics and Personalized Medicine. *Pharmacogenomics, 13*(5), 525–528. https://doi.org/10.2217/pgs.12.22(accessed on 17th July 2025).

11. Camilleri, A., Camilleri, G. E., Camilleri, J., et al. (2004). Dentistry. https://core.ac.uk/download/46601883.pdf (accessed on 17th July 2025).
12. Riezzo, I., Cantatore, S., DeCarlo, D., Fiore, C., Neri, M., Turillazzi, E., & Fineschi, V. (2015). Confocal laser scanning microscope, Raman microscopy and Western blotting to evaluate inflammatory response after myocardial infarction. *Current vascular pharmacology, 13*(1), 78–90. https://doi.org/10.2174/1570161113119990004(accessed on 17th July 2025).
13. Potikha, T., Ella, E., Cerliani, J. P., Mizrahi, L., Pappo, O., Rabinovich, G. A., Galun, E., & Goldenberg, D. S. (2016). Galectin-1 is essential for efficient liver regeneration following hepatectomy. *Oncotarget, 7*(22), 31738–31754. https://doi.org/10.18632/oncotarget.9194accessed on 17th July 2025).
14. Che, J., Yu, V., Dhar, M., Renier, C., Matsumoto, M., Heirich, K., Garon, E. B., Goldman, J., Rao, J., Sledge, G. W., Pegram, M. D., Sheth, S., Jeffrey, S. S., Kulkarni, R. P., Sollier, E., & Di Carlo, D. (2016). Classification of large circulating tumor cells isolated with ultra-high throughput microfluidic Vortex technology. *Oncotarget, 7*(11), 12748–12760. https://doi.org/10.18632/oncotarget.7220(accessed on 17th July 2025).
15. Chen, S., Saeed, A. F. U. H., Liu, Q., Jiang, Q., Xu, H., Xiao, G. G., Rao, L., et al. (2023). Macrophages in immunoregulation and therapeutics. *Signal Transduction and Targeted Therapy, 8*. https://doi.org/10.1038/s41392-023-01452-1 (accessed on 17th July 2025).
16. Collyar, D., Basila, D., Lynch, T., Schnitt, S. J., Marks, J., Strand, S. H., Hyslop, T., et al. (2024). Abstract PO4-13-04: Added value from patient advocates in a translational working group: The COMET study. *Cancer Research*. https://www.semanticscholar.org/paper/d2b1109cdb47e3a758118378b22431fe8cf438f5 (accessed on 17th July 2025).
17. Critchley, H., Babayev, E., Bulun, S. E., Clark, S., Garcia-Grau, I., Gregersen, P. K., Kilcoyne, A., et al. (2020). Menstruation: Science and society. *American Journal of Obstetrics and Gynecology, 223*, 624–664. https://doi.org/10.1016/j.ajog.2020.06.004 (accessed on 17th July 2025).
18. Wild, P. J., Ikenberg, K., Fuchs, T. J., Rechsteiner, M., Georgiev, S., Fankhauser, N., Noske, A., Roessle, M., Caduff, R., Dellas, A., Fink, D., Moch, H., Krek, W., & Frew, I. J. (2012). p53 suppresses type II endometrial carcinomas in mice and governs endometrial tumour aggressiveness in humans. *EMBO molecular medicine, 4*(8), 808–824. https://doi.org/10.1002/emmm.201101063 (accessed on 17th July 2025).
19. Guido, C. A., Zicari, A. M., Duse, M., & Spalice, A. (2019). Eye movement desensitisation and reprocessing (EMDR) treatment associated with parent management training (PMT) for the acute symptoms in a patient with PANDAS syndrome: a case report. *Italian journal of pediatrics, 45*(1), 74. https://doi.org/10.1186/s13052-019-0667-1 (accessed on 17th July 2025).
20. Kaufman, G. E., Epstein, J. H., Paul-Murphy, J., & Modrall, J. D. (2008). Designing graduate training programs in conservation medicine-producing the right professionals with the right tools. *EcoHealth, 5*(4), 519–527. https://doi.org/10.1007/s10393-008-0208-7(accessed on 17th July 2025).
21. Fernandes, E., Sores, J., Cotton, S., Peixoto, A., Ferreira, D., Freitas, R., Reis, C. A., et al. (2020). Esophageal, gastric, and colorectal cancers: Looking beyond classical serological biomarkers towards glycoproteomic-assisted precision oncology. *Theragnostic, 10*, 4903–4928. https://doi.org/10.7150/thno.42480 (accessed on 17th July 2025).

22. Fonseca e Fonseca, B. de P., Albuquerque, P. C., & Zicker, F. (2020). Neglected tropical diseases in Brazil: Lack of correlation between disease burden, research funding, and output. *Tropical Medicine & International Health, 25*, 1373–1384. https://doi.org/10.1111/tmi.13478 (accessed on 17th July 2025).

23. Gallucci, B., Bierut, M., & McCarthy, D. O. (1995). The immune system. https://core.ac.uk/download/213081395.pdf (accessed on 17th July 2025).

24. Halbrook, C. J., Lyssiotis, C. A., Pasca di Magliano, M., & Maitra, A. (2023). Pancreatic cancer: Advances and challenges. *Cell, 186*, 1729–1754. https://doi.org/10.1016/j.cell.2023.02.014 (accessed on 17th July 2025).

25. Laird, A., Thomson, J. P., Harrison, D. J., & Meehan, R. R. (2013). 5-hydroxymethylcytosine profiling as an indicator of cellular state. *Epigenomics, 5*(6), 655–669. https://doi.org/10.2217/epi.13.69 (accessed on 17th July 2025).

26. Hu, K., Zhang, X., Li, Y., Wang, Z., & Li, Y. (2025). Metabolite changes in oral tumors and cysts: A narrative review. *BMC Oral Health, 25*. https://www.semanticscholar.org/paper/1a9ba0d5d51c954a05c2bf79187a6cbd61e46aab (accessed on 17th July 2025).

27. Jäntschi, L., Diudea, M. V., Bălan, M. C., Sestras, R. E., & Bolboacă, S. D. (2010). Results of evolution supervised by genetic algorithms. http://arxiv.org/abs/1009.0915 (accessed on 17th July 2025).

28. Jones, E. M., & Tansey, E. M. (2014). Clinical molecular genetics in the UK c.1975-c.2000. https://core.ac.uk/download/30696934.pdf (accessed on 17th July 2025).

29. Koptyra, M. P., Rahti, K., Zhu, Y., Farrow, B. K., Miller, D. P., Kraya, A., Guo, Y., et al. (2023). Abstract 3566: Expansion of the Pediatric Brain Tumor Atlas: Children's Brain Tumor Network, Kids First Data Resource and Childhood Cancer Data Initiative Open Science effort. *Cancer Research*. https://www.semanticscholar.org/paper/922a70be27dec2c4ca37bba1cbf9e08f817e1bff (accessed on 17th July 2025).

30. Kotov, R., Krueger, R. F., Watson, D., Cicero, D. C., Conway, C., DeYoung, C. G., Eaton, N. R., et al. (2021). The Hierarchical Taxonomy of Psychopathology (HiTOP): A quantitative nosology based on consensus of evidence. *Annual Review of Clinical Psychology, 17*, 83–108. https://doi.org/10.1146/annurev-clinpsy-081219-093304 (accessed on 17th July 2025).

31. Watkins, J., Marsh, A., Taylor, P. C., & Singer, D. R. (2010). Personalized medicine: the impact on chemistry. *Therapeutic delivery, 1*(5), 651–665. https://doi.org/10.4155/tde.10.64(accessed on 17th July 2025).

32. Najjar, R. (2023). Redefining radiology: A review of artificial intelligence integration in medical imaging. *Diagnostics, 13*, 2760–2760. https://doi.org/10.3390/diagnostics13172760 (accessed on 17th July 2025).

33. Olorunsogo, T. O., Balogun, O. D., Ayo-Farai, O., Ogundairo, O., Maduka, C. P., Okongwu, C. C., & Onwumere, C. (2024). Bioinformatics and personalized medicine in the U.S.: A comprehensive review: Scrutinizing the advancements in genomics and their potential to revolutionize healthcare delivery. *World Journal of Advanced Research and Reviews, 21*, 335–351. https://doi.org/10.30574/wjarr.2024.21.1.0016 (accessed on 17th July 2025).

34. Otlowski M. (2006). Essentially yours: the protection of human genetic information in Australia. *Genewatch : a bulletin of the Committee for Responsible Genetics, 19*(1), 9–12. (accessed on 17th July 2025).

35. Pölcher, M., Wimberger, P., Meinhold-Heerlein, I., Runnebaum, I. B., Schüler-Toprak, S., Mahner, S., Grimm, C., et al. (2025). Intergroup statement: Opportunistic salpingectomy—molecular pathology, clinical outcomes and implications for practice (German Ovarian Cancer Commission, the North-Eastern German Society of Gynecologic Oncology (NOGGO), AGO Austria and AGO Swiss). *Archives of Gynecology and Obstetrics, 311*, 1451–1459. https://www.semanticscholar.org/paper/80f9ebb1257839cc0e055bfb48c21fac69698902 (accessed on 17th July 2025).

36. Samarkhanova, D., Zhabagin, M., & Nadirov, N. (2025). Reviewing the genetic and molecular foundations of congenital spinal deformities: Implications for classification and diagnosis. *Journal of Clinical Medicine, 14*. https://www.semanticscholar.org/paper/1831511ede66456d00cbd8d7429e07e194fb581c (accessed on 17th July 2025).

37. Shah, P., Kendall, F., Khozin, S., Goosen, R., Hu, J., Laramie, J. M., Ringel, M. S., et al. (2019). Artificial intelligence and machine learning in clinical development: A translational perspective. *npj Digital Medicine, 2*. https://doi.org/10.1038/s41746-019-0148-3 (accessed on 17th July 2025).

38. Struelens, M., Ludden, C., Werner, G., Sintchenko, V., Jokelainen, P., & Ip, M. (2024). Real-time genomic surveillance for enhanced control of infectious diseases and antimicrobial resistance. *Frontiers in Science, 2*. https://doi.org/10.3389/fsci.2024.1298248 (accessed on 17th July 2025).

39. Świątek, W., Kłodziński, O., Ciesielski, M., Adamkiewicz, Z., Podolak, M., Mozdziak, P., & Kranc, W. (2024). Glioblastoma: A molecular insight into current discoveries and treatment directions. *Medical Journal of Cell Biology, 12*, 1–20. https://www.semanticscholar.org/paper/3bc2f8548d5a7a178d30173b22003076358714a3 (accessed on 17th July 2025).

40. Virginia Commonwealth University. (2018). Virginia Commonwealth University Professional Bulletin. https://core.ac.uk/download/215485746.pdf (accessed on 17th July 2025).

41. Winkleman, Don, 1986. "**The Evolving Role of CIMMYT: Some Issues for World Food and Agriculture**," 1986: Trade and Development Meetinghttps://core.ac.uk/download/pdf/6383429.pdf (accessed on 17th July 2025).

42. Yang, C., Chen, F., Wang, S., & Xiong, B. (2019). Circulating tumor cells in gastrointestinal cancers: Current status and future perspectives. *Frontiers in Oncology, 9*. https://doi.org/10.3389/fonc.2019.01427 (accessed on 17th July 2025).

43. Yu, X., Qu, Z., Jian, C., Wang, Z., Jian, L., Jin, L., Pan, Y., et al. (2024). Deep learning application in prediction of cancer molecular alterations based on pathological images: A bibliographic analysis via CiteSpace. *Journal of Cancer Research and Clinical Oncology, 150*. https://www.semanticscholar.org/paper/398e74c4edb61cc26bcab881aadd7aab8267cbba (accessed on 17th July 2025).

44. Zyma, A., Skuratov, O. Iu., Huk, Y. M., Filipchuk, V., Cheverda, A., Kincha-Polishchuk, T., Melnyk, M., et al. (2025). Fibrous Dysplasia: From Historical Approaches to Modern Treatment Perspectives. *Terra Orthopaedica*. https://www.semanticscholar.org/paper/930c30d1eed0db2c3cf3dfc5e8611abf2bb21ad5 (accessed on 17th July 2025).

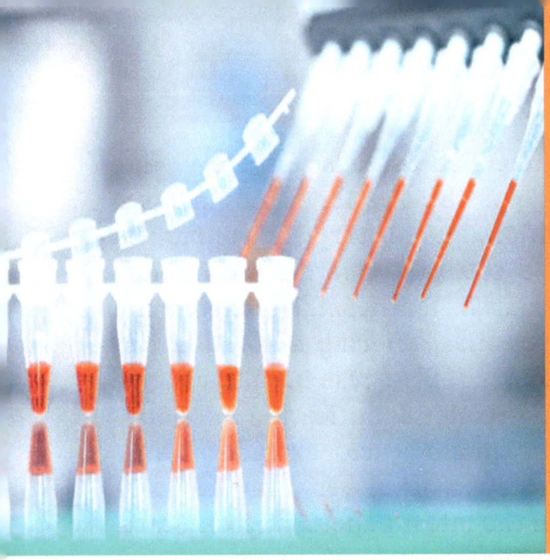

Chapter 2

NUCLEIC ACID EXTRACTION AND QUANTIFICATION

Contents

Introduction

Extraction and quantification of nucleic acids form the foundation of most applications in molecular biology, from genetic research, diagnostics, and forensic science. It all begins with the extraction of deoxyribonucleic acid (DNA) or ribonucleic acid (RNA) from various samples of biological material with extreme care. Good extraction procedures are important because the purity and yield of the nucleic acids directly impact downstream assays , such as polymerase chain reaction (PCR) and next-generation sequencing. With the progressing times, and in recent studies, the demand for effective nucleic acid extraction techniques increases with the rise in technological advancements and increased knowledge of genetic factors in disease and health. Hence, creating and perfecting these extraction techniques is crucial to guaranteeing accurate and effective molecular analysis, eventually leading to sound scientific conclusions and clinical decisions. Technological advances in the quantification of nucleic acids have greatly changed the character of molecular diagnostics. Modern methods have emphasized not only the sensitivity and specificity of detection but also the ease of use in the field. For instance, innovations , such as microfluidics create new possibilities for rapid analysis that allow for on-site testing, which can be performed outside traditional laboratory environments. This shift towards portability is necessary in resource-constrained settings, where conventional diagnostic tools may be less convenient. As shown by new research, isothermal nucleic-acid quantification technology functions well with unreliable power supplies, offering a solution for reliable diagnostics in poorly equipped health clinics (Cesarman et al., 2018). These breakthroughs confirm the necessity of ongoing innovation in nucleic acid extraction and quantification methods. Microfluidics has emerged as an essential element in enhancing nucleic acid extraction and quantitation processes. Microfluidics facilitates several analytical steps within very tiny devices, bundling processes and improving overall efficiency. As described in the latest papers, microfluidics allows for targeted sample preparation and immediate analysis, significantly reducing time to obtain results and improving sensitivity (Jayamohan et al., 2017). This technology not only enables more precise quantification of nucleic acids but also supports a range of applications , including infectious disease monitoring, environmental testing, and food safety screening. As the molecular diagnostics field continues to mature, no one can exaggerate the value that microfluidic devices bring to improving nucleic acid extraction processes and quantification, pledging an age of quicker and more dependable diagnostic capabilities in all industries (Figure 2.1).

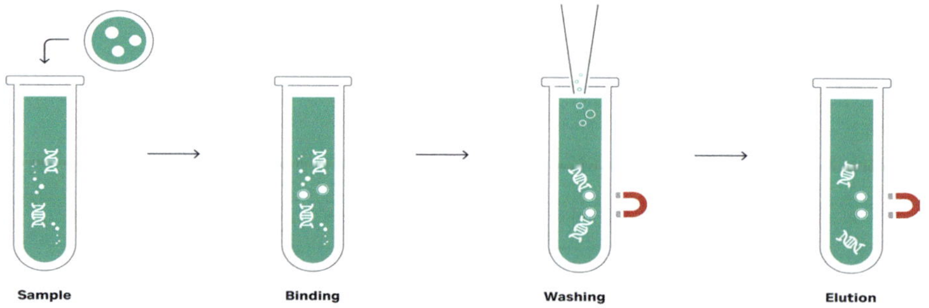

Figure 2.1. Introduction to nucleic acid extraction.

Source: https://www.geneture.com/uploadfile/ueditor/image/202209/1663558212b83286.jpg.

Definition of Nucleic Acids

Nucleic acids are macromolecules common to all living organisms and are centrally involved in the storage and transmission of hereditary information. They exist primarily in two forms: deoxyribonucleic acid (DNA) and ribonucleic acid (RNA). DNA serves as the blueprint for the growth, operation, and reproduction of an organism and contains the information necessary for the assembly of proteins. Conversely, RNA acts as a messenger that brings genetic information from DNA to ribosomes, where proteins are made. The structural organization of such nucleic acids, characterized by sequences of nucleotide monomers that are composed of a sugar, a phosphate group, and a nitrogenous base, allows them to act in highly complex ways in coding, decoding, regulation, and expression of genes. It is critical to understand these definitions for a variety of applications, particularly genetic engineering and molecular biology. Quantitation and nucleic acid extraction are crucial processes in molecular biology that facilitate a myriad of experimental techniques, such as polymerase chain reaction (PCR) and sequencing. Successful extraction is required for the purification of high-quality nucleic acids, which in turn is necessary for accurate downstream applications. Techniques can be fairly varied and can involve the use of chemical reagents to depolymerize cell membranes or enzymatic treatment aimed at freeing nucleic acids without destroying them from degradative activities. Such protocols must be followed strictly to maintain the integrity of the nucleic acids as well as yield sufficient amounts for subsequent analyses. The measurement of nucleic acid concentration and purity usually employs spectrophotometric methods or fluorescence technologies, yielding precise values that are crucial for successful experimental outcomes and conclusions. As a final point, the definition of nucleic acids includes their structural elements, biological functions, and extraction methods that render them accessible in scientific research. In addition to mere storage of genetic data, nucleic acids are critical to life processes, illustrating the precarious balance between structure and function in biology. As genetics and molecular biology continue to advance, so too do the methods for extracting and quantifying nucleic acids, with new possibilities and increasing ability for the study of genetic material. Therefore, it is critical for anyone pursuing genomic research or associated scientific disciplines to familiarize themselves with these basic concepts and methods, cementing their place as essential tools in contemporary biological science (Figure 2.2).

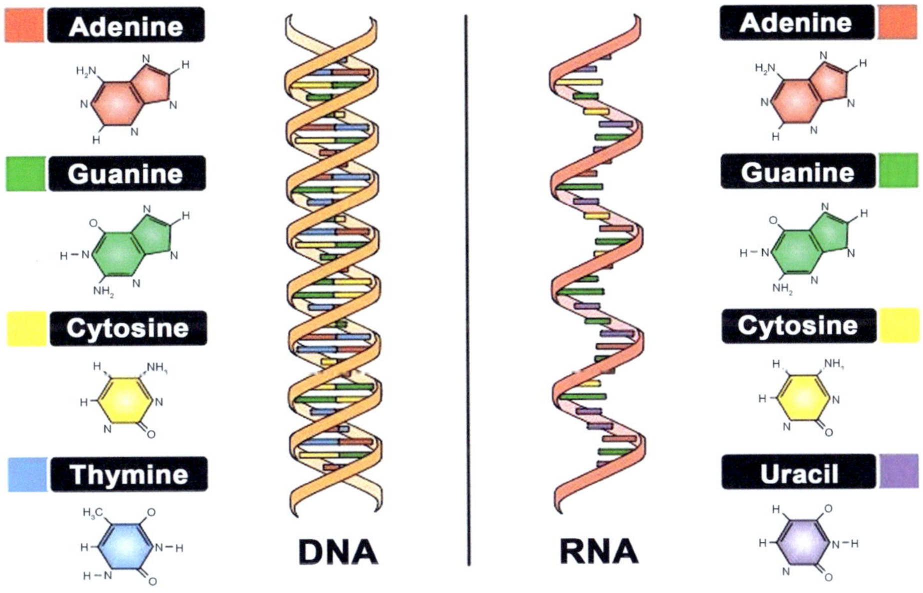

Figure 2.2. Nucleic acid.

Source: https://www.biologyonline.com/wp-content/uploads/2019/10/DNA.jpg.

Importance of Nucleic Acid Extraction

Nucleic acid extraction is a critical molecular biology technique, where DNA and RNA are separated from biological samples. It is a precursor to numerous applications, including genetic research, clinical testing, and drug development. The purity and concentration of isolated nucleic acids directly affect the validity of ensuing processes like PCR, sequencing, and gene expression analysis. As outlined in various studies, technological advancements in extraction processes have enabled the automation of these processes and efficiency enhancement while reducing exposure to contamination. An instance is the manner in which complete automation of equipment in rapid diagnostic methods has significantly shaped the detection of infectious diseases, which points to the role of nucleic acid extraction in the strengthening of public health responses. High-quality extraction upholds high standards to guarantee consistent data generation, a vital process for evidence-based decision-making during research and in clinical practice (Ince & McNally, 2009). Nucleic acid extraction in infectious diseases is additionally useful through application in viral pathogenesis and host response knowledge.

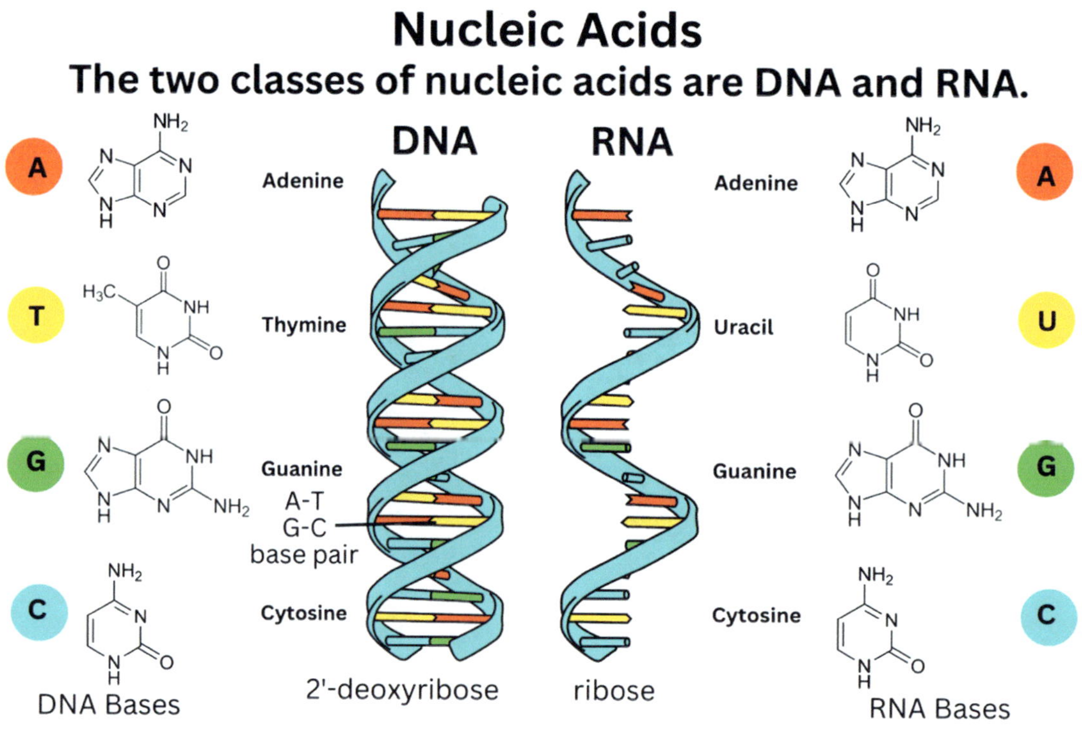

Figure 2.3. Importance of nucleic acid extraction.

Source: https://miro.medium.com/v2/resize:fit:700/1*6wVkxnxAgScRlFcalKb-Uw.png.

One of the best examples is the nucleic acid extraction from patient samples to identify the presence of certain viral agents, for instance, Parvovirus B19. Quantitation of viral load using nucleic acid extraction has been shown through research to be associated with the severity of diseases like inflammatory cardiomyopathy. In a single study, high B19V viral loads were measured in endomyocardial biopsies, pointing to the need for high accuracy in extraction methods to predict the dynamics of viral infection (D'Ambrosio et al., 2008). Such potentiality of extracting and quantifying nucleic acids with high accuracy is not only important for disease detection, but also for disease evolution and, perhaps, therapeutic responses monitoring. Finally, the significance of nucleic acid extraction is also relevant to personalized medicine, wherein the understanding of a person's specific genetic information is of prime significance. It becomes possible to study genetic variations through the possibility of extracting good-quality DNA and RNA, thus providing scope for customized treatment regimens based on a patient's genetic information. Since research is increasingly aimed at developing rapid diagnostic tools, the extraction of nucleic acids is at the center of such innovations. Better methods , such as biosensor-based immunoassays, leverage the nucleic acid extraction to ensure affordable and efficient diagnostics and hence transform the provision of healthcare (Ince & McNally, 2009). Therefore, constant development in extraction techniques is imperative not only in the formation of scientific research but also for clinical efficacy and personalized health strategies (Figure 2.3).

Overview of Quantification Methods

For nucleic acid extraction and analysis, a number of methodologies exist that have been established to meet specific research needs and technological advances. Traditional methods , such as spectrophotometry, yield a straightforward means of nucleic acid quantification via absorbance at certain wavelengths. While this has its built-in limitations regarding sensitivity and specificity, it has prompted the development of more advanced techniques. By applying fluorescence-based detection, methods like quantitative polymerase chain reaction (QPCR) have revolutionized the field by offering the capacity to amplify and quantify nucleic acids in real time. The methodological switch has resulted in greater accuracy and capacity to detect low-abundance targets, making it essential in a broad range of applications from genetics to clinical diagnostics. Microfluidic devices are the cutting edge of nucleic acid quantification and aim to make processes more efficient, decrease sample size, and increase sensitivity. Microfluidics enables small fluid volumes on a chip to be manipulated, making many assays extremely more efficient, like nucleic acid amplification and sequencing. By putting multiple steps on one device, microfluidics enables rapid results while minimizing the risk of contamination. Furthermore, advances in nanotechnology allow for the manufacture of highly sensitive biosensors capable of measuring to unparalleled precision. Such sophistication not only complements traditional approaches but also meets the growing need for point-of-care diagnosis, particularly in areas lacking material resources, as seen in recent breakthroughs where they utilize portable tools for isothermal nucleic acid quantification (Jayamohan et al., 2017). Innovative approaches in quantification methods are also being transformed, addressing the actual problem of accessibility and reliability in diagnostic tools. A decentralized diagnostic system has the potential to increase the speed of treatment, particularly for infectious diseases, without recourse to stationary power sources. New technologies have been invented to yield portable instruments that can conduct nucleic acid quantification using non-conventional energy sources, such as solar or combustion (Cesarman et al., 2018). This flexibility not only makes the operation survivable in the case of power failure but also enhances the use of diagnostics in diverse environments. Filling the gap between advanced laboratory practices and use in the field, these innovations promote health gains and demonstrate a paradigm shift in the domain of molecular diagnostics with specific implications for global health initiatives.

2.1. Types of Nucleic Acids

The different nucleic acids are focal in molecular biology, and they are primarily categorized under deoxyribonucleic acid (DNA) and ribonucleic acid (RNA). DNA is the substance passed on by nearly all living organisms, with the genetic code required for life. Its double helix structure, consisting of two coiled strands, can store genetic information safely. Conversely, RNA also plays a crucial role in translating these genetic codes into functional proteins, an activity central to cell functions. Specifically, messenger RNA (mRNA) carries genetic information from DNA to ribosomes for protein synthesis and is aided by transfer RNA (tRNA) and ribosomal RNA (rRNA). It is essential to understand these primary categories of nucleic acids, especially for the extraction procedures of nucleic acids in a way that preserves their integrity for subsequent applications , such as next-generation sequencing and quantitative PCR (Martins et al., 2023).

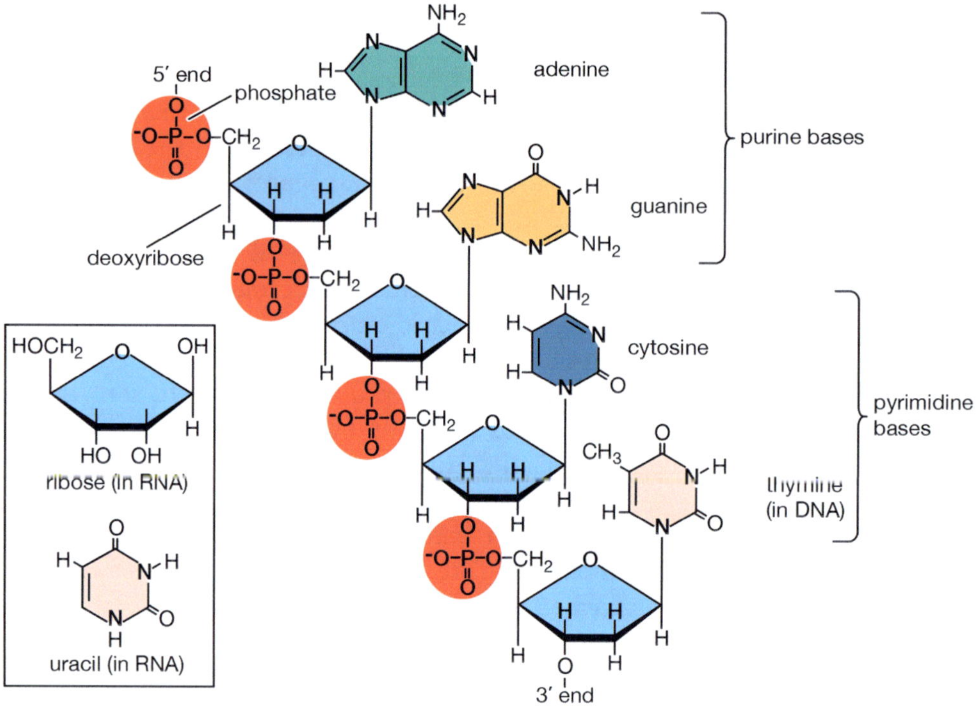

Figure 2.4. Types of nucleic acids.

Source: https://conductscience.com/wp-content/uploads/2021/07/A-representative-complete-structure-of-nucleic-acids-1024x701.png.

The extraction procedures for nucleic acids vary extensively depending on the nature of the sample and the nucleic acid that is to be extracted. For instance, phenol-chloroform extraction gives good-quality DNA but may not be so suitable for RNA, as it could be broken down. Alternatively, commercially purchased kits, e.g., silica membrane technology-based kits, can provide rapid and efficient extraction as well as high yield of DNA and RNA. It is important that extraction methods consider the inherent nature of the nucleic acids; for example, RNA is degraded more by ribonucleases and hence strict precautions must be observed during storage and extraction (Cesarman et al., 2018). Additionally, different nucleic acids require particular elution buffers and purification strategies, which add complexity to the utility of specialized methods to effectively recover these biomolecules and reach their full potential in research and clinical applications. Quantification of nucleic acids is also necessary as it is imperative for future applications. Techniques , such as fluorometry and spectrophotometry provide reliable means to quantify nucleic acid concentration and purity. Fluorometric assays, particularly intercalating dye-based assays, can provide higher sensitivity compared to UV absorption-based assays and are therefore important to quantify low levels of nucleic acids derived from multiplexed biological samples. In addition, accurate quantification can inform scientists on the optimal input for amplification reactions to ensure successful amplification in scientific fields like PCR and library preparation for sequencing. As the types of nucleic acids vary in properties and roles in cellular activities, understanding the nuances becomes essential in extraction and quantification techniques, which indirectly impacts the fidelity and reproducibility of molecular assays (Martins et al., 2023) (Figure 2.4).

2.1.1. DNA: Structure and Function

The double helix pattern of DNA, its most typical form, provides for the storage of genetic information. The DNA strand is a sugar-phosphate backbone and nucleotide bases (adenine, thymine, cytosine, and guanine) paired together in specific combinations: adenine with thymine and cytosine with guanine. Complementary base pairing is crucial for DNA replication, where it will provide for genetic information to be copied and transferred to daughter cells correctly. Besides, the antiparallel structure of the two strands provides a site for binding proteins that participate in replication and gene expression. The special shape of DNA with protein-binding grooves is essential for regulating gene operation such that cells can respond dynamically to internal and external factors without compromising the integrity of the genetic code (Groll et al., 2012). Aside from the structural make-up of DNA is the fact that it is the template for the synthesis of proteins. Transcribed out of DNA is messenger RNA (mRNA), which itself is translated into proteins that perform an array of tasks essential to the organism.

Transcription and translation represent the central dogma of molecular biology, invoking the passing of genetic information from DNA via RNA to protein. Moreover, variations in DNA sequences may also lead to variations in protein structure and function, reaffirming the significance of genetic variation in adaptation and evolution. Molecular technologies , such as the CRISPR-Cas tools, enhance our ability to manipulate DNA, providing avenues for novel advances in genetic engineering, such as targeted medicines and agricultural enhancements (Gleditzsch, 2020). To effectively utilize DNA in biotechnology and research, proper nucleic acid extraction and quantitation protocols are of the highest significance. These procedures are necessary to obtain high-quality DNA from various biological samples to enable downstream applications , such as cloning, gene expression, and sequencing. Purity and yield of purified nucleic acids directly determine the success of experiments and therefore optimal extraction protocol is crucial. Several techniques, including phenol-chloroform extraction and silica column-based protocols, have been developed to purify DNA with low contamination and degradation. Furthermore, accurate quantification techniques like spectrophotometry and fluorometry allow scientists to evaluate the concentration and purity of DNA before performing experimental manipulation (Groll et al., 2012). By providing high-quality nucleic acid preparations, scientists are better able to explore the intricate relationship between DNA structure and function, ultimately achieving a deeper understanding of molecular biology (Figure 2.5).

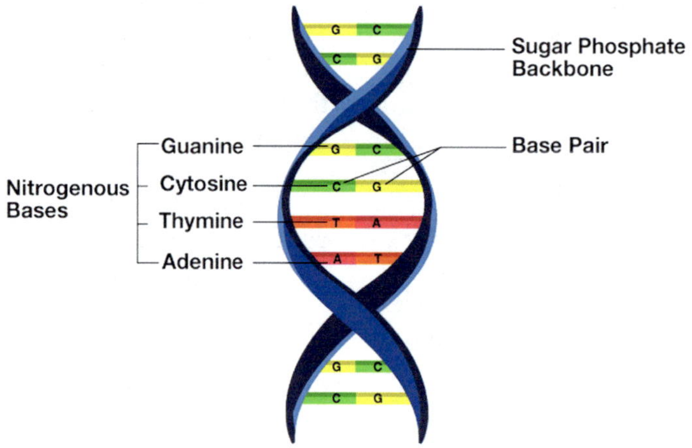

Figure 2.5. DNA: Structure.

Source: https://cdn1.byjus.com/wp-content/uploads/2018/12/DNA-Structure1.png.

2.1.2. RNA: Types and Roles

In molecular biology, ribonucleic acid (RNA) plays a vital role in the translation of genetic information as well as assisting with many cell processes. There are several varieties of RNA, and each performs specific functions essential for life. Messenger RNA (mRNA), which carries the genetic code from DNA to the ribosome where proteins are synthesized, is an essential process in gene expression. Transfer RNA (tRNA) and ribosomal RNA (rRNA) work together during the process of translation, tRNA delivering the appropriate amino acids and rRNA constructing the structural and functional core of the ribosome. Regulator RNAs , such as small interfering RNAs (siRNAs) and microRNAs (miRNAs), are also important for controlling gene expression and silencing specific targets to maintain cellular homeostasis and respond to environmental stress. An understanding of the functions of these kinds of RNA is significant when nucleic acid extraction and quantitation methods are being considered. Good RNA extraction is crucial in quantitative analysis in various areas of science, e.g., genomics and oncology. Standardized protocols ought to be able to be responsible for seeing to it that the RNA extracted is of adequate integrity and purity to give viable results. For instance, the quality of RNA recovered from formalin-fixed, paraffin-embedded (FFPE) samples has remained a significant challenge due to degradation and contamination. Recent advances in extraction protocols involving the incorporation of a micro-homogenizing device have provided evidence of the improvement of RNA recovery from such recalcitrant samples with higher integrity and longer RNA fragments (Adamian et al., 2016).

These developments in RNA purification techniques are vital not only in preserving accurate gene expression profiles but also in the ease of identification of disease state-associated biomarkers to enable advancements in the field of personalized medicine. Along with these developments in extraction techniques, quantification of RNA is equally vital in understanding its functions within cells. Methods , such as reverse transcription quantitative polymerase chain reaction (RT-qPCR) and next-generation sequencing (NGS) provide information regarding RNA dynamics that allow researchers to quantify expression levels and identify new transcripts. Of particular importance is the application of on-chip purification and amplification technologies for the rapid detection of RNA. Such innovations leverage the high stability, abundance of some forms of RNA, such as tmRNA (10Sa RNA), which could potentially help in raising the detection limit in the diagnosis of microbes (Antonio et al., 2008). Researchers are able to follow the changes in RNA more effectively as a result of environmental stimuli or disease progression, employing these advanced techniques, which points towards the importance of quantification and extraction of RNA for research and therapeutic applications.

2.1.3. Differences Between DNA and RNA

These distinctions between ribonucleic acid (RNA) and deoxyribonucleic acid (DNA) are more than structural components, symbolizing their exclusive functions in cellular function. DNA, or double helix in composition, is the predominant genetic material that contains hereditary information required for the development and functioning of organisms. RNA is typically single-stranded and serves various functions, such as messenger RNA (mRNA), which translates genetic information from DNA into proteins. This inherent disparity forms a basis for the understanding of the varied methodologies in nucleic acid extraction and quantification. Techniques should be tailored to these disparities to ensure the integrity and purity of the extracted nucleic acids, a consideration particularly essential in microbial dynamic research, as noted by the utilization of high-quality nucleic acids to provide accurate representation and analysis within ecological assessments (Aronson et al., 2014). For the purification of nucleic acids, there is a need to overcome the inherent challenges posed by the nature of both DNA and RNA. DNA purification often involves lysis buffers and precipitation methods that isolate the nucleic acid with minimal or no contamination with cellular residues. However, the extraction of RNA involves care to prevent degradation by ribonucleases and therefore, involves the use of special reagents to maintain RNA samples. Furthermore, the occurrence of RNA, especially in microbial-dense systems, can similarly complicate quantitation processes because total RNA includes mRNA, rRNA, and many others. Techniques , such as selective enrichment methods prove useful when isolating single species of RNA to be analyzed, highlighting the importance of understanding these differences in optimizing extraction protocols for the target type of nucleic acid, which ultimately enhances downstream analytical applications (Jue et al., 2020).

Further, quantitation methods for DNA and RNA differ considerably, which influences the choice of techniques employed in nucleic acid research. DNA quantitation is usually performed by spectrophotometric methods or fluorescence assays, in which concentration and purity can be determined rapidly. , such assays are made possible because of the relative stability of DNA due to its higher resistance to degradation than RNA. On the other hand, RNA quantification generally requires more challenging techniques due to its structural instability and sensitivity towards enzymatic degradation. Techniques , such as reverse transcription-quantitative polymerase chain reaction (RT-qPCR) become critical to accurately quantify RNA, for which thorough optimization becomes indispensable to remove inhibitors that can interfere with reaction efficiency. By recognizing these quantification strategy variations, researchers are able to customize the approach in response to the specific type of nucleic acid utilized in their study, providing reproducible and precise results (Aronson et al., 2014; Jue et al., 2020) (Figure 2.6).

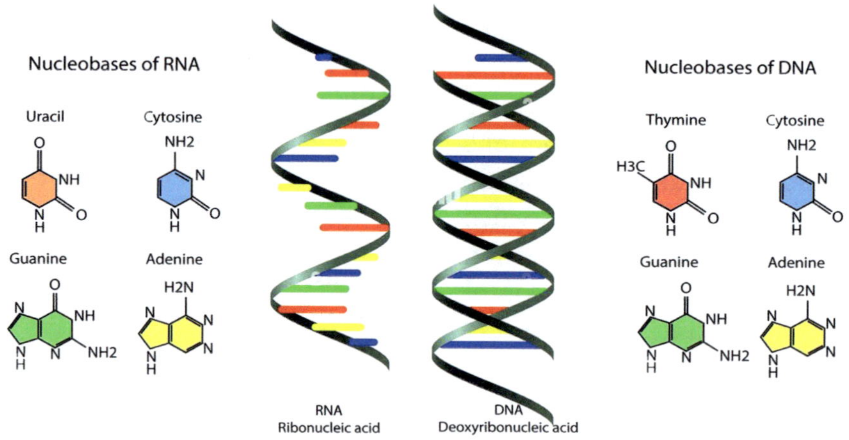

Figure 2.6. Differences between DNA and RNA.

Source: https://c8.alamy.com/comp/2R0WPEE/poster-showing-differences-between-rna-and-dna-on-white-background-illustration-2R0WPEE.jpg.

2.2. Common Methods of Nucleic Acid Extraction

Nucleic acid purification is a critical first step in most molecular biology protocols, ranging from gene cloning to PCR amplification. Silica-based nucleic acid extraction methods are one of the favorite techniques utilized, which avail themselves of the unique features of silica to have the capacity to bind nucleic acids under appropriate ionic conditions. Silica spin columns, for instance, make purification of DNA and RNA efficient after cell lysis. This technique typically involves the use of chaotropic salts that disrupt the hydrogen bonds and increase the binding of nucleic acids onto the silica matrix, permitting subsequent washes to remove the contaminants. These methods have been developed for a range of biological specimens and are therefore general in their capacity to address the needs of both fundamental research and clinical applications in genetic diagnosis. Other methods of nucleic acid extraction are the phenol-chloroform method and magnetic bead-based protocols. While the phenol-chloroform method has been the traditional default for many years, relying on phase separation with organic solvents, it produces potentially hazardous waste and is less suitable for high-throughput protocols. Magnetic bead protocols, however, have gained widespread popularity because they are amenable to automation of the extraction protocol and a significant reduction in time spent "hands-on." These methods utilize magnetic beads with immobilized nucleic acid-binding moieties that are easily recovered by a magnet, thus facilitating the purification of nucleic acids from complex biological samples. New advances have advertised the strength of such approaches, as extraction efficiency and purity studies are compared; incidentally, comparison studies of nucleic acid isolation kits show variations in performance depending on the sample source, indicating the need for tailored approaches (Kalmar et al., 2016). Moreover, for specific applications, recovery of nucleic acids from formalin-fixed paraffin-embedded (FFPE) tissues is especially demanding because of cross-linking and fragmentation of nucleic acids. Special extraction kits are formulated for this reason. The RNeasy FFPE kit from Qiagen, for instance, has been found to yield higher RNA levels and quality, and it is deemed an indispensable resource for cancer studies because tissue samples are frequently used. Methods should cater to the trade-off between yield and integrity, as described in comparative studies of commercial kits for DNA and RNA extraction from various sample sources (Böhner et al., 2024). Selecting the correct extraction protocol, in addition to its impact on the quantity and purity of the extracted nucleic acids, affects downstream procedures , such as sequencing and quantitative PCR, making it an important consideration in experimental design (Figure 2.7).

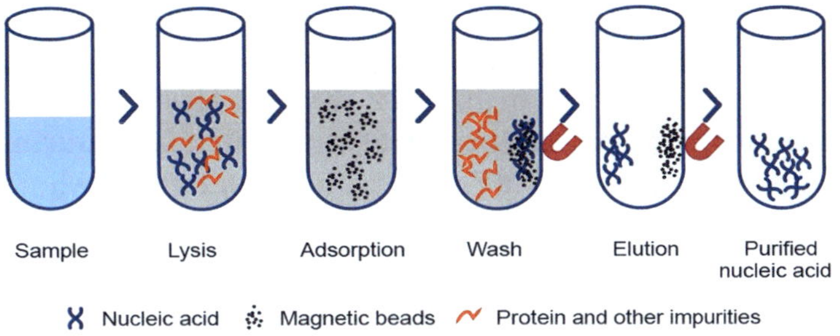

Figure 2.7. Nucleic acid extraction.

Source: https://www.vdobiotech.com/group1/ef/0ea2f870ecb247399850826bcdcb7ac2.jpg.

2.2.1. Phenol-Chloroform Extraction

Phenol-chloroform is one of the oldest and best-established procedures for nucleic acid isolation, particularly due to its effectiveness in recovering high DNA yields as well as RNA. By using a biphasic solvent system, this procedure permits the removal of nucleic acids from proteins and other cellular debris. Adding phenol, for denaturing protein, and chloroform increases the purification process and the quality of nucleic acids obtained by adding strength. Phenol-chloroform extraction has been demonstrated to yield concentrations of 50 100 ng/μL of DNA, a factor that makes its application highly valuable when downstream applications require high integrity of nucleic acids (Damian, 2025). However, despite its effectiveness, the method is not without its limitations, mainly in terms of safety hazards and the manpower-intensive nature of the protocol. While phenol-chloroform extraction has a good yield and purity, its application is accompanied by significant safety risks. Phenol is a toxic substance that is dangerous when exposed to it by inhalation or dermal absorption and requires careful attention to standard laboratory precautions. Furthermore, the multi-step extraction process makes laboratory workflows cumbersome, with a potential for inconsistency in results if not carried out carefully (Böhner et al., 2024). The process is likely to require additional purification to remove traces of chloroform and phenol, further contributing to the hindrances. Scientists will therefore have to weigh the benefits of high-yielding nucleic acids against the inherent risk and time needed in this process. Thus, alternative extraction methods , such as silica-based and magnetic bead-based, have gained popularity in laboratories due to their simplicity in handling and safety. Despite all the disadvantages, phenol-chloroform extraction still has unrivaled benefits, particularly when it comes to complex biological samples. For example, in tick-borne disease research, scientists have observed that this method is capable of yielding high-quality DNA from challenging samples like engorged ticks, which tend to contain PCR inhibitors due to their blood content (Böhner et al., 2024). The successful amplification of DNA prepared by this method is, at times, unpredictable and may require rigorous optimization of downstream processes, including PCR. With the recent comparative research, scientists have lobbied for the use of phenol-chloroform extraction in conjunction with high polymerase mixes to ensure maximum amplification efficiency. It is likely that standardization of extraction processes involving this traditional method might eventually provide better results in molecular diagnosis and research studies, bridging the current gaps in nucleic acid extraction methods (Damian, 2025).

2.2.2. Silica-Based Methods

The application of silica-based nucleic acid extraction has been of interest due to its efficiency and effectiveness. Silica possesses some properties that enable it to adsorb nucleic acids under specific conditions, particularly in combination with chaotropic salts during lysis. The adsorption enables the selective recovery of nucleic acids from proteins and other cellular components, thereby becoming a crucial component of most contemporary extraction kits. As noted in certain research, e.g., with Hepatitis B core Antigen (HBcAg) virus-like particles, silica spin column methods not only enhance nucleic acid yield but also purity levels, thus overall nucleic acid preparation quality for downstream application. The compatibility of silica extraction with stable analytical methods enables quantitation precision, an essential ingredient for application in gene delivery and other applications in molecular biology (Böhner et al., 2024). The second most notable feature of silica-based extraction techniques is that they can be applied to different types of nucleic acids and sample sources.

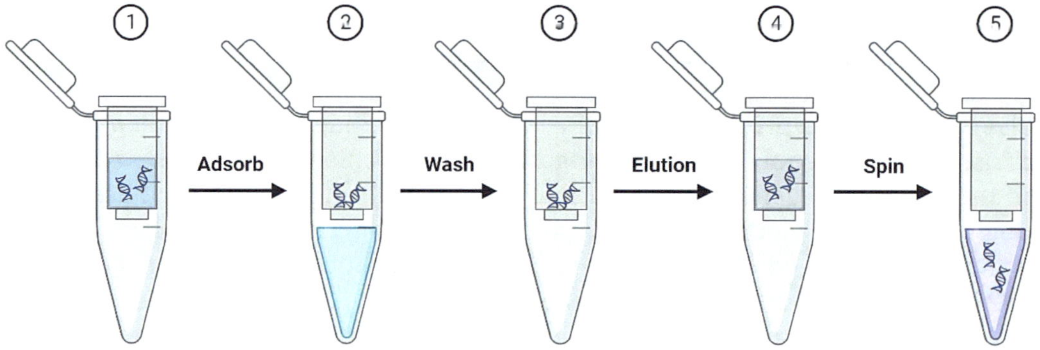

Figure 2.8. Silica-based methods.

Source: https://www.cd-bioparticles.com/upload/image/silica-spin-column.jpg.

They are versatile enough to process DNA and RNA from diverse matrices in the biological universe, including tissues, blood, and cell cultures. Nonetheless, the purity of purified nucleic acids is compromised by carryover of inhibitory buffers and contaminants. New developments have focused on solving these problems, as illustrated by a study in which improved procedures, such as a two-phase wash (TPW), were used to minimize buffer carryover with nucleic acid yield maintenance. These advancements point toward the refinement of extraction methods to ensure that the extracted nucleic acids are free of impurities that would affect downstream applications like PCR or sequencing. The ability to do so to enhance the reliability of nucleic acid quantification is a critical step toward enhancing accuracy in experimental findings (Jue et al., 2020). Silica-based methods, further, offer an organized approach to nucleic acid quantification. Through a series of lysis steps, silica adsorption, washing, and elution, researchers can maximize nucleic acid recovery while minimizing remaining contaminants to their lowest level. Large amounts of research have demonstrated that such protocols obtain an equilibrium among yield, purity, and efficiency in amplification and are particularly well adapted for sensitivity-based applications , such as single-cell genomics and the detection of pathogens. The effectiveness of silica-based kits and related protocols in the recovery of high-quality nucleic acids not only meets the immediate needs of experimental approaches but also opens doors to continuous research in nucleic acid research as well as application development. With advancing research, the integration of such methods will further improve the robustness of quantitative analysis as well as further our understanding of complex biological systems (Böhner et al., 2024) (Figure 2.8).

2.2.3. Magnetic Bead-Based Extraction

Among the procedures of nucleic acid extraction and quantification, magnetic bead-based extraction is a standout process, which is characterized by its versatility and efficacy in nucleic acid purification from a wide range of sample types. Magnetic bead-based extraction utilizes the superior quality of magnetic beads, which has the capability to bind nucleic acids selectively under specific conditions. The process involved lysing the cells to free nucleic acids and then adding magnetic beads to the sample and allowing their binding onto the nucleic acids by various interactions. The beads are then separated from the solution by applying a magnetic field that not only simplifies purification but also minimizes the risk of contamination. Due to its relatively uncomplicated protocol, magnetic bead extraction is a favored method by laboratories that target high-throughput scenarios and has become one of the main tools in molecular biology. Despite the apparent advantages of applying magnetic bead-based extraction, there are prevailing challenges, primarily the purity and concentration of the extracted nucleic acids. The occurrence of carryover inhibitory compounds from extraction buffers can pose tremendous effects on downstream applications, such as polymerase chain reaction (PCR) and quantitative PCR (qPCR). Recent research has revealed the effects of carryover buffer application when extracts were prepared using various extraction kits, often resulting in overall decreased performance (Jue et al., 2020). The careful process optimization, for example, through the addition of novel washing steps like the two-phase wash, can significantly reduce such issues. By improving the separation of carryover contaminants from the purified nucleic acids without yield loss, researchers can achieve higher sensitivity in their assays and enable gains in applications ranging from pathogen diagnostics to genomic sequencing. Moreover, the combination of microfluidic devices with magnetic bead-based extraction is a promising future for nucleic acid quantification. Microfluidic devices enable miniaturization of reactions and multiplexing, which significantly enhances throughput without wasting precious reagents (Jayamohan et al., 2017).

As scientists combine the technologies, they can streamline the process of extraction and amplification and get rapid results where environments like point-of-care diagnostics are in question. This synergy not only enhances the utility of nucleic acid analysis but also aligns with the growing demand for rapid and precise molecular diagnosis in the aftermath of infectious outbreaks and other medical emergencies. As developments continue, exploring new areas of application and integration of magnetic bead-based methodologies will be crucial in catering to the evolving demands of scientists and healthcare providers alike.

2.3. Factors Influencing Extraction Efficiency

The efficiency of nucleic acid extraction also relies on a number of factors, including the nature of the extraction procedure, the biological matrix employed to recover the nucleic acids, and the physical and chemical properties of the samples. The different methods of extraction, for instance, mechanical disruption, chemical lysis, and column-based methods, yield diverse amounts of yield and purity, thereby highlighting the need to select them accordingly based on the nature of the sample. For instance, silica-based procedures, while best for consistent use in most applications, will give suboptimal yields in highly microbially contaminated samples, as has been witnessed in studies that have shown wide variability between various tick species DNA preparations (Damian, 2025). This shows that the extraction procedure must be optimized to the biological nature of the sample to ensure maximum nucleic acid yield. The other highly significant factor influencing extraction efficiency is the condition of the sample when extracting. Such factors as pH, temperature, and incubation time could play a determining role in the binding of nucleic acids to extraction materials. The SHIFT-SP process, for example, illustrates that adjusting the pH and varying the binding time and temperature increases the rate of recovery with high yield in a short time—about six to seven minutes for samples (Vutukuru et al., 2025).

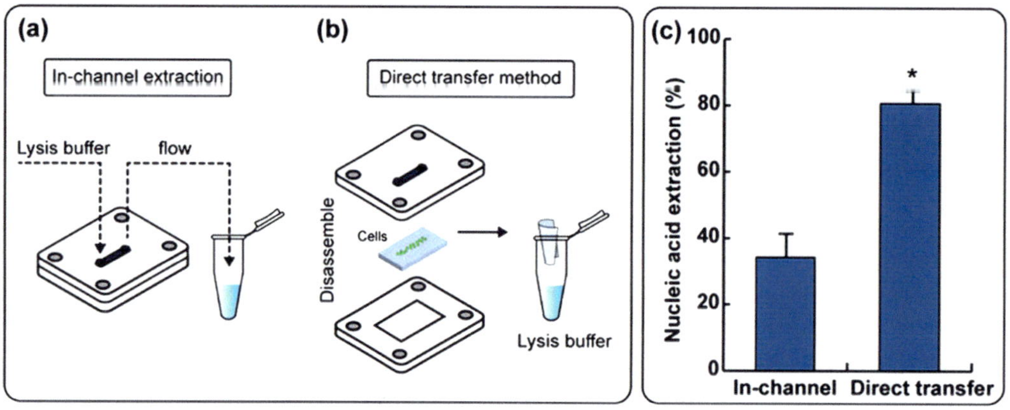

Figure 2.9. Nucleic acid extraction from captured cells.

Source: https://www.researchgate.net/publication/319432367/figure/fig6/AS:11431281211724558@1702478443806/a-Nucleic-acid-extraction-from-captured-cells-using-in-channel-lysis-The-dotted-line.jpg.

This rapid extraction can prove particularly useful in high-throughput settings where having effective use of time is paramount. Further, the study reveals that optimization of these conditions not only maximizes yield but also includes accommodation in automation, making it suitable for existing laboratory practice. Physical integrity of the biological material is another determining factor for extraction efficiency. Maintenance of nucleic acid stability against degradation in the course of extraction can significantly influence the result. For instance, tick exoskeletons can impede efficient lysis and DNA extraction, necessitating the use of methods involving chemical and mechanical disruption. Review also emphasizes the importance of using standardized protocols that may be varied to adapt to varying environmental conditions to improve reliability and reproducibility of extraction (Damian, 2025). Deflection of these variabilities by way of method refinement and optimization can lead to improvements in both the results of research and diagnostic application, once more highlighting the value of a differentiated understanding of extraction factors in nucleic acid quantification research (Figure 2.9).

2.3.1. Sample Type and Quality

In nucleic acid extraction and quantification, the type of sample has a significant impact on the yield and quality of the extracted nucleic acids. Different biological samples, i.e., whole blood, saliva, or tissue, contain varying concentrations of DNA and RNA. For instance, blood samples collected in special tubes can be utilized to recover circulating cell-free DNA (cfDNA), which is critically involved in cancer diagnosis based on non-invasive means. Also, sample handling time is critical in nucleic acid integrity determination. In a study, it was indicated that blood samples processed on the day of extraction deliver the best-sized cfDNA fragments compared to stored samples for many years. These nuances must be appreciated to enable the selection of proper samples to be used in molecular biology downstream applications and clinical diagnostics. Sample quality is also an important factor in evaluating nucleic acid extraction protocols. Pre-analytical processing, from collecting specimens, handling, and storage, all contribute significantly to the nucleic acid quality extracted. Adherence to standardized protocols is important in maintaining similarities between samples. Laboratory practice , such as control of tissue fixation for solid tumors and adherence to specific blood collection protocols, contributes to resilient nucleic acid yield and purity. The assessment of sample quality through techniques , such as multiplexed droplet digital PCR (ddPCR) would be capable of identifying potential contaminants and variations in cfDNA characteristics so that researchers and clinicians can confidently ensure that their nucleic acids isolated are of the best quality. Ultimately, rigorous quality control steps must be implemented to ascertain that the isolated nucleic acids are appropriate for proper molecular analysis. In addition, the chosen analytical methods for nucleic acid quantification must be able to respond to the inherent properties of the processed samples. The variations in nucleic acid yield and quality due to different extraction kits and protocols necessitate sound selection of methods that are amenable to clinical and research requirements. Institutions that perform molecular pathology should have clear guidelines for standardizing extraction and quantification procedures, such as regular inspection of the quality and quantity of extracted nucleic acids. This not only enhances the integrity of results but also ensures that samples are handled in a manner that will allow them to obtain reliable molecular diagnostics. Continuous refinement of procedures based on changing research results, such as those found in literature on pre-analytical variables, will further increase the efficacy of nucleic acid extraction and quantification procedures in the clinic (Edsj et al., 2014; Berens et al., 2018).

2.3.2. Extraction Method Selection

The choice of the correct extraction method for nucleic acids is a serious consideration for the success of subsequent molecular biology analysis. Various extraction procedures have varying efficiencies, yields, and purities of nucleic acids and can have a significant impact on experimental outcomes. Between manual and automated extraction protocols, for example, selection often hinges on the specific requirements of the sample type and required throughput. More recent comparisons of these techniques reveal that specialized extraction kits, made specifically for the type of samples , such as formalin-fixed paraffin-embedded (FFPE) tissues, may provide superior results. The assessment of these kits illustrates that geometric mean yield and nucleic acid purity are parameters that warrant greatest attention during the selection of an appropriate extraction protocol for different applications, exhibiting maximum success in personalized medicine and genomics studies (Kalmar et al., 2016). Moreover, advances in extraction technologies have introduced new protocols that enhance the sensitivity and productivity of nucleic acid purification.

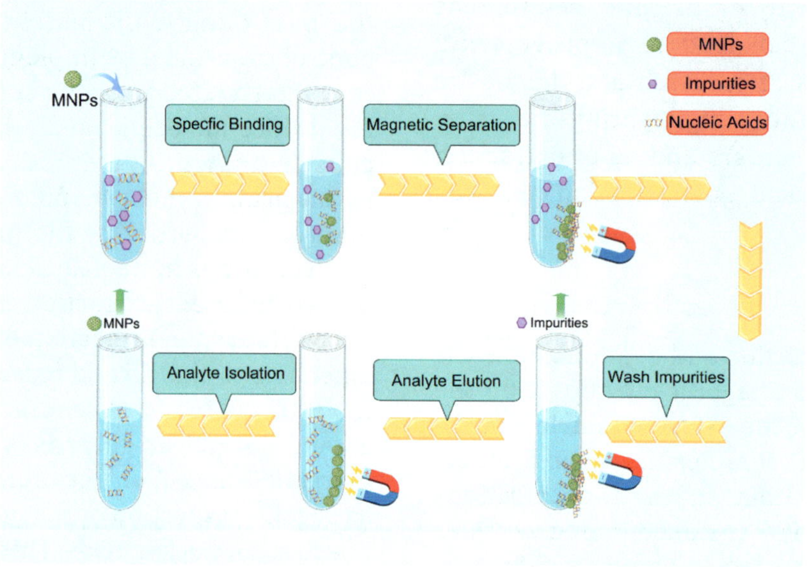

Figure 2.10. The extraction process of nucleic acids based on MNPs.

Source: https://www.researchgate.net/publication/366169457/figure/fig2/AS:11431281108335476@1671466688930/The-extraction-process-of-nucleic-acids-based-on-MNPs-, including-lysis-binding-washing.png.

The incorporation of microfluidics and nanotechnologies is a paradigm shift that enables the design of smaller, more efficient extraction platforms suitable for point-of-care diagnostics. Such technologies not only reduce the time and amount of resources utilized in conventional extraction processes but also improve the quality of nucleic acids isolated. The integration of microfluidic technologies and optimized protocols makes automated sample handling possible, thereby minimizing contamination and human error. As the demand for speed and efficacy in nucleic acid extraction increases, the selection of techniques that facilitate these new frontier technologies becomes a more critical requirement for researchers who endeavor to maintain high-quality standards in data quality and analysis (Jayamohan et al., 2017). In addition to the technology innovation, the preferred extraction method should also conform to the specific purposes of the research study. Factors , such as the source of nucleic acids—tissues, blood, or cultured cells—and the final downstream applications significantly influence the choice decision. For instance, gene expression profiling experiments might require greater RNA quality approaches, whereas other research studies might prioritize higher DNA yield. Experiments with commercial extraction kits have shown considerable differences in performance data, and certain kits work better under criteria pertaining to the aims of research. Lastly, it is required to have a strong awareness of the techniques that can be used and their individual strengths so that the most proper extraction technique may be selected, so that the nucleic acids obtained will be adequate enough to be analyzed (Kalmar et al., 2016) (Figure 2.10).

2.3.3. Environmental Conditions During Extraction

Environmental conditions during nucleic acid extraction have a drastic impact on the efficiency and integrity of molecular materials obtained. These conditions involve several parameters like temperature, pH ranges, and contaminants that may influence the yield and stability of extracted nucleic acids. For instance, high temperatures would enhance cellular structure degradation but otherwise degrade nucleic acids unless stringently regulated. In addition, extreme pH values influence the chemical composition of the nucleic acids and their recoverability and quality. Understanding these factors is critical as they have the potential to determine the success of subsequent applications like quantitative analyses and sequencing. Therefore, it is critical to optimize environmental factors during the extraction of nucleic acids to achieve a greater yield with purity of the end product, paving the way for reproducible results in molecular biology applications. The relationship between microbial communities and environmental conditions is also important under nucleic acid extraction protocols. The diversity and makeup of microbial populations are also very different among ecosystems, presenting varying challenges in extraction. For example, the existence of strong cell walls in certain microorganisms will prevent the lysis process, and nucleic acid recovery is then compromised. Moreover, microorganisms have the propensity to live in complicated groups that influence nutrient cycles and interactions, and potentially extend to influencing the extraction environment as well. Recent advances in molecular biology, as cited in the literature, suggest that reliance on culture-dependent approaches may not reflect the entire microbial richness, particularly when the majority of the species are in a viable but non-culturable state. Thus, the key environmental conditions must be accurately controlled and controlled to accurately trap and measure nucleic acids of various microbial communities (Aronson et al., 2014). Additionally, the method used to extract nucleic acids must be complemented with the environmental conditions to achieve maximum yields. Molecular processes, particularly polymerase chain reaction (PCR) for amplification, significantly aid in identifying specific nucleic acids in various samples. But as observed, such techniques also have associated biases that may originate from the habitat of extraction. For instance, differences in lysing efficiency among microbial species may lead to skewed representation of community members. Hence, researchers must sensibly evaluate their extraction techniques for their responsiveness to the specific environmental conditions from which samples are drawn. By understanding these parameters, scientists can optimize extraction techniques and overall nucleic acid quantification quality and thereby enhance the science of ecological microbiology and its applications (Saunders & Saunders, 1997).

2.4. Quantification Techniques for Nucleic Acids

Measurement of nucleic acids is important in most applications, from research to clinical diagnostics. Accurate measurement is dependent on solid procedures yielding reproducible and accurate determination of the concentration of nucleic acids. A popular method is spectrophotometry, which assesses absorbance at specific wavelengths to quantify nucleic acid concentration. Fluorometry, which quantifies fluorescent dyes selectively bound by DNA or RNA, is another. Fluorometric methods are usually desired because of their sensitivity and less interference from impurities. The preference, though, usually depends on sample quality since degradation and the presence of impurities affect readings considerably. This highlights the need for high-quality nucleic acid extraction that maintains integrity for accurate quantification. Cankar et al. (2006) observe that standardization of such processes, especially considering the heterogeneity of biological samples, is a key challenge in the quantification of nucleic acids. Among the emerging trends in nucleic acid quantitation is the use of high-tech methods , such as microfluidics. Such techniques enable high throughput with extremely small sample volumes and reduce cross-contamination hazards. Microfluidic chips allow control of reaction conditions with high precision and can accommodate several detection modalities in a single platform. Furthermore, sample preparation and analysis under continuous flow conditions enhance speed and efficiency in nucleic acid quantitation. This is particularly crucial for fields like infectious disease management, where reaction time plays a major role. Miniaturization of assays not only lowers the cost of reagents but also enables point-of-care testing, and molecular diagnostics are made feasible in resource-limited environments. By way of a discussion on applications of microfluidics for nucleic acid amplification and analysis, one can see how these technologies upend the conventional methods of quantification. Jayamohan et al. (2017) recognize this intersection of biology and technology as a paradigm-shifting field in molecular diagnostics. Lastly, nucleic acid estimation is highly dependent on the extraction method chosen and the matrix for nucleic acid extraction, as shown in different research studies. The sample type needs unique extraction methods to achieve optimal DNA quantity and quality, particularly when working with complex matrices like food samples. The presence of inhibitors or co-extracted materials can introduce quantitation biases in results, particularly in the case of PCR amplification, where small changes can affect the outcome. It is hence important to have stringent quality controls and an understanding of interactions between sample types and varying extraction protocols for minimizing these effects. As research advances, there is ever greater demand to have standardized protocols for extraction that preserve the integrity of the nucleic acids that are being extracted so that quantification outcomes are credible across an extensive array of uses. The demand for methodological strictness has been answered by the results, indicating the necessity for improved protocols in laboratory methodologies. Cankar et al. (2006) remind the importance of interdependence between extraction techniques and quantification precision in molecular studies (Figure 2.11).

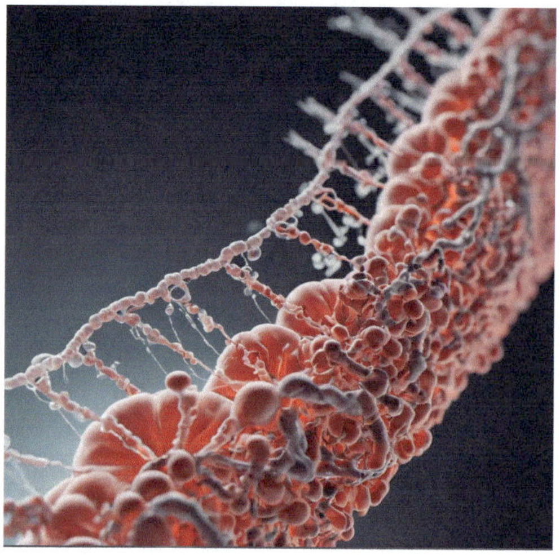

Figure 2.11. Nucleic acid quantification: Methods.

Source: https://biquantumarc.com/images/large/quantification-nucleic-acid-amplification-techniques.webp.

2.4.1. Spectrophotometry

Spectrophotometry is a general technique in nucleic acid extraction and quantification that provides a reliable method of assessing levels of

DNA and RNA content across various samples. The science is based on the principle of identifying the absorption of specified wavelengths of light by nucleic acids and the fact that the amount of absorbance is directly proportional to the concentration of molecules present. The spectrophotometric application allows researchers to quantify nucleic acid purity and integrity with precision, very crucial parameters in molecular biology applications. Second, since the technique is non-destructive, one can perform repeated tests in experiments without using up any sample. This feature proves handy when working with small or precious biological samples, allowing researchers to gain maximum utility while applying precise quantification methods crucial for successful downstream processes. In practice, spectrophotometric measurements are influenced by a number of factors, including the presence of impurities and sample composition. For instance, the protein and other biomolecule absorption characteristics can mask the absorbance values of nucleic acids at given wavelengths. To assist in overcoming this issue, it is common practice to measure the ratio A260/A280, which provides information regarding the purity of the nucleic acid sample. A value of about 1.8 for DNA and 2.0 for RNA is typically indicative of good purity and implies low levels of protein or phenol contamination. Understanding and interpreting this spectral information is therefore critical to enable researchers to accurately make choices on the quality of their sample so that further experiments can be performed on properly prepared nucleic acid extracts. Such rigorous testing is crucial to maintaining experimental integrity in applications , such as quantitative PCR and cloning. The versatility of spectrophotometry extends far beyond mere quantitative analysis; it plays critical roles in the design of portable diagnostic devices. Contemporary breakthroughs have put focus on the ability to implement spectrophotometric techniques into field-deployable devices, which can operate on alternative means of power. Such technologies are particularly relevant in resource-limited settings, where consistent access to electricity may be a problem. A good case is a portable nucleic acid quantifier system, which demonstrated performance equivalent to standard qPCR machines in clinic settings, including during power outages and varying energy supply conditions (Cesarman et al., 2018). These developments pinpoint the contribution of spectrophotometry in the facilitation of swift and cost-effective diagnostic techniques, ultimately resulting in effective disease management and improved public health outcomes worldwide. In addition, as validated by the preparation of plasmid solutions for quantitative PCR confirmation, reference material development also improves the reliability of spectrophotometric methods in nucleic acid quantitation (Cesarman et al., 2018) (Figure 2.12).

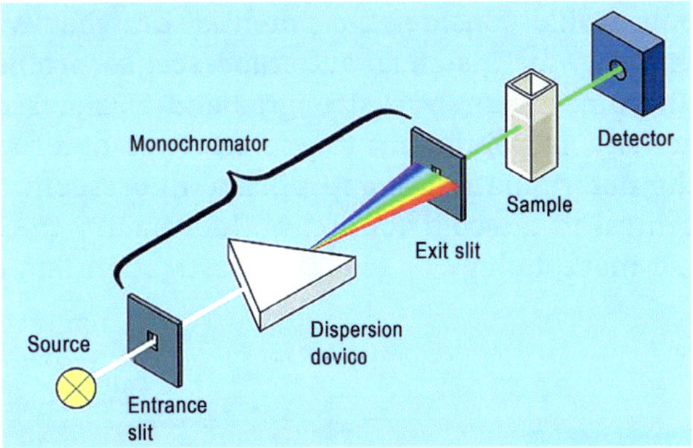

Figure 2.12. Spectrophotometry.

Source: https://biochemden.com/wp-content/uploads/2016/07/Spectrophotometer-Instrumentation.png.

2.4.2. Fluorometry

Fluorometry is an important technique in the extraction of nucleic acids and the quantification of DNA, which enhances the sensitivity and specificity of the detection of DNA. Fluorometry is basically the measurement of the fluorescence emitted by compounds, such as fluorescent dyes that bind to nucleic acids by intercalation, thereby enabling precise quantitation. One of the key developments in this field is the application of enzyme-free assays, which have been shown to be beneficial for the quick diagnostics of DNA mutation, as reported in recent research. An example is the incorporation of locked nucleic acids (LNA) probes, which greatly enhances the affinity of binding to targeted mutations, allowing for improved detection ability even at diluted template concentrations. Scientists can achieve detection levels orders of magnitude lower than those achieved with standard methods by utilizing fluorometric methods, thus hastening the search for mutations associated with various diseases, including cancer, and paving the way for new diagnostic tools in molecular biology (Astakhova et al., 2015). Not only does the use of fluorometric methods improve sensitivity, but it also allows the analysis of specific gene expressions and gene mutations. The use of intercalating dyes , such as EvaGreen, is another example of this, as they emit higher levels of fluorescence once they are bound to double-stranded DNA. This makes them better suited to detect even minute levels of nucleic acid, and thus, it remains a useful addition in assays for rare mutation detection. Further, the ease with which these assays can be performed in a high-throughput mode addresses the growing need for rapid analysis in both clinical and research settings. This capability to perform multiple assays simultaneously increases the efficiency of genetic research by enabling the thorough mapping of the genomic landscape and its clinical application within personalized medicine (Astakhova et al., 2015). Besides, fluorometry offers significant advantages aside from detection, particularly in establishing the efficacy of experimental models, for instance, reporter gene-based transgenic mouse models. These models utilize reporter genes, for instance, EGFP, that are quantified using fluorescence microscopy to measure promoter activity. However, one should consider the potential drawbacks associated with weaker promoters in fluorescence imaging, for instance, autofluorescence problems that could obscure results. The knowledge of fluorometric analysis strengths and weaknesses, for instance, in research on HERV-LTR promoter activity, is paramount to the effective determination of the results of experiments. Harmony in the determination of appropriate fluorescent markers and achieving accuracy in quantification is central to the contribution of fluorometry to exhaustive nucleic acid analysis and how this affects the methodology of genetic investigation and diagnostics (Figure 2.13).

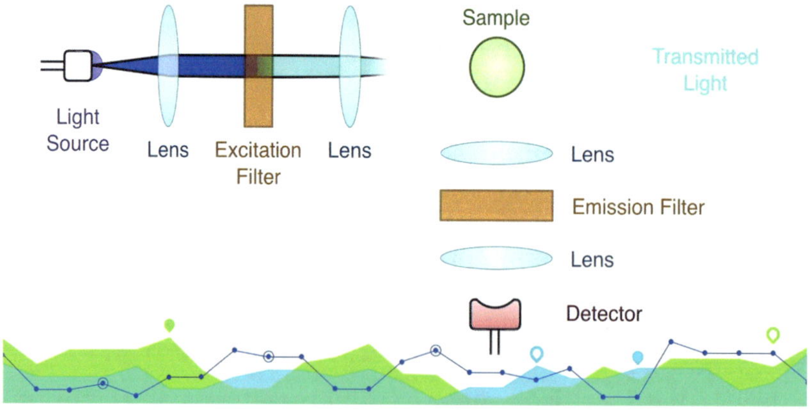

Figure 2.13. Fluorimetry pronunciation from the Sandra Moody blog.

Source: https://i.ytimg.com/vi/zGFQEbdeAF0/maxresdefault.jpg.

2.4.3. PCR-Based Methods

The evolution of PCR-based technologies has significantly transformed nucleic acid extraction and quantification protocols. Quantification of nucleic acids by older methods traditionally included the use of spectrophotometric and fluorometric approaches, each possessing distinct strengths and limitations. Spectrophotometric platforms , such as NanoDrop and DeNovix provide rapid DNA quantification through absorbance measurements, facilitating an effective laboratory workflow strategy. However, such methods risk supplying overestimates of DNA concentration, particularly in the presence of contaminants, a challenge that is forcefully demonstrated in experiments contrasting spectrophotometry against fluorometric assays like Qubit. This makes comparison show that Qubit tends to make more precise estimates of nucleic acid concentrations, particularly when determining levels of purity, providing a valuable insight into the basis for accuracy in downstream processes , such as library preparation for whole genome sequencing (Versmessen et al., 2024). The emergence of digital PCR (dPCR) has taken the quantification of nucleic acids to an even higher level by making it possible to accurately detect target molecules in complex biological samples. dPCR enhances the sensitivity and specificity of nucleic acid quantification by partitioning the sample into millions of tiny volumes where individual PCR amplification occurs. Notably, dPCR is particularly useful in applications where low-abundance targets have to be discovered, such as in viral diagnosis and mutation tracking. The new format presented for competitive PCR signifies a new method through the identification of limitations within traditional Poisson distribution models in quantitative accuracy. By utilizing the competitive DNA within the same PCR reaction, the quantification of the target nucleic acid is performed with more accuracy, producing robust results within less time and minimizing the requirement for complex post-PCR handling (Ganguly & Lee, 2024). In practice, the integration of multiplexing functions within PCR-based methods also enhances the analytical power of nucleic acid quantification methods. Multiplex PCR allows multiple target sequences to be amplified in a single reaction, dramatically increasing throughput and efficiency. It is especially useful in the clinical and research environments where time and resource constraints may threaten the viability of individual amplifications for each nucleic acid target. In addition, recent advances in microfluidic technologies have made possible the production of high-throughput platforms capable of processing several samples in parallel, including various PCR-based approaches, both in the conventional and digital versions. The careful application of these technologies not only enhances the process speed of quantification but also makes possible additional opportunities for real-time monitoring of nucleic acid, representing a significant step forward in the realm of molecular diagnostics as well as personal medicine.

2.5. Applications of Nucleic Acid Extraction and Quantification

The applications of nucleic acid extraction and quantification are extensive and cut across numerous disciplines and have important applications in biological research and medical diagnostics. In contemporary molecular biology, the efficiency to extract and quantify nucleic acids well is crucial for applications ranging from gene expression analysis to disease diagnosis. Successful nucleic acid extraction enables scientists to obtain high-purity DNA or RNA from complex biological samples for robust downstream applications. For instance, the developments in microfluidics and nanotechnology have revolutionized molecular diagnostics such that novel analyses are now feasible that are not only faster but also less expensive and more sensitive. The technologies allow for a wide variety of applications, including point-of-care testing, which is essential in infectious disease management and personalized medicine (Jayamohan et al., 2017). Although methodologies are enhanced, their application in investigation and diagnostics becomes complicated and offers new directions for investigation and intervention. Clinically, nucleic acid measurements are important in infectious disease diagnosis and assessing response to therapy. Proper measurement allows clinicians to determine the viral load of patients, which is essential in monitoring diseases , such as HIV and hepatitis. Advanced techniques, such as digital PCR, permit precise quantification of nucleic acids, thereby facilitating targeted treatments and improved patient care. However, the efficiency of these quantitative methods is contingent on the purity of isolated nucleic acids. Differing protocols employed in the extraction of nucleic acids can lead to a sample containing inhibitory compounds that hamper the precision of such quantifications. Therefore, techniques that reduce contamination and improve nucleic acid purity, such as the two-phase wash technique, are necessary for reproducible diagnostic outcomes (Jue et al., 2020). This requires constant innovation and validation of nucleic acid extraction techniques to yield high-quality diagnostic outcomes. Quantification of nucleic acids influences domains of clinical diagnostics and beyond, ranging from environmental science to food safety. In these areas, the presence of specific nucleic acids can identify pathogen contamination or genetic modification in crops. For example, in food safety, quantification using real-time quantitative PCR can identify the presence of foodborne pathogens to prevent outbreaks. Similarly, environmental monitoring can employ nucleic acid extraction techniques to quantify biodiversity or track the invasion of species by genetic material detection. With regulatory agencies more concerned with environmental and food safety, the necessity for precise nucleic acid extraction and quantification techniques becomes critical. These applications define the scope of nucleic acid technologies and exhibit their pivotal role in public health and environmental protection (Jayamohan et al., 2017). The rapid advancements in the subject area promise further improvements in research and applied science (Figure 2.14).

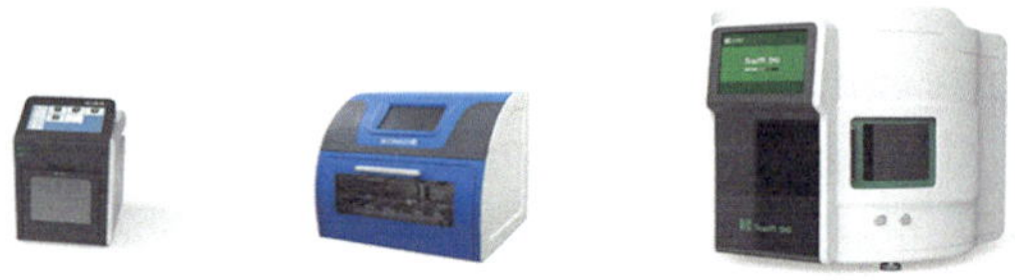

Figure 2.14. Principles and applications of nucleic acid extraction.

Source: https://en.daangene.com/uploads/image/20240115/daan-gene-nucleic-acid-extraction-machine-1.jpg.

2.5.1. Clinical Diagnostics

The role of clinical diagnostics in modern medicine has been revolutionized by advances in methods for extracting and quantifying nucleic acids. These technologies enable clinicians to accurately and rapidly diagnose disease, particularly infectious agents. Traditional infection diagnosis generally relies on culture-based techniques, which are time-consuming and potentially yield incorrect results. Conversely, molecular testing, particularly nucleic acid analysis tests, allows for the identification of causative agents at the genetic level. This capability not only streamlines diagnosis but also enhances the clinical handling of disease, which translates into less wasteful intervention and better patient outcomes. With the use of robust extraction processes, such as those involving microfluidics, the process is streamlined, hence bridging the gap between lab results and clinical interventions on time. Furthermore, the utilization of point-of-care diagnostic devices in resource-poor settings is a gigantic shift in the presence of specialized clinical diagnostics. Production of such equipment, which can operate on variable levels of power and is independent of stable electricity, has profound implications for health delivery in poor areas. For instance, a handheld nucleic acid quantifier was found to have promise for application in clinics in Uganda, where it performs consistently in spite of power shortages without compromising performance from that delivered by standard qPCR machines. This portability not only reduces treatment time but also provides health practitioners with the expertise they require to treat infectious diseases effectively, where traditional laboratory settings are not adequate (Cesarman et al., 2018). This technology, therefore, marks a significant milestone towards improvement in global health outcomes. The fusion of microfluidics and nucleic acid quantitation is also ushering in a new era of speed and sensitivity in molecular diagnostics. Microfluidic technology innovations enable the development of point-of-care devices that are low-cost and can generate fast and precise results from a small sample. Such technologies enhance the analytical capabilities of traditional lab procedures while reducing the time and cost of molecular diagnostics significantly. Tests range from nucleic acid amplification to next-generation sequencing, illustrating the versatility of these systems for the detection of other pathogens and disease markers (Jayamohan et al., 2017). As clinical diagnostics becomes more advanced, integration of these innovative techniques not only enhances the test menu but also inspires the development of personalized treatment plans, further solidifying the importance of early and correct diagnosis in patient management.

2.5.2. Genetic Research

Genetic studies have advanced a lot in the understanding of microbial genomes, particularly with the application of nucleic acid extraction and quantification techniques. With these genetic methods focused on, researchers can identify and isolate single genes responsible for adaptive traits, hence improving biomass yield in various microbial groups. Techniques like Polymerase Chain Reaction (PCR) can be applied to amplify nucleic acids purified from environmental samples and thus facilitate the examination of genetic loci that are involved in metabolic processes. These analyses give rise to the discovery of novel regulatory genes that hold great importance in terms of metabolic engineering and biotechnology. For instance, such methods can pick out genes that might serve as metabolic switches to enable adaptations under environmental stress and ultimately result in sustainable processes in bioenergy production (Astakhova et al., 2015). The impact in clinical laboratories is just as significant, particularly in cancer research. The ability to accurately quantify and characterize nucleic acids of various sample types, such as FFPE tissues and liquid biopsies, facilitates early cancer detection and patient monitoring. Automation of nucleic acid purification phases, as illustrated by the Genexus system, allows for rapid and reproducible analysis, streamlining workflow complexity and reducing turnaround time. This tool, through the Oncomine Precision Assay, can extract and profile significant oncogenic markers from limited DNA and RNA samples. The efficiency of such techniques not only eases laboratory operations but also enhances the precision of information obtained from genetic research, thereby making it an indispensable tool in translational genomics (Jayaweera et al., 2022). Lastly, ongoing advances in genetic research, particularly concerning nucleic acid extraction and determination, are going to transform both basic and applied scientific research. Once scientists succeed in further refining these tools, they will find usage in several fields , including microbial ecology and oncology. Incorporating automated platforms not only makes the process more reproducible but also allows for managing unprecedented amounts of data generated using high-throughput sequencing platforms. This new paradigm of the movement towards automation and efficiency reinforces the need for genetic studies in deciphering intricate biological mechanisms and diseases, leading to innovative treatments and eco-friendly environmental practices. Consequently, genetic research is increasingly becoming vital in solving significant global problems in ecology and health (Astakhova et al., 2015; Jayaweera et al., 2022) (Figure 2.15).

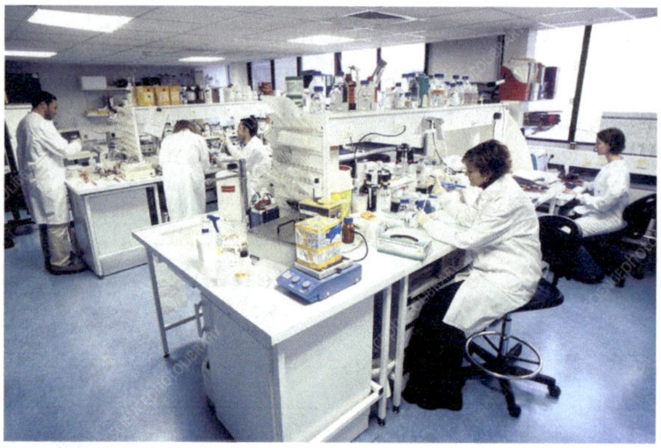

Figure 2.15. Genetic research

Source: https://media.sciencephoto.com/image/g2101210/800wm/G2101210-Genetic_research.jpg.

2.5.3. Forensic Analysis

Forensic analysis is an essential aspect of criminal investigation, particularly through the recovery and quantitation of nucleic acids, i.e., DNA. Integrity and reliability of extracted DNA are of utmost concern here. The inherent complexities posed by biological samples are inherent; biological samples typically contain inhibitors of subsequent applications. Recent studies have identified the impact of such contaminations, which have revealed that traditional methods have been known to lead to significant carryover of inhibitory buffers into the eluent. The carryover plays a significant role in affecting the sensitivity of most tests, such as polymerase chain reaction (PCR) when nucleic acid extraction is diluted for the analysis of low-template samples. Therefore, embracing improved extraction techniques that minimize contamination is key to enhancing the credibility of forensic DNA evidence and delivery of accurate results in courtrooms (Jue et al., 2020). New nucleic acid extraction technologies have revolutionized the process of forensic investigation, particularly when it comes to the reliability of DNA typing. Traditional protocols used to involve extensive physical handling of samples, which resulted in greater susceptibility for errors to be introduced through pipetting and transfers. Innovation , such as single-tube DNA extraction together with direct amplification approaches, has made it easier, decreasing pre-PCR sampling errors and enabling more fidelity in resulting DNA profiles. The forensicGEM® Saliva Kit is a strong example, as its high-efficiency cell lysis and minimal presence of inhibitory compounds that could interfere with subsequent PCR amplification make it ideal. By using procedures that eliminate the transfer steps, forensic testing can yield greater accuracy and prevent issues like allele drop-out and peak height imbalance associated with low-template usage (Nguyen, 2015). Assessment of the efficiency of such extraction and enrichment procedures is key to the maximization of forensic examination. Studies have demonstrated that minimizing pre-PCR sampling errors has a corresponding correlation with improved peak height ratios (PHRs) and, therefore, overall DNA profile quality. For example, using cell transfer procedures can result in higher mean PHRs than samples prepared via sequential steps of transfer. Furthermore, the application of carrier RNA has also been explored as a means of signal augmentation during amplification to guide optimization of forensic procedures. Evaluation of these approaches not only guides how stochastic effects inherent in low-template DNA amplification can be reduced but also reveals that forensic science requires continued development. By embracing innovative extraction and quantification techniques, the forensic quality of evidence can be significantly enhanced and it becomes simpler for criminal investigations to facilitate justice (Nguyen, 2015).

2.6. Challenges in Acid Extraction and Quantification

Extraction and quantification of the nucleic acids are bedeviled by a myriad of challenges, particularly sample quality and integrity. Environmental contaminants , such as lipids, proteins, and polysaccharides, will contaminate the purification process and lead to incorrect quantification. Sample preparation can also lead to nucleic acid breakage, thereby contaminating downstream processes like PCR and sequencing. As a result, the creation of perfect conditions for the conservation of nucleic acids during extraction is critical to the achievement of credible results. Furthermore, variations in nucleic acid recovery owing to the type of biological sample—either tissues, cells, or biological fluids—present additional challenges to the quantification process. These challenges render it necessary for the development of standard protocols that can accommodate various sample types and minimize contamination as well as nucleic acid degradation. The other significant challenge of nucleic acid extraction and quantification is the efficiency of extraction techniques. Various techniques, such as organic solvent-based extraction, silica-based procedures, and magnetic bead-based procedures, all have their own advantages and disadvantages in terms of yield and purity. The extraction procedure has the potential to directly affect the accuracy of downstream quantification. For instance, higher purity can be achieved through procedures that yield lesser quantities of nucleic acids or vice versa. Furthermore, microfluidic technologies have been promising to reduce extraction processes; however, such advanced systems have not yet achieved widespread application due to limitations in scalability and economy. Overcoming these challenges is necessary to enhance the reliability and performance of nucleic acid quantification such that the findings can be safely translated into meaningful applications in diagnostics and research (Jayamohan et al., 2017).

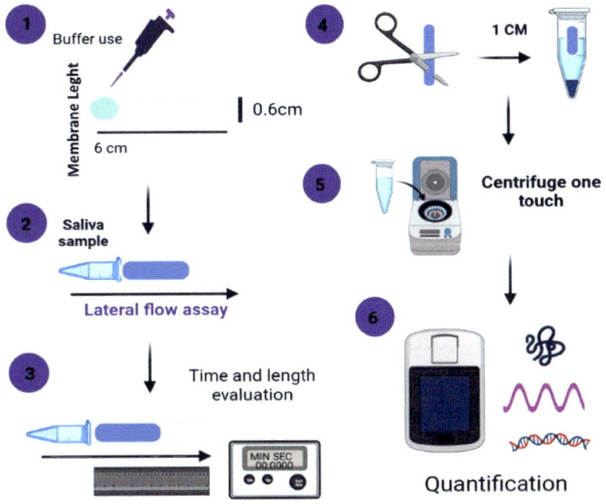

Figure 2.16. Schematic representation of paper-based nucleic acid extraction.

Source: https://www.researchgate.net/publication/366404667/figure/fig1/AS:11431281432489413@1746873612043/Schematic-representation-of-paper-based-nucleic-acid-extraction-assay-steps-1-3.tif.

Even extraction and quantification of extracted nucleic acids has inherent complexities based primarily on accuracy and specificity. Classical methods, such as spectrophotometry and fluorometry, are often variable in sensitivity and responsiveness to contaminants and may yield different measured concentrations. Distorted quantification data can be obtained by the presence of degraded nucleic acids or even minute reagents, making it impossible to determine the true nucleic acid concentration. New breakthroughs in biosensor technology and immunoassay approaches attempt to optimally achieve sensitivity and quantification precision, with a replacement for traditional methods. However, deployment of these sophisticated techniques is typically costly, either in terms of equipment or resources, and thus represents a limiting factor for most labs. Thus, there is a need to continually develop both extraction procedures and quantification assays to further enhance general diagnosis accuracy and credibility (Ince & McNally, 2009) (Figure 2.16).

2.6.1. Contamination Issues

In nucleic acid extraction and quantitation, the major issue of contamination can be a threat to the validity of findings. This can be due to reagents, laboratory environment, and cross-contamination between samples. One of the common issues is the presence of nucleases, which degrade nucleic acids and produce inappropriately low yield readings. Besides contamination due to human error, extraneous factors , such as aerosols and dust are also potential sources with the ability to introduce foreign DNA or RNA into the sample, complicating quantification. The intricacy of such impurities necessitates strict attention to laboratory procedures, where continuous monitoring and quality control validation must be maintained to keep nucleic acids unaltered. Stringent accuracy in controlling contamination can significantly enhance the purity of the recovered nucleic acids as well as the integrity of subsequent quantification procedures. Secondly, the method of extraction employed during the isolation of nucleic acids can also exacerbate contamination issues unless given due consideration. Traditional means of extraction usually involve the use of open systems that are more susceptible to foreign contaminants. Microfluidic technologies have been more recently developed that seek to minimize exposure to potential sources of contamination while optimizing extraction efficiency. These advances represent a shift in molecular diagnostics whereby the building of extraction protocols more and more comprises the incorporation of closed systems and minimized workflows, thus towards sample-in, answer-out functionality (Jayamohan et al., 2017). Such advances not only enhance the purity of extracted nucleic acids but also solve problems introduced by contamination, ultimately leading to more uniform diagnostic outcomes in various fields, for example, infectious disease management and biodefense. The effects of contamination extend beyond the laboratory to affect the broader field of research outcomes and clinical applications. Contaminated nucleic acid samples can lead to incorrect conclusions in research, defeating the purpose of the scientific research process. For instance, errors in the identification of pathogens or genetic mutations can hinder prompt medical intervention, having direct effects on patient outcomes. Therefore, one must adopt stringent contamination control practices at each step of the entire process from sample collection to final quantification. This entails not only continuous enhancement of extraction protocols but also maintaining laboratory practice to high standards (Groll et al., 2012). Through contamination control as a top priority, scientists can guarantee that nucleic acid extraction and quantification procedures produce reproducible and accurate results that are crucial for progress in biological research, public health, and safety applications.

2.6.2. Degradation of Nucleic Acids

The degradation of nucleic acids poses extreme challenges under the scenario of nucleic acid extraction and quantification. Many intrinsic and extrinsic factors are to blame for the cause of the degradation process, including fluctuations in temperature, pH, and nucleolytic enzyme exposure. RNases, for instance, are ubiquitous in biological samples and have the potential to degrade RNA rapidly if not properly contained. This vulnerability necessitates that stringent measures be implemented in all extraction protocols. Ideal measures , such as keeping in cold temperatures and using RNase inhibitors, are required to maintain nucleic acid integrity throughout the process of extraction. Furthermore, understanding why nucleic acid degrades can assist scientists in constructing more stable extraction protocols, ultimately making downstream application consistency , such as quantitative PCR and sequencing, more reliable. Efforts to surmount the issues associated with nucleic acid degradation have seen new extraction technologies emerge. For instance, advancements of extraction methods specifically optimized for formalin-fixed, paraffin-embedded (FFPE) samples indicate a remarkable improvement in recovering RNA, with a promise of obtaining high-quality RNA from degraded samples. One such study highlighted that the addition of a micro-homogenizing device to existing extraction methodologies is three times more efficient in recovering RNA, impressively improving A260/A280 ratios and RNA quality index (RQI) scores. These advancements facilitate more intimate recapitulation of the initial nucleic acid profile of the sample, which is pivotal in biomarker discovery and analysis. By overcoming the degradation challenge of FFPE samples, researchers can more firmly relate molecular signatures and clinical information, thereby opening the field to new innovations in cancer diagnostics and therapeutics (Adamian et al., 2016). In addition to methodological improvement, understanding of the molecular mechanisms of nucleic acid degradation can inform better practice in nucleic acid quantitation. For example, it is known that certain environmental conditions have a propensity to promote degradation and that skewed quantitation will be obtained if they are not controlled. Additionally, because nucleic acids are subject to enzymic activity, extraction protocols must include measures to inhibit nucleases. Techniques , such as the use of stabilizing agents or the rapid extraction of nucleic acids can reverse these risks. Moreover, as illustrated in the case of CRISPR-Cas systems, effective nucleic acid protection methods may involve the design of constructs that stabilize RNA against degradation. This observation brings to light the importance of not only being observant of extraction techniques but also understanding the critical role played by safety protocols in maintaining the integrity of nucleic acids throughout experiment procedures (Gleditzsch, 2020) (Figure 2.17).

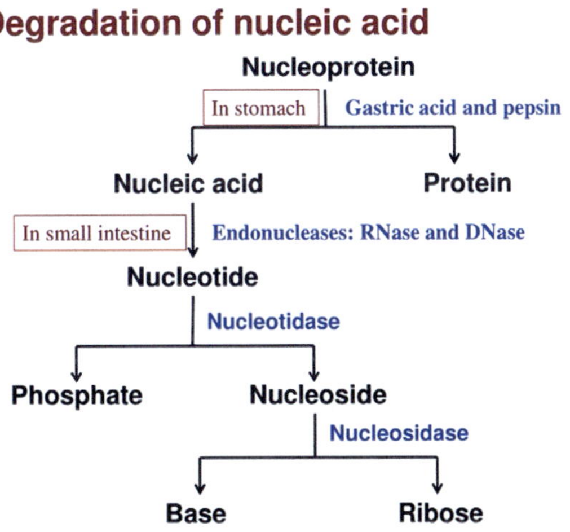

Figure 2.17. Degradation of nucleic acids.

Source: https://slideplayer.com/slide/13052601/79/images/10/Degradation+of+nucleic+acid.jpg.

2.6.3. Variability in Quantification Results

In the scenario of nucleic acid extraction and quantitation, within-laboratory variation of the results is of significant concern that needs to be met strictly. Factors , such as the choice of extraction kits significantly contribute to the purity and quantity of nucleic acids recovered. For instance, comparison of three commercial kits for SARS-CoV-2 viral RNA extraction demonstrated wide variations in yield and purity of the recovered RNA. The results indicated Kit C was better than its counterparts in yielding the highest total RNA and demonstrating enhanced linearity and reproducibility, showing how critical the choice of good methods is for accurate quantification (Sait et al., 2025). This heterogeneity is illustrative in that it shows extraction protocols are not created equal, pointing to the importance of using standardized methods so results between studies can be compared. On top of the variability issue comes the inherent sample type and concentration differences utilized in extraction. During a ten-different nucleic acid extraction protocols, researchers observed significant variability in the detection of antibiotic resistance genes (ARGs) in wastewater samples from aircraft, where it was demonstrated that extraction had an impact on the presence and concentration of target nucleic acids (Smith et al., 2024). This variation could be a result of biological sample complexity, e.g., concentration of nucleic acids, as well as the degree of inhibitors. This, in turn, renders quantitative outcomes unreliable, hence poised to misinform during the interpretation of data. The differences observed between extraction protocols call for personalized methods for every sample type, and this calls for validation studies considering the divergence in different methodologies. Also, the impact of sample volume and processing procedures on quantification results cannot be prevented. To put it simply, scaling down the sample volume to as low as 0.2 mL would still yield valid characterizations of the target genes, according to the said study on ARGs (Smith et al., 2024). However, sample complexity in biological matrices frequently requires careful control of processing steps like tissue homogenization and interference removal, interfering substances that can degrade extraction efficiency. Such factors are crucial for ensuring quantitative assays are as reproducible as well as accurate as possible. In conclusion, the discrepancy in quantification results underscores the intricacy of nucleic acid extraction that necessitates ongoing research and optimization to standardize methods across studies to uphold enhanced reliability of nucleic acid quantification across settings (FadL, 2022).

SUMMARY

In short, the effectiveness of nucleic acid extraction and measurement depends upon the purity and integrity of nucleic acids isolated from various biological samples. An elaborate examination of traditional extraction methods illustrates those commercial kits, being easy to operate, do not necessarily provide the high level of purity required for applications sensitive in nature. It is important to treat the carryover of inhibitory buffers, as shown by evidence indicating remarkable reaction inhibition in PCR and other amplification methods when dilutions of eluents are low, especially under high-sensitivity conditions like single-cell sequencing. The advancement of methodologies like two-phase wash (TPW) has been promising in restricting such contaminants while not interfering with the nucleic acid yield, underscoring methodological advancement as paramount in this field (Jue et al., 2020). Moreover, the importance of such research goes beyond laboratory effectiveness, drawing attention to the impact on research outcomes in genomics, diagnostics, and biotechnology. Problems regarding carryover effects and integrity of nucleic acids underscore the necessity of continuous optimization of extraction protocols, particularly for uses where detection limits must be nuanced. The aforementioned study illustrated that raising the quality of downstream processes like quantitative PCR and LAMP can be achieved by optimizing extraction conditions and employing TPW techniques. These advances not only improve reproducibility but might also increase the scope of research usable, such that results from nucleic acid analysis are robust and reliable (Jue et al., 2020). Ultimately, the science of nucleic acid isolation and quantitation stands at a place where the convergence of innovative strategies and meticulous quality control is imperative. Continued research into metabolomics and other analytical strategies enhances our understanding of biological processes engaged and underscores the function of nucleic acids in dynamic systems. The interplay among extracting protocols and resultant nucleic acid behavior represents the necessity of an integrated strategy to molecular biology encompassing both technical acumen and biological relevance. As emerging extraction technologies unfold, they might open up new avenues of research and improve our knowledge of the cellular building blocks relevant to life sciences.

Nucleic acid extraction and measurement are critical in various fields of biological science, such as transcriptomics, genomics, and molecular diagnostics. Effective extraction leads to high-quality nucleic acids that are amenable to downstream applications , such as PCR and sequencing. Various approaches , such as phenol-chloroform extraction and silica column-based approaches, offer varying benefits in terms of yield and quality of DNA and RNA. Understanding the principles of these procedures allows researchers to choose the most appropriate one for their specific use. Phenol-chloroform extraction, for example, is very effective in separating nucleic acids from lipids and proteins, but must be manipulated carefully due to its toxic reagents. On the other hand, silica-based methods are simpler and safer but may not always deliver the same level of purity as traditional methods, necessitating exact method selection based on research requirements. Quantitation of eluted nucleic acids is similarly important, allowing scientists to assess sample concentration and quality. Quantification is achieved using spectrophotometric methods, including absorbance at 260 nm to measure nucleic acid concentration and ratios of 260/280 nm and 260/230 nm to determine purity. The ratios provide an indication of interfering contaminants that will influence downstream processes. The inclusion of fluorometric methods provides additional accuracy because the methods will selectively measure nucleic acids, meaning that contaminants will be minimized in interference. The combination of spectrophotometric and fluorometric quantitation techniques allows scientists to attain a full picture of nucleic acid integrity and concentration, ensuring the downstream experimental protocols are conducted using quality inputs. Nucleic acid extraction and quantitation are significant to broader biological studies, such as microbial community and cellular response. For example, metabolomics in combination with nucleic acid analysis has been identified as key by recent research, demonstrating how intracellular metabolites are altered in response to varying environmental stresses. Such demonstrations highlight the interdependence between different biological macromolecules and their functions within cellular adaptation and activity, as demonstrated by research where metabolic alterations were witnessed during microbial death experiments (Longnecker & Kujawinski, 2020). Furthermore, the function of Polycomb Group proteins, which bind with nucleic acids, highlights the complex regulation of gene expression by both nucleic acids and RNA structures, pointing toward the complexity of cellular systems (Alecki et al., 2020). Combined, these findings further clarify the dynamic nature of biological systems and indicate the importance of nucleic acid extraction and quantification methods in investigating these complex pathways.

A LOOK TO THE FUTURE

NUCLEIC ACID MEASUREMENTS

Nucleic acids—primarily deoxyribonucleic acid (DNA) and ribonucleic acid (RNA)—are the fundamental carriers of genetic information in all living organisms. Accurate measurement of these molecules is central to modern molecular biology, biotechnology, and clinical diagnostics because nearly every downstream application—from polymerase chain reaction and cloning to next-generation sequencing and gene expression analysis—requires precise knowledge of nucleic acid concentration and quality. Quantifying nucleic acids ensures that experimental conditions are standardized, reduces variability between samples, and enhances the reproducibility and reliability of research findings. Small inaccuracies in measurement can compromise reaction efficiencies, skew analytical results, or lead to misinterpretation of biological phenomena.

Nucleic acid measurement encompasses both **quantification**—determining the amount of DNA or RNA in a sample—and **qualification**—evaluating purity and integrity. Historically, optical absorbance methods such as ultraviolet-visible (UV-Vis) spectrophotometry have been foundational. Nucleic acid molecules characteristically absorb ultraviolet light maximally near **260 nm** due to the electronic properties of purine and pyrimidine bases, allowing concentration to be inferred using Beer-Lambert's law. Ratios of absorbance at different wavelengths (e.g., A260/A280 or A260/A230) provide insight into contamination by proteins or chemical solvents that absorb at adjacent wavelengths, thereby flagging potential impurities that may affect downstream assays. While simple and rapid, absorbance-based approaches can lack sensitivity at low concentrations and cannot distinguish between DNA and RNA. As a result, **fluorescence-based techniques** using nucleic acid–selective dyes have become widely adopted, particularly in high-throughput environments. Fluorometric assays improve sensitivity and specificity by emitting a signal only when dyes bind to nucleic acids, enabling accurate quantitation even at low abundance and in complex mixtures.

Beyond optical methods, electrophoretic techniques such as gel electrophoresis separate nucleic acid fragments by size, offering both visual confirmation of integrity and semi-quantitative assessment of sample composition. Advanced technologies—including qPCR for targeted quantification, mass photometry for single-molecule sizing, and emerging methods that integrate mass spectrometry or microfluidics—expand the analytical toolkit for researchers probing nucleic acid structure, abundance, and modifications in greater depth and resolution.

Nucleic acid measurements form the analytical backbone of molecular life sciences. They ensure that genetic material is accurately characterized before further manipulation, provide essential quality control, and underpin ongoing advances in genomics, diagnostics, and therapeutic development. Continued improvements in measurement technologies promise greater sensitivity, throughput, and functional insight into the dynamic roles of DNA and RNA in health and disease.

REFERENCES

1. Jayamohan, Harikrishnan & Romanov, Valentin & Li, Huizhong & Son, Jiyoung & Samuel, Raheel & Nelson, John & Gale, Bruce. (2017). Advances in Microfluidics and Lab-on-a-Chip Technologies. 10.1016/B978-0-12-802971-8.00011-0. (accessed on 17th July 2025).
2. Adamian, Y., Bouvet, M., Brown, M., et al. (2016). A novel method for RNA extraction from FFPE samples reveals significant differences in biomarker expression between orthotopic and subcutaneous pancreatic cancer patient-derived xenografts. *Cancer Research, 76*(11), 3256–3264. https://core.ac.uk/download/323066094.pdf (accessed on 17th July 2025).
3. Alecki, C., Arias Pérez, O., Armache, K. J., et al. (2020). RNA-DNA strand exchange by the Drosophila Polycomb complex PRC2. *Nature Communications, 11*(1), 2934–2947. https://core.ac.uk/download/323310728.pdf (accessed on 17th July 2025).
4. Aronson, E., Izard, J., Klatt, C., et al. (2014). The unseen world: Environmental microbial sequencing and identification methods for ecologists. *Environmental Microbiology, 16*(6), 1234–1245. https://core.ac.uk/download/286364389.pdf (accessed on 17th July 2025).
5. Astakhova, K., Brewer, J., Ji, H., et al. (2015). Enzyme-free detection of mutations in cancer DNA using synthetic oligonucleotide probes and fluorescence microscopy. *Nature Methods, 12*(5), 408–413. https://core.ac.uk/download/pdf/50713073.pdf (accessed on 17th July 2025).
6. Baptista, V., Castanho, S., Cruz, J., et al. (2019). Swimming abilities of temperate pelagic fish larvae prove that they may control their dispersion in coastal areas. *Marine Biology, 166*(4), 1–12. https://core.ac.uk/download/288958418.pdf (accessed on 17th July 2025).
7. Berens, M. E., Borad, M. J., Bryce, A., et al. (2018). Evaluation of pre-analytical factors affecting plasma DNA analysis. *Journal of Translational Medicine, 16*(1), 87–95. https://core.ac.uk/download/323080502.pdf (accessed on 17th July 2025).
8. Böhner, N., Hubbuch, J., & Valentic, A. (2024). Absolute quantification of hepatitis B core antigen (HBcAg) virus-like particles and bound nucleic acids. *Journal of Virology Methods, 300*, 108411. https://core.ac.uk/download/604492518.pdf (accessed on 17th July 2025).
9. Cankar, K., Dreo, T., Gruden, K., et al. (2006). Critical points of DNA quantification by real-time PCR: Effects of DNA extraction method and sample matrix on quantification of genetically modified organisms. *Journal of Agricultural and Food Chemistry, 54*(7), 2579–2586. https://core.ac.uk/download/pdf/4050284.pdf (accessed on 17th July 2025).
10. Cesarman, E., Duru, J., Erickson, D., et al. (2018). A portable device for nucleic acid quantification powered by sunlight, a flame or electricity. *Scientific Reports, 8*(1), 7323. https://core.ac.uk/download/323063231.pdf (accessed on 17th July 2025).
11. Chung, P. Y. J., Corbisier, P., Emons, H., Kortekaas, A. M., Matrai, J., Mazoua, S., Scaravelli, E., et al. (2013). The preparation and characterization of three solutions of plasmid DNA containing a ruminant-specific fragment with defined copy number concentrations–Reference Materials: IRMM-AD482a, IRMM-AD482b, IRMM-AD482c. https://core.ac.uk/download/38626664.pdf (accessed on 17th July 2025).
12. D'Ambrosio, A., Isa, A., Caforio, A. L., Block, A., Ay, B., Lassner, D., Nixon, D. F., et al. (2008). NS1 specific CD8(+) T-cells with effector function and TRBV11 dominance in a patient with parvovirus B19 associated inflammatory cardiomyopathy. *Journal of Clinical Immunology, 28*(5), 557–563. https://core.ac.uk/download/2710425.pdf (accessed on 17th July 2025).

13. Donath, D. (2025). Methods for nucleic acid extraction from ticks: Challenges and potential for advancement. *Vector Borne and Zoonotic Diseases*. https://www.semanticscholar.org/paper/9b80e7341b3de6b9e2539ed980f65f60c763337c (accessed on 17th July 2025).

14. Edsjö, A., Baskovich, B., Cox, E., Schuuring, E., Dequeker, E., Thunnissen, E., et al. (2014). Guidance for laboratories performing molecular pathology for cancer patients. *European Journal of Clinical Pathology, 8*(2), 123–133. https://core.ac.uk/download/29190116.pdf (accessed on 17th July 2025).

15. Mostafa G. FadL. (2022). Characterization of Genetic Resources of Microorganism as Response of Climate Change. J Gene Engg Bio Res, 4(2), 175-182.(accessed on 17th July 2025).

16. Ganguly, R., & Lee, C. S. (2024). A Poisson-independent approach to precision nucleic acid quantification in microdroplets. *ACS Applied Bio Materials*. https://www.semanticscholar.org/paper/71a228862f464f61bf8d565c7a21b63710b01714 (accessed on 17th July 2025).

17. Gleditzsch, D. (2020). Production and analysis of synthetic Cascade variants. https://core.ac.uk/download/288436499.pdf (accessed on 17th July 2025).

18. Groll, A. H., Pham, A. S., De Pauw, B., Costa, C., Girmenia, C., Halliday, C., Mengoli, C., et al. (2012). A MIQE-compliant real-time PCR assay for Aspergillus detection. *Journal of Clinical Microbiology, 50*(10), 3303–3311. https://core.ac.uk/download/30696634.pdf (accessed on 17th July 2025).

19. Ince, J., & McNally, A. (2009). Development of rapid, automated diagnostics for infectious disease: advances and challenges. *Expert review of medical devices*, *6*(6), 641–651. https://doi.org/10.1586/erd.09.46(accessed on 17th July 2025).

20. Jue, E., Witters, D., & Ismagilov, R. F. (2020). Two-phase wash to solve the ubiquitous contaminant-carryover problem in commercial nucleic-acid extraction kits. *Scientific reports*, *10*(1), 1940. https://doi.org/10.1038/s41598-020-58586-3(accessed on 17th July 2025).

21. Jayaweera, T., Siepert, N., Hradecky, B., Ostrowska, E., Casuga, I., Lea, K., Kshatriya, P., et al. (2022). Abstract 2939: Automation meets reliability: Use of Oncomine™ precision assay on the Genexus™ system for accurate identification of cancer biomarkers in FFPE and liquid biopsy samples. *Cancer Research*. https://www.semanticscholar.org/paper/5ae156008bd3075d2d8ae4045af7b4858606f186 (accessed on 17th July 2025).

22. Kalmar, A., Ribeiro-Silva, A., Sharpe, A., Williams, C., Seiler, C., Harrington, E. A., Jones, E. V., et al. (2016). Nucleic acid extraction from formalin-fixed paraffin-embedded cancer cell line samples: A trade-off between quantity and quality? *BMC Research Notes, 9*(1), 1–9. https://core.ac.uk/download/83942099.pdf (accessed on 17th July 2025).

23. Longnecker, K., & Kujawinski, E. B. (2020). Intracellular Metabolites in Marine Microorganisms during an Experiment Evaluating Microbial Mortality. *Metabolites*, *10*(3), 105. https://doi.org/10.3390/metabo10030105(accessed on 17th July 2025).

24. Lynton-Jenkins, J. G., Chaine, A., Russell, A., & Bonneaud, C. (2023). Parasite detection and quantification in avian blood is dependent on storage medium and duration. *Ecology and Evolution, 13*. https://www.semanticscholar.org/paper/904cee8ec40840c3d751fc07fd3f5b06a439d21e (accessed on 17th July 2025).

25. Martins, L. A., Domingues, R. S., de Moraes, G. M., Penna, G. C., Zauli, D. A., & de Lima, A. B. (2023). B-392 standardization of nucleic acid extraction method from thyroid fine needle aspiration (FNA) cells on stained and fixed slides for next-generation sequencing protocols. *Clinical Chemistry*. https://www.semanticscholar.org/paper/17117e3162b5d759e69cfdb34b6dcd34db0e0b84 (accessed on 17th July 2025).

26. Nguyen, T. T. (2015). Examining peak height ratios in low template DNA samples with and without sampling using a single-tube extraction protocol. https://open.bu.edu/bitstream/2144/13979/8/Nguyen_bu_0017N_11545_web.pdf (accessed on 17th July 2025).

27. Reifenberger, G. C., Thomas, B., & Rhodes, D. (2022). Comparison of DNA extraction and amplification techniques for use with engorged hard-bodied ticks. *Microorganisms, 10*. https://www.semanticscholar.org/paper/a9641df4388968a519af7f956f9111d7f02e6aa8 (accessed on 17th July 2025).

28. Ricco, A. J., Breadmore, B. L., Lincoln, C., Cady, C., Viguier, C., Chen, C., et al. (2008). Integrated microfluidic tmRNA purification and real-time NASBA device for molecular diagnostics. *Analytical Chemistry, 80*(14), 5562–5570. https://core.ac.uk/download/19085589.pdf (accessed on 17th July 2025).

29. Sait, A., Korkmaz, S., Parmaksız, A., Bayraktar, B., & Aslan, İ. (2025). Assessment of nucleic acid extraction kits for SARS-CoV-2 surveillance in wastewater samples. *Mersin Üniversitesi Tıp Fakültesi Lokman Hekim Tıp Tarihi ve Folklorik Tıp Dergisi, 36*(2), 21–32. https://www.semanticscholar.org/paper/47aa4da26b3bc71d272c06c020c8745f5717f247 (accessed on 17th July 2025).

30. Saunders, J. R., & Saunders, V. A. (1997). The impact of molecular biology on assessment of water quality: Advantages and limitations of current techniques. https://core.ac.uk/download/11020751.pdf (accessed on 17th July 2025).

31. Schönfeld, R. M. (2003). Generation of transgenic mice to evaluate promoter activity and specificity of two human endogenous retrovirus long terminal repeats. *Untersuchungen zur Promotor-Aktivität Und -Spezifität Von Zwei Long Terminal Repeats Humaner Endogener Retroviren in Transgenen Mäusen*. https://core.ac.uk/download/11025988.pdf (accessed on 17th July 2025).

32. Smith, W., Liu, Y., Simpson, S. L., Bivins, A., & Ahmed, W. (2024). Assessment of nucleic acid extraction protocols for antibiotic resistance genes (ARGs) quantification in aircraft wastewater. *Human Genomics, 18*. https://www.semanticscholar.org/paper/47d0eeb8e96868939762ad778dcc7795bc39653b (accessed on 17th July 2025).

33. Versmessen, N., Van Simaey, L., Negash, A., Vandekerckhove, M., Hulpiau, P., Vaneechoutte, M., & Cools, P. (2024). Comparison of DeNovix, NanoDrop and Qubit for DNA quantification and impurity detection of bacterial DNA extracts. *PLOS ONE, 19*. https://www.semanticscholar.org/paper/adc2f16b3dc82674289aa924c3bc03aedd55d5b7 (accessed on 17th July 2025).

34. Vutukuru, M. R., Sharma, D. K., Chakraborty, I., Mukhopadhyay, D., & Mitra, N. (2025). A rapid and high-yield method for nucleic acid extraction. *Scientific Reports, 15*. https://www.semanticscholar.org/paper/e930fb2d072a2560c73311759814577f77ad09da (accessed on 17th July 2025).

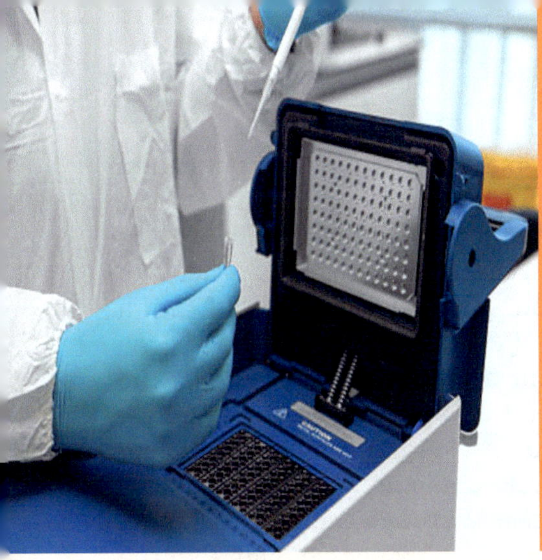

Chapter 3

POLYMERASE CHAIN REACTION (PCR) AND VARIANTS

Contents

Introduction

The Polymerase Chain Reaction (PCR) has revolutionized molecular biology, offering unprecedented levels of capability to amplify DNA sequences. Developed in the 1980s by Kary Mullis, PCR allows researchers to exponentially replicate targeted segments of DNA, facilitating detailed analysis of the genetic material much faster than previously possible. Its methodological simplicity, along with its capacity to generate millions of copies from an infinitesimally small sample, has made it widely applied in forensic analysis, medical diagnostics, and biological research. Not only has PCR expanded our knowledge of genetic material, but it's also a fundamental foundation to explore genetic variants, which play a dominant role in uses like pharmacogenomics and personalized medicine. It is important to understand the terminology of genetic variants, especially in PCR, to enhance clinical diagnostics. Genetic diagnosis is now among the most evolving areas of medicine, thanks to advances in technology that make it easier to identify variants capable of influencing disease susceptibility or drug response. As is defined in literature, the increasing demand for such genetic information compels the application of high-throughput diagnostic methods, hence fusing traditional PCR technologies with innovative approaches. This integration of diagnostic ability is imperative in the provision of effective patient care. As more genetic markers are discovered and confirmed by researchers, there is a need to realize the implications for clinical use and result interpretation, particularly if identification of variants tends to surpass our knowledge of their clinical use (Wiita & Schrijver, 2011). As well, the incorporation of new methodologies into PCR and variant discovery has broadened the scope of genetic studies. Techniques , such as gapped plasmids and others have been created as probes to study DNA polymerase fidelity *in vitro* replication and to provide information about the frequency of mutations and fidelity of the polymerase (Jozwiakowski & Connolly, 2009) and hold significant significance in understanding genetic variations in disease. Through the use of gapped plasmids, researchers not only explore the error rates of different DNA polymerases but also the functional consequences of specific genetic mutations. Incrementally, this process ultimately results in improved comprehension of how variations can affect gene function and interaction and thus opens the door for more specific diagnosis and treatment mechanisms in personalized medicine (Figure 3.1).

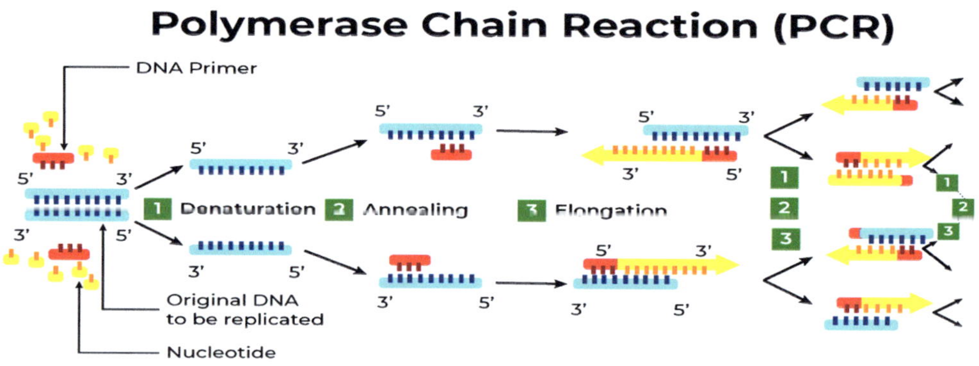

Figure 3.1. Polymerase chain reaction (PCR).

Source: https://media.geeksforgeeks.org/wp-content/uploads/20240122152308/Polymerase-chain-Reaction-768.png.

Definition of Polymerase Chain Reaction (PCR)

The Polymerase Chain Reaction (PCR) is a revolutionary molecular biology technique through which the duplication of specific DNA sequences is facilitated, enabling researchers to generate thousands to millions of copies of a single piece of DNA. The procedure plays a crucial role in genetics, forensic analysis, and medical diagnostics. PCR exploits the inherent character of DNA replication by employing heat-stable DNA polymerase enzymes, typically Taq polymerase, which are resistant to the high temperatures employed to melt DNA strands. The operation involves repeating cycles of denaturation, primer annealing, and extension, which progressively enhance the selectivity and efficiency of DNA amplification. The value of PCR is not only in its fundamental role in genetic analysis but also in its application in a broad category of scientific disciplines, demonstrating its far-reaching impact on modern bioscience research and clinical diagnostics. For clinical diagnostics, PCR application has been quite handy, particularly in infectious disease detection where accurate and rapid identification of pathogens is needed. One of the most significant advancements of PCR technology is the quantitative PCR (qPCR), a method that quantifies the DNA in a sample. It is particularly relevant for applications where the pathogen load may have implications for treatment. For instance, one study found that quantitative PCR of bronchoalveolar lavage fluid for the diagnosis of *Pneumocystis pneumonia* (PCP) among immunocompromised patients had a pooled sensitivity of 98.7% and specificity of 89.3% (Brown et al., 2024). PCR is therefore not only employed in diagnosing but also as a critical test that aids clinicians to make patient management decisions. Besides, new developments like allele-specific PCR (AS-PCR) show the utility of PCR in genetic studies, particularly in livestock genetics, where differentiation between allelic variants has significantly an impact on breeding programs. A study comparing the A1 and A2 allelic variants of the beta-casein gene in cattle employed AS-PCR to genotype and presented data on genetic diversity and genes related to milk quality (Safa et al., 2024). This depicts the extensive variety of PCR-based applications, from biomedical diagnosis to agricultural development. With the knowledge of genetic markers and hybridization studies, PCR is essential to enhance animal breeding regimes and productivity in agriculture for overall well-being in food security and economy (Figure 3.2).

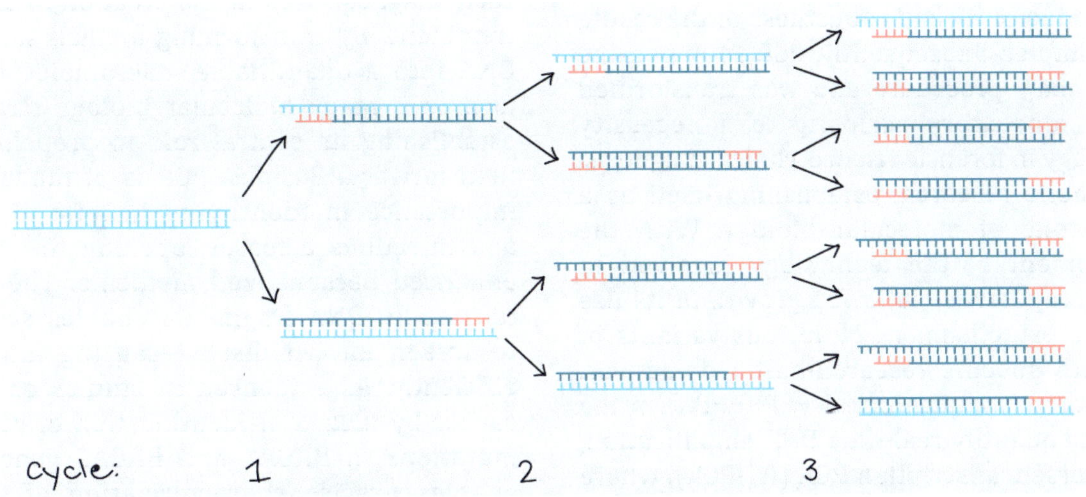

Figure 3.2. Definition of polymerase chain reaction (PCR).

Source: https://cdn.kastatic.org/ka-perseus-images/41f0e0fd8b49ba824db0eb707015557bb72ae72b.png.

Historical Background and Development of PCR

The history of Polymerase Chain Reaction, or PCR, dates back to the early 1980s when Kary Mullis, a Cetus Corporation biochemist, conceived a method to amplify specific DNA sequences. This discovery resulted from Mullis's observation of the need for a reliable method that would allow scientists to generate millions of copies of a target DNA fragment, thereby enabling further investigation. His initial experiments involved the use of DNA polymerases in conjunction with strategically designed primers to propel the synthesis of DNA. The earliest form of PCR was a time-consuming and labor-intensive process, but it it laid the foundation for a pioneering approach that would change the face of genetics and molecular biology. The simplicity and efficiency of PCR allowed it to quickly become accepted by scientists, sparking a new era of innovation in DNA manipulation and analysis. The identification of the thermostable DNA polymerases, notably Taq polymerase isolated from *Thermus aquaticus*, was a landmark event in the history of PCR. The previous DNA polymerases used to be denatured when exposed to high temperatures, crippling the process of amplification. Taq polymerase, however, could endure thermal cycling demanded by denaturation, annealing, and extension phases of PCR and hence enabled automated, high-throughput application of the technique. Here was the avoidance of the need to replenish the enzyme during amplification that made execution of the protocol, as well as reproducibility and robustness of the result, much simpler. Subsequently, PCR soon became a customary procedure and was transformed from a laboratory curiosity to a necessity technology in forensic science, clinical diagnosis, and genetic research, establishing itself as a cornerstone of molecular biology. With the development of the technology involved in PCR, there likewise followed growth in its use with the establishment of various variants of PCR with specific research-based objectives. Among these are quantitative PCR (qPCR), or the ability to quantify real-time DNA amplification, and reverse transcription PCR (RT-PCR), where RNA is examined by being reverse transcribed into complementary DNA. Such developments as multiplex PCR, in which multiple targets are amplified within one reaction, have also further extended the scope of PCR applications. This versatility has made PCR indispensable in contemporary genetic research and diagnostics. Particularly, as we enter an era where genomic data are at the center of unlocking disease mechanisms and the design of tailored therapies, the versatility and usefulness of PCR are even greater, placing it among the most significant techniques used in molecular biology today (Li et al., 2020; Wang et al., 2021).

Importance of PCR in Molecular Biology

It is the Polymerase Chain Reaction (PCR) that occupies a key position in amplifying specific DNA sequences in molecular biology, which makes deep studies into genetic information possible. Using the technique, researchers are able to generate millions of copies of an isolated DNA fragment from an initial minimum amount, thereby enabling diverse applications ranging from cloning to the study of gene expression and mapping genes. PCR sensitivity makes it critical for the study of mutations and variations encountered in genetic material. For instance, in cancer studies, PCR facilitates the detection of specific genomic alterations in association with tumorigenesis that may aid in early diagnosis and in the creation of targeted treatment. By transforming a small sample of DNA into a quantifiable macromolecule, PCR facilitates many molecular biology strategies, establishing its central role in propelling the field forward. Besides, PCR is of fundamental importance in identifying genetic disorders and infectious diseases, opening the way for enhanced personalized medicine. The ability to amplify DNA fragments enables scientists to screen known disease-causing mutations efficiently. As evidenced in studies on breast cancer by means of identification of germline mutations in BRCA1 and BRCA2 genes, PCR enables precise characterization of genetic variation in populations. PCR in such situations not only enables direct visualization of mutation but also assists in disease course monitoring and treatment response. New variant generation through differential splicing, as observed in analogous studies, points to the importance of PCR not only as an amplification technique but as a diagnostic tool that determines therapy. The clinical impact of PCR is tremendous and profound. Moreover, the functional diversity of PCR technologies, including quantitative PCR (qPCR) and reverse transcription PCR (RT-PCR), enhances its functional diversity in molecular biology. Such sophisticated forms of PCR entail real-time detection of amplification of DNA or RNA, providing quantitative information regarding levels of gene expression and dynamics of viral load in infectious diseases. The application of PCR in mutation detection, such as that revealed in breast cancer research, illustrates its function in translating genetic diversity in different populations (Yassaee et al., 2002). Additionally, the capacity to investigate splice variants, as illustrated in the identification of CEA family proteins using PCR, signifies its fundamental function in uncovering complex genetic interactions and processes (Nagel et al., 1993). As PCR continues to develop, its fundamental importance to research and clinics is never lost, allowing breakthroughs to inform the genomics of the future (Figure 3.3).

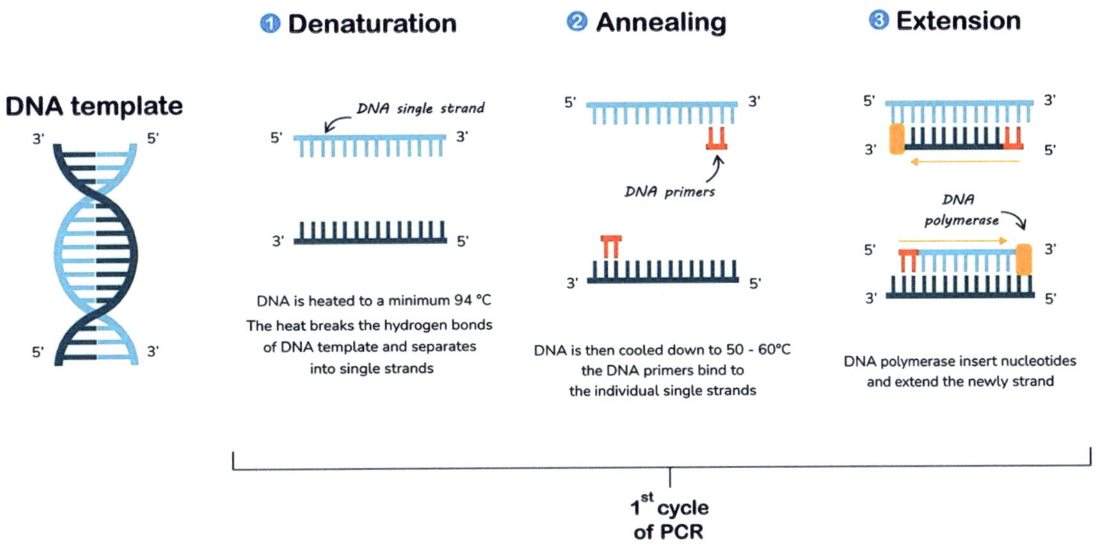

Figure 3.3. PCR in molecular biology.

Source: https://static.vecteezy.com/system/resources/previews/009/890/932/non_2x/molecular-biology-present-principle-and-process-of-polymerase-chain-reaction-or-pcr-technique-for-dna-amplification-vector.jpg.

3.1. Mechanism of PCR

The mechanism of polymerase chain reaction (PCR) is mainly based on the enzymatic copying principles and thus allows for the amplification of target DNA sequences. The process begins with denaturation, in which the double-stranded DNA template is heated, most commonly to 94–98 C, to separate the strands. Single-stranded DNA molecules are generated through this heat denaturation, which are used as templates for the subsequent synthesis processes. Once the DNA has been denatured, the temperature is lowered to about 50–65°C in the annealing process to enable the primers to bind to the complementary strands of their own on the target DNA. Precision in designing the primers is important since it also directly influences the specificity and the efficiency of the amplification, thereby setting the stage for the final yield of the copies of the DNA in the reaction.

Following annealing, the procedure proceeds into the extension phase, in which new DNA strands are synthesized by DNA polymerase. This is typically done at a temperature of approximately 72 C to allow for optimal enzyme activity. Taq polymerase enzyme, or occasionally standard Taq polymerase, appends nucleotides that are complementary to the primers to build a new DNA strand. The fidelity of the polymerase is highly crucial because any errors that are committed will result in mutations in the amplified target DNA. Therefore, advancements have led to the development of high-fidelity polymerases whose accuracy has improved during amplification. This potential to produce numerous copies of a target DNA sequence allows for subsequent uses, like cloning, sequencing, and diagnostics, and demonstrates the clinical utility of PCR and its derivatives in health care and scientific investigations. In addition, PCR is an ultrasensitive assay that can amplify trace amounts of DNA, a valuable commodity in numerous fields, including forensic science and molecular biology. The capability of PCR to recognize particular DNA sequences renders it absolutely essential in the determination of pathogens in clinical samples, the clarification of genetic mutations in cancer diagnostics, and the investigation of gene expression. Furthermore, the development of different PCR variants, including quantitative PCR (qPCR) and reverse transcription PCR (RT-PCR), attests to the versatility of this method in current genomics. For instance, RT-PCR allows the reverse transcription of RNA to DNA before amplification so that researchers can quantify the expression of genes upon various stimuli. This flexibility also underlines the immense contribution of PCR technologies towards enhancing our understanding in the field of genetic material and their applications in many fields, thereby making it a cornerstone technique in molecular biology research (Figure 3.4).

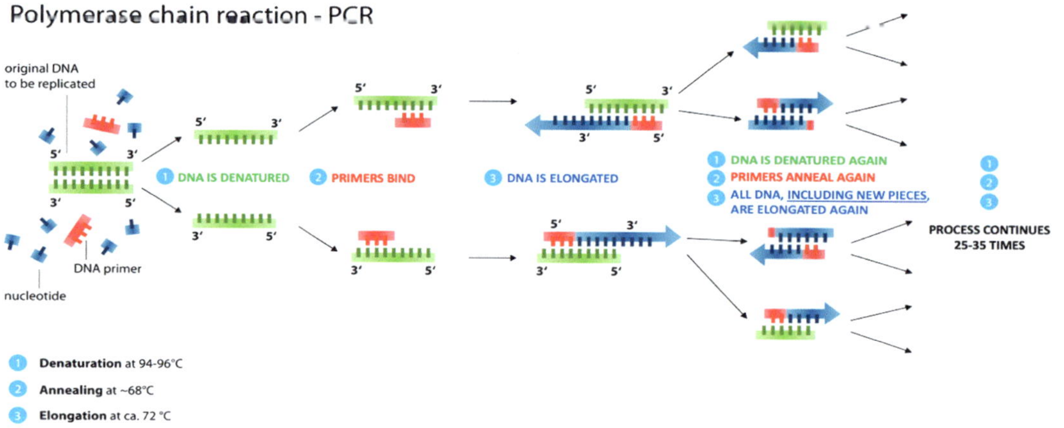

Figure 3.4. Polymerase chain reaction steps.

Source: https://d3rw207pwvlq3a.cloudfront.net/attachments/000/118/700/original/image.png?1594577977.

3.1.1. Components Required for PCR

Polymerase chain reaction (PCR) is fundamentally reliant on a series of critical factors to make it effective and precise in amplifying target DNA sequences. At the center of this is the DNA template from which the sequence of interest is amplified. In addition, two primers, also referred to as forward and reverse primers, are needed since they hybridize to the DNA template and specify the target region for amplification. The specificity of PCR is highly dependent on the annealing temperature and the design of these primers. Moreover, the incorporation of the deoxynucleotide triphosphates (dNTPs), which are the building blocks of the DNA strands, supports the amplification cycle in the formation of new DNA strands and, since a high-fidelity DNA polymerase is needed to reproduce the DNA fragments with accuracy, increases the yield and minimizes errors during amplification. The reaction buffer is also an essential ingredient that assists in providing the proper conditions for the PCR process to occur. This buffer typically consists of salts and stabilizers, which optimize the ionic environment for enzymatic activity. Most crucially, the pH of the buffer must be optimally adjusted to facilitate optimal polymerase activity under thermocycling conditions. The buffer can also contain additives, such as bovine serum albumin (BSA), which can desensitize the inhibition of DNA polymerase and optimize reaction performance. The quality and make-up of these buffer materials can have a significant impact on the specificity and efficacy of PCR, and thereby on the success of the ultimate experiment. So, not only are the fundamental materials but also the precise conditions under which PCR is carried out extremely important in determining the outcome. The application of these materials has ramifications far greater than their mere amplification; they play an important part in the advancement of PCR's downstream applications. For instance, primer design variations or polymerase fidelity differences can influence diagnostic results, for instance, in detecting infectious agents or genetic mutations. In a research article describing the diagnostic performance of PCR, different types of respiratory tract specimens were subjected to it, which indicated how sample type variation may influence sensitivity and specificity (Brown et al., 2024). Similarly, the impact of PCR on treatment and diagnosis in infectious uveitis highlights the importance of proper determination of pathogen existence using PCR, with a notable distinction being observed in findings when the diagnosis was unknown or known previously (Fallon et al., 2022). Thus, the purity, selection, and handling of PCR reagents enhance the technique itself as well as enhance its application in clinical practice (Figure 3.5).

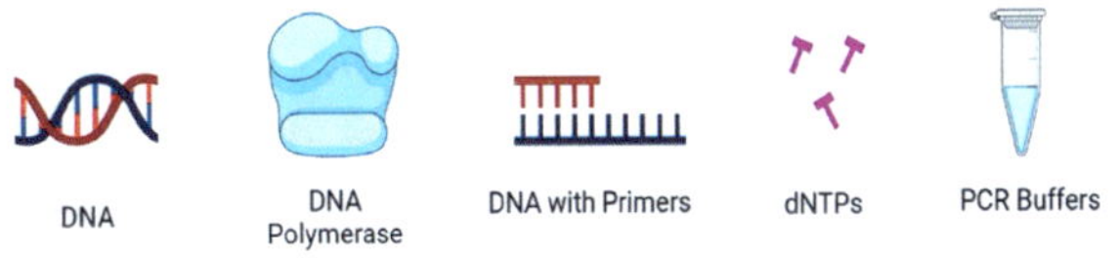

Figure 3.5. Components required for PCR.

Source: https://microbenotes.com/wp-content/uploads/2022/09/PCR-Components-PCR-reagents.jpg.

3.1.2. Steps Involved in the PCR Process

The Polymerase Chain Reaction (PCR) process entails several significant steps that amplify specific DNA sequences and thus enable extensive analysis and manipulation of the gene material. Denaturation is the initial step when the reaction mixture is subjected to a temperature of approximately 94–98°C. This heat denatures hydrogen bonds among complementary strands, causing the double-stranded DNA to separate into two single strands. This denaturation of the DNA structure, which is critical, comes first, as it makes the target sequence accessible to amplification in subsequent steps and thus forms the basis of the entire PCR process. Without effective denaturation, the targeted gene's structure is interrupted, leading to submaximal results in amplification and subsequent analyses. In the second step, following the denaturation step, is the annealing of the primers, which occurs at a temperature below denaturation, typicaly 50–65°C. Short nucleotide sequences called primers bind to the complementary areas of the single-stranded DNA templates. This is a crucial process because it will determine the specificity of the PCR amplification by defining the start and end points of the target DNA region exactly. The success of primer annealing can be influenced by several factors, including primer length and primer composition, and overall melting temperature of the regions in question. These considerations emphasize the importance of good primer design for optimal successful amplification, which may include consideration of regional genetic polymorphism in the sequences of interest, as discussed in recent advances in genetic assessments (Srivastava et al., 2020). The final phase of the PCR cycle is elongation, usually at an enzyme DNA polymerase-optimized temperature of about 72°C. In this step, the polymerase builds new strands of DNA by adding nucleotides that are complementary to the template strands, constructing a new strand that corresponds to each single-stranded template. This elongation phase is where the actual amplification occurs, as phosphodiester bonding is initiated by the enzyme DNA polymerase to form a large quantity of target DNA fragment. Through a cycle of denaturation, annealing, and elongation repeated numerous times, typically between 25 and 35 cycles, the PCR process creates millions to billions of copies of the target sequence for future genetic examination and applications. PCR accuracy and efficiency are enhanced by using high-fidelity DNA polymerases that ensure accurate replication irrespective of potential errors that might be present in the process of DNA synthesis, a process critical to the integrity of genetic information (Bolger et al., 2014) (Figure 3.6).

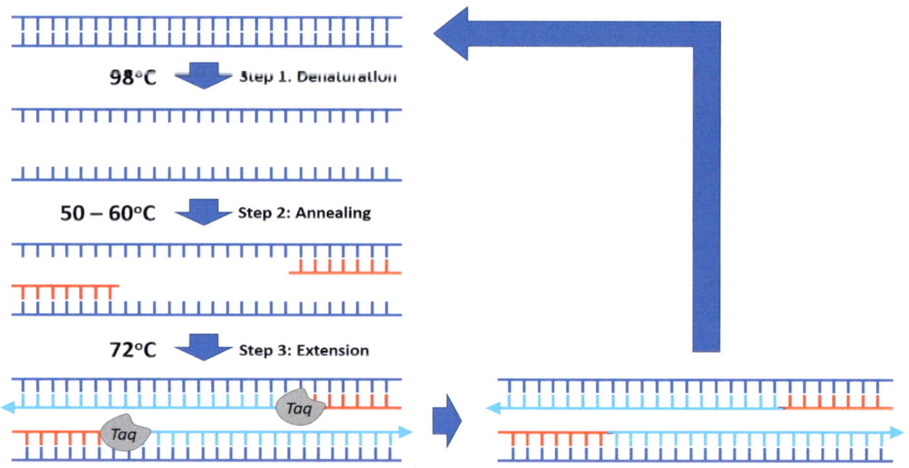

Figure 3.6. Steps and procedure of polymerase chain reaction (PCR).

Source: https://overallscience.com/wp-content/uploads/2018/07/PCR-cycle-overview.jpg.

3.1.3. Role of Temperature Cycles in Amplification

Polymerase Chain Reaction (PCR) success also relies heavily on its carefully designed temperature cycles, permitting amplification of the desired DNA sequence. The reaction begins with the denaturation stage, in which the reaction mixture is kept around 94–98°C for a brief period, denaturing the double-stranded DNA into individual strands. This first critical step serves as a basis for the rest of the steps since it makes the template DNA available to bind with primers. Temperature precision is important since a low temperature might be too little to achieve full denaturation, or too much of the temperature might damage the DNA or the enzyme. The denaturation cycle, in that case, serves not only a purpose but also a critical function and that is determining the final PCR product yield. Following denaturation, the temperature is lowered to around 50–65°C during the annealing process so that primers can identify their complementary sequences in the single-stranded DNA templates. Efficiency and specificity of this annealing are critical; improper temperatures can lead to non-specific binding, which will reduce the yield of the desired product. The temperature needs to be tailored for each specific primer pair to develop high fidelity in the amplification process. High temperatures of annealing may stop primer binding, while low temperatures may cause inadequate annealing or primer binding to undesired sequences. Hence, the correct calibration of this temperature cycle is an essential factor for the generation of specific and robust amplification in PCR. The final step is extension, which is usually carried out at 72°C, the optimal temperature for Taq polymerase activity. During this phase, DNA polymerase adds newly synthesized DNA strands from the annealed primers, hence doubling the target sequences exponentially. The efficiency of this temperature is crucial as low temperature may hinder the activity of the polymerase, and high temperature would inactivate the enzyme. In addition, variability due to factors like the size of the target sequence and the reaction conditions can influence extension efficiency. Lastly, the thermal cycle balance—extension, annealing, and denaturation—is the backbone of PCR and governs both amplification yield and the quality of the produced DNA and is therefore a linchpin in the success of this molecular biology mechanism (Ullah et al., 2006; Walsh et al., 2013).

3.2. Applications of PCR

Applications of Polymerase Chain Reaction (PCR) are widespread and vital, spanning numerous sciences. The most vital application is in medical diagnostics, namely the detection of infectious diseases. PCR can amplify specific sequences of DNA, which enables one to rapidly detect pathogens, i.e., bacteria and viruses. For instance, in the case of the COVID-19 pandemic, the utility of PCR was illustrated as it enabled quick and accurate diagnosis of SARS-CoV-2. Studies have highlighted the manner in which PCR, particularly its reverse transcription version RT-PCR, could be employed for the detection of the virus among patients, providing valuable information towards informing public health interventions and policy (Colac et al., 2024). Its ability to identify trace levels of viral RNA in biological samples says a lot about PCR's role as a pillar method in modern medicine, furthering the integration of molecular techniques into health care processes. Diagnostics of infectious diseases is not the only area where PCR has become a pillar technology, but oncology as well. Liquid biopsy is a new technology employing PCR for analysis of ctDNA found circulating in the bloodstream for noninvasive diagnosis and monitoring of cancer. This technique significantly enhances the potential to detect genetic changes associated with various cancers, treatment resistance, and metastasis. Digital PCR (dPCR) has enhanced these applications, allowing clinicians to quantify some genetic variants in real-time, thereby individualizing personalized treatment strategies for cancer patients (Ho et al., 2024). The liquidity of liquid biopsy not only allows for the detection in early stages but also ongoing tracking of disease status, which aids in improved prognostic outcomes. Thus, the convergence of PCR technology and oncology is a testament to the revolutionary impact of molecular biology on contemporary medical practice. The effects of PCR applications further extend to epidemiological research and public health, particularly in understanding and tracking viral variants. The continuous mutation of viruses , such as SARS-CoV-2 demands sophisticated genomic surveillance to monitor new strains and the impact that they can exert. Using PCR in addition to sequencing methods, researchers are able to identify mutations of the viral genome, elucidating patterns of transmission and variation with time (Colac et al., 2024). This real-time genomic data is essential to design successful vaccines and therapeutic treatments, demonstrating the fundamental role PCR plays in safeguarding public health. Detection of novel genetic variants guarantees that health agencies make educated choices, thereby maximally optimizing containment procedures. Through its diverse applications in diagnostics, cancer research, and epidemiology, PCR remains at the forefront of scientific advancements, triggering revolutionary advancements in diverse areas.

3.2.1. Use of PCR in Medical Diagnostics

The technology for polymerase chain reaction (PCR) has yielded a sea change in medical diagnosis with unparalleled sensitivity and specificity in the identification of various pathogens and genetic variants. Its ability to amplify trace DNA has made it an asset in detecting infectious diseases, where treatment hinges on the early diagnosis. In clinical laboratories, PCR techniques enable rapid disease screening for diseases , such as HIV, tuberculosis, and pulmonary infections, which has transformed the area of traditional diagnostic tools.

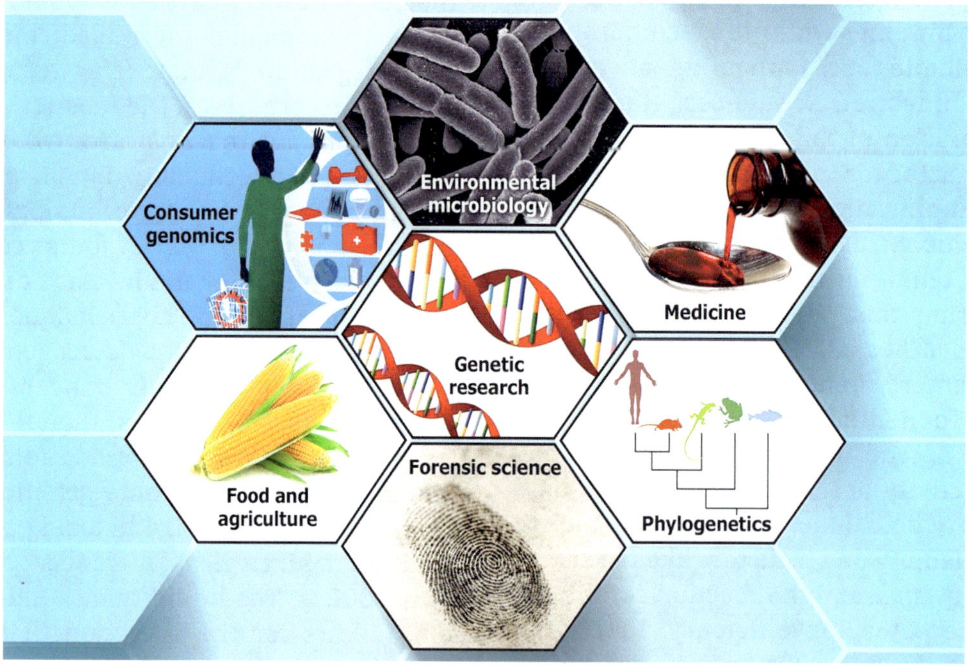

Figure 3.7. Use of PCR in medical diagnostics of polymerase.

Source: https://external-content.duckduckgo.com/iu/?u=https%3A%2F%2Fstatic.sciencelearn.org.nz%2Fimage_maps%2Fimages%2F000%2F000%2F035%2Foriginal%2FPCR_ITV_WhatIsPCR_UsedFor_BG-Plate_Final_v4.jpg%3F1522282461%261633578319804&f=1&nofb=1&ipt=1922b4f1685f48ccdb5cb10cde8af166a79c439d7d5f0065dcb8676047cd16bc.

The inclusion of high-throughput systems has further increased these efforts, with the ability to monitor a number of different genetic variants in a single assay at once. This is particularly important in the area of personalized medicine, where it is imperative to be aware of an individual's genetic makeup to tailor treatment and intervention (Wiita & Schrijver, 2011). Furthermore, the role of PCR in pharmacogenomic testing cannot be overstated. As our understanding of genetic determinants influencing drug metabolism expands, PCR has become a needed tool in determining some of the genetic variants that make an individual susceptible to drug response. This capacity allows doctors to make informed prescribing choices, decreasing drug side effects and optimizing therapeutic efficacy. The rapid expansion of genetic testing, as mentioned in recent publications, has a price, with great difficulty involving the interpretation of the clinical importance of detected variants. The ability to identify a genetic variant is not necessarily the same as understanding the implications this carries in biology, necessitating strong interpretation frameworks to direct healthcare professionals in the best way to apply this knowledge (Wiita & Schrijver, 2011). In addition to its use in genetic diagnosis, PCR has gained more adoption in infectious disease diagnosis, particularly in times of global health emergencies. Over the past two years, funding for research to spur advanced rapid diagnostic technologies for significant infectious pathogens has increased considerably. Among the significant advances are fully automated systems for real-time PCR-based testing, which have the capacity to accelerate pathogen detection methods and improve turnaround times for diagnostic purposes. It is important during outbreaks, when early identification has the ability to make a huge impact on public health interventions. In addition, researchers are exploring the potential to combine traditional immunoassays with advanced biosensor technology to enhance diagnostic accuracy at less cost than molecular testing. This transdisciplinary method of diagnosis demonstrates the evolving nature of medical testing and the vital role PCR technology still plays in addressing present-day health challenges (Figure 3.7).

3.2.2. Role of PCR in Forensic Science

The advent of polymerase chain reaction (PCR) technology has revolutionized forensic science by allowing unprecedented capability to analyze DNA evidence. PCR allows for amplification of minute DNA quantities, allowing for analysis of materials previously too degraded or insufficient for profiling. This technology has dramatically enhanced the precision and reliability of DNA examination in forensic analysis to the point that it is currently possible to obtain genetic profiles from trace evidence, such as hair, saliva, or blood that would otherwise not be identifiable under traditional examination. These advancements point to the revolutionary contribution of PCR to forensic procedures towards a deeper understanding of the contribution of DNA evidence to legal cases (Raju et al., 2025). While extremely influential, the application of PCR in forensic science is not without challenges. Inhibitors in biological samples can affect reaction efficiency, hence making it impossible to amplify degraded DNA. Further, the integrity of the original evidence can also dictate the quality of the findings, as older or contaminated samples may yield non-specific amplification or poor-quality profiles. With forensic scientists facing such constraints, ongoing innovation in PCR methods continues to advance the fidelity and sensitivity of the process. Attempts at maximizing cycling conditions and utilizing advanced primer design have had potential in maximizing the yield of valuable information from compromised samples, illustrating an evolving dynamic in the potential of PCR for forensic applications (McDonald et al., 2024). The use of PCR in forensic science not only enables criminal identification but also has a significant bearing on cases of exoneration. As increasing numbers of people are mistakenly convicted, the mechanism of re-evaluating evidence by PCR technology has become imperative in the quest for justice. The ability of the technology to unlock new information from previously gathered evidence can uncover the innocence of the wrongly accused. In addition, advances like multiplex PCR, which enables the amplification of multiple DNA targets at once, equip forensic analysts with means to enhance efficiency and extend the purview of investigations. As the future of forensic science lies before them, the versatility of PCR guarantees it will continue to be a pillar in the pursuit of justice and establishment of codes of conduct within the criminal justice system (Raju et al., 2025) (Figure 3.8).

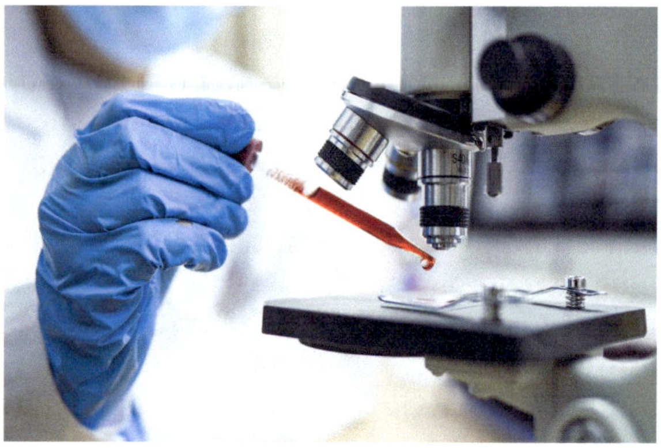

Figure 3.8. PCR in forensic science.

Source: https://cropper.watch.aetnd.com/cdn.watch.aetnd.com/sites/4/2022/06/AE-Crime-Blog-GettyImages-1211487998.jpg.

3.2.3. Applications in Genetic Research and Biotechnology

Polymerase chain reaction (PCR) has become a classic in genetic research and biotechnology, enabling numerous applications that were previously unfeasible. Because it can amplify specific DNA sequences, PCR makes it easy and accurate for scientists to analyze genetic material. This capability is crucial in fields , such as forensic science, where sufficient DNA samples are generated from limited biological traces to aid criminal investigations. Furthermore, PCR is an important tool in the diagnosis of genetic disorders by amplifying target sequences, which can lead to the identification of mutations associated with a variety of diseases. With progression in genetic research, the need for accurate and efficient tools in studying DNA sequences becomes heightened, underscoring PCR's importance in contemporary scientific inquiry and use. Additionally, the validity of PCR-based techniques is progressively enhanced by innovations aimed at minimizing sources of error that would invalidate experimental results. One such development is the blocker method, which aims to address issues like mishybridization that can lead to false positives in viral detection. The technique uses a mixture of blocker sequences to suppress contaminating DNA amplification, thus boosting the quality of PCR assays. These advances are necessary, as increased sensitivity of PCR can also raise the risk of mispriming and contamination, potentially obscuring the correct interpretation of results (Takahashi et al., 2024). With the advancement of such methods, researchers are able to employ PCR safely in its myriad applications, from genome editing and RNA interference to wider access in synthetic biology and therapeutic drugs. Genetically engineered DNA polymerases have greatly improved the accuracy and efficiency of PCR and further expanded its application in genomics and biotechnology in the past few years. For instance, Pfu-Sso7d, a fusion polymerase, exhibits excellent processivity and high fidelity and is therefore a highly sought-after polymerase for high-accuracy amplification purposes (Mahboob et al., 2024). Despite the numerous commercial options available, the cost of these polymerases is often beyond the budget of the average researcher. As a result, new processes for purifying and optimizing the enzymes have been developed, such as a cost-effective process using ethanol or acetone as the purification medium. This innovation not only makes high-performance polymerases more accessible to everyone but also optimizes PCR buffer solutions to better enhance the overall performance of PCR applications in genetic science and biotechnology. All these make it feasible for scientists to pursue the vast potential of PCR without interruption while maintaining high levels of accuracy and reliability.

3.3. Variants of PCR

Polymerase Chain Reaction (PCR) has also undergone significant advancements since its discovery, with various forms of PCR being developed with enhanced application in a variety of uses. One such prominent form is real-time PCR, also known as quantitative PCR (qPCR), which provides qualitative data regarding the amount of DNA in a sample while being amplified. This method employs fluorescent dyes that react proportionally to the levels of target nucleic acids and allow scientists to monitor reactions in real time.

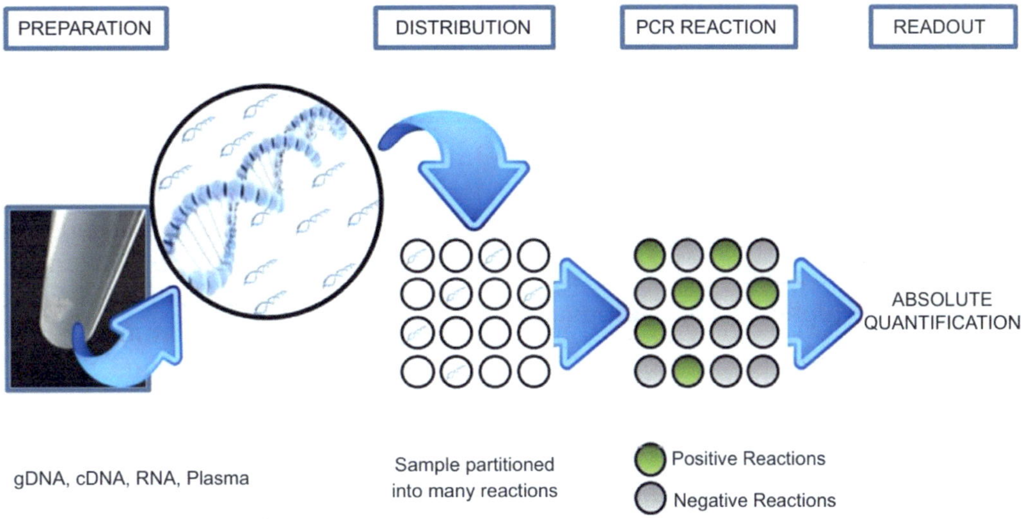

Figure 3.9. Types of PCR.

Source: https://www.mybiosource.com/learn/wp-content/uploads/2023/04/3.2.jpg.

Thus, while qPCR detects pathogens, it also plays a significant role in gene expression profiling and researching genetic differences. This kind of capability finds a vital application in clinical diagnostics, where proper quantification can lead to treatment, hence better patient outcomes for many areas of medicine. Another PCR variant is the Reverse Transcription PCR, also known as RT-PCR, and it has come into prominence especially during global health crises , such as the COVID-19 pandemic. The process enables RNA amplification by first converting it into complementary DNA (cDNA) through reverse transcription, rendering it invaluable for the identification of RNA viruses. Although RT-PCR is the conventional standard for the diagnosis of COVID-19, concerns have been raised regarding sensitivity and the risk of false negatives, particularly in the context of rapidly evolving viruses. The demand for increased diagnostic specificity has fueled interest in the use of Artificial Intelligence in RT-PCR protocols, enhancing the detection profile and clinically responding to the limitations imposed by emerging virus variants. This integration of technology and molecular biology reveals the ongoing evolution of PCR technologies as a consequence of emergent health issues. In addition, advances in many PCR methodologies continue to expand research strategies across genomics, transcriptomics, and beyond. Multiplex PCR is a variant of this kind that can provide simultaneous amplification of numerous targets in one reaction, which significantly increases throughput and reduces the cost of resources. This technique is particularly useful in applications , such as pathogen identification and genetic profiling where detection of multiple genetically important markers or organisms is imperative. While scientists keep pushing the boundaries of what is achievable with PCR technology, nanopore sequencing technologies (NST) have emerged as an adjunct, allowing for sequencing without the application of traditional amplification steps (Lang et al., 2023). This extensive variety of PCR variants, ranging from multiplex to NST, underlines the flexibility of PCR techniques, so that they still dominate molecular biology and clinical diagnostics as the biological research environment continues to evolve (Figure 3.9).

3.3.1. Real-Time PCR (qPCR) and Its Advantages

Real-time polymerase chain reaction, or qPCR, has become a necessary molecular biology technique because of its several benefits over traditional PCR. It is perhaps the most significant benefit that it enables real-time detection of the amplification of DNA, and this allows one to precisely measure nucleic acid concentration throughout the whole process of PCR. This capability is critical in clinical diagnostic use, for instance, where the amount of viral load of infective pathogens should be known for therapeutic procedures. Experiments have demonstrated the effectiveness of qPCR for detecting pathogens, such as in the study of infectious bronchitis virus (IBV) among chicken flocks, with real-time qPCR showing the presence of certain viral strains and their quantitative levels, proving its precision in identifying likely outbreaks (Currie et al., 2016). Sensitivity and qPCR efficiency are further enhanced through the use of fluorescent dyes or probes, enabling detection of the amplified product directly without post-amplification manipulation, such as gel electrophoresis. This not only saves time for the entire procedure but also reduces contamination, a common problem in molecular biology. Furthermore, qPCR allows for high-throughput screening since several samples can be screened simultaneously in one assay. The scalability of this method is especially useful in research laboratories where many samples need to be processed quickly and precisely. For instance, qPCR has been employed in teleost fish immune response research comparing immune-related gene expression levels in various tissues subjected to various experimental treatments, showing its applicability in comparative immunology (Bas et al., 2008). In addition, the ease of qPCR is also due to its applicability in other fields like pharmacogenomics, environmental monitoring, and forensic analysis, making it a one-size-fits-all molecular diagnosis instrument. Its ability to quantify low concentrations of DNA with high specificity and sensitivity has made it possible to advance in gene studies and personalized medicine. As researchers continue to place their confidence in the precise measurement of nucleic acids and the level of gene expression, the role of real-time qPCR in actionable information cannot be overemphasized. Its integration into routine laboratory protocols underlines its significance in furthering our understanding of complex biological processes and developing effective therapeutic interventions. Altogether, the advantages of qPCR, including speed, sensitivity, and flexibility, have rendered it an indispensable weapon in the arsenal of modern molecular biology techniques.

3.3.2. Reverse Transcription PCR (RT-PCR) for RNA Analysis

Reverse transcription polymerase chain reaction (RT-PCR) is an important technique applied in the analysis of RNA, enabling scientists to reverse transcribe RNA into complementary DNA (cDNA) that is amenable to amplification afterward. RT-PCR plays a crucial role in quantifying the levels of gene expression, detecting viral RNA, and studying alternative splicing events.

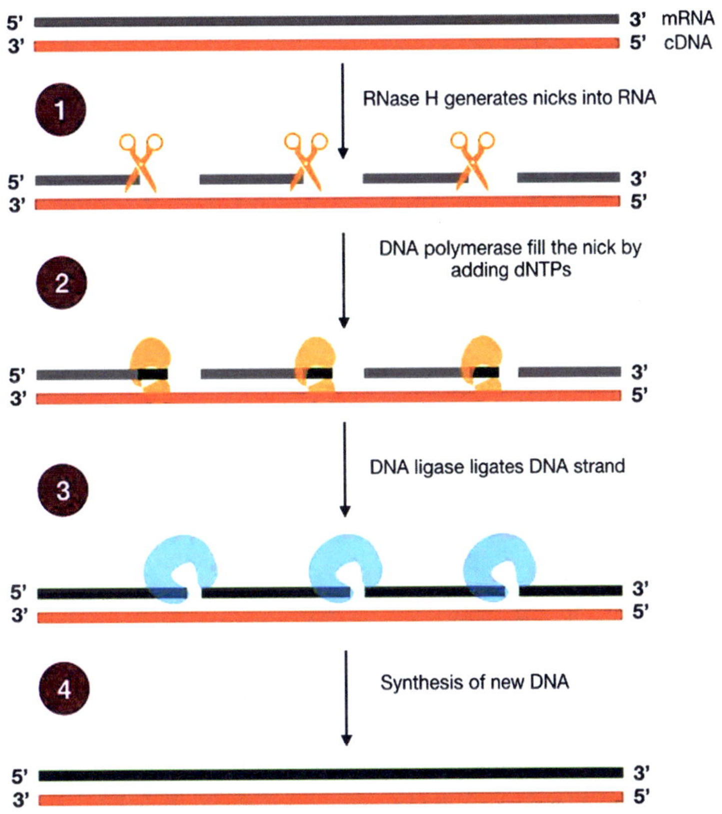

Figure 3.10. Reverse transcription PCR.

Source: https://geneticeducation.co.in/wp-content/uploads/2019/04/RT-qPCR.009-e1554278126197.jpeg.

One of the special advantages of RT-PCR is that it will amplify single RNA transcripts, making the investigation of splicing variants possibly associated with genetic disorders or disease conditions possible. By enabling the detection of low-abundance transcripts, RT-PCR illuminates the mysteries of RNA biology, with important potential implications for diagnostics and therapy in the future." Hence, RT-PCR is not only an immensely valuable tool for fundamental research but also an important ingredient in clinical applications to determine the functional significance of RNA variants in disease. The utility of RT-PCR is of great importance clinically when handling variants of uncertain significance (VUS) that arise during genetic testing. As has been suggested in the latest studies, RNA splicing defects, which are often present with inherited diseases, can be effectively screened for utilizing targeted RT-PCR assays along with high-complexity sequencing techniques. To illustrate, blood RNA samples that are analyzed via RT-PCR might elucidate how VUSs impact splicing and facilitate better interpretation of genetic testing. Notably, research has established that most clinically confirmed variants have a high association with abnormal splicing, an observation that underscores the importance of RNA analysis in the determination of the functional impact of VUSs. Inclusion of RT-PCR in the diagnostic process enables researchers to better establish the pathogenicity of genetic variants and formulate personalized treatment strategies based on patients' individualized RNA profiles, thereby leading to better patient outcomes (Htoo et al., 2020). Furthermore, advances in high-resolution RT-PCR techniques have improved the accuracy of transcript quantification derived from RNA sequencing (RNA-seq) datasets. Development of comprehensive reference transcript databases , such as the *Arabidopsis* reference transcript dataset (At RTD) has provided valuable resources to analyze alternative splicing between organisms. When combined with HR RT-PCR, RNA-seq provides precise splicing ratio measurement, a robust tool for validation of computational predictions of transcript abundance. Comparative analyses, as evident from the results, demonstrate a sharp correlation between the analysis of RNA-seq data and HR RT-PCR measurement, confirming the utility of such tools in examining complex gene expression dynamics. These synergies among RNA-seq and RT-PCR technologies highlight the potential of general gene expression analysis complementing our understanding of molecular mechanisms involved in various biological processes (Zhang et al., 2015) (Figure 3.10).

3.3.3. Multiplex PCR for Simultaneous Detection of Multiple Targets

The recent advances in multiplex polymerase chain reaction (PCR) technology have highly enhanced the detection of multiple genetic targets in a single assay. The new technology enables researchers and clinicians to identify various pathogens or genetic markers simultaneously, hence saving time and resources in diagnostics. Multiplex PCR works by using more than one pair of primers to target distinct sequences so that numerous targets are amplified in a single reaction. The process is of particular utility within the clinical setting where rapid and accurate identification of pathogens is needed, e.g., during infectious disease or genetic disease. For instance, the ability to detect more than one transgene in blood samples using multiplex PCR can be a game-changer in sports doping control since it assists in detecting several substances that can erode competition integrity (Yuen et al., 2025).

Furthermore, the integration of multiplex PCR with advanced analytical methods is proving essential to streamline the accuracy and sensitivity of target detection. Techniques like liquid chromatography high-resolution tandem mass spectrometry (LC-HRMS/MS) can be used in complement with multiplex PCR to check the presence of detected transgenes and therefore preclude false positives or false negatives in analysis. Multiplex PCR assay design also involves optimization of amplification conditions under strict scrutiny to prevent inhibition of amplification by primer-primer interactions for any target. As depicted in recent studies, the use of internal controls in multiplex PCR reactions increases assay reliability, increasing detection limits for all targets (Yuen et al., 2025). The integration of multiplex PCR with other emerging technologies therefore, remains to inform better molecular diagnostics practices. In the recent past, the development of data-driven approaches integrated with multiplex PCR has revealed new avenues of advanced pathogen detection and discrimination. Techniques , such as Amplification Curve Analysis (ACA) apply machine learning to calculate the amplification curves generated during qPCR to allow for the detection of multiple targets within one simultaneous reaction. Issues existregard to discrepancies among sources of data that can impact classification accuracy. This has led to new innovations like the application of transformer-based conditional domain adversarial networks (T-CDAN) to eliminate these disparities in distributions, resulting in improved classification performance in multiplex scenarios. These advancements suggest the importance of continuous improvement in techniques to maximize the effectiveness of multiplex PCR applications in real-world clinical settings. With the combination of classical PCR techniques and machine learning together with sophisticated analysis tools, the field of rapid, accurate diagnostics ever expands.

3.4. Advantages of PCR

The PCR has transformed molecular biology with the power to amplify short, specified DNA sequences, garnering it one of the most powerful methods used in a wide array of disciplines , including genetics, diagnostics, and forensic science. One of the greatest advantages of PCR is that it can produce a million copies of a fragment of DNA from a starting minute quantity, thus enabling scientists to try out very small samples. This function is particularly significant in clinical practice when it may not be possible to obtain sufficient genetic material. In research involving rare genetic mutations, such as those for thalassemia, the higher sensitivity of the PCR enables one to detect low-abundance sequences, an aspect of paramount significance in correct diagnosis and patient-specific treatment plans (Huang et al., 2025). Therefore, the mechanism of amplification is critical in the early detection of genetic diseases, allowing for therapeutic intervention and management. Other than its high sensitivity, PCR is also notorious for its quick turnaround time, which makes it an invaluable tool in research and clinical diagnostics. Traditional methods of gene analysis tend to be slow, taking days or even weeks to give results. By contrast, PCR is able to produce massive amounts of amplified DNA within a few hours, which is especially critical for situations where quick decisions need to be made, such as the diagnosis of infectious diseases.

Furthermore, real-time PCR, or quantitative PCR (qPCR), has also become increasingly useful with the capability to track the amplification process in real-time. This innovation not only increases the accuracy of nucleic acid measurement but also makes the procedure simpler by eliminating the need for post-amplification gel analysis (El-Tholoth & Bau, 2024). Hence, PCR really adds to the efficiency of lab procedures while being very accurate and reliable. Its flexibility and versatility in usage across a broad array of scientific and medical disciplines are another distinct advantage of PCR. PCR not only has been the backbone of genetic research but has emerged as a standard component of pathogen detection, forensic analysis, and environmental analysis. By being capable of amplifying the entire range of targets—be it genetic mutations, viral RNA, or bacterial DNA—the method can be fashioned to meet the needs of scientists and medical practitioners alike. The use of PCR-based diagnostic tools in the diagnosis of avian respiratory diseases, for example, highlights their utility in veterinary medicine, where rapid and reliable diagnosis of disease-causing pathogens is imperative for avoiding disease outbreaks (El-Tholoth & Bau, 2024). With future advancements in PCR, the emergence of new variants and techniques will further bolster its applications and highlight its continued role in scientific research and clinical practice (Figure 3.11).

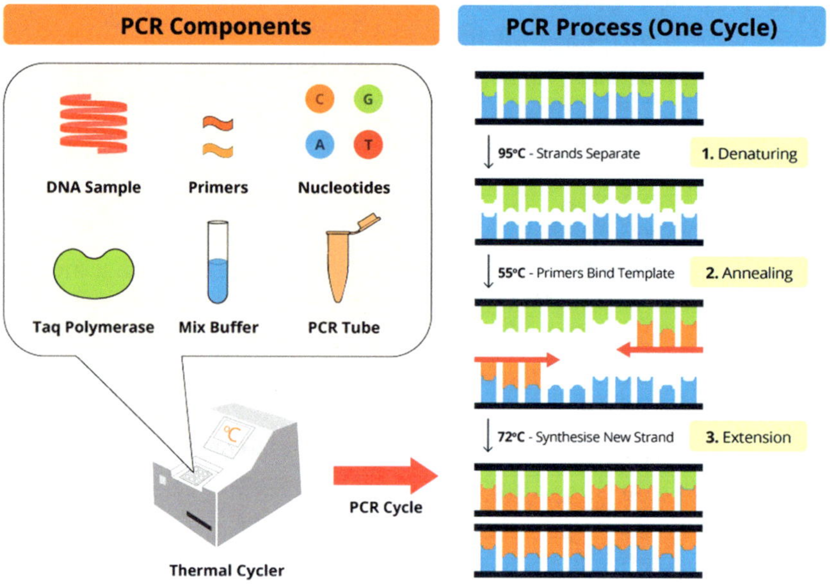

Figure 3.11. Scientech biology: Polymerase chain reaction (PCR).

Source: https://microbenotes.com/wp-content/uploads/2018/09/Polymerase-Chain-Reaction.jpeg.

3.4.1. Sensitivity and Specificity of PCR

Specificity and sensitivity of Polymerase Chain Reaction (PCR) are the determining factors of its utility in molecular diagnostics, particularly in infectious diseases. Sensitivity describes the assays ability to identify positive cases correctly, whereas specificity represents the assay's capability to identify negative cases correctly. High-sensitivity PCR assay minimizes false negatives to a significant degree and allows detection of low-abundance targets when present in large amounts of background noise. Conversely, high specificity ensures that the amplification process will not yield false positives, which can lead to misdiagnosis and inappropriate treatment. Getting an optimal balance between sensitivity and specificity is most important for PCR assays used in clinical applications, as the implications of diagnostic mistakes can have severe impacts on patient outcomes. Evolution and refinement of PCR tests have shown specificity to often be enhanced by altering reaction conditions, such as by varying the annealing temperatures or employing more specific primers. Recent advances have emphasized the utility of employing highly complementary primers to target sequences to prevent the likelihood of off-target amplification. Further, the application of high-fidelity engineered enzymes can also contribute to specificity, thus minimizing non-specific binding during amplification. The fine-tuning not only improves the dependability of the PCR product but also addressing the challenges posed by genetic variants, which may have subtle sequence changes. Therefore, the tricky balancing act between sensitivity and specificity remains a significant issue in the design of solid PCR protocols. Economical solutions like those found in evolutionary studies of transcriptional regulators like LuxR indicate an intrinsic flexibility that could be applied in the development of PCRs. In sensory systems, variants were observed which exhibited increased sensitivity and specificity to various acyl-homoserine lactones, which implied the capacity to evolve rapidly to recognize new substrates (Collins et al., 2005). Similarly, PCR technologies can also leverage the theme of directed evolution to adapt assay parameters to optimize them so that assays continue performing at an optimal level even as target sequences mutate. For example, while in research, LuxR variants were made more sensitive to specific signals; the modified systems show how customized adaptations can tighten sensitivity and specificity (Hawkins et al., 2007). Thus, evolutionary biological findings can drive innovative solutions to improve PCR diagnostic tests so that there can be elasticity when confronting new variants and pathogens (Figure 3.12).

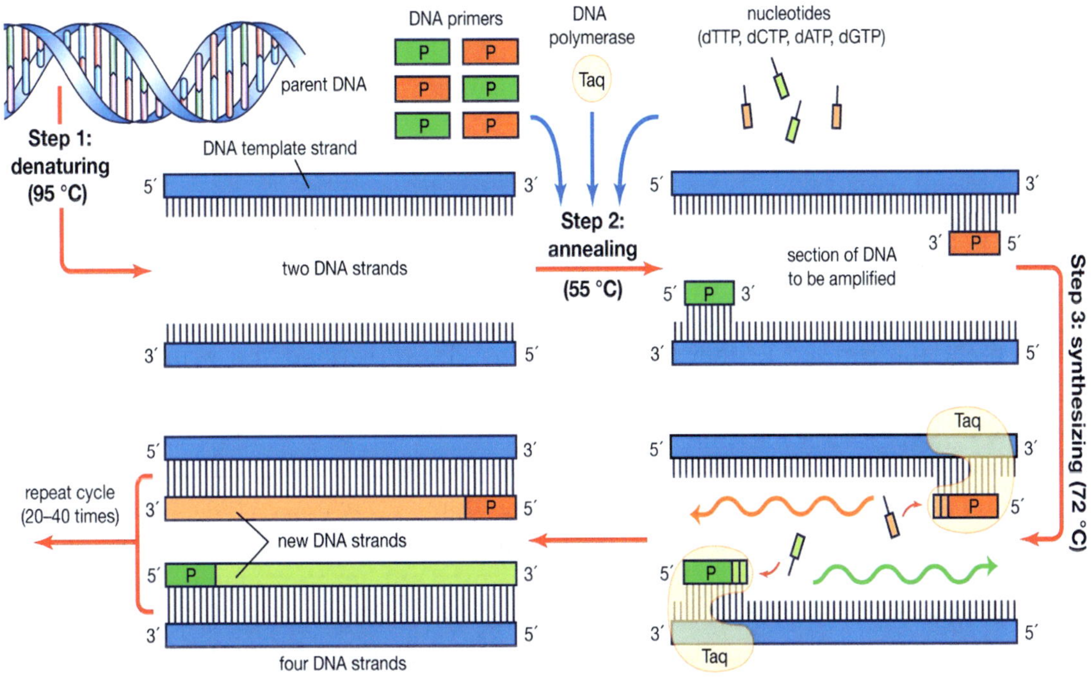

Figure 3.12. Specificity and sensitivity of conventional polymerase chain reaction.

Source: https://cdn.britannica.com/77/22477-050-16EFB7B3/process-polymerase-chain-reaction.jpg.

3.4.2. Speed and Efficiency of the Amplification Process

The process of PCR amplification is dependent on speed and efficiency, both of which are crucial for its applications in areas , such as genetic research and diagnostics. Speed is particularly crucial where early results could lead to early intervention, as in the case of disease identification. Advances , such as the All-In-One Dual CRISPR-Cas12a (AIOD-CRISPR) assay emphasize the potential for speeding up detection processes. This method, which is able to detect SARS-CoV-2 in 20 minutes, is one of a trend towards quicker amplification times without loss in sensitivity and specificity. By providing a streamlined, instrument-independent means of detecting nucleic acid, such methods demonstrate the potential of PCR-based approaches for performing well without taking the long time normally allocated to conventional amplification and processing, eventually leading to clinical decision-making and public health action (Ding et al., 2020). Efficiency is equally important in the amplification process, with a bearing on PCR application utility, especially in high-throughput applications. Proper primer design is a major consideration to gain the highest efficiency in PCR, optimizing the likelihood of successful amplification.

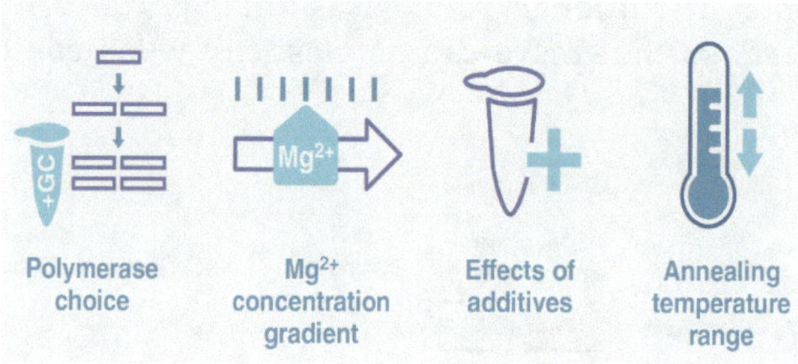

Figure 3.13. PCR amplification.

Source: https://www.neb.com/-/media/nebus/page-images/blogs/blog-posts/4-tips-for-gc-rich-pcr-amplification/nebinspired_gcrichpcr_blog_considerations_0822.png?la=en&rev=6900482a7d074d27a3f7f0f6c9d369ec&hash=A0B9391EFEAF9C30CF2EB14C9043A4AA.

Software technologies like Primer3 have broadened and refined the primer design process, enabling better control over melting temperatures and reducing the prevalence of unwanted secondary structures , such as hairpins or dimers. Such advancements enable primers not only to work well but also to be specific, thereby providing more precise results during amplification. The capacity to create primer sequences based on whole-genome information also maximizes efficiency by the potential for more flexibility in use across many genomic contexts. These advancements are obviously an effort made to maximize PCR protocols to be applicable to high-throughput analysis, maximizing overall experimental throughput and reliability (Untergasser et al., 2012). The synergism of speed and efficiency in PCR cannot be overemphasized because they assist in maximizing the technique's applicability across disciplines. In the context of healthcare, where early pathogen detection can prevent outbreaks, the addition of rapid amplification technology is groundbreaking. The ability of the AIOD-CRISPR assay, for instance, to deliver results in minutes directly addresses the urgent need for emergency diagnostics during public health emergencies. Meanwhile, advances in primer design and thermodynamic modeling lead to more effective amplification processes, further establishing PCR as a method of identifying genetic variation and conducting genomic studies. Consequently, the ability to perform fast and efficient PCR not only offers real-time utilization in disease management but also promotes research and biotechnology development. Through such advances in technologies that are still unraveling, the amplification process is poised to take a more pivotal position in science (Untergasser et al., 2012; Ding et al., 2020) (Figure 3.13).

3.4.3. Versatility in Various Fields of Study

The virtue of versatility is highly entrenched in the realms of scientific inquiry, particularly in the case of the Polymerase Chain Reaction (PCR). The process has undergone refinement from its initial use in molecular biology to assume an unstoppable influence on various fields like forensic science, medical diagnostics, and environmental monitoring. As scientists utilize the potency of PCR, they are presently able to amplify trace amounts of DNA, making genetic material identifiable even within challenging samples. Amplification not only enhances genetic identification in forensic analysis but also spurs advances in personalized medicine through the ability to precisely test unique genetic profiles. The versatility of PCR in these contexts is typical of the flexibility of the technology, seamlessly aligning with the evolving demands of different scientific pursuits and giving rise to innovations outside traditional discipline boundaries. In the field of environmental science, the flexibility of PCR is exemplified in uses from biodiversity estimation to pollution monitoring. By characterizing environmental samples, scientists can identify and count a specific microorganism or quantify genetic diversity in ecosystems. For instance, amplification of ribosomal RNAs by genes has proved to be essential in monitoring microbial populations as a reaction to changes in the environment and ultimately toward the management of ecosystems. Additionally, uses of PCR extend to the detection of pathogens and toxins in environmental matrices, demonstrating the use of the technique for public health protection. PCR's versatility in environmental applications is symptomatic of a broader trend of integrating molecular techniques and ecology, characteristic of an interdisciplinary approach that promotes innovative solutions to pressing environmental concerns. Beyond its applicability, the methods underlying PCR have enabled us to attain many of the achievements in biochemistry and genetics, enhancing our understanding of the molecular underpinnings of life. Techniques , such as CRISPR-Cas9 genome editing and gel electrophoresis have become pivotal to this paradigm, providing access to new techniques of gene manipulation and expression. The study of DNA interactions has been transformed by bringing together methodologies , such as PCR, where the amplification of specific segments of DNA provides increased study of gene function and regulation. As we examine the overall uses of PCR and its variants, it is evident that such techniques are not standalone techniques but a part of complete components of a broad set of tools to innovate in various domains, and accentuating the role of interdisciplinary thinking in modern scientific research (Choi et al., 2017; Rahul, 2023).

3.5. Limitations of PCR

Polymerase Chain Reaction (PCR) has revolutionized molecular biology, but with a caveat; its application is not without limitations. The primary limitation arises from the requirement of high precision in the process of amplification. Contamination by extraneous DNA leads to false positives that undermine the validity of test results. In a clinical setting, it can have far-reaching implications, particularly in the case of disease diagnoses , such as skin infections, where precise identification is critical. The traditional diagnostics, including culture tests, usually have the same disadvantages, but the need for dedicated laboratories and sophisticated protocols in PCR increases the obstacle of correct and prompt diagnoses. Alternatives that combine new methods may simplify the obstacles, offering innovation in the technique of detection without invasion, as recent studies evaluating new CRISPR technology to detect pathogens from sweat samples, as van Dongen et al. (2024) have suggested. Another drawback is the pre-known DNA sequence dependency. PCR is programmed beforehand to amplify known target sequences;

thus, any new mutations or gene variations not discovered beforehand can be overlooked. This is where it comes into focus with special significance in genetic trait research, such as the A1 and A2 allelic variants of the CSN2 gene of livestock animals. In employing allele-specific PCR (AS-PCR) for genotyping, researchers should exercise caution to possess substantial insight into the allele sequences before analysis to avoid excluding crucial variants (Safa et al., 2024). Thus, the use of PCR is restricted in the case of looking for unidentified genetic modifications, requiring the employment of complementary approaches able to identify broader genetic diversity or mutations. Finally, PCR's efficiency reduces in complicated samples marked by numerous competing templates, with the consequence of unequal amplification. In biological fluids like blood or environmental samples, multiple nucleic acid sources can substantially hinder PCR performance. Under these circumstances, elements , such as primer specificity and reaction conditions need careful optimization for the generation of consistent results. While PCR's versatility enables varied modifications, e.g., multiplexing, such additions can also introduce supplementary issues, e.g., increased potential for primer-dimerization and non-specific amplifications. The variation in sample composition therefore, underlines an intrinsic limitation of PCR, which requires continued refinement and integration of complementary techniques to extend its usefulness in a variety of situations (Figure 3.14).

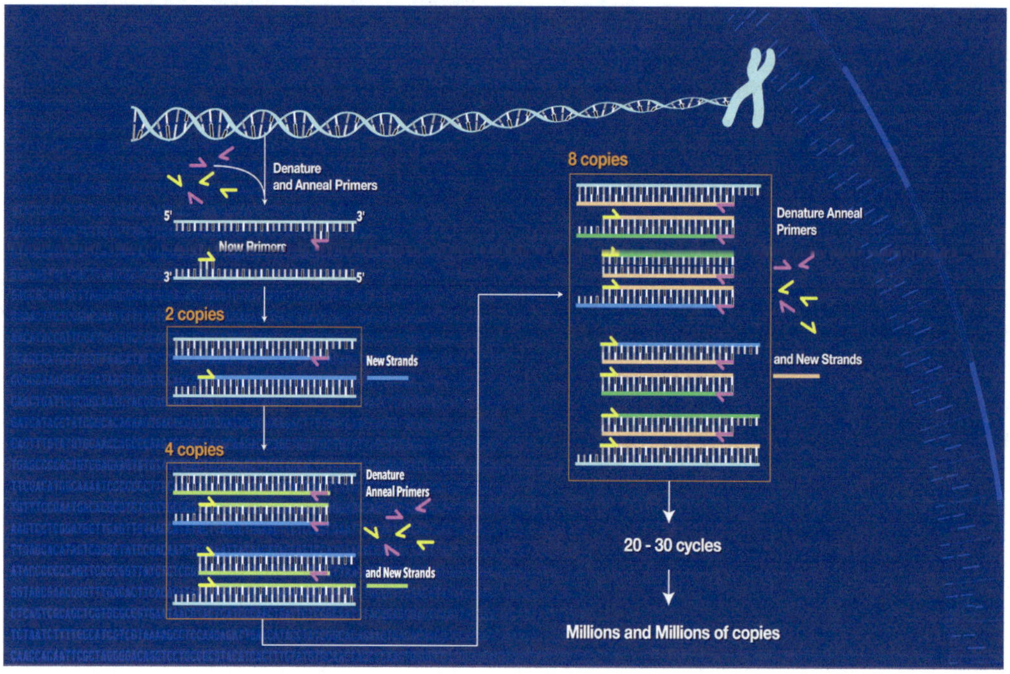

Figure 3.14. Polymerase chain reaction (PCR) – In vitro biotechnology.

Source: https://www.genome.gov/sites/default/files/inline-images/PCR_Fact-sheet2020.jpg.

3.5.1. Potential for Contamination and False Positives

The Polymerase Chain Reaction (PCR) is best known for its unmatched sensitivity in detecting nucleic acids, which also allows for real risks of contamination and false positives. Because it can amplify minute traces of DNA, even trace amounts of contaminants—of reagents, hardware, or surroundings—can trigger false positives. This is particularly risky in clinical situations where accurate detection of pathogens is crucial. For instance, Duane et al. (2025) highlight that the traditional methods struggle to distinguish between non-viable and viable pathogens, thus making it challenging to interpret the result of the PCR. The possibility of misleading results through contamination helps reinforce the necessity of strict procedural controls in PCR applications, particularly when examining environmental samples or clinical specimens within health care facilities. Another crucial consideration is the specific technical challenge of susceptibility to contamination. False positives can result through a variety of different pathways, including aerosol contamination during sample handling or cross-contamination from other amplified products. These are exacerbated when endpoint detection is employed, in which the presence of a non-target product can have a significant impact on results. Developments in recent years have sought to circumvent these issues, such as with more advanced methods of reaction setup and template preparation. In the case in question, Lin et al. (2021) illustrate a novel CRISPR/Cas9 eraser method that targets and annihilates contamination in PCR processes, ultimately bringing into focus the need to devise new methods for enhancing the specificity and reliability of PCR results. Additionally, the development of best practices regarding how to limit contamination is essential in ensuring integrity in PCR analysis. Using rigorous laboratory protocol, such as maintaining dedicated equipment for PCR preparations and installation of physical barriers that prevent airborne contamination, can reduce the likelihood of false positives by a wide margin. Having these practices consistently demonstrated to laboratory personnel is equally critical because human error is typically a risk of contamination. Also, the addition of emerging technologies like CRISPR/Cas9, as suggested by Lin et al. (2021), is a possible thrilling future direction for PCR technology advancement, ultimately boosting detection fidelity and producing more reliable results in clinical and research contexts. Continued reliance on PCR implies that combating contamination and reducing false positives are still among the most crucial considerations for further improving this essential diagnostic tool.

3.5.2. Limitations in Detecting Low-Abundance Targets

Low-abundance target detection remains a problem area in the application of polymerase chain reaction (PCR) methods, particularly concerning the successful quantification. Traditional PCR protocols are often hampered by sensitivity since they are unable to detect low-copy-number sequences accurately. This imbalance can have serious consequences in oncology, where it is critical to detect circulating tumor DNA to make an early diagnosis and target treatment. Moreover, conventional PCR effectively amplifies the target sequences without adequately compensating for the presence of background noise, which obscures low-abundance signals. In this way, this highlights the need for novel methodologies that will enhance detection capability and provide increased specificity to detect low-abundance nucleic acids in complex biological samples, being an essential factor towards the quest for improving molecular diagnostics. The advent of digital PCR (dPCR) aimed to alleviate some of these limitations that accompany traditional PCR approaches. While dPCR allows absolute quantification and improved sensitivity, it is not entirely problem-free, particularly in low-abundance target detection. For example, the precision of dPCR quantitation can still be compromised by such factors as the sample matrix and inhibitors. While its capacity to split samples into numerous compartments, hence theoretically raising the chance of encountering rare sequences, would in theory increase the sensitivity, its own sensitivity in practice can be significantly different depending on assay conditions and make-up. Recent improvements, such as those presented by Xu et al. (2021), have brought into question protocol differences of dPCR that could enhance sensitivity, but reproducible detection of low-frequency alleles remains a very significant challenge to address. With these issues in mind, new technologies , such as real-time digital PCR have been suggested as solutions to the limitations of the conventional detection systems. With their ability to use cycle-based amplification plots, these new systems increase sensitivity while decreasing false negatives that are particularly problematic when using liquid biopsies and low-abundance targets. The finding that a lowered threshold for baseline detection can significantly enhance the detection of mutations is particularly encouraging, as hypothesized by Xu et al. (2021). Such detection refinement not only holds promise of enhanced diagnostic precision but also underscores the persistent need for innovation in PCR protocols. As the field of molecular diagnostics continues to change, it is certain that addressing these limitations will be instrumental in achieving the fullest potential of PCR in clinical applications, ultimately impacting patient outcome in cases like cancer treatment (Figure 3.15).

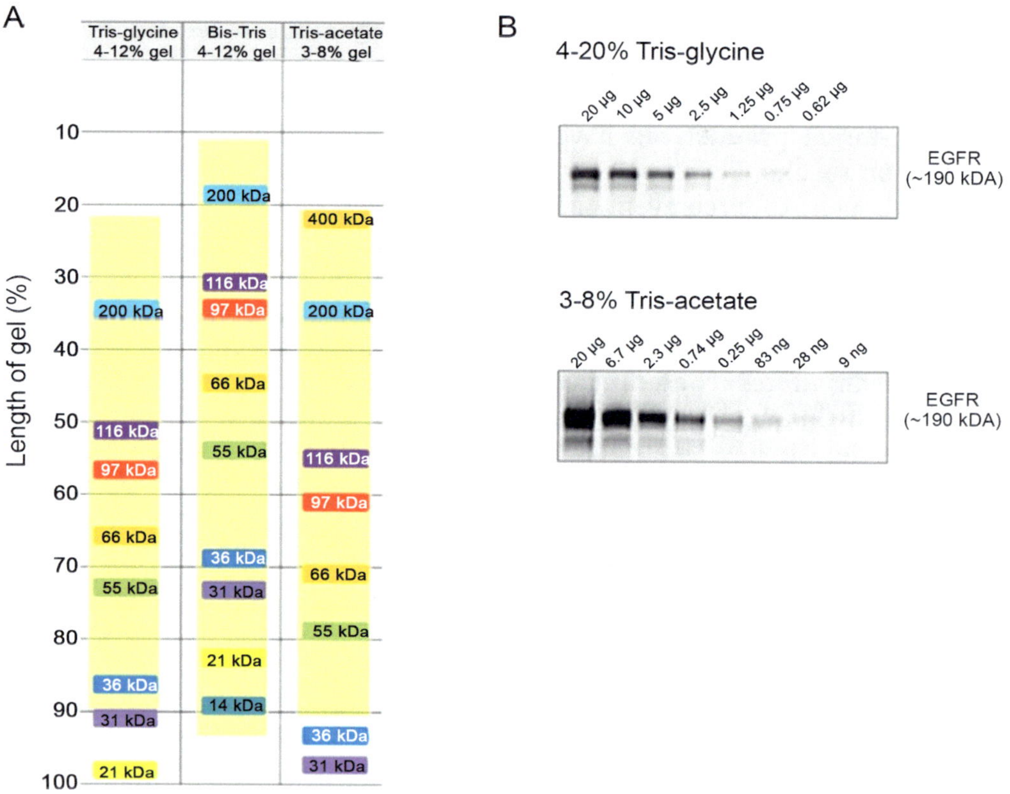

Figure 3.15. Low-abundance targets in polymerase chain reaction (PCR).

Source: https://www.thermofisher.com/kr/ko/home/life-science/protein-biology/protein-biology-learning-center/protein-biology-resource-library/pierce-protein-methods/detecting-low-abundance-proteins-in-western-blotting/jcr:content/MainParsys/image_17d5/foregroundimg.img.620.high.jpg/1637589050597.jpg.

3.5.3. Challenges in Quantification and Interpretation of Results

Quantification and interpretation of results using polymerase chain reaction (PCR) methods are increasingly being viewed as the key bottlenecks in genetic analysis. The primary source is that analytical thresholds (AT) are used to determine true signals from noise, particularly when testing samples of low-template DNA (LT-DNA). Research indicates that ATs that are currently in use lack efficiency in differentiating signal from noise, making it challenging to interpret PCR results. For example, the LT-DNA sample noise distribution would often display behavior that defies typical models, and this implies that threshold calibration should be adjusted to compensate for differential baseline noise due to various DNA template masses and injection times (Wellner, 2016). This ubiquitous uncertainty calls for a rethinking of prevailing practices to enable proper interpretation, thus reinforcing the need to be aware of the intricacies involved in PCR result readings. Furthermore, the complexities of electron capillary electrophoresis (CE) as used in PCR create additional realms of challenge regarding quantification of outcomes. Variability in sample preparation can lead to differences in baseline noise between different electropherograms. From research evidence, comparative capillary lot, amplification batch, and injection time conditions incorporate significant variations in distributions of noise and therefore compromise the reliability of detected peaks. The shift in noise distribution by variation in kit lots and resultant peak height discrepancies can hide intrinsic results, necessitating fine-tuning in the optimization of PCR protocols. Accurate probabilistic approaches for profile interpretation are based on a complete understanding of the underlying noise dynamics so that misinterpretation would not be followed by wrong conclusions regarding the presence or absence of genetic variants (Wellner, 2016). In recent years, the topic of rapid diagnostic testing has similarly endured the same quantification and interpretation problems, particularly with the additional funding for the development of sophisticated diagnostic technology. Automated real-time PCR platforms promise greater efficiency but likely overlook the fine details of noise handling and quantification challenges that exist in more conventional methods. The issue is not only in the automation of the process but also in ensuring that such machines can accurately differentiate between genuine signs of pathogenicity and artifacts generated by background noise. Furthermore, as biosensor-based immunoassay technologies evolve, the requirement for strong data interpretation frameworks becomes increasingly stringent. Without a critical focus on these interpretative challenges, there is the risk that speeded-up diagnostic methods will yield untrustworthy results, ultimately influencing the effectiveness of medical interventions.

3.6. Recent Advances in PCR Technology

Improvements in the polymerase chain reaction (PCR) technology of the past several years have significantly widened its application in many fields, particularly in genetics and molecular diagnostics. One notable development is the invention of multiplex PCR protocols, which allow for the amplification of several DNA targets within a single reaction. This innovation improves efficiency and reduces cost, particularly in hospitals where numerous genetic variants need to be screened. For instance, a cystic fibrosis-specific multiplex PCR assay panel has been found to perform superbly, with 92% coverage of disease-causing CFTR mutations in ethnically diverse U.S. populations. Such versatility not only enhances carrier detection rates but also addresses the previous gaps in ancestry-specific testing, indicative of PCR's larger ability to endure global genetic diversity (Hall et al., 2024). Another significant development in PCR technology is its integration with liquid biopsy approaches. Liquid biopsy, which includes circulating tumor DNA and other biomarkers isolated from body fluids, is a noninvasive approach to cancer diagnosis and monitoring. The development of PCR-based technologies, in combination with improvements in next-generation sequencing technologies, has enabled simpler processing of these biomarkers' analysis in a timely and precise fashion for molecular tumor profiling. New technologies , such as droplet-based microfluidics, support traditional PCR methods to facilitate high-throughput and sensitive single-cell and exosome detection, with capacities of addressing cell heterogeneity challenges as well as sample preparation-related challenges. This union of PCR technology and liquid biopsy is reflective of a paradigm shift towards precision medicine in which treatment plans are tailored based on solid genetic data (Shi et al., 2024). The constant evolution of PCR technology includes advancements in automation and digital PCR systems, delivering unparalleled accuracy and reproducibility. Digital PCR quantifies target DNA molecules with high precision, enabling scientists to detect low-frequency variants and enhance the sensitivity of genetic analysis. Automation of PCR protocols has also enhanced laboratory processes, reduced human errors and maximized throughput. These advances are particularly important in the field of forensic science, where precise DNA quantification and identification are of paramount concern. With the increasing utility and sophistication of PCR technology, the necessity for ongoing research and development to meet the evolving demands of genetic diagnostics and beyond becomes paramount. The convergence of these technologies positions PCR at the forefront of contemporary molecular biology, painting the crucial position that PCR occupies in the evolution of healthcare and medical science (Hall et al., 2024; Shi et al., 2024) (Figure 3.16).

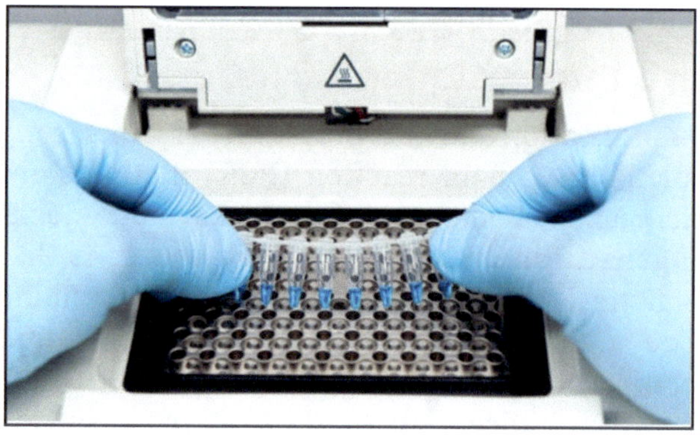

Figure 3.16. PCR technology research diagnostics.

Source: https://www.xlbiotec.com/wp-content/uploads/2023/08/1692691642577.jpg.

3.6.1. Development of High-Fidelity Polymerases

The development of high-fidelity polymerases has seen significant advances in the Polymerase Chain Reaction (PCR) and its applications. Traditional DNA polymerases possessed some serious shortfalls in terms of fidelity, which caused them to introduce erroneous nucleotides in DNA amplification reactions. These errors had the potential to significantly affect downstream applications, particularly in sensitive contexts , such as medical diagnostics and research. The evolution of high-fidelity (HiFi) polymerases, which are engineered with increased proofreading capacity, is an important breakthrough. With a 50- to 250-fold greater fidelity than wild-type polymerases, HiFi variants minimize misincorporation, thereby optimizing the accuracy of PCR assays. Such increased precision is paramount when detecting low-abundance targets that may be pivotal in early cancer diagnosis or the detection of drug-resistance mutations. In addition, the introduction of HiFi polymerases into PCR technologies becomes increasingly relevant to the detection of rare DNA-sequence variants. As highlighted in recent studies, conventional quantitative polymerase chain reaction (qPCR)-

based variant detection methods are often limited by sensitivity shortfalls caused by misincorporation rates of commercial DNA polymerases. This shortfall diminishes diagnostic value where early and precise detection is most important for patient health. Hence, the employment of HiFi polymerases addresses this issue by improving the overall limit of detection (LoD). With the advent of novel constructions , such as the occlusion system, which includes altered primers and target probes, multiplexing capability is enhanced in HiFi qPCR, encouraging more reliable identification of genetic variants at the same time boosting detection sensitivity as indicated in recent studies (Zhang et al., 2022). The implications of high-fidelity polymerases extend to real-world uses that find a profound impact in many areas, including clinical diagnosis and genetic analysis. The stability of HiFi polymerases stabilizes the PCR reaction by retaining the integrity of genetic material under repeated cycles of amplification. This stabilization comes in handy while analyzing samples that could contain trace amounts of nucleic acids, such as in certain instances of onychomycosis, where PCR has documented improved rates of detection compared to traditional culture methods (Aditya et al., 2023). The promise of high-fidelity polymerases thus goes beyond mere error minimization, opening a new frontier for genomic research in which accurate detection of mutations is able to catalyze breakthroughs in personalized medicine and targeted therapy protocols. Improved precision by HiFi polymerases is a basis change that leads to more precise diagnoses and new therapeutic interventions.

3.6.2. Innovations in PCR Instrumentation

The rapid expansion of PCR technology has significantly transformed the practice of molecular diagnostics. One of these is real-time PCR, or quantitative PCR (qPCR), which allows for amplification and measurement of DNA simultaneously. The technique has been proven to be instrumental in most applications, such as the identification of agents of disease, such as SARS-CoV-2, where proper diagnosis at the earliest possible opportunity is necessary in managing patients and public health interventions. Even more sophisticated thermal cycling equipment has also enhanced reaction speed and trustworthiness, enabling laboratories to test large numbers of samples in minutes as opposed to the hours previously required. Integration of microfluidics with PCR has facilitated high-throughput, miniaturized usage, reducing the consumption of reagents and cost considerably while increasing scalability in clinical settings, hence paving the way for broad utilization of QPCR techniques in many real-time diagnosis applications amidst dynamic health issues, e.g., the COVID-19 pandemic (Dutta et al., 2022). Besides, advancements in PCR instrumentation have enabled digital PCR (dPCR) to be a more sophisticated method that provides absolute nucleic acid quantification with unwavering sensitivity and precision. The technology divides the PCR reaction into small partitions so that single amplification events can be quantified, thus eradicating imprecision characteristic of traditional methods. dPCR sensitivity is of vital value in cancer studies, where low-abundance mutations may play a role in treatment. Their application in ovarian cancer, for instance, highlights the value of dPCR in identifying novel biomarkers that complement clinical assessments and improve patient management (Xiao et al., 2022). Progress in dPCR is not only to the benefit of various fields of research but also advances the potential for delivering personalized medicine through ensuring targeted therapies are informed by accurate genetic profiles. Further, PCR instrumentation development is facilitated by the use of artificial intelligence (AI) and machine learning in PCR workflows. Algorithms with the ability to analyze complex data sets allow the assessment of results at unprecedented speed and accuracy, facilitating the translation of results into useful information with greater efficiency. Cloud-based platform advancements provide remote access to PCR data, facilitating collaborative opportunities among clinicians and researchers globally. Such advancements promise to bring the entire process of PCR-based diagnosis, from sampling through to result sharing, together under one roof, and hence enhance disease surveillance and outbreak response. Such fusion of innovation represents a gigantic leap forward for PCR application, and indeed for the broad discipline of molecular biology and infectious disease control, and is a testament to the staggering potential of PCR instrumentation innovation for reshaping the health sciences (Figure 3.17).

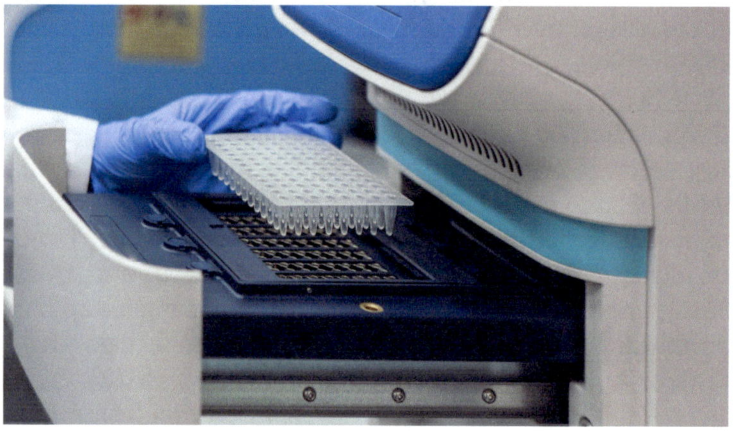

Figure 3.17. PCR instrumentation.

Source: https://www.igenels.com/wp-content/uploads/2022/03/pcr-machine_igene-labserve.jpeg.

3.6.3. Emerging Techniques Such as Digital PCR

The advances in molecular biology have inspired various new approaches that enhance the roles of the standard polymerase chain reaction (PCR). One of the most important developments is digital PCR (dPCR), which revolutionizes the quantification and detection of nucleic acids. While standard PCR provides quantitative data based on threshold cycles, dPCR offers absolute quantification by partitioning the sample into thousands of single reactions. This method reduces the amplification bias and error effects to a minimum, enabling researchers to detect rare variants in heterogeneous samples with unprecedented precision. Consequently, dPCR is of greatest use in oncology and infectious disease diagnosis, where it is imperative to identify low-frequency mutations or pathogens with precision. Thus, dPCR is a significant development in PCR technology that provides a more sensitive and trustworthy research and clinical diagnostic instrument. Later developments in PCR technology are focused on making procedures easier to enhance sensitivity and specificity for nucleic acid detection. Technologies , such as multiplex PCR are now widely accepted, allowing multiple targets to be amplified within a single reaction. But new technologies are pushing the boundaries even further, employing microfluidics and automated platforms to minimize human handling. By employing high-throughput analysis, these platforms decrease the time needed for results while maximizing reproducibility. Adding artificial intelligence and machine learning algorithms to interpret complex data sets can potentially unlock even greater insights from PCR data, allowing the identification of variants that are typically not detected. Cumulatively, the technologies are constructing the future of applications for PCR, from simple amplification to sophisticated analytical processes that can address complex biomedical questions. Emerging developments also emphasize the utility of dPCR in tackling important public health concerns, such as antibiotic resistance and invasive fungal infections. By detecting genetic variants involved in mechanisms of resistance with speed, dPCR facilitates clinicians in providing more targeted antibiotic therapies. Furthermore, with the advancements of fungal diagnostics, the marriage of dPCR and other molecular techniques and biosensors can enhance the sensitivity and efficacy of the detection of pathogens, ultimately leading to better patient outcomes. Moreover, novel applications for dPCR are gaining strength in a number of avenues, including personalized medicine and epidemiological surveillance, thereby affirming its status as a valuable resource in the arsenal of diagnostics. With continued research, it is without a doubt that the progress towards increasingly precise and sophisticated techniques, such as digital PCR, is crucial in addressing current health concerns and forms the basis of future innovation for the sector of PCR and its variants.

SUMMARY

In short, the Polymerase Chain Reaction (PCR) emerged as an essential molecular biology technique that has achieved unprecedented precision in copying any DNA sequence. Its use crosses various disciplines, particularly clinical diagnosis, gene studies, and forensic examination. The ability of PCR to amplify tens of millions of copies of DNA from minute samples makes it possible to detect genetic variations, which are vital in disease mechanism understanding and the provision of personalized care. As evidenced in genetic disease research—, such as studies of interleukin-1 receptor antagonist gene mutations in aphthous stomatitis and beta-globin mutations in sickle cell patients, PCR has proved useful for examining the genetics of illness and wellness. The advances underscore its significance not only as a lab technique but also as an inspiration to innovation in clinical research and therapeutic strategies. Moreover, the uses of PCR technology are not limited to amplification. The method can detect single-nucleotide polymorphisms (SNPs) and variants that are found to influence the susceptibility to disease and response to treatment. For instance, the findings concerning the IL-1Ra VNTR variant and its lack of association with recurrent aphthous stomatitis indicate the importance of genetic screening in assessing the risk for a disease. Even though no meaningful correlation was detected, this study serves as an indicator of the pivotal role of PCR in genomics and the relentless quest for the deciphering of intricate genetic architecture. Likewise, research on beta-globin variation among Palestinian refugees demonstrates how PCR facilitates the discovery of uncommon genetic variants that are responsible for different phenotypic expressions, which ultimately contribute to clinical interventions and sickle-cell disease management. The future prospects of PCR technology and its use are promising as we keep expanding and refining its functionality. Technologies , such as digital PCR and multiplex PCR are opening new avenues for improved and more efficient identification of genetic variants. The greater sensitivity and specificity offered by these next-generation PCR technologies will be instrumental in tackling complex health conditions with more studies on the genetic map of diseases. In the future, it is crucial to address the ethical considerations of genetic testing and the availability of these technologies among various populations. The ongoing development of PCR and its application in achieving personalized medicine continues to be a priority in genetics and health care, with the promise to revolutionize disease control and prevention on a worldwide scale.

The polymerase chain reaction (PCR) is a revolutionary technique that has transformed molecular biology and genetics. Through the ability to amplify a specific DNA sequence, PCR allows for the analysis of minute traces of genetic material for applications from diagnostics and forensic studies to research. Its significance stems from its ability to perform qualitative and quantitative analysis of DNA, thus being very essential in the diagnosis of genetic disorders, tracking infectious diseases, and deciphering genetic susceptibility. Furthermore, advances in techniques of PCR variants , such as quantitative PCR (qPCR) and reverse transcription PCR (RT-PCR), have also enhanced its utility, enabling more sophisticated studies of gene expression and RNA analysis. These advances not only make the genetic tests more sensitive and specific but also faster and more precise in speed and accuracy, thereby placing useful information about the genetic etiology of disease in the hands of scientists and clinicians. The application of PCR extends beyond amplification as its variants have found use in detecting cancer early and personalized medicine. For example, RT-PCR is of growing significance in oncogenic mutations detection in genes found to be breast cancer-related, such as

BRCA1 and BRCA2. The ability to analyze these specific genes can lead to early treatment and customized treatment options for high-risk patients. In a study of early-onset breast cancer among Iranian women, PCR was instrumental in identifying several sequence forms of the BRCA1 and BRCA2 genes, which underscored the significance of the method in genetic screening programs. Not only did the findings contribute to breast cancer genetics information in certain populations, but they also helped to reinforce the significance of establishing mutation databases for effective cancer screening. Thus, PCR variants are essential for filling the gap between genetic knowledge and beneficial healthcare use. Moreover, the significance of PCR and its variants is that they have broad application in a number of fields, including virology, microbiology, and environmental science. In virology, for instance, PCR has proven to be a useful tool for the rapid detection of viruses, such as those associated with outbreaks. The precise amplification of DNA or RNA viruses enables a quick public health response and disease control. PCR is applied in microbiology to detect microorganisms in clinical samples with high diagnostic specificity as compared to traditional culture methods. Environmental scientists apply PCR in monitoring microbial diversity and assessing the prevalence of genetically modified organisms within ecosystems to guide policy regulations and ecological studies. Thus, the value of PCR and its analogues is not so much in their technical complexity as in the potential to address key problems in a swide variety of scientific disciplines, underpinning their central place in modern biology and medicine.

A LOOK TO THE FUTURE

PUBLIC HEALTH EMERGENCIES:

Public health emergencies represent some of the most profound challenges facing societies in the modern era. At their core, these events reflect situations in which the health of populations is threatened in a way that overwhelms ordinary public health capacities and necessitates urgent, coordinated action. Whether arising from infectious disease outbreaks, natural disasters, chemical exposures, or other hazards, public health emergencies share a common feature: they demand rapid mobilization of resources and innovative responses to protect life, prevent disease transmission, and mitigate social disruption. Such crises can strain health systems, disrupt economies, and expose underlying vulnerabilities in preparedness and health equity.

A public health emergency is distinguished from routine health issues by its scale, speed, and potential for widespread impact. It may be defined operationally as an occurrence or imminent threat of illness or harm that poses significant risk to public welfare and exceeds the capacity of routine health infrastructures to manage effectively. These emergencies may emerge suddenly—for example, through a previously unknown infectious disease—or build gradually, as with slow-onset environmental health threats that accumulate over time. Notably, the International Health Regulations (IHR) 2005 provide a formal framework for declaring a Public Health Emergency of International Concern (PHEIC), emphasizing serious, unusual, or unexpected events that carry implications beyond national borders and may warrant coordinated international action.

Public health emergencies extend well beyond the realm of infectious diseases, encompassing natural disasters, technological accidents, and socio-environmental crises that jeopardize health and safety on a community or global scale. Their impacts are multifaceted, affecting not only morbidity and mortality but also access to health services, economic stability, and societal well-being. The COVID-19 pandemic, for instance, underscored how a novel virus can upend daily life worldwide, revealing both the strengths and limitations of global surveillance, preparedness, and response systems.

In response, public health systems have increasingly embraced a holistic approach to emergency preparedness and response, integrating surveillance, risk assessment, communication, and cross-sector partnerships to build resilience. International cooperation, strategic planning, and investment in robust health infrastructures are critical to mitigating the impacts of emergencies and safeguarding vulnerable populations.

Thus, the study of public health emergencies occupies a central place in contemporary public health scholarship and practice. It invites not only analysis of acute crisis responses but also reflection on ethical decision-making, equity, and sustainable readiness. In understanding and preparing for these emergent threats, public health professionals and policymakers contribute to the broader goal of protecting communities, reducing avoidable harm, and strengthening global health security for the future.

REFERENCES

1. Antonarakis, E. S., Lu, C., Wang, H., Luber, B., Nakazawa, M., Roeser, J. C., Chen, Y., et al. (2014). AR-V7 and resistance to enzalutamide and abiraterone in prostate cancer. *New England Journal of Medicine, 371*, 1028–1038. https://doi.org/10.1056/nejmoa1315815 (accessed on 17th July 2025).
2. Collins, C. H., Arnold, F. H., & Leadbetter, J. R. (2005). Directed evolution of Vibrio fischeri LuxR for increased sensitivity to a broad spectrum of acyl-homoserine lactones. *Molecular microbiology*, *55*(3), 712–723. https://doi.org/10.1111/j.1365-2958.2004.04437.x(accessed on 17th July 2025).
3. Hawkins, A. C., Arnold, F. H., Stuermer, R., Hauer, B., & Leadbetter, J. R. (2007). Directed evolution of Vibrio fischeri LuxR for improved response to butanoyl-homoserine lactone. *Applied and environmental microbiology*, *73*(18), 5775–5781. https://doi.org/10.1128/AEM.00060-07(accessed on 17th July 2025).
4. Bas, A., Radonic, A., Szabo, A., Zapata, A., Filby, A. L., Liss, B., Ramakers, C., et al. (2008). Housekeeping genes for quantitative expression studies in the three-spined stickleback *Gasterosteus aculeatus*. https://core.ac.uk/download/pdf/11444551.pdf (accessed on 17th July 2025).
5. Jozwiakowski, S. K., & Connolly, B. A. (2009). Plasmid-based lacZalpha assay for DNA polymerase fidelity: application to archaeal family-B DNA polymerase. *Nucleic acids research*, *37*(15), e102. https://doi.org/10.1093/nar/gkp494(accessed on 17th July 2025).
6. Bolger, A., Lohse, M., & Usadel, B. (2014). Trimmomatic: A flexible trimmer for Illumina sequence data. *Bioinformatics, 30*, 2114–2120. https://doi.org/10.1093/bioinformatics/btu170 (accessed on 17th July 2025).
7. Brown, L., Rautemaa-Richardson, R., Mengoli, C., Alanio, A., Barnes, R., Bretagne, S., Chen, S. C. A., et al. (2024). Polymerase chain reaction on respiratory tract specimens of immunocompromised patients to diagnose pneumocystis pneumonia: A systematic review and meta-analysis. *Clinical Infectious Diseases: An Official Publication of the Infectious Diseases Society of America, 79*, 161–168. https://www.semanticscholar.org/paper/3ab9b8f319befeeb785eb74fb250817db3a05dcf (accessed on 17th July 2025).
8. Colac, S., Burduniuc, O., & Apostol, M. (2024). Genetic significance and tracking of circulating SARS-CoV-2 variants in the Republic of Moldova. *Romanian Archives of Microbiology and Immunology*. https://www.semanticscholar.org/paper/662aecf20222182e9016b65eac24e039a2f1f826 (accessed on 17th July 2025).
9. Currie, R., De Gussem, M., De Herdt, P., et al. (2016). Infectious bronchitis virus infections of chickens in Belgium: An epidemiological survey. https://core.ac.uk/download/84043316.pdf (accessed on 17th July 2025).
10. Yassaee, V. R., Zeinali, S., Harirchi, I., Jarvandi, S., Mohagheghi, M. A., Hornby, D. P., & Dalton, A. (2002). Novel mutations in the BRCA1 and BRCA2 genes in Iranian women with early-onset breast cancer. *Breast cancer research : BCR*, *4*(4), R6. https://doi.org/10.1186/bcr443(accessed on 17th July 2025).
11. Davies, N. G., Abbott, S., Barnard, R. C., Jarvis, C. I., Kucharski, A. J., Munday, J. D., Pearson, C. A. B., et al. (2021). Estimated transmissibility and impact of SARS-CoV-2 lineage B.1.1.7 in

England. *Science, 372.* https://doi.org/10.1126/science.abg3055 (accessed on 17th July 2025).

12. Choi ES, Min K, Kim GJ, Kwon I, Kim YH. Expression and characterization of Pantoea CO dehydrogenase to utilize CO-containing industrial waste gas for expanding the versatility of CO dehydrogenase. *Sci Rep.* 2017;7:44323. Published 2017 Mar 14. doi:10.1038/srep44323(accessed on 17th July 2025).
13. Ding, X., Yin, K., Li, Z., Lalla, R. V., Ballesteros, E., Sfeir, M., Liu, C., et al. (2020). Ultrasensitive and visual detection of SARS-CoV-2 using all-in-one dual CRISPR-Cas12a assay. *Nature Communications, 11.* https://doi.org/10.1038/s41467-020-18575-6 (accessed on 17th July 2025).
14. Dongre, S. B., Pugazhendy, K., Pandit, R. N., Sukaiya, G., & Vamanrao, K. (2023). Unlocking the secrets of DNA - A study of biochemical techniques in genetic research. https://core.ac.uk/download/603896960.pdf (accessed on 17th July 2025).
15. Duane, E., Sharma, A., Oldenburg, E., Barrett, A., Fils-aime, G., Graves, A. M., Anderson, D. J., et al. (2025). P-252. Culture-based viability PCR: Strategies to harness its sensitivity and minimize false positives. *Open Forum Infectious Diseases, 12.* https://www.semanticscholar.org/paper/53bc0a9b07d443cc3020437b81bc87ebe8d252ea (accessed on 17th July 2025).
16. Dutta, D., Naiyer, S., Mansuri, S., Soni, N., Singh, V., Bhat, K. H., Singh, N., et al. (2022). COVID-19 diagnosis: A comprehensive review of the RT-qPCR method for detection of SARS-CoV-2. *Diagnostics, 12*, 1503–1503. https://doi.org/10.3390/diagnostics12061503 (accessed on 17th July 2025).
17. El-Tholoth, M., & Bau, H. (2024). Molecular detection of respiratory tract viruses in chickens at the point of need by loop-mediated isothermal amplification (LAMP). *Viruses, 16.* https://www.semanticscholar.org/paper/2db489c54dc74f66536dfb48af8d64b4ce33d0ad (accessed on 17th July 2025).
18. Fallon, J., Narayan, S., Lin, J. L., Sassoon, J., & Llop, S. (2022). The impact of polymerase chain reaction (PCR) on diagnosis and management of infectious uveitis at a tertiary care facility. *Journal of Ophthalmic Inflammation and Infection, 12.* https://www.semanticscholar.org/paper/f555d90f617cb9c50d18a5ed1fdffdff02a57c1f (accessed on 17th July 2025).
19. Fang, W., Wu, J., Cheng, M., Zhu, X., Du, M., Chang, C., Liao, W., et al. (2023). Diagnosis of invasive fungal infections: Challenges and recent developments. *Journal of Biomedical Science, 30.* https://doi.org/10.1186/s12929-023-00926-2 (accessed on 17th July 2025).
20. Gupta, A. K., Cooper, E., Wang, T., Lincoln, S. A., & Bakotic, W. L. (2023). Single-point nail sampling to diagnose onychomycosis caused by non-dermatophyte molds: Utility of polymerase chain reaction (PCR) and histopathology. *Journal of Fungi, 9.* https://www.semanticscholar.org/paper/5042be9ee2abc71c0072a7dcebb762f6b7e85055 (accessed on 17th July 2025).
21. Nagel, G., Grunert, F., Kuijpers, T. W., Watt, S. M., Thompson, J., & Zimmermann, W. (1993). Genomic organization, splice variants and expression of CGM1, a CD66-related member of the carcinoembryonic antigen gene family. *European journal of biochemistry, 214*(1), 27–35. https://doi.org/10.1111/j.1432-1033.1993.tb17892.xpdf (accessed on 17th July 2025).
22. Hall, B., Milligan, J. N., Kelnar, K., Hallmark, E., Ashton, J. D., Parker, C. A., Filipovic-Sadic, S., et al. (2024). Multisite verification of a targeted CFTR polymerase chain reaction/capillary electrophoresis assay that evaluates pathogenic variants across diverse ethnic and ancestral groups. *Archives of Pathology & Laboratory Medicine.* https://www.semanticscholar.org/paper/475ee55e9a13bc8fb641824634b41ce07650ab68 (accessed on 17th July 2025).

23. Ho, H. Y., Chung, K. S. (Kasey), Kan, C., & Wong, S. (2024). Liquid biopsy in the clinical management of cancers. *International Journal of Molecular Sciences, 25*. https://www.semanticscholar.org/paper/acfea334b166eb9816095f76c54d5709a24ad5d6 (accessed on 17th July 2025).

24. Huang, M., Huang, J., Yu, L., & Lin, K. (2025). Enhancing thalassemia diagnosis: Advantages of third-generation sequencing. *Clinical Laboratory, 71*(1). https://www.semanticscholar.org/paper/6676e903547a4e59052d59cb3fd066de3eef9992 (accessed on 17th July 2025).

25. Ince, J., & McNally, A. (2009). Development of rapid, automated diagnostics for infectious disease: Advances and challenges. https://core.ac.uk/download/30633630.pdf (accessed on 17th July 2025).

26. Khanna, V., Chadaga, K., Sampathila, N., Prabhu, S., Chadaga, R., & Umakanth, S. (2022). Diagnosing COVID-19 using artificial intelligence: A comprehensive review. *Network Modeling Analysis in Health Informatics and Bioinformatics, 11*. https://www.semanticscholar.org/paper/8fce12e02bb974155f03c80fda53332ee6744183 (accessed on 17th July 2025).

27. Lang, J., Yang, J., & Xu, M. (2023). Editorial: Bioinformatics analysis tools for nanopore sequencing and applications. *Frontiers in Bioengineering and Biotechnology, 11*. https://www.semanticscholar.org/paper/d7bf1bb7f43f6e819c736ca865be72f723f3037e (accessed on 17th July 2025).

28. Li, H., Yang, Y., Hong, W., Huang, M., Wu, M., & Zhao, X. (2020). Applications of genome editing technology in the targeted therapy of human diseases: Mechanisms, advances, and prospects. *Signal Transduction and Targeted Therapy, 5*. https://doi.org/10.1038/s41392-019-0089-y (accessed on 17th July 2025).

29. Lin, W. J., Tian, T., Jiang, Y., Xiong, E., Zhu, D., & Zhou, X. (2021). A CRISPR/Cas9 eraser strategy for contamination-free PCR end-point detection. *Biotechnology and Bioengineering, 118*, 2053–2066. https://www.semanticscholar.org/paper/3b56f5063afb04883531893a3643948741e89b63 (accessed on 17th July 2025).

30. Mahboob, A., Fatma, N., & Husain, A. (2024). In-house extraction and purification of Pfu-Sso7d, a high-processivity DNA polymerase. *Bio-protocol, 14*. https://www.semanticscholar.org/paper/1a94d795fca86b439efaecc8ab9db138737d4539 (accessed on 17th July 2025).

31. Mao, Y., Xu, K., Miglietta, L., Kreitmann, L., Moser, N., Georgiou, P., Holmes, A. H., et al. (2023). Deep domain adaptation enhances amplification curve analysis for single-channel multiplexing in real-time PCR. *IEEE Journal of Biomedical and Health Informatics, 27*, 3093–3103. https://www.semanticscholar.org/paper/07c61a46c393aa34a55a1dde57375990b4b52d78 (accessed on 17th July 2025).

32. McDonald, C., Taylor, D., & Linacre, A. (2024). PCR in forensic science: A critical review. *Genes, 15*. https://www.semanticscholar.org/paper/d5b82d1acbbfe85ca6b5fc0e0793adbb79dda181 (accessed on 17th July 2025).

33. Moussa, E. Y., Yassine, N., & Borjac, J. M. (2018). New variants in beta-globin gene among the Palestinian refugees with sickle cell disease in Lebanon. *Saudi Medical Journal, 39*, 1253–1258. https://www.semanticscholar.org/paper/9906bc155563d6732b69033a232fd650e325ce43 (accessed on 17th July 2025).

34. Muteeb, G., Rehman, M. T., Shahwan, M., & Aatif, M. (2023). Origin of antibiotics and antibiotic resistance, and their impacts on drug development: A narrative review. *Pharmaceuticals, 16*,

1615–1615. https://doi.org/10.3390/ph16111615 (accessed on 17th July 2025).

35. Raju, T., Prakash, S., & M. L., L. P. (2025). Polymerase chain reaction: An efficient tool for genotypic studies. *World Journal of Biology, Pharmacy, and Health Sciences*. https://www.semanticscholar.org/paper/62221234931f631dfee958a6824334631c241ff6 (accessed on 17th July 2025).

36. Safa, M., Mou, M., Hridoy, M., Siddiqua, S., Bhuiyan, A., & Bhuiyan, M. (2024). Analysis of β-casein gene for A1 and A2 allelic variants in Holstein-local crossbred cattle of Bangladesh using allele-specific PCR. *Journal of Advanced Biotechnology and Experimental Therapeutics*. https://www.semanticscholar.org/paper/e6ed072ee8c94146b89a19cd4adf216b1b35e72a (accessed on 17th July 2025).

37. Wiita, A. P., & Schrijver, I. (2011). Clinical application of high throughput molecular screening techniques for pharmacogenomics. *Pharmacogenomics and personalized medicine, 4*, 109–121. https://doi.org/10.2147/PGPM.S15302 (accessed on 17th July 2025).

38. Shi, J., Zhang, Y., Fan, Y., Liu, Y., & Yang, M. (2024). Recent advances in droplet-based microfluidics in liquid biopsy for cancer diagnosis. *Droplet*. https://www.semanticscholar.org/paper/2071809a37d4fb532a1e6f7090bfdbbf1cf6dcc0 (accessed on 17th July 2025).

39. Srivastava, A., Santagostino, E., Dougall, A., Kitchen, S., Sutherland, M. L., Pipe, S. W., Carção, M., et al. (2020). WFH guidelines for the management of hemophilia, 3rd edition. *Hemophilia, 26*, 1–158. https://doi.org/10.1111/hae.14046 (accessed on 17th July 2025).

40. Takahashi, T., Aoyanagi, H., Pigolotti, S., & Toyabe, S. (2024). Blocking uncertain mispricing errors of PCR. *bioRxiv*. https://www.semanticscholar.org/paper/5a6eb03cd957ef76c9a000508adfe3de0172bf20 (accessed on 17th July 2025).

41. Tekcan, A., Yıgıt, S., Nursal, A., Tumer, M., Yerliyurt, K., & Kuruca, N. (2020). Analysis of interleukin-1 receptor antagonist variable number tandem repeat variant in recurrent aphthous stomatitis. *Endocrine, Metabolic & Immune Disorders Drug Targets*. https://www.semanticscholar.org/paper/098d4c6fc2ef2053b23eace2e298caa1de329129 (accessed on 17th July 2025).

42. Ullah, M. S., Davies, A., & Halestrap, A. P. (2006). The plasma membrane lactate transporter MCT4, but not MCT1, is up-regulated by hypoxia through a HIF-1α-dependent mechanism. *Journal of Biological Chemistry, 281*, 9030–9037. https://doi.org/10.1074/jbc.m511397200 (accessed on 17th July 2025).

43. Untergasser, A., Cutcutache, I., Kõressaar, T., Ye, J., Faircloth, B. C., Remm, M., & Rozen, S. (2012). Primer3—new capabilities and interfaces. *Nucleic Acids Research, 40*, e115–e115. https://doi.org/10.1093/nar/gks596 (accessed on 17th July 2025).

44. van Dongen, J. E., Moonen, E. J. M., Segerink, L. I., & den Toonder, J. M. J. (2024). CRISPR/Cas Enabled Sweat Analysis Paving the Way for Non-Invasive Point-Of-Care Detection of Pathogens by Analyzing Cas12a Trans-Cleavage Performance in Human Sweat. In 2024 IEEE BioSensors Conference, BioSensors 2024 IEEE. https://doi.org/10.1109/BioSensors61405.2024.10712662(accessed on 17th July 2025).

45. Wai, H. A., Lord, J., Lyon, M., Gunning, A. C., Kelly, H., Cibin, P., Seaby, E. G., et al. (2020). Blood RNA analysis can increase clinical diagnostic rate and resolve variants of uncertain significance. *Genetics in Medicine, 22*, 1005–1014. https://doi.org/10.1038/s41436-020-0766-9 (accessed on 17th July 2025).

46. Walsh, P. S., Metzger, D. A., & Higuchi, R. (2013). Chelex 100 as a medium for simple extraction of DNA for PCR-based typing from forensic material. *Biotechniques, 54*, 134–139. https://doi.org/10.2144/000114018 (accessed on 17th July 2025).

47. Wang, Z., Schmidt, F., Weisblum, Y., Muecksch, F., Barnes, C. O., Finkin, S., Schaefer-Babajew, D., et al. (2021). mRNA vaccine-elicited antibodies to SARS-CoV-2 and circulating variants. *Nature, 592*, 616–622. https://doi.org/10.1038/s41586-021-03324-6 (accessed on 17th July 2025).

48. Wei, C., Yu, C., Li, S., Meng, J., Li, T., Cheng, J., Pan, F., et al. (2022). Easy-to-operate co-flow step emulsification device for droplet digital polymerase chain reaction. *Analytical Chemistry*. https://www.semanticscholar.org/paper/16bdfe30c0a7508870191820cecc8998e99add96 (accessed on 17th July 2025).

49. Wellner, G. A. (2016). The examination of baseline noise and the impact on the interpretation of low-template DNA samples. https://open.bu.edu/bitstream/2144/14939/1/Wellner_bu_0017N_10536.pdf (accessed on 17th July 2025).

50. Xiao, Y., Bi, M., Guo, H., & Li, M. (2022). Multi-omics approaches for biomarker discovery in early ovarian cancer diagnosis. *EBioMedicine, 79*, 104001–104001. https://doi.org/10.1016/j.ebiom.2022.104001 (accessed on 17th July 2025).

51. Xu, J., Duong, K., Yang, Z., Kaji, K., Ou, J., Head, S., Crynen, G., et al. (2021). Real-time digital polymerase chain reaction (PCR) as a novel technology improves limit of detection for rare allele assays. *Translational Lung Cancer Research, 10*, 4336–4352. https://www.semanticscholar.org/paper/bc92971b2a69a9e26bc269807a567db8ac93fbdf (accessed on 17th July 2025).

52. Yuen, B. P. N., Wong, K. S., So, Y. M., Kwok, W. H., Cheung, H. W., Wan, T. S. M., Ho, E., et al. (2025). Multiplex PCR-liquid chromatography high-resolution tandem mass spectrometry for simultaneous detection of multiple transgenes in equine plasma. *Analytical Chemistry*. https://www.semanticscholar.org/paper/05657f9dd82686b2eec9103a14c81c5c59042a30 (accessed on 17th July 2025).

53. Zhang, K., Pinto, A., Cheng, L., Song, P., Dai, P., Wang, M., Rodriguez, L., et al. (2022). Hairpin structure facilitates multiplex high-fidelity DNA amplification in real-time polymerase chain reaction. *Analytical Chemistry*. https://www.semanticscholar.org/paper/1bad5f96e26fe9a2f120c3fda1dc5c1feb7cc81a (accessed on 17th July 2025).

54. Zhang, R., Calixto, C. P. G., Tzioutziou, N. A., James, A. B., Simpson, C. G., Guo, W., Márquez, Y., et al. (2015). AtRTD–a comprehensive reference transcript dataset resource for accurate quantification of transcript-specific expression in *Arabidopsis thaliana*. *New Phytologist, 208*, 96–101. https://doi.org/10.1111/nph.13545 (accessed on 17th July 2025).

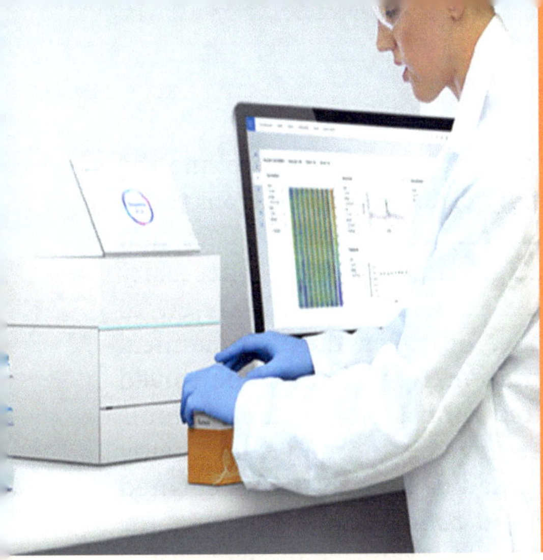

Chapter 4

NEXT-GENERATION SEQUENCING (NGS) TECHNOLOGIES

Contents

Introduction

The advent of next-generation sequencing (NGS) technologies is a paradigm shift in genomics, revolutionizing the analysis and interpretation of genetic data. Compared to the old, labor-intensive, scalable-limited sequencing methods, NGS allows for parallel sequencing of multiple DNA strands at a high-throughput rate that dramatically reduces costs and turnaround times. This technological advancement has established new avenues of research and clinical application, particularly in the elucidation of complex diseases. The integration of NGS into genomic studies enables the identification of genetic variation and mutation pertaining to various conditions, such as cancer, for an enhanced understanding of disease mechanisms and targeted therapy. The clinical applications of NGS are vast, particularly for cancer genomics. With the promise of sequencing entire genomes or hitting regions of interest, researchers are learning about the genetic alterations that drive tumorigenesis. The discovery of cancer genomics has revealed that numerous genes undergo mutation, copy number alteration, or structural rearrangement across different tumor subtypes, ultimately controlling the growth and progression of cancer. Notably, it has become increasingly clear that aside from those genes that are commonly mutated, there is also a "long tail" of less frequently altered genes that might also play crucial oncological functions. This multi-faceted insight emphasizes the necessity for ongoing integration of NGS into cancer diagnosis and personalized medicine, with a view to individualizing treatments based on genetic profiles (Elaine, 2014). However, the astronomical rise in data generated by NGS platforms creates large-scale computational problems to be solved to tap its potential. The sheer volume of genomic data necessitates robust bioinformatics tools that can handle and analyze this data efficiently. Several approaches have been brought into being to overcome the challenges like distributed parallel computing and dedicated hardware designed for genomic analysis. While such advances enable more scalability and computation efficiency for analyzing data, they generate challenges in algorithmic design, handling data, and distributing computational resources. Thus, the same balancing act marrying advances in computing with genomics biology is needed to facilitate the evolution of bioinformatics tools that are essential to the comprehensive assessment of large-scale genomics data (Shi & Wang, 2019) (Figure 4.1).

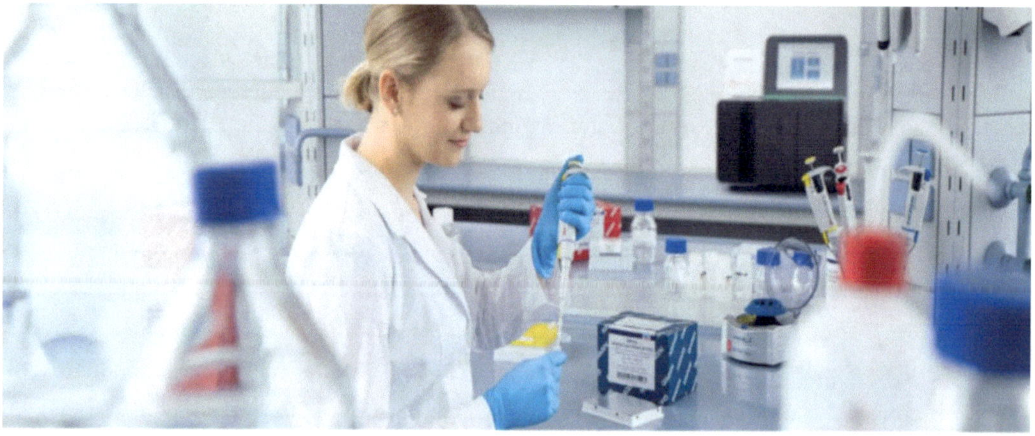

Figure 4.1. Next-generation sequencing (NGS).

Source: https://image.slidesharecdn.com/prom-10329ngstechnologyintroductionww2016-161114192446/75/Introduction-to-Next-Generation-Sequencing-NGS-Technology-1-2048.jpg.

Definition of Next-Generation Sequencing

Next-generation sequencing (NGS) is a revolutionary technology in genomic analysis that allows for the simultaneous sequencing of millions of DNA fragments. Traditional sequencing technologies, such as Sanger sequencing, are time-consuming and have low throughput. However, NGS involves massively parallel sequencing techniques, which allow for the acquisition of vast genomic information at high speed. This not only enhances the productivity of genomic studies but also reduces overall expenses significantly, making high-throughput sequencing accessible to a broader range of scientific studies. The ability to sequence whole genomes or specific areas at heretofore unimaginable speeds offers an understanding of genetic variations, particularly single-nucleotide polymorphisms (SNPs) and haplotypes, which are required to understand disparate biological phenomena and disease mechanisms. The key applications of high-throughput sequencing technologies are analyzed below.

The maturity of NGS technologies is underscored by their reliance on sophisticated statistical models to analyze data. As an example, the statistical aspects of fragment coverage in sequencing experiments are critical to ensure data completeness and accuracy. One advancement achieved in NGS is the addition of fragment length distributions, which possess a high potential to influence the coverage within a genome. As shown in extensions of the standard Lander-Waterman model, randomness of site initiation of fragments can offer new insights into coverage aberrations potentially lost by standard methods.

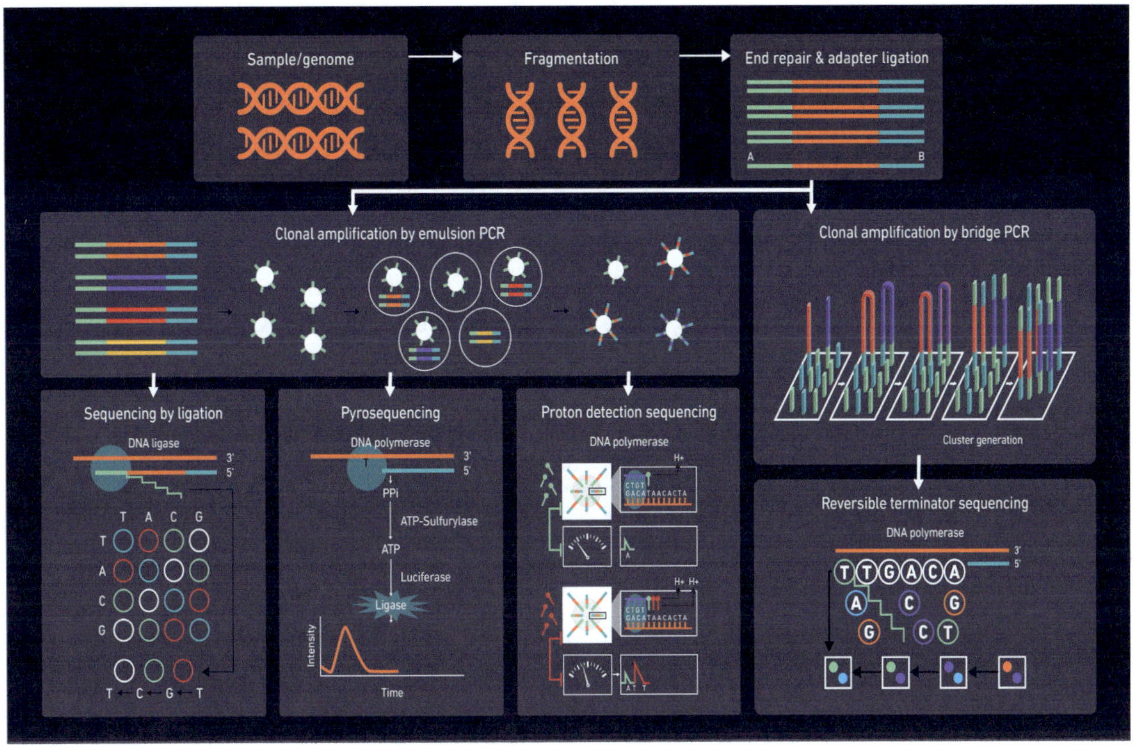

Figure 4.2. Next-generation sequencing (NGS): Definition.

Source: https://cdn.technologynetworks.com/tn/images/body/ngsseo31615391054366.png.

This information serves scientists in the form of detecting variation from typical coverage patterns, thus making genomic outcomes more credible and the integrity of resulting data procured through NGS methods more enhanced (Evans et al., 2010). The haplotype assembly procedure yet again illustrates the innovations and challenges of NGS. Haplotype, or a specific allele sequence on chromosomes, is invaluable information for disassembling the genotype-phenotype relationship complex. However, processes like Minimum Error Correction (MEC) haplotype reconstruction can lead to inconsistencies, particularly when utilizing error-prone long-read technologies. This variation affects reconstructed haplotype quality, as revealed by comparisons of various NGS platforms, including those from Illumina and Pacific BioSciences (Majidian et al., 2020). As continuous progress is made on improving the algorithms for haplotype assembly and error correction techniques, high coverage levels become a requirement. These technical challenges are being overcome and are not only advancing NGS technologies but also raising awareness about genetic architectures, paving the way for personalized medicine and targeted therapeutics (Figure 4.2).

Historical Context and Development

The background to next-generation sequencing (NGS) technologies is a tale of dizzying advances in genomics. Original sequencing was laboriously slow and relied heavily on Sanger sequencing, developed in the 1970s, a method accurate but notoriously slow and only able to process a small number of sequences. Human genome sequencing, completed in 2003, was a milestone that defined the need for greater efficiency. While researchers grappled with growing genomic complexity and volume of data, radical developments in sequencing technologies began to emerge. This technology not only facilitated the rapid formation of massive datasets but also allowed applications in many areas, from medicine and targeted treatment to monitoring public health, ushering in a new era in genetic diagnostics and research. The development of NGS technologies throughout the early 21st century has revolutionized the science of microbial genomics, particularly in public health applications. A systematic review of the literature on NGS cites instances where methods like whole-genome sequencing (WGS) have become a necessary tool in outbreak investigations to facilitate quick detection and tracing of pathogens. Source tracing and early outbreak detection have been enabled through the use of WGS, and epidemiologists have been provided with tools to decipher transmission dynamics and trace drug resistance patterns effectively. As emphasized in studies, integration of NGS with high-quality contextual data enhances its worth, evoking the significance of interdisciplinary collaboration in public health interventions. This development in microbial genomics is a shift towards breaking away from conventional methods and embracing a more holistic approach in disease control and surveillance (Van Goethem et al., 2019). In addition to its medical and public health uses, NGS technologies have enabled deeper biological understanding through comparative genomics and evolutionary biology. Deep homology, which was first explored through the study of conserved gene expression among diverse organisms, has become more powerful because of high-throughput sequencing strategies. This approach has revolutionized evolutionary developmental biology with the capacity for transcriptome-wide comparisons and not just using gene-by-gene studies. Hence, NGS facilitates maximum understanding of anatomical characters that do not have phylogenetic affiliations clearly defined, providing improved context to morphology evolution. The significance of such technological advancement not only establishes the capabilities of NGS technologies but also their role in broader scientific discussion, opening avenues for future research endeavors (Tschopp & Tabin, 2017) (Figure 4.3).

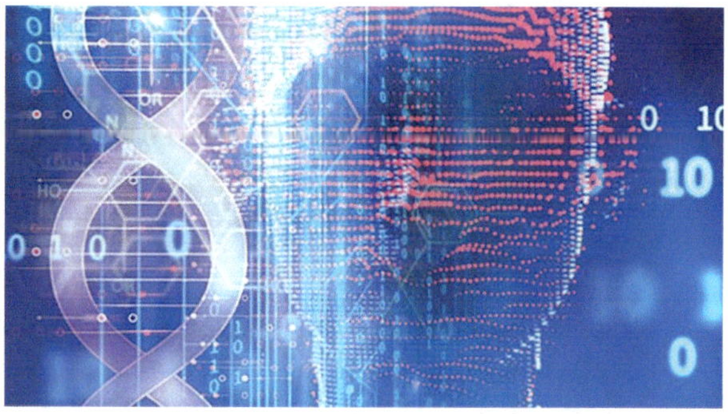

Figure 4.3. A brief history behind the next-generation sequencing.

Source: https://thrivearticles.weebly.com/uploads/1/4/0/0/140060710/next-generation-sequencing-market_orig.jpg.

Importance of NGS in Modern Genomics

The evolution of next-generation sequencing (NGS) technologies has revolutionized modern genomics, allowing rapid advances in our understanding of genetic diseases and the development of target-based therapeutics. NGS allows for the analysis of multiple genes or the entire genome simultaneously, significantly increasing the efficiency of genomic investigation and clinical diagnosis. By providing total comprehension of the genetic origins of disease, NGS enables scientists and doctors to tailor treatments to the individual patient, a notion inscribed in the yet-emerging discipline of precision medicine. With the rising frequency of utilization of NGS in the clinic, particularly with initiatives like the 100,000 Genome Project, it is increasingly obvious that this technology is the future of enhancing diagnostic accuracy and therapeutic outcome in cancer and more (Jones et al., 2018).

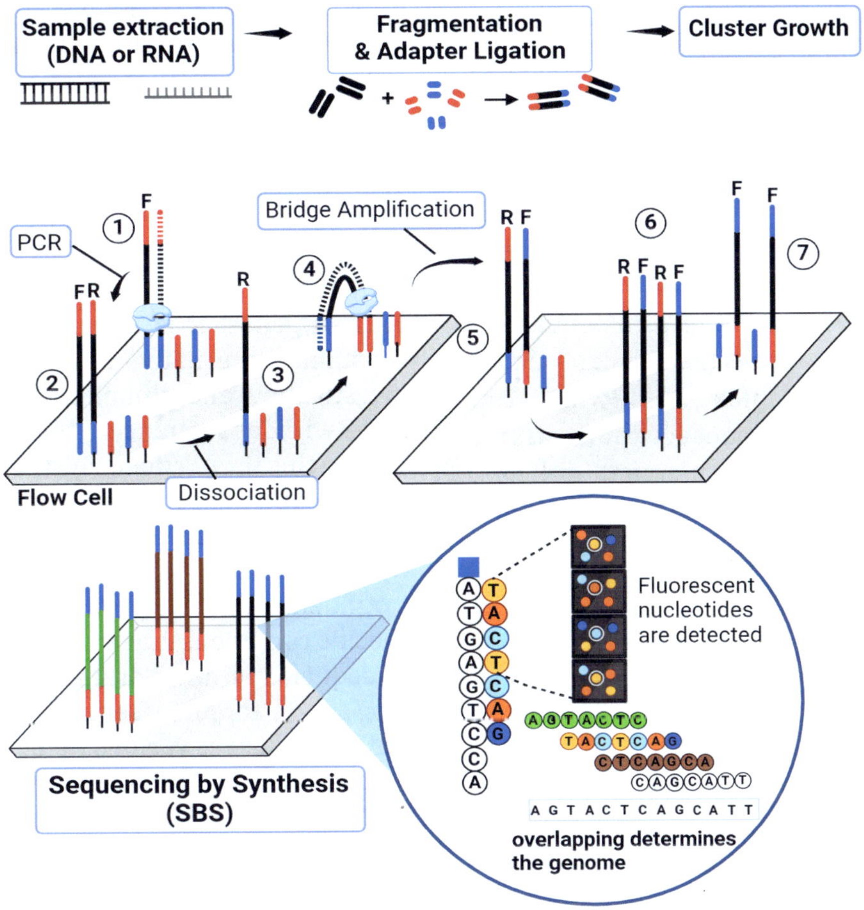

Figure 4.4. Next-generation sequencing (workflow).

Source: https://cdn.prod.website-files.com/621e95f9ac30687a56e4297e/6616e431969cb09a484ad825_V2_1710736280155_6bea9c2c-7e31-4b5c-8d1b-ef5863d5d6af_HIGH_RES.png.

In addition, NGS technologies play a pivotal role in bridging existing gaps among medical specialties, particularly pathology. The convergence of cellular pathology and molecular characterization is increasingly important in the management of cancer. New integrative pathology, fueled by NGS, ensures that morphological and genomic information are interpreted within a unified context, thus making the overall diagnostic process more valuable. This has led to an inclusion of NGS, which has urged upskilling within pathology training to fill knowledge deficits and enhance interdisciplinarity. This combined strategy not only preserves the relevance of classical cellular pathology but also favors morphomolecular pathology advances, which contribute significantly to patient management improvement (Jones et al., 2018). Besides patient management, NGS also has extensive impacts on evolutionary biology and species conservation. With high-quality reference genomes—for example, the recent release of EquCab3.0 for the horse—scientists can now more effectively investigate genetic diversity and ancestral lineages. The construction of whole-genome sequences (WGS) from different breeds and ancient horses demonstrates how NGS can facilitate groundbreaking studies on population genetics. Such data allows the breaking down of Mendelian and complex traits, which can be applied to inform conservation efforts and improve species management policies. In addition, the results obtained from equine genome research not only benefit horse health and performance but also serve as models for elucidation of complex diseases in various species, highlighting the central position of NGS in contemporary genomics (Figure 4.4).

4.1. Types of Next-Generation Sequencing Technologies

The next-generation sequencing (NGS) technology landscape is controlled by several technologies that are appropriate for different scientific and clinical applications. Whole-genome sequencing (WGS) stands out among them due to the capability it holds to provide an all-encompassing view of an organism's full genomic profile. Single-nucleotide polymorphisms (SNPs), structural variations, and copy number variations throughout the genome can be identified using this technique. In the clinical setting, WGS is key to the understanding of genetic diseases, tumor genomics assessment, and facilitation of personalized medicine. However, the sheer amount of data output, as well as the analytical complexity inherent in WGS, creates challenges in interpretation, and therefore robust bioinformatics tools and experts are key. In spite of this, the intensity of information that WGS provides makes it a cornerstone of research and clinical applications of NGS technologies. Another interesting NGS approach is targeted sequencing, where emphasis is put on specific genomic regions of interest, i.e., exomes or known disease-causing genes. It is a cost-effective and time-consuming alternative to WGS in that it enables investigators and clinicians to identify crucial areas without sequencing the genome. Targeted sequencing is particularly useful in inherited disease and cancer studies because it enables the thorough analysis of pertinent mutations without increasing the amount of data produced. Optimizing the choice of genes important in specific conditions maximizes both the efficiency of sequencing and variant detection accuracy. The use of targeted sequencing has expanded across numerous various fields, including in the fields of oncology and cardiology, as seen in the study of congenital heart defects, where the precise diagnosis of genetic variants is important for therapy advancement (Touma et al., 2017). Metagenomic next-generation sequencing (mNGS) has also been a groundbreaking technique to study microbial communities in a sample, expanding the scope of NGS beyond traditional genomic sequencing. mNGS allows for simultaneous detection of a wide variety of pathogens in complex samples, particularly valuable in clinical diagnosis of infectious diseases. Through the sequencing of microbial and host genomic and/or transcriptomic content, the technology offers insights into host-pathogen relationships, antimicrobial resistance, and the overall microbiome's role in disease and health. However, the adoption of mNGS into clinical practice is fraught with serious hurdles like bioinformatics complexity and barriers to interpretation. To maximize its contribution to patient care and population health, these challenges should be addressed as mNGS can revolutionize infectious disease diagnosis and treatment by more effective and streamlined methods (Chiu & Miller, 2019) (Figure 4.5).

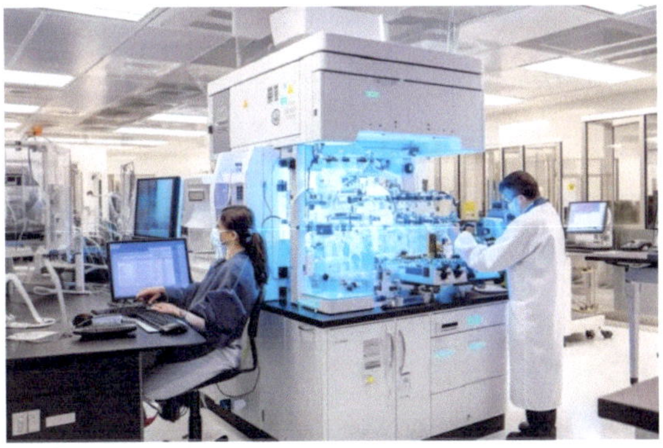

Figure 4.5. Next-generation sequencing technologies.

Source: https://genomic.news/wp-content/uploads/2023/07/Decoding-the-Genome-The-Rise-of-Next-Generation-Sequencing-Technologies-670x446.webp.

4.1.1. Illumina Sequencing

Illumina sequencing has revolutionized the landscape of next-generation sequencing (NGS) technology, making high-throughput genome analysis a possibility in many fields. Sequencing by synthesis is the method applied in this platform, where millions of fragments of DNA are read in parallel. Illumina sequencing reduces the cost of genomic data acquisition with increased throughput through the use of small flow-cell chip sizes. Consequently, researchers are now able to carry out extensive research with whole-genome sequencing, transcriptomics, and epigenomics and thereby derive insights that were previously unattainable. Notably, the versatility of Illumina technologies makes it possible for them to be applied in a wide variety of areas, ranging from clinical diagnosis to environmental studies, showing their potential in expediting biomedical and ecological understanding. Illumina sequencing is also pivotal to clinical metagenomic applications, namely, infectious disease diagnosis. This groundbreaking technology allows complete examination of host and microbiome genetic material from patient samples, thereby making it possible for the quick identification of pathogens. Such capabilities are especially crucial in resolving antimicrobial resistance problems and improving patient care outcomes. The range of applications is reflective of Illumina's integration within clinical laboratories, where it assists in the identification of infectious agents and informs therapeutic protocols. With the incorporation of massive datasets now becoming standard in clinical settings, the forthcoming medical interventions hold a serious implication of supplying physicians with more timely and precise information to guide patient care, as outlined in the findings of Chiu & Miller (2019). Apart from clinical use, Illumina sequencing has significant contributions in ecological science, particularly in aquatic biodiversity studies. Through the help of NGS, researchers can investigate the molecular past of water animals, thus addressing key environmental conservation issues. The large amount of genomic data generated requires sophisticated bioinformatics tools for assessing and interpreting the results in a useful manner. This interaction of sequencing technologies and bioinformatic strategies is at the heart of unlocking the evolutionary histories of the varied species, informing conservation and policy in the conservation of endangered ecosystems. What is revolutionary about Illumina and bioinformatics is their ability to mediate the urgent need to preserve species amid the accelerated pace of environmental change, as documented in the academic literature by Tan et al. (2019) (Figure 4.6).

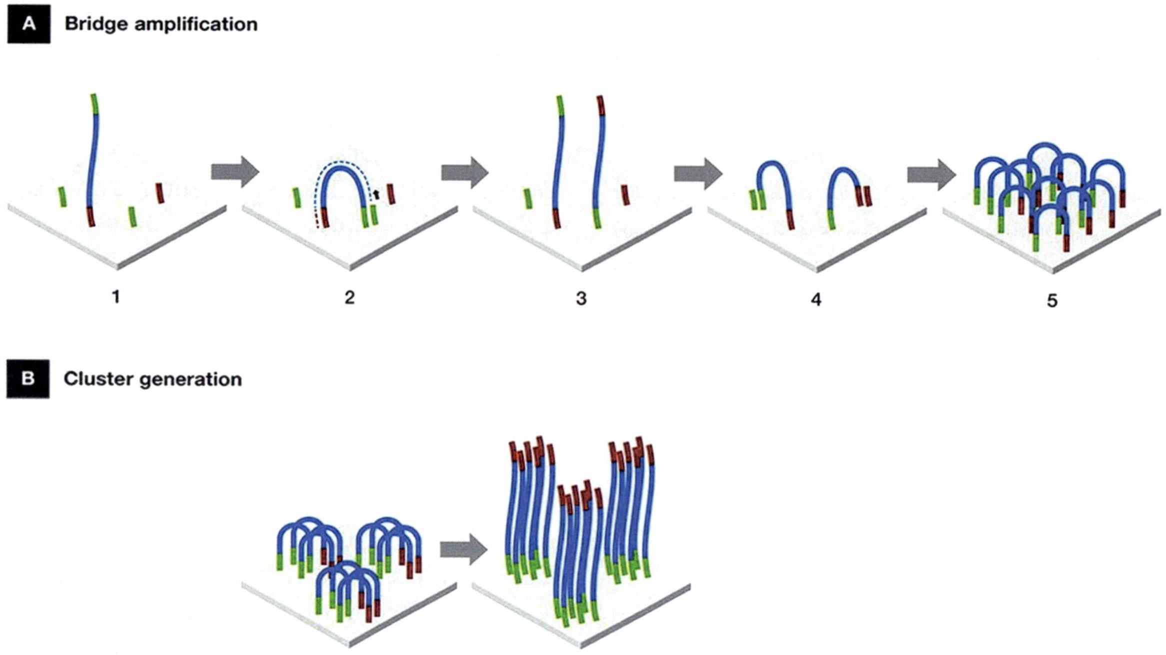

Figure 4.6. Next-generation sequencing Illumina workflow – four key steps.

Source: https://www.thermofisher.com/us/en/home/life-science/cloning/cloning-learning-center/invitrogen-school-of-molecular-biology/next-generation-sequencing/illumina-workflow/jcr:content/MainParsys/textimage_1d51/image.img.480.high.jpg/1626791434214.jpg.

4.1.2. Ion Torrent Sequencing

Among the next-generation sequencing technologies, Ion Torrent sequencing is a strong contender because it relies on a different method of reading DNA sequences. As opposed to the traditional methods that involve optical detection of fluorescence signals, this technology employs a semiconductor platform that reads the pH changes as nucleotides are incorporated during the process of sequencing. The Ion Torrent technology has some advantages, including quick turnaround times and lower cost per base sequenced, which have driven its expanding application in clinics and research labs. The ability of the technology to perform targeted sequencing with speed makes it particularly well-suited for applications , such as cancer genomics, where mutation detection is crucial for personalized therapeutic strategies. The application of Ion Torrent sequencing is not only limited to basic genomic studies but also has immense applications in the field of microbial ecology studies. For instance, on the 2013 Southern Line Islands Research Expedition, researchers efficiently used the Ion Torrent PGM platform to sequence 26 real-time marine microbial genomes. This pioneering effort combined field research with genomic sequencing, enabling scientists to explore microbial contributions to coral reef biology without the usual delay in sequencing. Immediate capability for sequencing gave a glimpse of phosphonate as the key phosphorus source, illustrating how field sequencing can facilitate accelerated hypothesis formation and experimental design, thus maximizing the productivity of research expeditions (Akhter et al., 2014). Moreover, Ion

Torrent sequencings versatility serves numerous genomic applications by showing its capability to accept a variety of research needs. By application of the technology in single-marker tests as well as whole-genome profiling, researchers have a reliable approach for managing various objectives in plant breeding and other genetic studies. The combined approach allows targeted genotyping while also offering total genomic information, providing efficient research and development across a variety of industries. Such flexibility not only streamlines workflow but also aids in cost reduction, rendering it an essential instrument for genomics advancement. Through the capability to enhance genetic studies in numerous fields, Ion Torrent sequencing is an amazing revolution in next-generation sequencing technologies (Rife et al., 2015) (Figure 4.7).

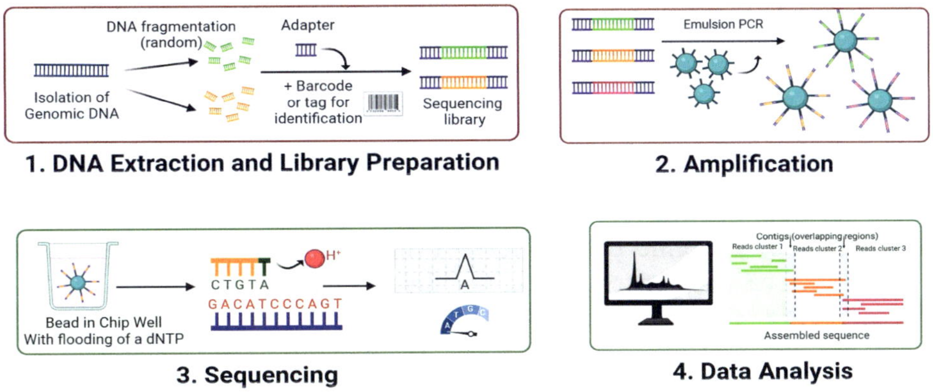

Figure 4.7. Ion Torrent sequencing.

Source: https://microbenotes.com/wp-content/uploads/2024/10/Steps-of-Ion-Torrent-Sequencing.jpeg.

4.1.3. PacBio and Oxford Nanopore Technologies

The emergence of long-read next generation sequencing technologies, characterized by Pacific Biosciences (PacBio) and Oxford Nanopore Technologies (ONT), has revolutionized the genomic study arena in the setting of Next-Generation Sequencing (NGS). The technologies enable sequencing of longer stretches of DNA than the traditional short-read technologies, hence making it simpler to resolve complex genomic areas that have a tendency to elude shorter reads. Long-read sequencing technology is particularly valuable for de novo genome assembly, the detection of structural variants, and the understanding of repetitive genomic regions, now broadly recognized to be fundamental components of genomic architecture. Unbroken stretches of DNA sequence data allow for more precise reconstructions of the genome and allow researchers to unravel the complexity of genetic information with greater precision. However, despite these advances, the heavy computational demands of the long-read technologies remain a significant barrier to effective sequencing workflows. While PacBio and ONT have pushed the limits of sequencing accuracy and speed, their operational mechanics are distinctly different, generating different strengths and weaknesses. PacBio employs the Single Molecule, Real-Time (SMRT) sequencing technique, producing high-quality reads that are particularly suited to addressing challenging genomes and enabling enhanced variant discovery. ONT, however, employs a nanopore-based approach, where it performs real-time sequencing at a lower cost per base and with rapid turnaround times. However, the high quality of ONT reads is generally difficult to attain and, in most cases, is dependent on hybrid sequencing approaches incorporating the strengths of both platforms. Recent studies highlight the importance of using hybrid approaches in maximizing contiguity and completeness of genomic assemblies and limiting the restrictions of native inaccuracies from individual platforms, which demonstrates the value of combined methods in genomic research (Sevim et al., 2019). Thanks to developments in the genomics field, researchers are now confronted with the intimidating challenge of choosing a diverse array of sequencing technologies and bioinformatics software to achieve high-quality genome assemblies for specific research objectives. The sequencing platform chosen—either PacBio or ONT—will dictate the quality of genomic data that they obtain. Furthermore, the intersection of different sequencing technologies and sequencing depth determination, combined with the implementation of innovative assembly strategies, presents an intricate web of variables influencing downstream analysis as well as result interpretation. These dynamics must be understood to realize the maximum potential of genomic research, especially with the challenges of intricate genomic architecture as well as variant detection. Last but not least, ongoing enhancement of both ONT and PacBio technologies and their use in holistic sequencing strategies will increasingly refine the tools of genetic analysis and widen the frontiers of genetic understanding in the full breadth of biological contexts (Espinosa et al., 2024).

4.2. Applications of NGS in Medicine

Advances in next-generation sequencing (NGS) technologies have transformed the field of oncology, shifting the manner in which clinicians understand and treat cancer. The treatment of cancer used to rely upon single biomarker testing to diagnose a specific mutation. These traditional methods, however, could not capture the immense genomic heterogeneity within the tumors. By applying NGS, it is now feasible to perform whole-genome or whole-exome sequencing that scrutinizes a vast array of genetic mutations as a single test. This broad platform permits the detection of novel therapeutic targets and biomarkers that could render treatment optimized and inform individualized medicine approaches. As highlighted in recent studies, NGS technologies play a vital role in improving diagnostic precision, enabling clinicians to tailor interventions ideally to the patient's individual genomic profile and thereby improve patient outcome and prognosis (Paolillo et al., 2016). The uses of NGS extend beyond cancer into other medical disciplines, such as infectious disease and genetic diseases. In the treatment of infectious diseases, NGS allows for quick sequencing of pathogens to identify genetic alterations associated with antibiotic resistance or virulence. This is especially true in the case of emerging infectious diseases, in which rapid detection will have a significant impact on treatment plans as well as on public health strategies. Likewise, in genetic disease, NGS can analyze several genes in parallel, revealing mysterious hereditary diseases that were not characterized before. This complete analysis not only helps in diagnosis but is also useful in genetic counseling as families get to know the possible risks and how the disease passes down, thus making informed health decisions. The adaptability of NGS technologies reflects their intrinsic capacity to propel the advancement of precision medicine in diverse medical situations (Marquardt et al., 2012). In addition, the integration of NGS and other molecular analysis techniques offers promising prospects for the improvement of clinical workflows and patient outcomes. With an increasing number of laboratories incorporating these technologies into their offerings, the potential for developing rich databases of genomic information grows. Such databases can facilitate mass data mining, potentially revealing pathophysiological patterns and biomarkers previously not detected. Second, the integration of NGS into clinical trials enhances patient stratification based on genetic profiles, maximally increasing recruitment while yielding more homogeneous trial results. This shift towards evidence-based decision-making is a landmark instance of the paradigm-shifting nature of NGS, providing clinicians with ways to not just enhance therapeutic development but also to adapt diagnostic protocols to various diseases. The continuous evolution in NGS technologies forms a revolution in modern medicine, enabling an era of patient-centric care (Marquardt et al., 2012; Paolillo et al., 2016) (Figure 4.8).

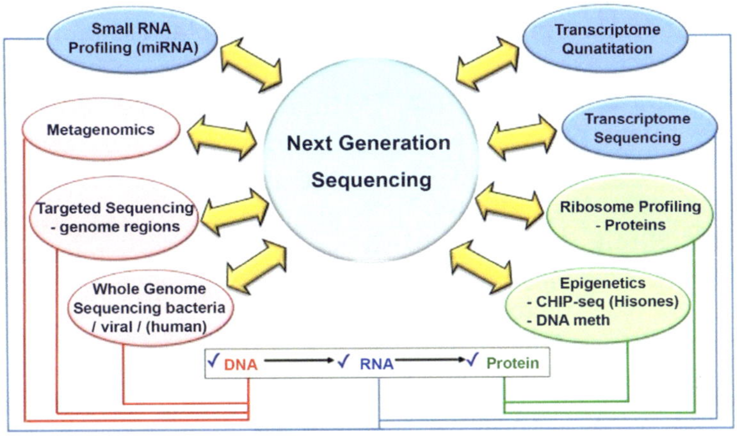

Figure 4.8. Applications of NGS.

Source: https://external-content.duckduckgo.com/iu/?u=https%3A%2F%2Fwww.europeanpharmaceuticalreview.com%2Fwp-content%2Fuploads%2FFig22-600x360.jpg&f=1&nofb=1&ipt=6a132d03d9827904c82c69356453a8dd123518fc9c3fa6e88a513e2fc8a92c02.

4.2.1. Cancer Genomics and Personalized Medicine

Technical breakthroughs in cancer genomics are revolutionizing the field of personalized medicine, particularly with Next-Generation Sequencing (NGS) technologies. With the technologies, it is feasible to thoroughly study the genomes of tumors, which can exhibit genetic mutations, copy number variations, and structural modifications that are accountable for the growth of cancer. By using NGS, physicians can obtain a detailed genomic snapshot of the cancer of a patient, which facilitates treatment strategies to be specially designed. This precision approach goes beyond the old one-size-fits-all therapy regimens to tailored therapies aimed at the unique molecular makeup of a tumor. With cancer treatment increasingly data-driven, insights based on genomic profiling are essential in guiding the right course of treatment, thus optimizing the impact of interventions and mitigating the side effects of conventional therapy. Pharmacogenomic testing within the healthcare system demonstrates the significance of cancer genomics in individualized treatment. The ability to detect a range of genetic variants among patient samples allows for early optimization of treatment by healthcare providers. Defined by Wiita & Schrijver (2011), the rapid expansion of knowledge regarding clinically important genetic variants necessitates the adoption of high-throughput diagnostic methods, which are essential to employing precision medicine strategies effectively. However, with growing access to these technologies, finding solutions to their economic and clinical impacts will be required. Effective management of pharmacogenomic markers needs to take into account the complexity that is required for sound interpretation of genetic information within a clinical environment. This fineness matters when it comes to enhancing patient care and when it comes to ensuring safe translation of genomics into daily clinical practice. The future of laboratory medicine is not clear, but trends are towards expanding roles for molecular pathology and cancer genomics within personalized treatment paradigms. As documented by Kricka et al. (2015), historical projections highlight the need for laboratory practices to remain flexible in view of technological, economic, and societal pressures. Ongoing improvement of NGS technologies will undoubtedly transform cancer diagnostics and therapeutics, instigating a new era of targeted therapy and improved patient care. As researchers advance the frontiers of knowledge regarding genomic alterations and therapeutic response, findings from novel biomarkers are likely to trigger more vigorous models of clinical decision-making. This advance validates the strength of a firm basis in cancer genomics as the key to unlocking the full potential of individualized cancer therapy.

4.2.2. Infectious Disease Diagnostics

The face of infectious disease diagnosis is being revolutionized with improvements in Next-Generation Sequencing (NGS) technologies. The conventional diagnostic approaches tend to be based on culture-based methods, which are time-consuming and can provide inconclusive outcomes. However, NGS provides a swift and inclusive approach by simultaneously analyzing a wide range of microbial and host genetic material. This paradigm shift not only hastens diagnosis but also makes diagnosis more accurate, allowing a wide range of pathogens, including those resistant to standard testing methods, to be identified. As clinical labs begin adopting these technologies, the potential for improved patient outcomes and targeted treatment protocols increases more clearly, hence ratifying the role of NGS as an essential tool in infectious disease diagnosis today (Chiu & Miller, 2019).

Further, the use of metagenomic NGS is particularly significant in addressing antimicrobial resistance issues. They enable clinicians not only to identify the pathogens in a sample but also their resistance, and hence it becomes simpler for them to make the right decisions on treatment. They are significant in an era when antimicrobial resistance poses one of the greatest threats to public health. In addition, employing NGS in the clinical setting uncovers the complex interplay among infectious pathogens and their host in humans, thereby providing a better holistic understanding of disease dynamics. With clinicians exposed to these findings, they can design interventions more effectively and also bring about significant impacts on infection control measures and treatment regimens (Chiu & Miller, 2019). The integration of microfluidics with NGS technology further enhances the capability of infectious disease diagnosis. Microfluidics allows for miniaturization and automation of the diagnostic process, the ability to conduct complex analyses with small sample volumes, and reduced assay times. The invention is especially valuable in point-of-care settings, where prompt diagnosis matters. The complementarity of NGS with microfluidics not only offers improved sensitivity and specificity but also streamlines workflows, curtailing time and the cost of traditional molecular diagnostic processes. In turn, as microfluidic technologies advance, they will increasingly contribute to taking the breadth of NGS to the next level, ultimately improving diagnostic convenience and efficacy in infectious disease (Figure 4.9).

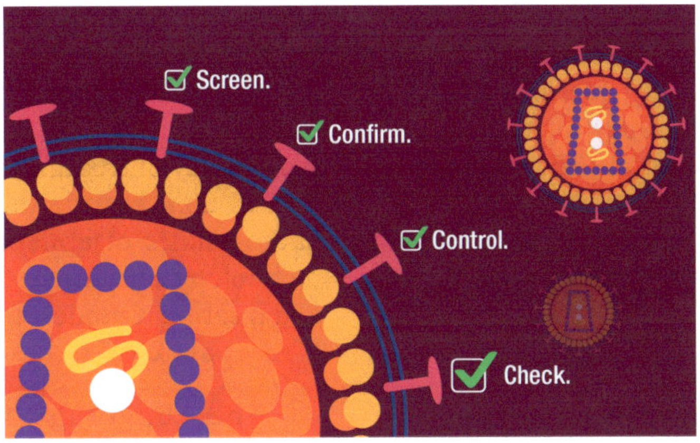

Figure 4.9. Infectious diseases diagnostics.

Source: https://www.bio-rad.com/sites/default/files/2023-04/DG23-0117-Specialties-InfectiousDisease-US-Images-02.jpg.

4.2.3. Genetic Disorder Analysis

Technological progress in Next-Generation Sequencing (NGS) has revolutionized the study of genetic disorders by significantly enhancing our understanding of the complex genetic etiology of most inherited diseases. Heterogeneity that is typical of genetic disorders, with typically more than one gene and pathways, makes it typically challenging to apply conventional diagnostic approaches. NGS allows for the complete sequencing of multiple genes simultaneously, which makes the detection of causative variants significantly more effective. For instance, in Fanconi anemia, a clinically heterogeneous disorder involving at least 17 genes, the NGS technologies allow the identification of novel mutations that might go undetected by standard methods. By applying high-throughput sequencing strategies, researchers can detect significant genetic information, which allows for early and accurate diagnosis and informs treatment plans for the patients (Nicchia et al., 2015). The adaptation of NGS technology in clinical labs has shifted the focus away from single-gene analysis towards more sophisticated methods like whole-exome and whole-genome sequencing. These methods not only expand the number of genetic tests but also offer complete coverage for potential pathogenic variants responsible for genetic diseases. With the reduced cost of these sequencing technologies, they are now more accessible to clinical use, thus enabling broader applications to be feasible in diagnosing genetic disorders. However, the use of whole-exome and whole-genome sequencing demands rigorous validation studies in the interest of guaranteeing the quality and reproducibility of outcomes. In this manner, laboratories become highly standardized while screening enormous volumes of data for germline variants linked to inherited diseases, ultimately leading to accurate diagnoses and evidence-based clinical decision-making (Hegde et al., 2017). In addition, the adoption of NGS can enhance our approach to genetic disease analysis with increased variant filtration and annotation protocols. Effective filtration allows the laboratories to filter through the hundreds of thousands of variants generated by sequencing to pick the most likely to result in disease. The integration of phenotypic information into the interpretation of sequencing results is central to making correct diagnoses. The adaptability of NGS to handle diverse genetic disorders is accompanied by the responsibility that clinical laboratories also remain alert to the ethics of their discovery, i.e., incidental mutations. As NGS continues to advance, the need for laboratories to continuously refine their techniques will remain so as to deliver robust and quality analyses, thereby guaranteeing the full potential of NGS technology for diagnosing genetic disorders (Hegde et al., 2017).

4.3. NGS in Research and Development

Next-Generation Sequencing (NGS) technologies have revolutionized research and development across most scientific fields, including medicine and environmental science. NGS is now a technology that can determine water quality and allow scientists to investigate the complexities of microbial communities. Scientists can identify microbial species and gene sequences indicating the health status of the environment and contamination levels using NGS methods , such as amplicon sequencing and metagenomics. The detailed information yielded by these tools is basic to the development of bioindicators of sewage pollution and tracking microbial causative organisms of pollution, thus informing water resource management practice. The use of NGS in microbial ecosystem science, as referenced in literature, not only enhances our comprehension of ecological relationships but also offers the technology with which gaps in environmental analysis can be filled (Tan et al., 2015). In the clinical sphere, NGS has made a remarkable impact on neurological and genetic studies, elucidating the underlying pathogenesis of such multifactorial conditions as epilepsy. The ability of NGS to sequence vast tracts of genetic data enables researchers to analyze genetic variations in sporadic instances of epilepsy, which provides an insight into their etiology and pathogenesis. Furthermore, this high-throughput sequencing technique allows one to identify epigenetic modifications that are accountable for the excitability of the neural tissue, thereby revealing the multi-factorial etiology of seizure disorders. These improvements in genetic research technologies encourage the development of targeted therapies and personalized medicine approaches, which can significantly enhance patients' outcomes and the efficacy of treatment. The foundation laid by NGS in demarcating the genetic and molecular pathogenesis of epilepsy bears witness to the technology's potential for advancing neurology and treatment models for challenging conditions (Tan et al., 2015).

The ongoing integration of NGS technologies into R&D also extends far beyond environmental and medical sciences, providing significant benefits to a host of disciplines ranging from agriculture and biotechnology. NGS enables researchers to analyze plant and animal genomes comprehensively, with the consequence that disease-resistance and crop-yield characteristics have been mapped. Such genetic information enables the production of genetically modified organisms capable of living under changed environmental conditions, thus addressing the problem of food security. Further, with researchers continuing to upgrade NGS platforms, reducing the cost and the time it takes to sequence genes is revolutionizing how research is conducted. Together, the advances in NGS are a testament to the revolutionary impact that NGS has had on scientific research and its enduring consequences for enhancing human health and environmental stewardship (Tan et al., 2015) (Figure 4.10).

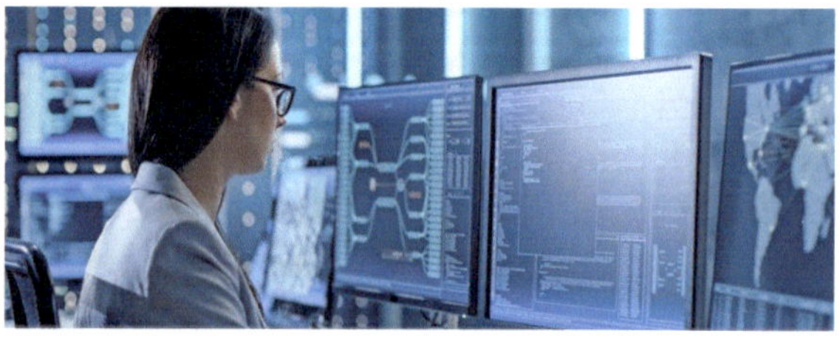

Figure 4.10. Custom NGS software development.

Source: https://eleks.com/wp-content/uploads/3840x1300_Custom-Software-Development-1024x347.jpg.

4.3.1. Role in Evolutionary Biology Studies

In recent years, next-generation sequencing (NGS) technologies have revolutionized evolutionary biology by allowing scientists to acquire enormous volumes of genetic data at unprecedented speed and accuracy. As a result of having the capacity to sequence genomes, scientists have been in a position to study the genetic diversity and evolutionary history of species at the molecular level, which makes it possible to gain a better comprehension of evolutionary processes. NGS technologies provide insight into speciation, adaptation, and the effects of environmental pressures on genetic diversity. Evolutionary biologists can now access detailed genomic information which now makes it possible to create detailed phylogenetic trees that describe the evolutionary past of organisms from various ecosystems. Moreover, NGS platforms have played pivotal roles in elucidating the evolutionary past of aquatic organisms, with erstwhile challenging-to-answer questions in the realm of molecular evolution being explored. Scientists, for example, have employed the platforms to understand the effects of environmental and anthropogenic stressors on aquatic biodiversity. The generated genomic data facilitate the application of bioinformatics platforms to determine evolutionary trends in the organisms, giving insights into their adaptation to new habitats. By examining such genetic variation, scientists are able to trace evolutionary lineages and assess the resilience of populations, thus aiding the conservation of threatened aquatic habitats (Tan et al., 2019). Such conclusions have implications that go beyond mere research and reach policy and management plans towards conserving biodiversity. With future development in NGS technologies, the application of bioinformatics software will be crucial in handling the complexities of the humongous datasets being produced. The combination of genomic data and bioinformatics enables more nuanced comprehension of evolutionary processes and more efficient drawing of valid conclusions from the data. But it is all a big challenge, and first and foremost in data analysis and interpretation, with more computational method development and interdisciplinarity needed. To maximize these technological advances, research endeavors must pursue further development of the bioinformatics platform and push current data analysis constraints (Buggs et al., 2010). With this, the scientific community is further empowered to optimize the contribution of NGS technologies towards understanding the nuanced dynamics of evolution, and hence towards optimized biodiversity conservation efforts.

4.3.2. Applications in Agricultural Genomics

Next-generation sequencing (NGS) technologies have made revolutionary advances possible in the field of agricultural genomics, enabling studies of plant and animal genomes at unprecedented resolution and speed. With the help of these technologies, scientists are able to conduct comprehensive genome analyses, significantly increasing our understanding of genetic traits in terms of crop yield, disease resistance, and climate tolerance. For example, NGS can identify single-nucleotide polymorphisms (SNPs), which are linked with desirable agronomic traits. This makes it possible for GMOs that are of improved performance across a variety of conditions to be produced. Incorporating NGS into breeding programs accelerates the selection process, which leads to more efficient cultivation methods, thus affecting food security. In animal genomics, NGS applications are also important in optimizing breeding strategies and animal health. With genome sequencing of various breeds, scientists can identify genetic markers associated with traits , such as growth rate, meat quality, and disease resistance. Genetic data not only assists breeders in selecting improved breeding animals but also enhances our ability to manage inherited disease in herds. Further, the implementation of genomic selection tools using NGS information is also capable of reducing the generation interval in breeding programs and thus facilitating faster genetic improvement. These changes make the agricultural livestock farming systems resistant to the effects of climate change as well as those of disease epizootics and hence support sustainable agriculture. The use of NGS technologies in genomics for agriculture also serves a critical role to facilitate conservation efforts for aquatic species, as has been highlighted in recent studies. Information regarding the genetic diversity and evolutionary history of aquatic species is critical to their conservation and management, particularly against stressors caused by humans , such as pollution and destruction of habitats. With the aid of advanced bioinformatics technology along with NGS data, researchers can map the genetic adaptations of aquatic animals and identify the mechanisms by which they respond to environmental stress. These genomic data not only assist in preserving biodiversity but also optimize the efficiency of breeding programs for enhancing resilience in aquaculture. Such polyvalent uses, as noted by Tan et al. (2019), reflect the revolutionary impact of NGS technologies on plant genomics and highlight the importance of continued investment in this area to address global agricultural needs.

4.3.3. Contributions to Microbiome Research

Next-generation sequencing (NGS) technology has revolutionized microbiome research, allowing for a comprehensive understanding of microbial populations and their roles in health and disease. One of the essential advances facilitated by NGS is the ability to study complex microbial communities with higher resolution than previously possible. Traditional culturing methods have difficulty capturing the diversity of microbes that are present in a given environment. However, NGS enables scientists to profile vast quantities of microbes from environmental and host samples, thereby unveiling new, unknown species and their dynamics. This feature is critical in research , such as preterm birth, where it takes hundreds of thousands of datasets in the context of genomic, transcriptomic, immunology, and microbiome data to uncover the mechanisms of complex conditions (Sirota et al., 2018). The use of such heterogeneous data sets not only enhances our understanding of microbial dynamics but also informs the development of innovative diagnostic and therapeutic strategies. The utilization of clinical metagenomic next-generation sequencing (mNGS) has accelerated the use of NGS technologies from the research field to facilitate the clinical laboratory. Through enabling comprehensive examination of microbial and host-derived genetic material in patient samples, mNGS is transforming the diagnosis and treatment of infectious diseases. Empowered by the potential to examine all this data as a whole, clinicians can diagnose causative pathogens more quickly and reliably than traditional diagnostics, taking antimicrobial resistance and the intricate human microbiome interactions into account (Chiu & Miller, 2019). Further, the knowledge gained from mNGS can also be applied to individualize therapy because the individual's own microbial composition could influence treatment success and disease outcome. In response, ongoing innovation and integration of mNGS into practice will raise patient care to a new level by allowing for more precise and informed interventions. The future of microbiome research is also secured by ongoing advancements in NGS technologies, enhancing precision and accessibility. Ongoing progress, utilizing increases in sequencing depth and bioinformatics capability, is empowering scientists with the technologies to study microbial communities in real-time at resolutions previously inaccessible. These improvements are critical for large-scale research into demarcating the role of microbiota in health and disease, notably in chronic disease and its correlation with microbial dysbiosis. With data sources like the March of Dimes Database for Preterm Birth Research becoming freely accessible and integrating staggering amounts of 'omics' data, scientific collaborations will accelerate microbiome research findings. This convergence of next-generation sequencing tools and data sharing is reflective of the promise of NGS to make a profound impact on our understanding of microbial impacts on human health and to provide novel therapeutic interventions (Sirota et al., 2018) (Figure 4.11).

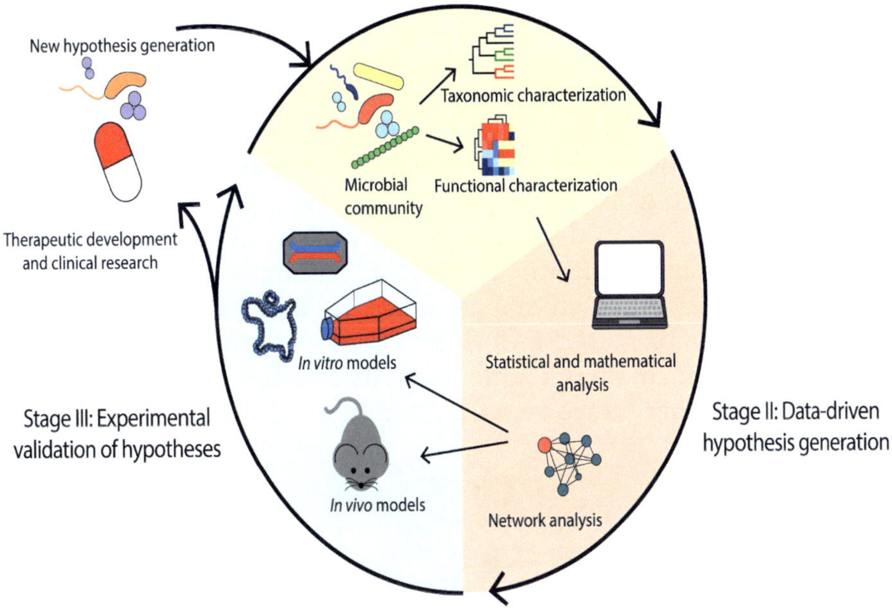

Figure 4.11. Contributions to microbiome research.

Source: https://www.frontiersin.org/files/Articles/685935/fmicb-12-685935-HTML/image_m/fmicb-12-685935-g001.jpg.

4.4. Data Analysis and Bioinformatics

The arrival of next-generation sequencing (NGS) technologies has required big changes in data analysis and bioinformatics, transforming our strategy to genomic research. Since NGS generates massive amounts of data, the issue arises in processing, analyzing, and interpreting that data efficiently. This has favored the creation of high-level bioinformatics tools that support the analysis of genomic sequences, transcriptomics, and epigenomics. Importantly, the integration of bioinformatics in NGS allows scientists to identify genetic variation, understand gene expression patterns, and examine the nuances of molecular interactions, thereby enhancing our understanding of biological systems. The development of bioinformatics techniques is pivotal, as it translates raw sequence information to meaningful biological insights, directly influencing fields , such as personalized medicine, evolutionary biology, and conservation genetics, which concentrate on the dramatic aspect of genetic variation in various contexts as evidenced by NGS studies (Kulski, 2016). Bioinformatics not only facilitates the analysis of NGS data but also enhances the accuracy and reliability of the findings derived from massive-scale genomic studies. Advances in computational power and storage devices have created high-throughput bioinformatics tools capable of handling the sophisticated data sets produced by NGS. This is especially relevant since the sheer volume generated—over 100 times that which is produced by traditional sequencing methods like Sanger sequencing (Pareek et al., 2011)—gives scientists gigantic datasets. Scientists can explore complex patterns in genomic data through machine learning algorithms and statistical modeling, allowing them to detect mutations, genetic disease susceptibility, and explore structural variation. In addition, bioinformatics facilitates collaboration across disciplines so that multi-omics can compile data from genomics, proteomics, and metabolomics and provide a broader perspective of organismal function and health. As NGS technologies evolve, so does the bioinformatics landscape guide future research and applications. Large-scale population genomics and individualized medicine approaches can be taken more seriously due to the availability of sequencing technologies. Consequently, bioinformatics has to evolve quite rapidly to keep pace with these trends, requiring constant improvement both in analytical methods and software design. Its impact on the processing and interpretation of NGS data is clear, facilitating critical applications in clinical diagnosis and analysis of complex traits in human as well as animal genomes. As underscored by recent studies in the sector, the combination of bioinformatics and NGS is central to the unlocking of not just genetic data but also to addressing fundamental health concerns and comprehending species diversity at a broader scale, hence influencing future research initiatives (Kulski, 2016) (Figure 4.12).

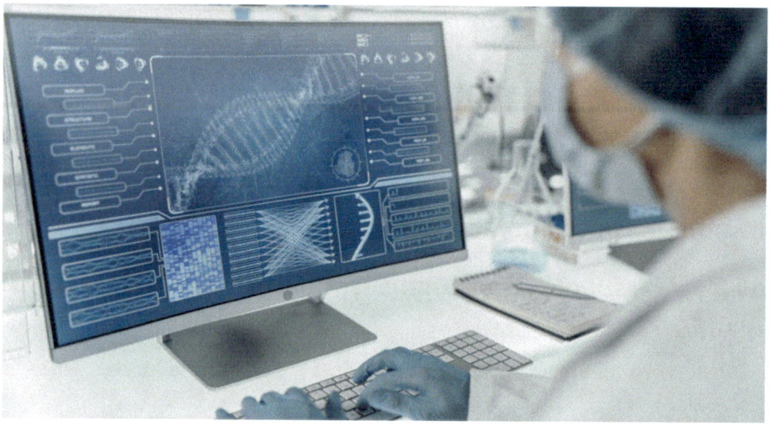

Figure 4.12. Data analysis and bioinformatics.

Source: https://www.novogene.com/amea-en/wp-content/uploads/sites/7/2022/05/one.png.

4.4.1. Overview of NGS Data Generation

The Next-Generation Sequencing (NGS) ecosystem is defined by its capacity to generate data speedily and in large detail, transforming the genomics era. NGS approaches allow for parallel sequencing of millions of DNA fragments, thereby allowing scientists the potential to generate huge amounts of data in a compact duration and effectively. This high-throughput capability is important for numerous applications, ranging from whole-genome sequencing to resequencing targeted and transcriptome analysis. Scientists can screen hundreds of samples in one experiment for genetic differences using massively parallel sequencing platforms, and so they are significantly faster and less expensive than earlier sequencing technology. This ability to make large sets of data has opened the door to unprecedented advances in genetics and molecular biology, enabling us to gain insights into complex biological systems and disease mechanisms. The NGS process of generating data includes several key stages that all add to the fidelity and usefulness of the eventual sequence data. First, the DNA or RNA is extracted and fragmentized so that it can be readied for library construction, where adapters are added to the ends of the fragments. These adapters are necessary for the amplification and sequencing to come, as they make the fragments compatible with the sequencer. Once library preparation has been completed, sequencing takes over, in which fragments get amplified and sequenced in parallel using various mechanisms, such as sequencing by synthesis or semiconductor ion sequencing. All these processes must be accurate to a very high degree, as the quality of data generated has a direct impact on subsequent analyses , such as variant detection and functional genomics. Finally, these advances in data generation technologies provide the foundation for the speedy progress of NGS applications in the fields of personalized medicine and oncology, among others. Furthermore, the integration of advanced computational capabilities becomes necessary to address the tremendous amount of data produced by NGS technologies. As the genomics data are in extremely prolific production, comes the issue of analysis and interpretation of data. Bioinformatics pipelines are used for the analysis of raw sequence data, facilitating alignment to reference genomes and identification of genetic variants. These analytical modalities not only enhance the value of the data, but also facilitate researchers to execute advanced analysis , such as gene expression profiling and epigenomic changes. With advancements in the field, integration of multi-omics data, including genomics, transcriptomics, and epigenomics, is increasingly being recognized for its utility in the elucidation of complex biological processes. This convergence is very promising in fields , such as cancer research, where more profound insight into genotype-phenotype correlations can result in new forms of therapeutic interventions as well as biomarkers. With ongoing developments in NGS technologies, the data generated will progressively influence our concept of health and disease (Turner et al., 2009; Marquardt et al., 2012).

4.4.2. Bioinformatics Tools for Data Analysis

The advent of Next-Generation Sequencing (NGS) technologies has revolutionized the field of genomics to enable researchers to generate unprecedented amounts of data in a shorter amount of time. With this rise in data generation comes the need to develop and utilize sophisticated bioinformatics tools for assisting in thorough data analysis. These tools are crucial in managing raw sequencing data, quality control, and read alignment to reference genomes. One of the major improvements is the TRAPID software, specifically designed for the quick analysis of RNA-Seq data, which addresses the need to handle large data sets while providing useful features like frameshift correction and open reading frame identification. Not only does the use of bioinformatics tools like TRAPID enhance data handling efficiency, but it also enables researchers to extract useful biological information from their results, further helping to create a better understanding of genomics in other organisms (Van Bel et al., 2013). As developments in bioinformatics continued side by side with NGS technologies, the creation of metagenomics further emphasized the necessity of tailored analysis programs. Metagenomics—the study of genetic material directly removed from environmental samples—requires the use of a variety of bioinformatics approaches to manage complex microbial communities without the need to culture organisms. In this context, various statistical and computational methods have been developed to decipher metagenomic data. These enable taxonomic and functional profiling, providing data on the diversity and ecological roles of microorganisms in their environments. Besides, there is a need for data handling and integration advancements in performing comparative metagenomic analysis because more than one dataset, which is obtained from credible databases, is used by scientists. These advancements highlight the core role of bioinformatics in advancing microbial ecology (Oulas et al., 2015). Apart from gene expression and metagenomic analysis tools, bioinformatics offers a variety of platforms specifically designed to cater to the many challenges posed by analysis of NGS data. Such platforms encompass features like data visualization, annotation, and multi-omics data integration, hence offering a complete solution for genomic research. Through the application of pipeline software that programs various stages of data analysis, scientists can shorten the time and effort devoted to result interpretation. Continuous improvement of bioinformatics software, as well as open community initiatives for collaborative software and methodology, is the way to make cutting-edge genomic research more accessible and affordable. With bioinformatics becoming more and more incorporated into standard experimental practice, the potential impact on our knowledge of biology, medicine, and ecology will be immense, setting the stage for novel breakthroughs in the post-genomic era (Figure 4.13).

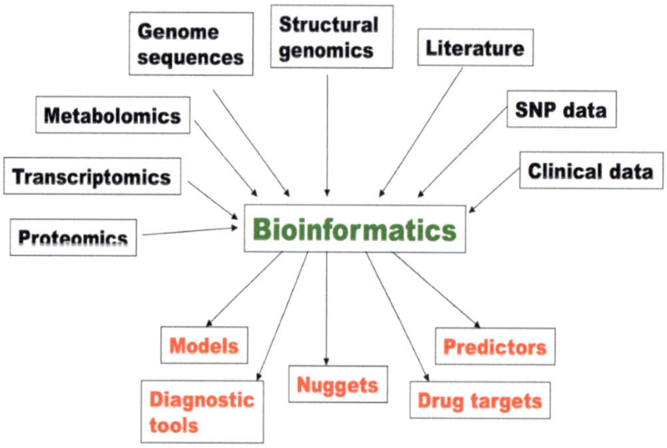

Figure 4.13. Bioinformatic tools useful in data analysis.

Source: https://www.uib.no/sites/w3.uib.no/files/media/bioinfo.png.

4.4.3. Challenges in Data Interpretation

Analysis of information that is drawn from next-generation sequencing (NGS) platforms poses a challenge with multiple implications for their medical usability. Although NGS platforms provide huge amounts of genetic data, the physician can be challenged to distinguish real clinically important mutations from innocuous ones. Adding complexity to this challenge is that incidental findings are alterations that are not clinically significant in the immediate future but could be a risk factor for future disease. For instance, myelodysplastic syndromes studies highlight the difficulty practitioners are facing in coming up with clinical evidence of mutations established, which is critical in making decisions on treatment strategies. Moreover, data interpretation processes standardization remains a concern, with there being no uniformity between laboratories regarding analysis approaches and reporting trends that facilitate potential variability in the treatment of patients and outcomes (Palomo et al., 2019). The biggest challenge in interpreting NGS data lies in the inherent nature of the complexity of the genetic information on which these instruments disentangle. The extremely complex nature of microbial communities and their interaction with the environment complicates it for us to derive definitive conclusions. For example, in water quality assessment, the complex relationships between microbial species call for advanced analytical models that can handle the immense data produced by metagenomic analysis. Researchers not only need to interpret the various species present but also assess their functional abilities, interactions, and implications on ecosystem health. This enhanced complexity brings along the need for robust bioinformatics tools to sort through very high levels of data, and this points out an important knowledge gap in existing methodologies, limiting useful interpretation and application of findings to real-world situations (Tan et al., 2015). Finally, the fast-paced development of NGS technologies contributes another level of sophistication in data handling. With the improvement in technology, the platforms and technologies employed are constantly changing, resulting in variation in the data quality as well as the analysis technique. One of these is heterogeneity among sequencing depth, read length, and error rates across platforms, which can significantly influence the results and conclusions drawn from the data. Also, as researchers strive to utilize these evolving technologies for many uses, including cancer genomics and environmental monitoring, they are confronted with the challenges of these changes to long-term comparability and reproducibility of findings. Hence, ensuring that data analysis remains in tandem with technological progress and is aligned with rigorous analytical standards is a condition precedent to the realization of full end-use of NGS in clinical and research use (Tan et al., 2015; Palomo et al., 2019).

4.5. Ethical Considerations in NGS

The increasing integration of Next-Generation Sequencing (NGS) technologies into the clinical setting brings a host of ethical concerns that need to be carefully considered. With increasing capabilities to rapidly sequence genomes, issues regarding genetic privacy and informed consent have come to the forefront. Individuals generally do not understand how their genetic data might be applied and have fears about third-party misuse by entities such as insurance companies or employers. Furthermore, there is an ethical imperative to ensure that individuals are fully informed of the implications of their genomic information, including those risks tied to family genetic information. As presented by Lyon & Segal (2013), the responsibility of protecting patient data is not only a question of regulatory adherence but also an ethical one, so that personalized genomic medicine benefits society and is not an instrument of discrimination or injustice. Beyond the data of patients, the ethics of NGS technologies encompass larger societal issues. The potential for unequal access to genomic services is a severe problem of justice and equity in health care. Specific worry is that advancements of genomic medicine may deepen existing differences between affluent and poor communities, leading to the establishment of a two-level health care system. Fair distribution of resources, like access to NGS technologies, becomes vital as advancement is made. As indicated by Lyon & Segal (2013), the health community has to become a champion for policies that promote technological advancement but also social justice, such that the benefits of genomics innovations are made accessible to the whole of the population and not merely a privileged few. Furthermore, the ethical concerns raised by NGS are not purely privacy and access concerns but also interpretation and utilization of genetic data. The subtleties underlying the interpretation of genomic information can lead to overinterpretation or misinterpretation of clinical findings, and both pose challenges to patients and clinicians. When clinicians are faced with decisions about the reporting of incidental findings that might be uncovered by sequencing, ethical issues are created. The impact of revelation of unexpected genetic information can be profound, leading to psychological distress or unnecessary treatment in families and patients. Hence, the formation of proper guidelines regarding the communication of genetic results is important in making sure there is an ethical reaction to NGS so that there are effects favorable to patient care amidst the complexities of genetics in various settings (Figure 4.14).

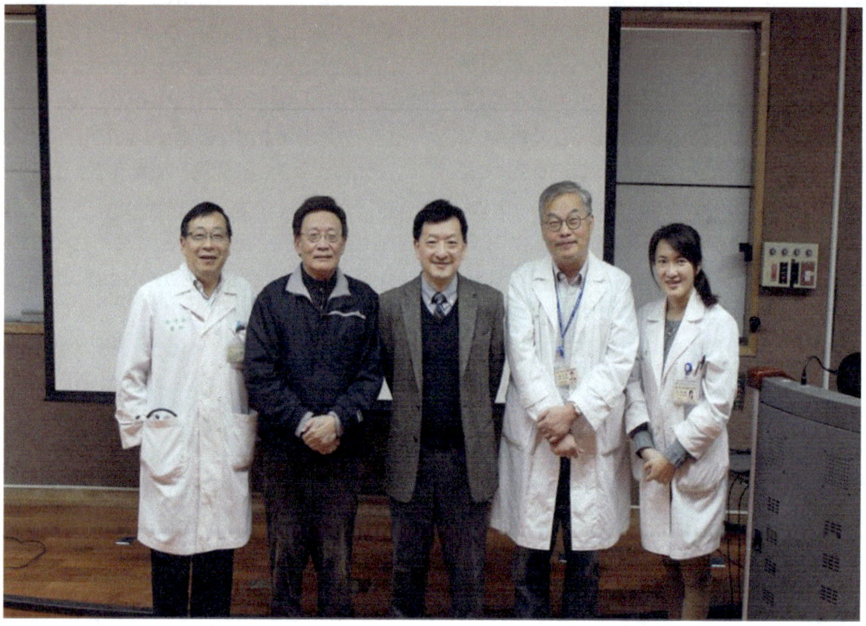

Figure 4.14. Ethical consideration in NGS.

Source: https://www.cbme.ntu.edu.tw/wp-content/uploads/2020/12/IMG_6350.jpg.

4.5.1. Privacy Concerns Regarding Genetic Data

The introduction of next-generation sequencing (NGS) technologies has indeed transformed the practice of genetic research and individual medicine but, in doing so, raised critical issues of privacy in the handling of genetic information. With genetic information providing increasing levels of direct access, particularly by direct-to-consumer tests, there lies greater potential for abuse. Of specific concern is the setting of testing children, whose genetic details can be assessed without their express permission. Opponents argue that children's right of opt-out—the said right not to know—is compromised when there is early genetic information acquisition, limiting later autonomy in matters of personal health decisions (Borry et al., 2014). This dilemma is a case of a broader ethical paradox: balancing the benefits of genetic information against people's natural privacy rights. Furthermore, storage and distribution of large-scale genomic data pose a myriad of legal and ethical concerns that mirror the urgent need for incorporating regulatory frameworks. The majority of institutions involved in whole genome and exome sequencing (WGS/WES) struggle to articulate clear-cut policies on data retention and access by individuals, necessary to ensure individuals' confidentiality and enhance scientific discovery. Scholars have noted that despite compliance with national guidelines, the lack of homogeneous practice is a factor leading to inconsistency in handling personal genomic data requests. The vagueness can lead to mistrust in genomic studies because individuals fear that their confidential information would be leaked, divulged without consent, or diverted to unwanted uses (Narayanasamy et al., 2020). Hence, the development of robust guidelines that honor individual rights is crucial. Furthermore, the impact of genetic data privacy goes beyond personal concerns to extend into societal and familial contexts. Genetic data usually relates not just to the tested individual but also to their family members, with serious issues being raised regarding the confidentiality of common genetic traits. The potential that these hereditary genetic susceptibilities could be disclosed unauthorizedly is extremely important and presents significant ethical issues, especially with respect to the increasing application of genetic testing across various portions of the population. Public attitudes regarding these dangers can deter individuals from employing NGS technologies, which may eventually hamper advancements in precision medicine. Thus, as NGS technology continues to advance, it is essential that policymakers, scientists, and ethicists have ongoing discussions to ensure the protection of genetic privacy and equal access to genomic progress for all members of society.

4.5.2. Implications of Genetic Information on Insurance

The consequences of genetic data on insurance are multifaceted and constitute a profound ethical and practical challenge for insurers. With advances in next-generation sequencing (NGS) technologies, insurers now have access to large amounts of genetic data that can ascertain the risk of an individual for particular disease conditions. This new technology raises issues of genetic discrimination in which individuals with genetically determined markers can be charged higher premiums or even denied insurance coverage. The moral implications are substantial as the practices may perpetuate current health inequalities among already vulnerable groups. Secondly, the risk of misuse of genetic information not only infringes on individual privacy but also undermines public confidence in the healthcare system. To address these challenges, there is a call for collaboration between stakeholders to create policies that protect against discrimination while allowing individuals to access the benefits of advances in genetic research and personalized medicine. Furthermore, genetic application in insurance can play a significant role in shaping the determination of coverage structure and risk. For instance, customized insurance policies become a standard, with premiums varying based on genetic predisposition to particular ailments. While this might, in theory, lower premiums for individuals with lower risk profiles, it would also raise suspicions about fairness and justice. Insurers must balance the demand for customized policies against potential public backlash against practices that, inadvertently, discriminate against those with genetic risks, raising their insurance premiums while impacting vulnerable groups. This tension is further exacerbated by the lack of overarching rules guiding the use of genetic data within the industry, and therefore, it requires legislative frameworks guaranteeing fair treatment but retaining flexibility within the regulatory regime for adaptation to evolving genomic information. Moreover, the connection between genetic data and social effects needs to be exaggerated. The revelations brought about by NGS technologies are not only affecting the individual but also have the potential to resonate in whole populations. Insurance providers must navigate the intricate web of public sentiment, regulatory environments, and growing ethical standards to draw equitable procedures for genetic information. As aptly expressed in the Global Risks report, knowledge of the interconnections between various types of risks can prove helpful in shaping the way such dangers are being addressed (Narayanaswamy et al., 2020). The ability to effectively analyze and react to such matters is key to ensuring that governments, businesses, and civil society unite in the creation of a responsible insurance ecosystem in the age of genetic information. These collaborative approaches will guarantee that the inherent benefits of the NGS technologies are realized without eroding equity and justice in health care treatment and access (Figure 4.15).

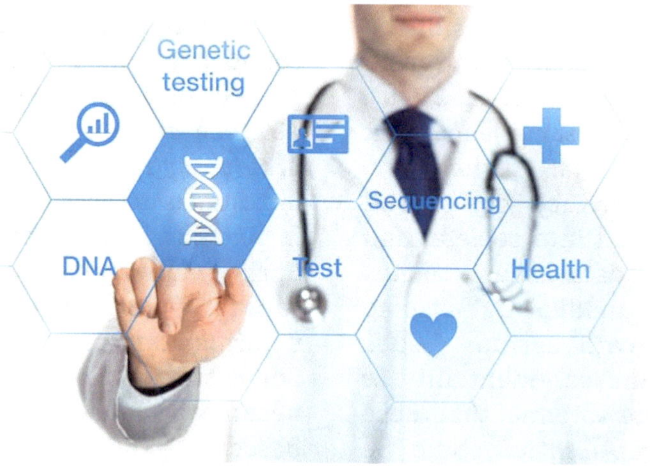

Figure 4.15. Insurance genetic testing.

Source: https://i.pinimg.com/originals/3d/e6/f5/3de6f54c36c46992de4c663f0396cc93.jpg.

4.5.3. Ethical Dilemmas in Genetic Editing

With the quickly evolving genetic editing tools, such as CRISPR-Cas9, society is confronted with extremely ingrained ethical difficulties for existing moral attention frameworks and regulative norms. With these tools, one can edit the genetic code of an organism, so raising the question of what it means to tamper with nature. Problems are generally couched in terms of matters of worry over long-term implications of germline editing, where such genetic alterations can be passed on to future generations. Others contend that germline modification violates natural boundaries inherent in the human species and inspires fear of creating so-called designer babies. Furthermore, the regulatory framework, as criticized by the guidelines of the European Society of Human Reproduction and Embryology and the European Society of Human Genetics, demonstrates that the majority of countries still prohibit germline gene editing on grounds of ethics related to safety and social impact of these technologies (De Wert et al., 2018). Furthermore, the differences in access to genetic editing technology raise additional ethical issues. The potential benefits of next-generation sequencing and gene editing could disproportionately inure to the rich or privileged groups, thereby solidifying existing inequalities in medical care. When advancements are being made, these technologies need to be made accessible to various populations, particularly those with genetic diseases like congenital heart defects (CHDs) (Touma et al., 2017). Without fair access, the promise of precision medicine risks becoming a luxury available to an elite class, disadvantaging marginalized populations. This is why the ethical imperative to develop competent frameworks that advocate for equity and espouse competent guidelines for safe use of genetic editing is so central. By wrestling with these ethical dilemmas, the importance of competent public discourse emerges as necessary for shaping the future of genetic editing. Engaging different stakeholders is one of the ways of looking at the complete picture of the consequences of genetic technologies. Developing regulations that are impactful enough needs to be tied with societal values and ethical attitudes so that the concerned communities' voices are heard and addressed. By having frank discussions about the values that are associated with genetic editing, society can all walk together to address the complex landscape of bioethics and balance issues with generating innovation in the interests of the public. Such discussion is most important to counter consequentialist reasons, e.g., safety and well-being for future generations, highlighted in the ethics assessments of germline interventions (De Wert et al., 2018).

4.6. Future Trends in NGS Technologies

The next-generation sequencing (NGS) technology field is evolving rapidly, driven by advances in computing processes and the diffusion of big data analytics. Shaping trends are likely to see enhanced data processing capacity that is able to process the increased level of genomic data. Advances in technology in the guise of artificial intelligence and machine learning are likely to enable data analysis to be done automatically, which will allow scientists to derive insights from sophisticated data at a quicker pace. For instance, as NGS becomes increasingly integrated into all fields of research, from clinical genomics to personalized medicine, the demand for sophisticated bioinformatics tools is higher. These trends underscore the requirement to overcome data storage and retrieval challenges, as well as the requirement for standard protocols to facilitate collaboration in diverse scientific fields to enable NGS technologies to be applied efficiently to real-world contexts, for instance, parasitology, as revealed in recent studies (Zarlenga & Gasbarre, 2009). A second important trend for the future of NGS technologies is the adoption of single-cell sequencing techniques. As scientists consider examining the genetic composition of single cells, this capability will revolutionize our understanding of cellular heterogeneity in complicated tissues. Single-cell sequencing will illuminate cellular behavior in a wide variety of biological contexts, such as tumor microenvironments or immune systems, thus enabling therapeutic intervention with greater accuracy. One significant implication of this trend is the prospect of more specific public health interventions, leading to more individualized treatment regimens based on the patient's genomic information. Additionally, as access to NGS technologies simplifies, we anticipate the analysis of genomic data to democratize, not just accessible to well-funded laboratories but also for small-scale research facilities and the developing world, therefore aligning with the global health agenda as part of the United Nations Sustainable Development Goals (Latif et al., 2017). Lastly, the emerging convergence of NGS technologies with changing connectivity paradigms , such as 5G, is likely to unlock hitherto unprecedented possibilities in healthcare and bioscience research. The higher bandwidth and reduced latency offered by 5G can offer for real-time transmission of genomic data, facilitating open-ended collaboration under global research programs. This connectivity has the potential to enable telemedicine solutions, which can be applied by healthcare professionals to facilitate NGS information leveraging in remote settings, enhancing patient care. When such technologies converge, we expect tremendous progress in addressing various healthcare challenges, ranging from infectious diseases to cancer genomics. It is, however, critical that we determine the corresponding ethical implications, particularly with regard to data privacy as well as the fair access to healthcare innovations. Prior planning for such futuristic scenarios, therefore, necessitates that we embrace a collective effort targeting ethical aspects as much as developing technology in NGS (Zarlenga & Gasbarre, 2009) (Figure 4.16).

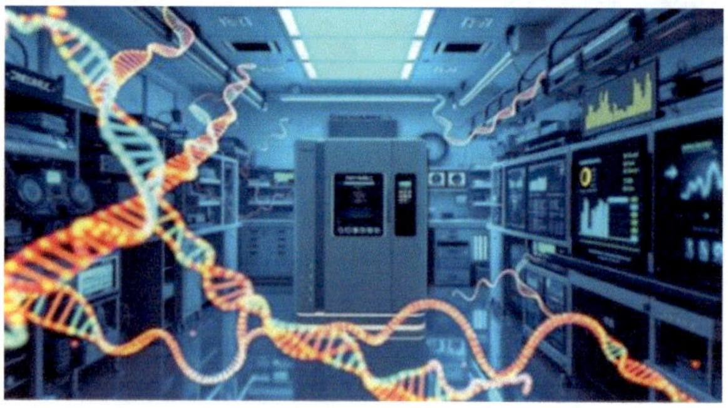

Figure 4.16. The rise of next-generation sequencing technologies (NGS).

Source: https://external-content.duckduckgo.com/iu/?u= https%3A%2F%2Ftse2.mm.bing.net%2Fth%2Fid%2FOIP.FA8k42mtMQpLYFcj1Bg46QHaEO%3Fpid% 3DApi&f= 1&ipt= 8823ac62d63f149cdcff3232afdcbe55fd3c87fa2dd12f15a14a6289dfd74829.

4.6.1. Advances in Sequencing Speed and Accuracy

The development of next-generation sequencing (NGS) technologies has transformed genomic analysis primarily by way of enormous advances in speed and precision of sequencing. Continual platform advances enable the generation of colossal volumes of data in incredibly short time frames. Rapid data generation is of special significance for applications , such as personalized medicine and infectious disease surveillance, where prompt information impacts treatment strategies. Recent technologies, including the integration of microfluidics and nanotechnologies, have increasingly reduced sequencing process time and expense. These advances not only ease sample preparation procedures but also enhance the sensitivity and specificity of molecular diagnostics, trending strongly towards more effective genetic analysis (Jayamohan et al., 2017). Despite the dramatic advance in speed, sequencing accuracy is still a top concern, particularly with genomic analyses trending towards high-coverage areas like cancer genomics and whole-genome sequencing. High-coverage sequencing is meant to provide full genomic information; however, it can impose significant errors in variant calling due to the complexity. Experiments have also indicated that intrinsic errors are primarily caused by the hardness of low-complexity genomic regions and reference genome incompleteness used in sequencing analysis. Recent reports indicate that the error rate of genotype calling can be up to 1 in 10–15 kb in raw data, but that filtering can reduce this rate significantly to 1 in 100–200 kb without severely impacting sensitivity (Li, 2015). This emphasizes the ongoing need for robust methodologies to enhance sequencing accuracy. With each advance in science, the quest for higher sequencing accuracy prompts researchers to develop bioinformatics tools and variant calling approaches better suited to overcome existing challenges. The interdependence of advances in sequencing speed and accuracy is of critical significance because, collectively, they define the feasibility and reliability of genomic research. Ongoing algorithmic advancements are indispensable to the enhancement of sequencing artifact understanding and reducing numbers of false positives in variant detection. For instance, identifying spurious calls in haploid genomes illuminates one regarding the complexities of realignment processes and highlights the importance of an extensive examination of genomic segments. By filling in these gaps, researchers are not only in a position to improve the precision of future sequencing technologies but also pave the way for their application in the broader area of biology and medicine (Jayamohan et al., 2017).

4.6.2. Integration of NGS with Artificial Intelligence

The marriage of Next-Generation Sequencing (NGS) technologies with artificial intelligence

(AI) has been a decisive advancement in genomic science and personalized medicine. NGS enables one to sequence complete genomes on an unprecedented scale within a brief span of time, providing informative insight into genetic variations causing diseases. However, the gigantic amount of data generated by NGS is a challenge, which can be met only with sophisticated analytical tools. Artificial intelligence techniques, such as machine learning algorithms, are increasingly used to address this problem through improvement of data processing and more accurate predictions of genetic vulnerabilities and response to treatment.

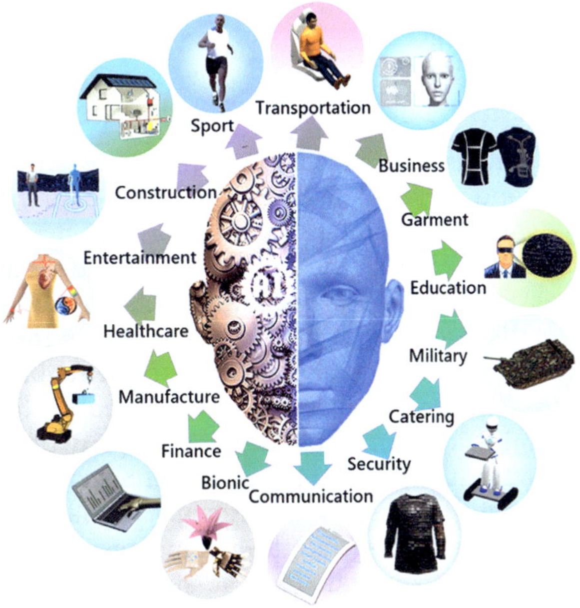

Figure 4.17. Artificial intelligence and database for NGS.

Source: https://www.researchgate.net/publication/334712951/figure/fig19/AS:11431281173283419@1688815191315/Promising-application-fields-of-NGs-in-artificial-intelligence-AI-For-example.png.

This convergence not only improves the analytical value of genomic data but also aids in evidence-based clinical decision-making, ultimately leading to customized therapeutic strategies. Also, the integration of AI with NGS can enhance the classification and interpretation of genomic alterations. Traditional methods of analysis of genetic data are inclined to apply pre-defined criteria that might not always capture the complexity of genetic interactions. AI-based models, however, can identify patterns and correlations in the data that may lie masked from traditional analysis. With the aid of advanced algorithms, the models facilitate better comprehension of the functional relevance of numerous genetic variations. The approach accommodates the overall movement toward more responsive and adaptive manufacturing systems, as discussed for artificial intelligence in manufacturing (Meziane et al., 2000). With healthcare networks embracing NGS technologies increasingly, the necessity for adaptive AI systems to continuously learn is most critical for optimized patient care. Also, the future prediction of the consequences of using AI on NGS should consider potential future developments in laboratory medicine. Historical predictions of technological advancement are an expression of the uncertainty characterizing scientific progress and socio-economic factors determining it (Kricka et al., 2015). With the advancement of AI capabilities, collaboration with NGS will become more sophisticated, driving innovation in precision medicine. This evolution has the potential to enhance the efficacy of diagnostic practices and lengthen the ability of health practitioners to provide customized treatments with genomic information. This ongoing dialogue among genomics, artificial intelligence, and clinical practice will then be the driver in setting future directions for healthcare while also enhancing patient care. The transformative potential of this integration reveals the need for researchers and health practitioners to remain attuned to emerging technologies (Figure 4.17).

4.6.3. Potential for Real-Time Sequencing Applications

The potential of real-time sequencing uses in Next-Generation Sequencing (NGS) technologies is a significant advance in genomics and personalized medicine. With emerging sequencing technologies, the potential of generating genomic data in real-time could transform clinical diagnostics and therapeutic strategies. Of special relevance is the fact that real-time sequencing can facilitate instant detection of genetic differences, facilitating timely clinical decision-making, particularly in oncology, infectious disease, and genetic disease. For instance, implementing the technologies in emergency settings can facilitate healthcare providers to customize treatments based on precise genetic data, thereby improving patient care. There continues to be an urgent call for error correction methods to be enhanced as sequencing mistakes can invalidate the integrity of real-time uses, necessitating improved algorithms and computational resources (Wiita & Schrijver, 2011). Application of real-time sequencing in a clinical environment can significantly enhance the speed and accuracy of genetic testing. New high-throughput next-generation sequencing platforms can analyze genomic sequences rapidly, and it is feasible to conduct large-scale testing under clinically applicable conditions. This capability has significant uses in pharmacogenomic testing, in which information regarding an individual's genetic profile can be used to inform drug selection and dosing regimens. Furthermore, advances in genomic databases, which enhance understanding of clinically relevant genetic variants, provide the potential for these technologies to be rapidly transferred to clinical contexts. However, discrepancies between our ability to recognize variants and our ability to identify their clinical significance are reflective of the shortfalls in real-time utility. As research advances, these technologies may bring not just speed; they may also provide more insight into disease pathophysiology and treatment response, thereby determining the future agenda of personalized medicine (Wiita & Schrijver, 2011). Despite the bright future of real-time sequencing uses, there are a number of challenges that currently lie in the path to their widespread use in clinical practice. One of the biggest challenges is the requirement for robust error correction software to correct faults built into today's NGS technologies. Software , such as RACER, a high-end error correction software tailor-made for Illumina sequencers, demonstrates the potential to increase sequencing accuracy dramatically. Correcting significantly more errors than conventional techniques, software , such as RACER has the potential to increase the reliability of real-time sequencing outcomes. Yet their adoption will rest on the extent to which they can demonstrate not only enhanced performance but also pragmatism in clinical practice. As NGS technologies develop, overcoming the technical and interpretative barriers will be required if one wishes to realize the revolutionary promise of real-time sequencing in health care settings (Molnar, 2012).

SUMMARY

The technological innovations in the next-generation sequencing (NGS) technologies introduce a new epoch of genomics with novel resolution and efficiency for the analysis of genes. Similar to the innovations in tools like REDHORSE, NGS not only assists in enhancing the ability to generate vast datasets of genes but also introduces sophisticated methodologies for the analysis of data. Algorithm design to transform genomic alignments into multiple sequence alignments is crucial for the application of existing recombination detection tools. Integration of such enables proper detection of genetic recombination events, which describes the revolutionary position NGS has taken in genetic research. Further, the capacity of REDHORSE to identify crossovers accurately in complex datasets indicates the promise of deeper insights into genetic and evolutionary diversity and cementing NGS as a non-negotiable tool in modern biological research (Shaik et al., 2015). Research into genomic datasets generated by NGS technologies extends to other organisms, and this underscores the breadth of uses in ecological and evolutionary studies. As shown through research on *Ostreococcus tauri*, it has been possible to reveal extensive genetic diversity and, at the same time, keep examining organismal evolution with high-quality NGS-derived genome assemblies. Genome stability across thousands of generations, supported by exhaustive assembly strategies, portrays both the robustness of NGS as an approach to research and its potential for longitudinal genetic research. These results further enhance the comprehension of the way genetic traits are transmitted and organisms evolve over the years, cementing the role of NGS in interpreting complicated biological mechanisms (Blanc-Mathieu et al., 2014). In conclusion, the extensive innovations brought by next-generation sequencing technologies are both evident in methodological progress and in universal access to genetic information. The ability to produce immensely accurate genomic datasets opens up new research avenues, ranging from population genetics to evolutionary biology. By incorporating reliable software tools and advanced sequencing methods, scientists can probe the complexity of genomes more accurately and effectively. This synergy fuels not only scientific inquiry but also ushers in a deeper insight into genetic processes that govern life. Finally, the future of genomics, fueled by NGS, holds the potential to clarify the intricacies of biology, enabling revolutionary discoveries that might redefine our knowledge of genetics and evolution.

The advent of Next-Generation Sequencing (NGS) technologies ushered in a revolutionary era of genomics with unprecedented scale and cost-effectiveness of DNA sequencing. By enabling the analysis of vast amounts of genetic information, NGS provides biologists with the capability to conduct sound experiments and make sense of complex biological processes. This capability is well beyond mere sequencing, as software , such as BamView exists to inspect and review aligned sequences against reference genomes. This software allows scientists to look at data in varying magnifications, such that nucleotide-level quality can be thoroughly examined, as well as genomic coverage overall. The interaction between sequencing technology and analytical software greatly improves result interpretation, facilitating the detection of key variations like single-nucleotide polymorphisms (SNPs) and the assessment of structural variation affecting biological interpretation and clinical outcomes (Carver et al., 2012). NGS technologies have also driven metagenomics breakthroughs, revolutionizing our knowledge of microbial populations and their functions in health and disease. The degree of sequencing enabled through NGS enables researchers to examine not only what microorganisms are present in a sample, but also how relevant they are functionally across scenarios. This shift from merely exploring abundance measures to understanding the complexity of microbial interaction fortifies the narrative that human beings and their individual microbiota act as super-organisms. This idea calls for the exploration of biomarkers that will support proof of disease states, particularly in the prevention of chronic disease, where proof of microbial contributions may elucidate prevention and treatment strategies (Izard, 2015). With developments in NGS technology, its role in public health and disease control becomes increasingly important. Moreover, the multidisciplinary applications of NGS are not just confined to the health of human beings but also have implications in the intricate ecosystems of the biosphere, impacting agriculture, ecology, and environmental sciences. The capability to perform cultivation-independent analysis widens our ability to discover ecological interactions as well as the genetic diversity of microbial organisms in a specific environment. The very complex associations between microbes and their environments necessitate novel techniques and paradigms for understanding these phenomena at large. This holistic strategy is essential to the study of complex biomes on Earth because genetic information from NGS has the potential to inform conservation and protection of biodiversity. Through deciphering microbial genomes, NGS tools make it possible for scientists to take a more holistic approach to viewing life on the planet and consequently inform future research and interventions in pursuit of preserving ecological balance (Rivera & Izard, 2015).

A LOOK TO THE FUTURE:

LARGE-SCALE POPULATION GENOMICS:

Over recent decades, large-scale population genomics has emerged as a transformative field at the intersection of genetics, evolutionary biology, and public health. Unlike traditional studies that focus on a limited number of genetic markers or individual genomes, population genomics leverages genome-wide genetic information across many individuals to characterize genetic variation at an unprecedented scale. This approach enables researchers to explore how evolutionary forces shape genetic diversity, to uncover the demographic history of populations, and to identify genetic factors associated with health, disease, and adaptation. Such genome-level analyses provide a depth and resolution that were previously unattainable, offering new insights into biological systems across species. At its core, large-scale population genomics involves the systematic collection, sequencing, and analysis of genetic data from hundreds to thousands—or even millions—of individuals. High-throughput sequencing technologies have been pivotal in driving this shift, as they dramatically reduce cost and increase throughput, making it feasible to generate comprehensive genomic datasets at the population level. These data enable the study of genome-wide patterns of variation, including single nucleotide polymorphisms (SNPs), structural variants, and other forms of genetic diversity, across large cohorts. As a result, scientists can disentangle the relative effects of mutation, natural selection, gene flow, and other evolutionary processes on the genome.

Large-scale population genomics has broad and growing applications across biology and medicine. In human health, population genomic data have been essential for mapping genetic risk factors for complex diseases, developing polygenic risk scores, and informing precision medicine initiatives that tailor prevention and treatment strategies to genetic backgrounds. These studies help address questions about how genetic variation influences disease susceptibility, drug response, and health outcomes across diverse populations. In ecological and evolutionary sciences, population genomics sheds light on speciation, adaptation to environmental change, and conservation genetics, providing tools to assess genetic resilience and guide biodiversity protection strategies.Despite these advances, the field continues to confront challenges. Ensuring representative sampling of diverse populations remains critical to avoid biases that can affect the interpretation and generalizability of findings. Additionally, the sheer volume of genomic data demands sophisticated computational methods and robust statistical frameworks to extract meaningful patterns. Future progress will likely depend on continued innovations in sequencing technology, bioinformatics, and collaborative data sharing across global research communities.

Large-scale population genomics represents a paradigm shift in how we study the genetic fabric of populations. By integrating comprehensive genomic data with phenotypic and environmental information, this field not only enriches our understanding of fundamental biological processes but also holds immense promise for improving human health, guiding conservation efforts, and unraveling the complexity of genetic diversity across the tree of life.

REFERENCES

1. Palomo, L., Ibáñez, M., Abáigar, M., Vázquez, I., Álvarez, S., Cabezón, M., Tazón-Vega, B., Rapado, I., Fuster-Tormo, F., Cervera, J., Benito, R., Larrayoz, M. J., Cigudosa, J. C., Zamora, L., Valcárcel, D., Cedena, M. T., Acha, P., Hernández-Sánchez, J. M., Fernández-Mercado, M., Sanz, G., ... Spanish Group of MDS (GESMD) (2020). Spanish Guidelines for the use of targeted deep sequencing in myelodysplastic syndromes and chronic myelomonocytic leukaemia. *British journal of haematology*, *188*(5), 605–622. https://doi.org/10.1111/bjh.16175(accessed on 17th July 2025).

2. Jayamohan, Harikrishnan & Romanov, Valentin & Li, Huizhong & Son, Jiyoung & Samuel, Raheel & Nelson, John & Gale, Bruce. (2017). Advances in Microfluidics and Lab-on-a-Chip Technologies. 10.1016/B978-0-12-802971-8.00011-0. (accessed on 17th July 2025).

3. Tan B, Ng C, Nshimyimana JP, Loh LL, Gin KY, Thompson JR. Next-generation sequencing (NGS) for assessment of microbial water quality: current progress, challenges, and future opportunities. *Front Microbiol*. 2015;6:1027. Published 2015 Sep 25. doi:10.3389/fmicb.2015.01027(accessed on 17th July 2025).

4. Buggs, R. J., Chamala, S., Wu, W., Gao, L., May, G. D., Schnable, P. S., Soltis, D. E., Soltis, P. S., & Barbazuk, W. B. (2010). Characterization of duplicate gene evolution in the recent natural allopolyploid Tragopogon miscellus by next-generation sequencing and Sequenom iPLEX MassARRAY genotyping. *Molecular ecology*, *19 Suppl 1*, 132–146. https://doi.org/10.1111/j.1365-294X.2009.04469.x(accessed on 17th July 2025).

5. Tan, M. P., Wong, L. L., Razali, S. A., Afiqah-Aleng, N., Mohd Nor, S. A., Sung, Y. Y., Van de Peer, Y., Sorgeloos, P., & Danish-Daniel, M. (2019). Applications of Next-Generation Sequencing Technologies and Computational Tools in Molecular Evolution and Aquatic Animals Conservation Studies: A Short Review. *Evolutionary bioinformatics online*, *15*, 1176934319892284. https://doi.org/10.1177/1176934319892284(accessed on 17th July 2025).

6. Akhter, J., Altschul, S. F., Aziz, A., Aziz, A., Aziz, A., Ben-Haim, G., Breiman, D., et al. (2014). Sequencing at sea: Challenges and experiences in Ion Torrent PGM sequencing during the 2013 Southern Line Islands Research Expedition. https://core.ac.uk/download/pdf/26959884.pdf (accessed on 17th July 2025).

7. Sirota, M., Thomas, C. G., Liu, R., Zuhl, M., Banerjee, P., Wong, R. J., Quaintance, C. C., Leite, R., Chubiz, J., Anderson, R., Chappell, J., Kim, M., Grobman, W., Zhang, G., Rokas, A., Muglia, L. J., Ober, C., England, S. K., Macones, G., Driscoll, D., ... March of Dimes Prematurity Research Centers (2018). Author Correction: Enabling precision medicine in neonatology, an integrated repository for preterm birth research. *Scientific data*, *5*(1), 3. https://doi.org/10.1038/s41597-018-0004-3(accessed on 17th July 2025).

8. Oulas, A., Pavloudi, C., Polymenakou, P., Pavlopoulos, G. A., Papanikolaou, N., Kotoulas, G., Arvanitidis, C., & Iliopoulos, I. (2015). Metagenomics: tools and insights for analyzing next-generation sequencing data derived from biodiversity studies. *Bioinformatics and biology insights*, *9*, 75–88. https://doi.org/10.4137/BBI.S12462(accessed on 17th July 2025).

9. Pareek CS, Smoczynski R, Tretyn A. Sequencing technologies and genome sequencing. *J Appl Genet*. 2011;52(4):413-435. doi:10.1007/s13353-011-0057-x(accessed on 17th July 2025).

10. Espinosa, E., Bautista, R., Larrosa, R., & Plata, O. (2024). Advancements in long-read genome sequencing technologies and algorithms. *Genomics*, *116*(3), 110842. https://doi.org/10.1016/j.ygeno.2024.110842(accessed on 17th July 2025).

11. Sevim, V., Lee, J., Egan, R. *et al.* Shotgun metagenome data of a defined mock community using Oxford Nanopore, PacBio and Illumina technologies. *Sci Data* **6**, 285 (2019). https://doi.org/10.1038/s41597-019-0287-z(accessed on 17th July 2025).

12. Becker, A. J., Rossignol, E., Loeb, J. A., Vinet, K., Kobow, K. L., Gilby, M., Simonato, L., et al. (2014). WONOEP appraisal: New genetic approaches to study epilepsy. https://core.ac.uk/download/54709926.pdf (accessed on 17th July 2025).

13. Bellone, R., Finno, C., Petersen, J., Raudsepp, T., et al. (2019). Ten years of the horse reference genome: Insights into equine biology, domestication, and population dynamics in the post-genome era. https://core.ac.uk/download/323069762.pdf (accessed on 17th July 2025).

14. Carver, T., Harris, S. R., Otto, T. D., Berriman, M., Parkhill, J., & McQuillan, J. A. (2013). BamView: visualizing and interpretation of next-generation sequencing read alignments. *Briefings in bioinformatics*, *14*(2), 203–212. https://doi.org/10.1093/bib/bbr073(accessed on 17th July 2025).

15. Shaik JS, Khan A, Beverley SM, Sibley LD. REDHORSE-REcombination and Double crossover detection in Haploid Organisms using next-geneRation SEquencing data. *BMC Genomics*. 2015;16(1):133. Published 2015 Feb 26. doi:10.1186/s12864-015-1309-7(accessed on 17th July 2025).

16. Blanc-Mathieu, R., Verhelst, B., Derelle, E., Rombauts, S., Bouget, F. Y., Carré, I., Château, A., Eyre-Walker, A., Grimsley, N., Moreau, H., Piégu, B., Rivals, E., Schackwitz, W., Van de Peer, Y., & Piganeau, G. (2014). An improved genome of the model marine alga Ostreococcus tauri unfolds by assessing Illumina de novo assemblies. *BMC genomics*, *15*(1), 1103. https://doi.org/10.1186/1471-2164-15-1103(accessed on 17th July 2025).

17. Narayanasamy, S., Markina, V., Thorogood, A., Blazkova, A., Shabani, M., Knoppers, B. M., Prainsack, B., & Koesters, R. (2020). Genomic Sequencing Capacity, Data Retention, and Personal Access to Raw Data in Europe. *Frontiers in genetics*, *11*, 303. https://doi.org/10.3389/fgene.2020.00303c(accessed on 17th July 2025).

18. Van Goethem, N., Descamps, T., Devleesschauwer, B., Roosens, N. H. C., Boon, N. A. M., Van Oyen, H., & Robert, A. (2019). Status and potential of bacterial genomics for public health practice: a scoping review. *Implementation science : IS*, *14*(1), 79. https://doi.org/10.1186/s13012-019-0930-2(accessed on 17th July 2025).

19. Borry, P., Howard, H., & Shabani, M. (2014). Is there a right time to know? The right not to know and genetic testing in children. https://core.ac.uk/download/237011214.pdf (accessed on 17th July 2025).

20. Rife, T. W., Wu, S., Bowden, R. L., & Poland, J. A. (2015). Spiked GBS: a unified, open platform for single marker genotyping and whole-genome profiling. *BMC genomics*, *16*(1), 248. https://doi.org/10.1186/s12864-015-1404-9(accessed on 17th July 2025).

21. Nicchia, E., Greco, C., De Rocco, D., Pecile, V., D'Eustacchio, A., Cappelli, E., Corti, P., Marra, N., Ramenghi, U., Pillon, M., Farruggia, P., Dufour, C., Pallavicini, A., Torelli, L., & Savoia, A. (2015). Identification of point mutations and large intragenic deletions in Fanconi anemia using next-generation sequencing technology. *Molecular genetics & genomic medicine*, *3*(6), 500–512. https://doi.org/10.1002/mgg3.160c(accessed on 17th July 2025).

22. Chiu, C. Y., & Miller, S. A. (2019). Clinical metagenomics. *Nature reviews. Genetics*, *20*(6), 341–355. https://doi.org/10.1038/s41576-019-0113-7(accessed on 17th July 2025).

23. De Wert, G., Heindryckx, B., Pennings, G., Clarke, A., Eichenlaub-Ritter, U., van El, C. G., Forzano, F., Goddijn, M., Howard, H. C., Radojkovic, D., Rial-Sebbag, E., Dondorp, W., Tarlatzis, B. C., Cornel, M. C., & European Society of Human Genetics and the European Society of Human Reproduction and Embryology (2018). Responsible innovation in human germline gene editing: Background document to the recommendations of ESHG and ESHRE. *European journal of human genetics : EJHG*, *26*(4), 450–470. https://doi.org/10.1038/s41431-017-0077-z (accessed on 17th July 2025).

24. Marquardt JU, Andersen JB. Next-generation sequencing: application in liver cancer-past, present and future?. *Biology (Basel)*. 2012;1(2):383-394. doi:10.3390/biology1020383(accessed on 17th July 2025).

25. Majidian, S., Kahaei, M. H., & de Ridder, D. (2020). Minimum error correction-based haplotype assembly: Considerations for long read data. *PloS one*, *15*(6), e0234470. https://doi.org/10.1371/journal.pone.0234470(accessed on 17th July 2025).

26. Van Bel M, Proost S, Van Neste C, Deforce D, Van de Peer Y, Vandepoele K. TRAPID: an efficient online tool for the functional and comparative analysis of de novo RNA-Seq transcriptomes. *Genome Biol*. 2013;14(12):R134. Published 2013 Dec 13. doi:10.1186/gb-2013-14-12-r134(accessed on 17th July 2025).

27. Evans, S. N., Hower, V., & Pachter, L. (2010). Coverage statistics for sequence census methods. https://core.ac.uk/download/pdf/81886397.pdf (accessed on 17th July 2025).

28. Latif, S., Qadir, J., Farooq, S., & Imran, M. A. (2017). How 5G Wireless (and Concomitant Technologies) Will Revolutionize Healthcare? Future Internet, 9(4), 93. https://doi.org/10.3390/fi9040093(accessed on 17th July 2025).

29. Hegde, M., Santani, A., Mao, R., Ferreira-Gonzalez, A., Weck, K. E., & Voelkerding, K. V. (2017). Development and Validation of Clinical Whole-Exome and Whole-Genome Sequencing for Detection of Germline Variants in Inherited Disease. *Archives of pathology & laboratory medicine*, *141*(6), 798–805. https://doi.org/10.5858/arpa.2016-0622-RA(accessed on 17th July 2025).

30. Kricka, L. J., Polsky, T. G., Park, J. Y., & Fortina, P. (2015). The future of laboratory medicine - a 2014 perspective. *Clinica chimica acta; international journal of clinical chemistry*, *438*, 284–303. https://doi.org/10.1016/j.cca.2014.09.005(accessed on 17th July 2025).

31. Paolillo, C., Londin, E., & Fortina, P. (2016). Next generation sequencing in cancer: opportunities and challenges for precision cancer medicine. *Scandinavian Journal of Clinical and Laboratory Investigation*, *76*(sup245), S84–S91. https://doi.org/10.1080/00365513.2016.1210331(accessed on 17th July 2025).

32. Zarlenga, D. S., & Gasbarre, L. C. (2009). From parasite genomes to one healthy world: Are we having fun yet?. *Veterinary parasitology*, *163*(3), 235–249. https://doi.org/10.1016/j.vetpar.2009.06.010(accessed on 17th July 2025).

33. Izard, J. (2015). Steps in metagenomics: Let's avoid garbage in and garbage out. https://core.ac.uk/download/286028026.pdf (accessed on 17th July 2025).

34. Rivera, Maria C. and Izard, Jacques, "Promises and Prospects of Microbiome Studies" (2015). Department of Food Science and Technology: Faculty Publications. 332. https://digitalcommons.unl.edu/foodsciefacpub/332 (accessed on 17th July 2025).

35. Jones, J. L., Lee, J. L., Moore, D. A., Morris, et al. (2018). Time for change: A new training programmed for morpho-molecular pathologists? https://core.ac.uk/download/132211774.pdf (accessed on 17th July 2025).

36. Meziane F, Vadera S, Kobbacy K, Proudlove N (2000), "Intelligent systems in manufacturing: current developments and future prospects". Integrated Manufacturing Systems, Vol. 11 No. 4 pp. 218–238, doi: https://doi.org/10.1108/09576060010326221(accessed on 17th July 2025).

37. Kulski, J. K. (2016). Next-generation sequencing–An overview of the history, tools, and "omic" applications. https://core.ac.uk/download/322425754.pdf (accessed on 17th July 2025).

38. Li, H. (2015). Towards better understanding of artifacts in variant calling from high-coverage samples. http://arxiv.org/abs/1404.0929 (accessed on 17th July 2025).

39. Lyon, G. J., & Segal, J. P. (2013). Practical, ethical and regulatory considerations for the evolving medical and research genomics landscape. *Applied & translational genomics*, *2*, 34–40. https://doi.org/10.1016/j.atg.2013.02.001(accessed on 17th July 2025).

40. Mardis, E. R. (2014). The translation of cancer genomics: Time for a revolution in clinical cancer care. https://genomemedicine.biomedcentral.com/track/pdf/10.1186/gm539?site=genomemedicine.biomedcentral.com (accessed on 17th July 2025).

41. Molnar, M. Z. (2012). Error correction in next-generation DNA sequencing data. https://core.ac.uk/download/61636305.pdf (accessed on 17th July 2025).

42. Turner, D. J., Keane, T. M., Sudbery, I., & Adams, D. J. (2009). Next-generation sequencing of vertebrate experimental organisms. *Mammalian genome : official journal of the International Mammalian Genome Society*, *20*(6), 327–338. https://doi.org/10.1007/s00335-009-9187-4(accessed on 17th July 2025).

43. Touma, M., Reemtsen, B., Halnon, N., Alejos, J., Finn, J. P., Nelson, S. F., & Wang, Y. (2017). A Path to Implement Precision Child Health Cardiovascular Medicine. *Frontiers in cardiovascular medicine*, *4*, 36. https://doi.org/10.3389/fcvm.2017.00036 (accessed on 17th July 2025).

44. Wiita, A. P., & Schrijver, I. (2011). Clinical application of high throughput molecular screening techniques for pharmacogenomics. *Pharmacogenomics and personalized medicine*, *4*, 109–121. https://doi.org/10.2147/PGPM.S15302(accessed on 17th July 2025).

45. Shi, L., & Wang, Z. (2019). Computational Strategies for Scalable Genomics Analysis. *Genes*, *10*(12), 1017. https://doi.org/10.3390/genes10121017(accessed on 17th July 2025).

46. Strathdee, D., & Whitelaw, C. B. A. (2013). TT2013 meeting report: The transgenic technology meeting visits Asia for the first time. https://core.ac.uk/download/16459953.pdf (accessed on 17th July 2025).

47. Tschopp, P., & Tabin, C. J. (2017). Deep homology in the age of next-generation sequencing. *Philosophical transactions of the Royal Society of London. Series B, Biological sciences*, *372*(1713), 20150475. https://doi.org/10.1098/rstb.2015.0475(accessed on 17th July 2025).

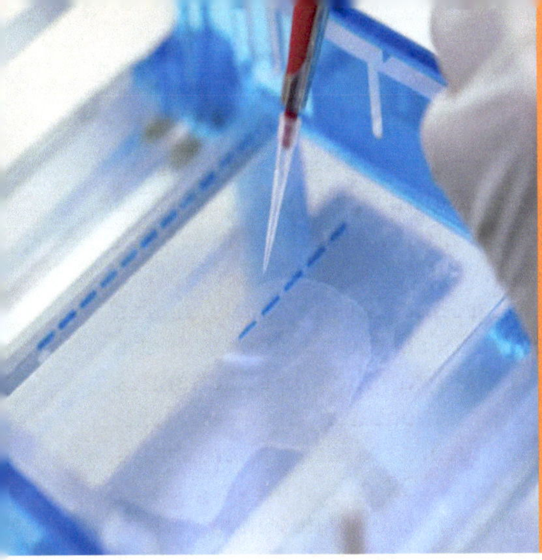

Chapter 5

MICROARRAYS AND GENE EXPRESSION PROFILING

Contents

Introduction

Gene expression lies at the center of unraveling the biological pathways underlying disease and developmental processes. Microarray technology is now an invaluable tool for quantifying gene expression on a genome-wide scale and allows thousands of genes to be surveyed in parallel. The high-throughput nature of this technology not only facilitates the identification of differentially expressed genes across conditions but also in interrogating the complex interplay in biological networks. With the rise in microarray application, it has become imperative to test the methods used to analyze data acquired so that conclusions drawn are valid and informative. Such methodologies have been exemplified in studies that utilize advanced statistical models and machine learning approaches in a bid to battle noise and variability inherent in high-dimensional data (Chu et al., 2014). The importance of microarray technology is again testified by its applications in a variety of model organisms, such as the chicken, which have a central position in biological research. When the sequence of the chicken genome was completed, microarray research has cast light on numerous facets of gene expression regulation and evolutionary biology. To give an example, long oligonucleotide microarray studies have enabled genome-scale surveys of gene expression between embryonic and adult tissues. Such research findings reveal intricate patterns of transcriptional regulation and reveal the conservation of gene expression in vertebrates (Nie, 2010). The context of this background not only underscores the significance of microarrays in the explosion of genetic studies but also the capability of the technology to be utilizable in various biological systems, rendering it highly applicable to genomics and bioinformatics. With the advent of gene expression profiling, complementarity between next-generation sequencing (NGS) and microarray technology bodes well for future research. Microarrays have already provided important data regarding the transcriptome, but NGS can achieve greater depth of coverage and more accuracy, and thus might surpass some of the issues involved in hybridization-based methods. Comparative analysis of microarray and NGS gene expression data highlights the strength and weakness of each method, paving the way to new research directions in transcriptional regulation (Nie, 2010). Thus, not only does technology development enhance our understanding of gene function and regulation, but it also sets the stage for revolutionary advances in personalized medicine and drug discovery. Overall, microarrays remain a focal resource in the elucidation of gene expression and its role in disease and health (Figure 5.1).

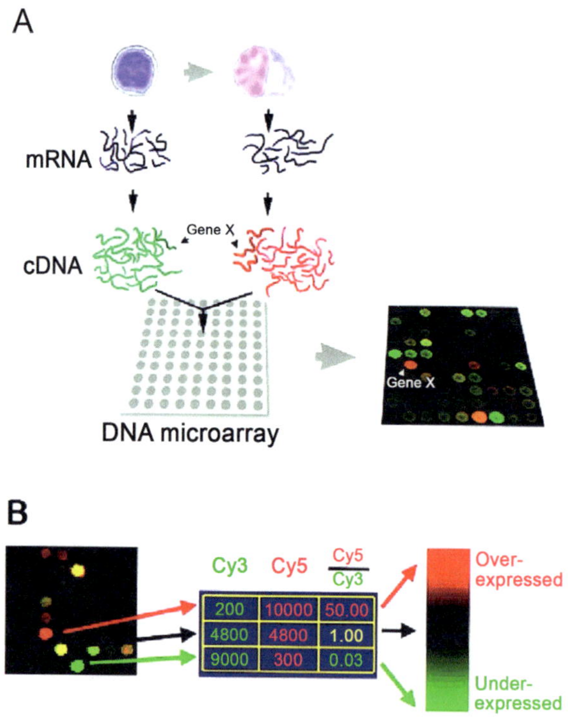

Figure 5.1. Microarrays and gene expression profiling.

Source: https://www.researchgate.net/profile/Patrick-Brown-23/publication/12481354/figure/fig2/AS:669633665331202@1536664515164/A-Schematic-of-cDNA-microarray-gene-expression-analysis-In-this-illustration-the.png.

Definition of Microarrays

Microarrays are advanced machines that are employed in molecular biology to quantify levels of gene expression across thousands of genes at the same time. Microarray essentially involves a small glass or silicon chip with a grid of microscopic dots, each carrying a specific DNA sequence or a probe. These probes hybridize to fluorescently labeled complementary DNA or RNA from cells or tissue so that researchers can quantify gene expression as the amount of fluorescence at each spot on the array. This high-throughput approach gives a good means of achieving a whole snapshot of gene expression under various conditions so that the multidimensional biological question of what occurs at the cellular level after exposure to drugs or environmental stimuli can be answered. The precision with which microarrays determine gene expression profiles greatly enriches our understanding of genomic regulation. By analyzing the hybridization patterns, researchers can identify which genes are induced or silenced in individual cell types or disease states. This feature is especially valuable in comparative analysis, such as comparisons between healthy and diseased tissues of diseases like cancer. The elucidation of regulatory modules and elements by integrative epigenomic mark analyses deconvolutes intricate gene regulation networks that significantly contribute to the explanation of developmental processes and diseases. As evidenced in large-scale studies, disease-associated genetic variants are enriched with particular epigenomic marks, and this presents the potential for using microarrays in the direction of the therapeutic strategy and understanding of disease mechanisms (Kundaje et al., 2015). Moreover, integrating epigenomic data with microarray technology widens its application to cancer biology and personalized medicine. For instance, studies based on whole-genome bisulfite sequencing coupled with high-definition microarrays have revealed important epigenetic alterations in pediatric B-cell acute lymphoblastic leukemias (B-ALLs). The studies show the complex interaction between DNA methylation levels and gene expression, revealing tumorigenesis mechanisms. By linking these epigenetic changes to specific regulatory contexts, researchers find out about the changes that regulate silencing and activation of genes in different cellular environments. Such comprehensive profiles can potentially unlock the door for treatment targeting that addresses the root-cause epigenetic contributions to disease, hence guiding our comprehension towards gene expression profiling and diagnostic applications of microarrays (Lee et al., 2015) (Figure 5.2).

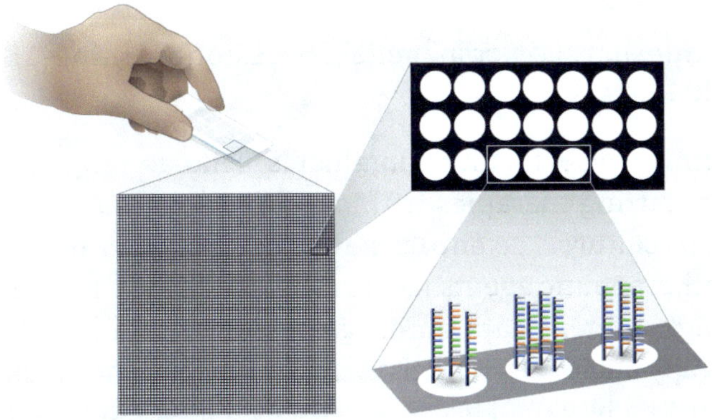

Figure 5.2. Microarray technology.

Source: https://www.genome.gov/sites/default/files/media/images/2022-05/Microarray-technology.jpg.

Importance of Gene Expression Profiling

Understanding gene expression profiling is a key foundation in modern molecular biology and its application in clinical and medical research. The ability to quantify the expression of thousands of genes simultaneously with technologies , such as microarrays allows researchers to elucidate complex biological mechanisms of disease, particularly cancer. In oncology, as previously emphasized in research on high-grade serous ovarian cancer (HGSOC), gene expression profiling captures typical molecular signatures separating malignant tissue from normal tissue. Profiling not only aids in the identification of possible early detection biomarkers but also identifies tumorigenesis pathways, allowing for targeted therapies and personalized treatment regimes. These results emphasize the value of gene expression profiling in unraveling the complexity of cancer biology, ultimately resulting in innovations in precision medicine tailored specifically to the requirement of individual patients (Hoffmann et al., 2020).

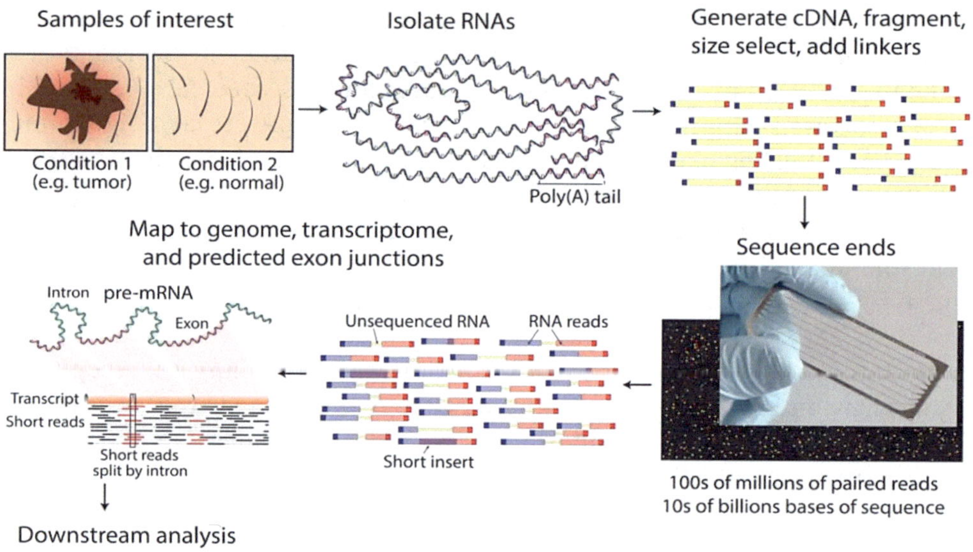

Figure 5.3. Gene expression profiling.

Source: https://image.slidesharecdn.com/geneexpressionprofiling-181013111841/75/Gene-expression-profiling-16-2048.jpg.

Gene expression profiling also further illuminates cellular responses to multiple therapies, which are essential for optimizing therapies within a clinical setting. For instance, through the use of patient-derived organoid cultures, scientists have demonstrated how some mutational profiles affect responses to chemotherapeutic agents like carboplatin. These models effectively mimic *in vivo* conditions and provide high-content data on drug sensitivity and resistance. By correlating gene expression patterns to therapy outcomes, scientists are able to identify which patients would be helped by certain therapies or, conversely, would be toxic. This level of personalized medicine is increasingly important in treating the risks posed by disease heterogeneity , such as cancer and ensuring therapeutic procedures are as effective and minimally invasive as possible to the patient (Zhou et al., 2019). Lastly, the integration of gene expression profiling into systems biology methodologies strengthens global insight into the molecular basis of diseases. By employing tools like Metascape, researchers can perform functional enrichment analysis through the simultaneous application of several biological databases, enhancing the interpretability of gene expression data. By doing this, the researchers are able to simplify massive datasets into interpretable biological findings, linking deregulated gene expression to physiological processes and disease pathology. By leveraging integrated analyses and network-based approaches, researchers try to decode intricate signaling pathways and biological processes.

Thus, gene expression profiling is no longer merely a tool for data accumulation; it becomes a necessary platform for hypothesis generation, biological interaction validation, and the guide for additional experimental strategies. This emphasizes the role of gene expression profiling as a platform that can drive us further in our overall understanding of cellular behavior under health and disease conditions (Hoffmann et al., 2020) (Figure 5.3).

5.1. History of Microarray Technology

The origins of microarray technology date back to the late 1980s, when researchers first began exploring mechanisms to examine numerous genes simultaneously. The innovation occurred in the aftermath of the Human Genome Project, which significantly positioned genomic data within reach. With the discovery and characterization of more human genes, it was apparent that transcriptomic level gene expression was required to reveal complex biological processes. It is the incorporation of these pieces of evidence that gave rise to microarray technology as a critical tool in molecular biology. Over the years, the technology has advanced significantly, from basic hybridization techniques to sophisticated platforms capable of capturing high-resolution gene expression profiles and thus transform the paradigm of genetic research and promote the magnitude of genomics research (Kulikov et al., 2023). With microarray technology advancing, so were its applications expanded from basic research into clinical oncology, and tumor genetics insight was accrued that was not possible earlier. This flexibility enabled scientists to analyze thousands of genes simultaneously, making it possible to study differential gene expression patterns in various cancers. Microarrays for expression were utilized to find molecular biomarkers that can be employed for cancer diagnosis and prognosis and ultimately aid personalized treatment approaches.

Furthermore, advancements in computer algorithms and statistical analysis techniques have enhanced the ability to comprehend intricate data from microarrays, underpinning their usefulness in clinical as opposed to research settings. The application of microarray technology in oncology represented a fundamental advancement toward personalized medicine, hence bridging the gap between genomic studies and implementation in real healthcare (Kulikov et al., 2023). Continuous technology development in microarray technology has enabled future enhancement in gene expression profiling, particularly with the development of new genomic tools and methodologies. Recent developments have included the optimization of probe design, array formats, as well as multiplexing capacity, which has all enhanced sensitivity and specificity of microarray assays. Notably, combining microarrays with other omics technologies, i.e., metabolomics and proteomics, has led to increased holistic insights into biological systems. The advances have made microarrays an essential tool in various fields, e.g., toxicology and environmental monitoring, as revealed by studies that utilize microarray profiling to establish the effect of pollutants on organisms. As research improves, the uses of microarrays keep expanding, and they are now a cornerstone in gene expression and molecular biology research (Figure 5.4).

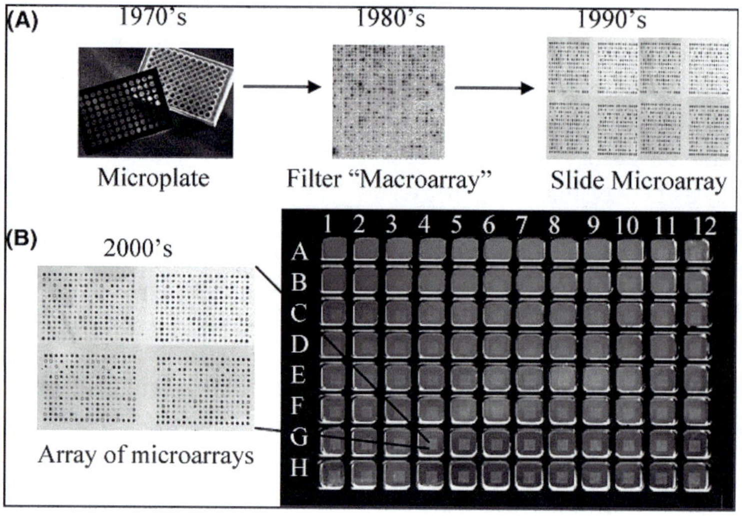

Figure 5.4. Evolution of array technology over the past 30 years.

Source: https://www.researchgate.net/publication/8559577/figure/fig1/AS:271563589156866@1441757213079/Evolution-of-array-technology-over-the-past-30-years-A-The-advent-of-microplate-based.png.

5.1.1. Development of Early Microarray Techniques

The development of early microarray techniques established a revolution phase in genomics and molecular biology and revolutionized the gene expression profiling landscape. Developed in the late 1980s, these techniques allowed analysis of thousands of genes in parallel, presenting a snapshot of their expression levels under various biological conditions. By applying a two-dimensional array format, researchers were able to hybridize labeled cDNA or RNA samples onto specially designed chips, allowing them to give a quantitative estimate of expression for the entire genome. The new technique not only speeded up research that had previously been slow and laborious, but it also gave a high-throughput process that allowed gene function and interaction to be studied on an unimaginable scale previously. The accuracy and reliability of early microarray technique were significantly enhanced by advancements in both probe design and analysis strategies. Initial microarray experiments, while revolutionary, were hindered by background noise and cross-hybridization problems and often yielded confounding interpretation of results. Improvements in biomolecular probes, such as the transition from cDNA to oligonucleotide arrays, increased specificity and sensitivity. With the evolution of new computational algorithms for expression data analysis, these advancements facilitated more sensitive identification of differentially expressed genes and therefore made microarrays increasingly valuable for clinical and research use. Microarrays subsequently became pivotal to the dissection of complex diseases like cancers and autoimmune diseases. The influence of the initial microarray techniques on disease diagnosis and comprehension cannot be overemphasized. For instance, research using high-throughput technologies was capable of detecting accurate gene biomarkers for inflammatory diseases and cancers, demonstrating the use of microarrays in personalized medicine. In cervical cancer, for example, the early detection through gene expression profiling has been linked to improved patient outcome, as seen in research examining machine learning application together with microarray data. By integrating the gene expression profiles and complex prediction models, researchers have made possible the construction of models predicting accurately patient survival rates, which mapped the clinical relevance of microarrays in enabling timely interventions. Thus, the development of early microarray techniques not only contributed to advancing basic research but also paved the way for revolutionary diagnostic and therapeutic strategies that expand in scope even now (Figure 5.5).

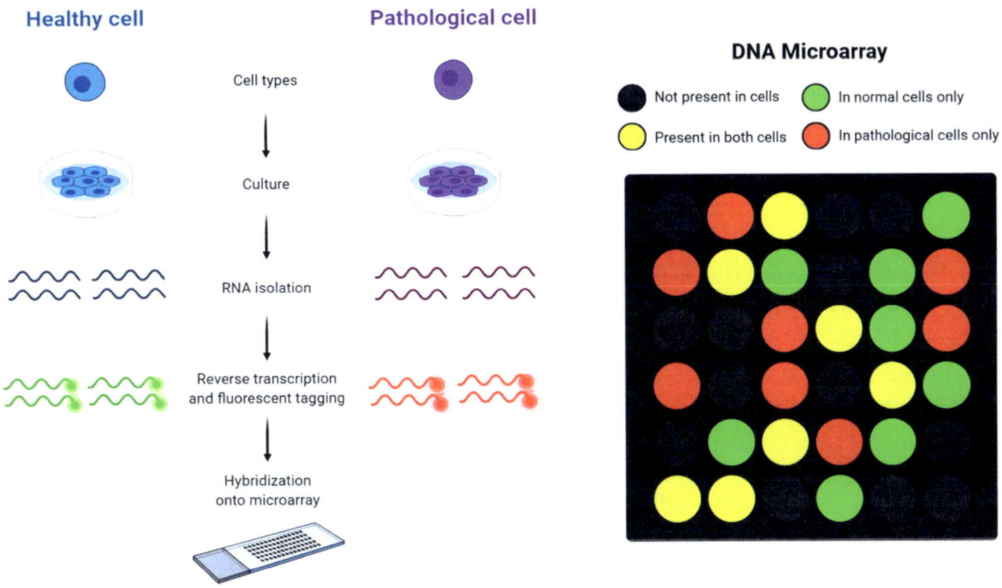

Figure 5.5. DNA microarray technology.

Source: https://thesciencenotes.com/wp-content/uploads/2023/04/Steps-Involved-in-cDNA-based-Microarray-1024x683.webp.

5.1.2. Key Milestones in Microarray Research

The history of microarray research has seen a significant transformation in the field of molecular biology, that is gene expression profiling. One of the pivotal turning points was the development of cDNA microarrays in the 1990s, which enabled researchers to screen thousands of genes at once for their expression level. This development opened the gates for large-scale gene expression research and gave the tools for powerful probing into cell functions as well as disease mechanisms. The collaborative efforts of scientists, including those located at the Massachusetts Institute of Technology and Stanford University, drove the technology mainstream so that it became applicable in cancer studies, drug discovery, and diagnostics. As high-throughput techniques picked up pace, data analysis as well as microarray design had to advance so that these techniques became more sensitive and specific, ultimately leading to refined methodologies further advancing the field of genomics. Yet another important milestone in microarray science was the introduction of oligonucleotide microarrays, where resolution and specificity were higher than with their previous versions. The early 2000s saw the change brought about by technological advancements in the synthesis technique, which enabled arrays of greater spot density and more accurate detection of genes. This advance enabled it to pursue large-scale comparative studies of gene expression in different tissues or states and reveal pathophysiology. Furthermore, the use of bioinformatics tools became a necessity for interpreting the vast amount of data generated by such microarrays. Machine learning algorithms improved the interpretation of such complex data significantly and identified patterns of correlation in the gene expression profiles. These advancements, besides making microarrays increasingly useful, also laid the groundwork for further progress in personalized medicine and targeted therapies. During the last couple of years, the incorporation of artificial intelligence (AI) and big data analysis has been yet another milestone in microarray research.

These technologies have transformed traditional methods to enable researchers to tap into the large volumes of data generated from microarrays. AI approaches, combined with network biology, provide quantitative models for the identification of novel anticancer targets and the design of upcoming drug candidates, as highlighted in recent studies on the topic (You et al., 2022). Additionally, the increasing focus on big data in healthcare is evidence of a deeper movement toward research that relies more on data, especially genomic data and its relevance to personalized medicine. As further advancements are made, the use of robust algorithms helps navigate the intricacies of biomolecular datasets, effectively addressing challenges in this complex research field, as noted in current debates concerning big data's role in healthcare (Hassan et al., 2022). These milestones characterize the ongoing progress of microarrays toward a new period of precision and individualization of gene expression profiling.

5.1.3. Evolution of Applications in Genomics

The generation of genomics applications has, in turn, been strongly impelled by the progress of high-throughput technologies, particularly in the case of microarrays and gene expression profiling. Microarrays originally provided scientists with the option to take into account the expression levels of thousands of genes simultaneously, enabling better comprehension of complex biological processes. With the advancement of technology, more recent methods , such as RNA sequencing, have emerged that offer even more precise and detailed information about gene expression patterns. In contrast to microarrays, with the drawback of pre-existing knowledge of gene sequences, RNA sequencing enables one to detect novel transcripts and splicing events, thus broadening the scope of genomic studies. This transition shows how technology development enables deeper biological inquiry, transforming raw genetic data into interpretive models of biology needed to dissect multilayered cellular mechanisms. Emerging from these technological foundations, spatially resolved transcriptomics has evolved into a critical innovation enabling researchers to map gene expression in the spatial context of tissues. This new approach combines single-cell RNA sequencing; its high-throughput capability with positional data obtained with techniques like *in situ* hybridization. Through such techniques, researchers can now investigate cellular heterogeneity and microenvironmental contributions to gene expression more thoroughly. For instance, novel imaging technologies allow for targeting of gene transcripts to specific cellular compartments, elucidating functional relationships that were previously obscured. This innovation not only enhances the resolution at which genomic data is read but also bridges the gap between abstract genomic data and functional biological networks, showcasing dynamic interaction between genes and their spatial environment within a living organism (Liao et al., 2020).

Furthermore, the use of genomics tools within clinic settings showcases the revolutionary ability of these technologies. For example, single-cell RNA sequencing has been employed to delineate tumor microenvironments and identify significant transcriptional heterogeneity between cancer cells and interaction with the surrounding stroma and immune cells (Tirosh et al., 2016). Such data are significant for the development of targeted therapies and the improvement of patient outcomes by refining therapies based on the individual tumor environment. This development highlights the move from conventional population-based genomic methods to the more sophisticated, single-cell view that addresses within-individual variation in the processes of disease. With advancements in techniques ongoing, the fusion of multi-omics data, where genomic, transcriptomic, and proteomic data are integrated, will improve our understanding of complex biological systems further, benefiting research as well as clinical applications in genomics (Figure 5.6).

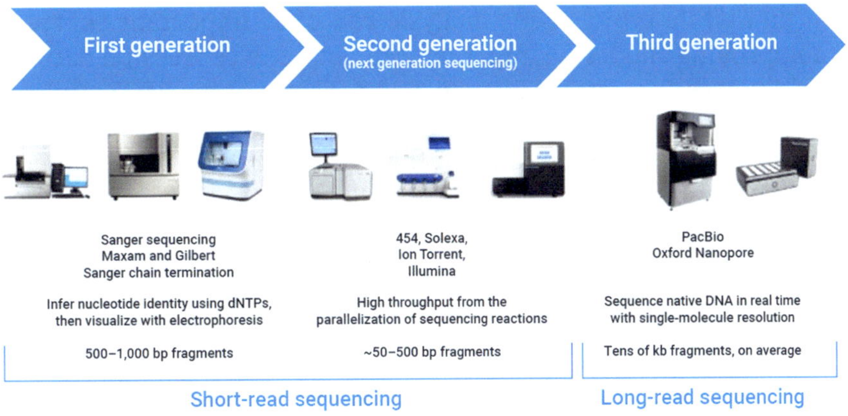

Figure 5.6. The evolution of DNA sequencing tools.

Source: https://www.pacb.com/wp-content/uploads/img_evolution_of_sequencing_technology-1.png.

5.2. Principles of Microarray Functionality

Microarray operation is based on the ability to conduct demanding gene expression profiling for thousands of genes simultaneously. This high-density tool enables researchers to determine differential expression of genes among a series of biological samples under a variety of experimental conditions. Labeled cDNA or RNA hybridization to a microarray with probes complementary to specific genes enables researchers to measure the intensity of fluorescence corresponding to the level of gene expression. The key to microarray activity is in its design, which is usually comprised of hundreds of thousands of oligonucleotide probes that enable the simultaneous examination of many genes, ultimately determining patterns of gene expression that reflect cellular response to environmental stress or state of disease. Microarrays have therefore become an indispensable item in genomics, allowing for the understanding of biological complexity and pathophysiology. One of the most important elements of microarray data analysis is the discovery of differentially expressed genes (DEGs), which seeks to enlighten the researcher regarding particular pathways or biological processes under stress within the conditions being investigated. Techniques , such as statistical analysis are employed to discover significant alterations in gene expression, which typically utilize a threshold of parameters , such as fold change and p-value thresholds. Interestingly, in studies of illnesses like repeated benign paroxysmal positional vertigo (BPPV), microarray experiments have isolated groups of DEGs that are useful in the study of disease mechanisms. For instance, one such study identified 39 DEGs with particular biological functions related to metabolic processes and immune responses, noting the utility of microarray technology to unravel complex disease pathways (Oh et al., 2023). It guides downstream research work by propelling hypothesis creation and further experimental validation. Besides, the analytical phase of microarray work tends to rely on sophisticated bioinformatics tools to unravel the extensive datasets generated via experimentation. Exploratory statistical methods, involving multivariate techniques , such as PCA, are used in dimensionality reduction of microarray data and thus the complex gene expression profiles into interpretable conclusions. By clustering genes based on expression patterns, researchers can identify correlations between clusters and the biological processes they represent. For example, studies have shown that while typical gene analysis can offer important expression changes, PCA application helps in improving clustering interpretation for gene expression data sets, particularly in the case of yeast gene expression during diauxic shifts (Sahoo et al., 2023). In the end, microarray functionality methodology represents a synergistic blend of computational and experimental approaches that is directed at refining valuable biological information, thus validating the core position of microarrays in modern genomic science (Figure 5.7).

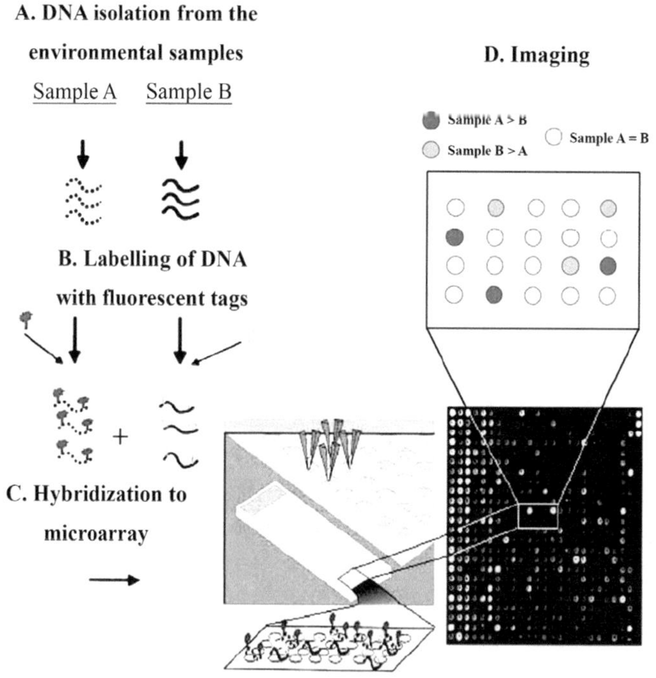

Figure 5.7. Principle of a microarray.

Source: https://www.researchgate.net/profile/Charles-Greer/publication/225557613/figure/fig4/AS:302858818867205@1449218577267/Principle-of-a-microarray.png.

5.2.1. Basic Components of a Microarray

Microarrays are the standard tools for gene expression profiling, which consist of thousands of DNA probes placed in a highly ordered manner on a solid surface. The probes are specially designed to hybridize with complementary sequences from RNA or cDNA samples. The two principal types of microarrays are cDNA microarrays and oligonucleotide microarrays, which differ primarily in their probe content. cDNA microarrays employ longer fragments of cDNA that can be up to whole genes, which is helpful when probing the expression of genes at a greater level. Oligonucleotide microarrays employ brief, man-made DNA molecules, which give greater specificity and allow greater precision in the detection of individual gene transcripts. This structural foundation is what enables microarrays to cope with large datasets, allowing for the examination of gene expression under numerous conditions and treatments all at the same time.

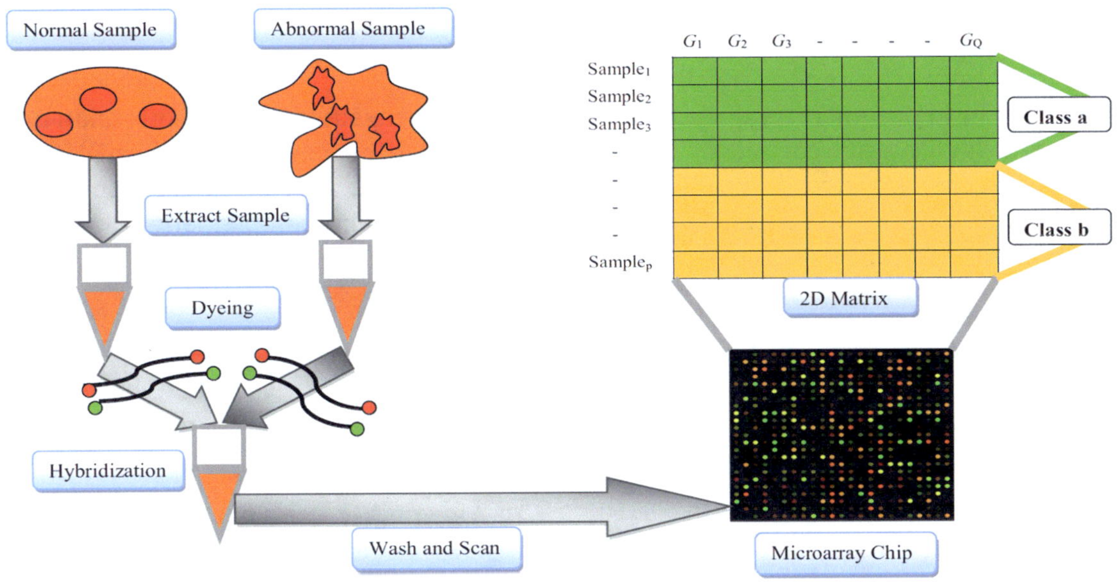

Figure 5.8. Basic concept of microarray chip formation and microarray extraction.

Source: https://www.researchgate.net/profile/Pratyay-Kuila/publication/363798250/figure/fig4/AS:11431281128954828@1679454734245/Basic-concept-of-microarray-chip-formation-and-extraction-of-microarray-data.png.

The functional component of the microarray is also equally significant, as it addresses the methods of sample preparation, hybridization, and detection. After the probe-carrying surface is created, the sample RNA is reverse-transcribed into labeled cRNA or cDNA, where targeted tagging optimizes detection. Unbound molecules are washed away after hybridization and the remaining hybridized strands are analyzed using fluorescence or other detection methods. This quantification step, based on how strong the received signal is, aids in the determination of levels of expression for the genes of interest. Technological innovations in imaging have also improved this step further to enhance the resolution and sensitivity of the outcomes. The combination of these factors ensures microarrays can provide accurate and high-throughput data used to analyze complex biological systems. Microarray technology is extremely challenging within the field of data analysis, primarily the interpretation of vast amounts of data generated through gene expression profiling. Probably one of the most significant steps in the analysis is the application of bioinformatics tools and statistical methods in the identification of differentially expressed genes that are critical to applications in biomarker identification and cancer diagnosis. Classical statistical analysis has been employed to analyze the data; nonetheless, applications of machine learning algorithms are on the rise as a means of enhancing accuracy in classification and reducing classification time. These sophisticated techniques, through the support of advanced algorithms, are capable of dealing with the dimensionality inherent in microarray data and thus enable a more sophisticated understanding of gene interaction and expression patterns. With improvements in microarray technology, so does data analysis for ensuing data, which holds immense promise for genomics and personalized medicine research in the future (Zhang et al., 2021; Hatim, 2022) (Figure 5.8).

5.2.2. Mechanism of Hybridization

Hybridization is the key to microarray operation, the essential reagents for gene expression profiling. Hybridization is the genetic reaction by which single-stranded nucleic acids, either DNA or RNA, anneal to complementary strands under right conditions. Target sequences are immobilized on a solid support, usually a glass slide, in microarray technology, and complementary fluorescently labeled probes are added.

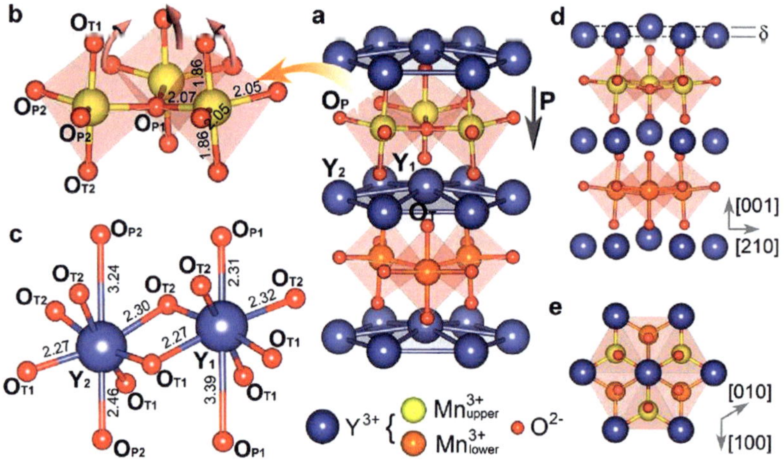

Figure 5.9. Atomic mechanism of hybridization.

Source: https://external-content.duckduckgo.com/iu/?u=https%3A%2F%2Fth.bing.com%2Fth%2Fid%2FOIP.UXWxvZZ1IczZUUPO_KY1xgHaEV%3Fr%3D0%26cb%3Dthvnextc1%2 6pid%3DApi&f=1&ipt=4ed6d1eb046382af54 62cddbde1231360536170 2e28c9bda7f2dfe8717f0d5c4.

The extent of hybridization is regulated by the specificity and stability of the binding interactions. Temperature and ionic conditions are tightly regulated to permit hybridization only by complementary sequences and reduce non-specific contacts. Thus, successful nucleic acid hybridization underlies the reliability of microarray data, enabling one to accurately quantify gene expression levels under varied conditions and time points. In applied research, hybridization is crucial to analyze gene expression profiles against various stimuli or environmental pressures. For instance, studies of microRNA expression are able to elucidate plant development and stress-response mechanisms. In a fascinating example, arsenic-stressed *Brassica juncea* microarray profiling indicated 69 miRNAs belonging to 18 families demonstrated differential expression based on hybridization findings (Srivastava et al., 2012). The results demonstrate the significance of hybridization in defining the ways individual miRNAs affect significant developmental processes and stress reactions. By being able to effectively use hybridization to quantify gene expression changes, researchers can uncover intricate networks of regulation in cells, providing valuable information regarding plant biology and stress resistance. In addition, the interaction of the hybridization mechanism with epigenetic alterations further illustrates the intricacy of gene regulation. For example, investigations of early-life trauma have found that DNA methylation patterns regulate gene expression, which can be quantitated by microarray hybridization techniques (Benoît et al., 2012). In these experiments, some level of promoter methylation correlates with alterations in gene expression genome-wide, due to the sophisticated role of hybridization in studying not only pure genetic sequences but their epigenetic regulation. Such findings underscore the utility of hybridization as a broad-purpose methodology in molecular biology, allowing researchers to examine the dynamic interplay between genetic and epigenetic factors that affect organism development and environmental challenge response (Figure 5.9).

5.2.3. Data Acquisition and Analysis Methods

Data acquisition is at the core of successful microarray and gene expression profiling usage. Given the high levels of gene expression data generated using different experimentation techniques, the challenge really lies in how this data can be organized systematically and combined. Public databases , such as the NCBI Sequence Read Archive (SRA), are valuable repositories where raw reads of RNA-sequencing experiments are kept. But it becomes even more complex when dealing with microarray data, as the absence of standardized submission protocols leads to a variety of data formats. This complicates the process even further, necessitating specially crafted instruments to ease the process of acquiring data. The development of software like COMMAND_> is an option, making the process of searching, downloading, and re-annotating gene expression experiments and preparing them for extensive analysis simpler. Following effective data acquisition, the analysis phase becomes a focal point and assists in the extraction of relevant information from complex gene expression profiles. This comprises rigorous statistical tests for the identification of differentially expressed genes and conducting functional analysis, all of which are quality-dependent on the data acquired. Novel advanced methods , such as single-sample gene set enrichment analysis (ssGSEA), have been devised to identify the biological significance of gene expression profiles. By avoiding limitations in background noise and cross-correlation between genes, such methods enhance the promise to acquire functional gene expression signatures (FGES). Not only do these act as disease biomarkers, for instance, cancer, but they also provide useful information on cellular processes. The validation of FGES by established criteria emphasizes the demand for quality control within the data analysis pipeline. The increasing heterogeneity of gene expression data necessitates the development of high-level analysis platforms that can handle diverse research questions. While scientists are grappling with the heterogeneity of data formats and methodology, it is more necessary to integrate gene expression datasets. Advances that facilitate such integration over recent periods have the tendency to draw on specialized software that is able to handle heterogeneity of data formats, thereby making them compatible for comparative analysis. Surpassing the acquisition itself, emphasis on bioinformatics tools streamlining the integration process also reflects a greater realization of the importance of merging holistic datasets into biological inquiry. As highlighted by studies, extensive scrutiny of signature quality by technical and biological standards provides a solid basis for taking the transcriptomics discipline forward to enable researchers to tackle increasingly demanding biological queries with assurance (Moretto et al., 2019; Shi, 2024) (Figure 5.10).

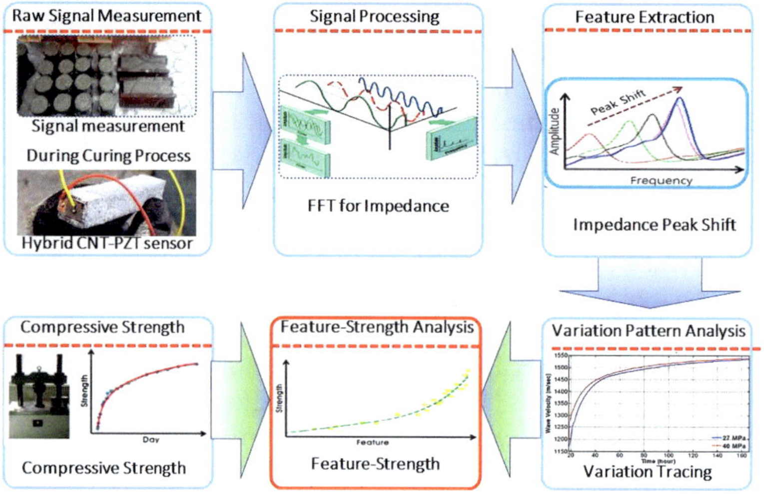

Figure 5.10. Data acquisition and analysis process.

Source: https://www.researchgate.net/publication/351998375/figure/fig4/AS:11431281406617051@1745736443998/Data-acquisition-and-analysis-process.tif.

5.3. Types of Microarrays

Microarrays are also critical tools in genomic studies, which enable one to analyze up to thousands of genes at once. Among all microarrays, the expression microarray is a core use of gene expression profiling. Microarrays play a key role in the quantification of mRNA, hence helping to unveil underlying biological processes governing cellular response. Using complementary DNA (cDNA) or oligonucleotide probes, expression microarrays are capable of detecting gene activities under various conditions, such as disease conditions or developmental stages. Furthermore, the inclusion of big data, like that in the Chinese Glioma Genome Atlas (CGGA), enhances the study of gene regulation and expression nuances between some tumor subtypes, aiding researchers further in their understanding of glioma biology and possible treatments (Zhao et al., 2021). Another important category of microarray is comparative genomic hybridization (CGH) microarray, which is particularly valuable for the detection of genomic aberrations , such as copy number variations (CNVs) and chromosomal deletions or duplications. Unlike expression microarrays that quantify gene expression, CGH microarrays are used to detect differences in DNA content between normal and disease tissue. This feature is critical in oncogenomics as it allows scientists to identify genetic alterations that relate to cancer formation. Advanced bioinformatics software, such as the limma package, facilitates the analysis of CGH microarray data using various statistical models and visualization strategies (Matthew et al., 2015). With these technologies, scientists are capable of making comprehensive maps of genomic alterations, which lead to a better understanding of disease mechanisms as well as possible drug targets. Finally, microRNA (miRNA) microarrays have become extremely popular during the past decade due to the fact that they are involved in post-transcriptional gene expression regulation. They can be employed for profiling miRNA expression levels, which will uncover the biological processes and pathologies that these small non-coding RNAs participate in. As they are involved in metabolic control, cell proliferation, and apoptosis, it is essential to explore their expression as a tool to understand complex pathologies like cancer. The combination of miRNA microarrays with expression microarrays has the potential to generate a more complete view of gene regulatory networks, ultimately enhancing the interpretation of gene expression data in terms of global regulatory processes. As researchers continue to uncover the complexity of gene regulatory processes, miRNA microarrays will undoubtedly be an integral part of developing personalized medicine and therapeutic strategies (Figure 5.11).

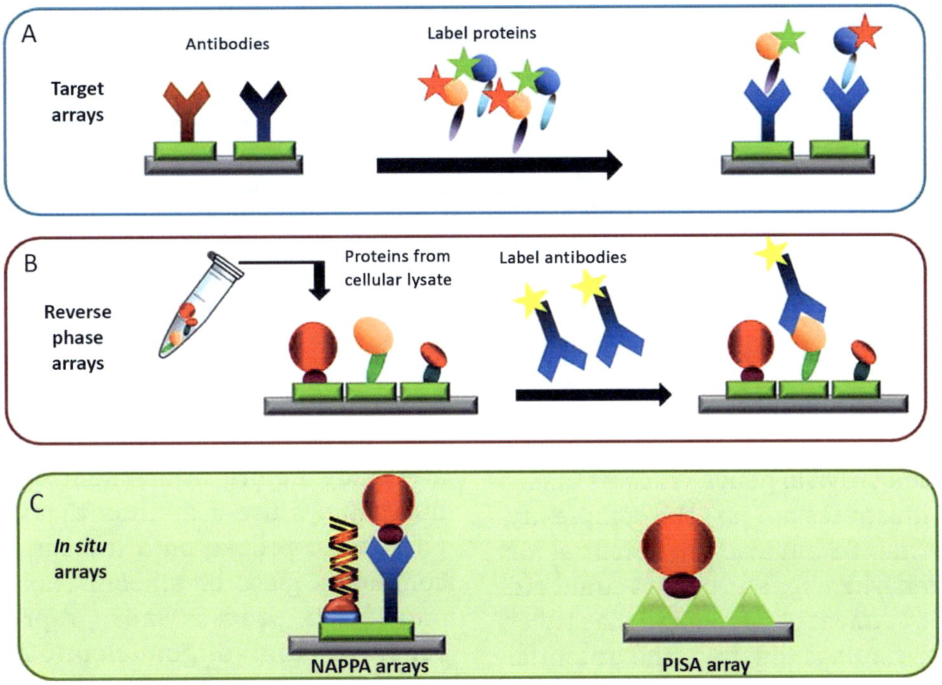

Figure 5.11. Major types of microarrays.

Source: https://www.researchgate.net/profile/Paula-Diez-3/publication/287308382/figure/fig2/AS:667601432768514@1536179993096/Major-types-of-protein-microarrays-A-targeted-protein-arrays-B-reverse-phase.png.

5.3.1. cDNA Microarrays

The advent of cDNA microarrays has revolutionized gene expression profiling so that scientists can assess the expression level of hundreds of genes simultaneously. The high-throughput system employs complementary DNA (cDNA) that has been synthesized from messenger RNA (mRNA) to generate a global profile of gene activity in a sample. Among the key aspects of cDNA microarray technology is the attention to detail in designing and assembling the arrays themselves, such attention being equally given in the selection of target genes and the fabrication processes adopted. Experimental design is necessary because it determines the conditions of the experiment through which the gene expression data are gathered and influences subsequent data analysis. This advanced approach demonstrates how cDNA microarrays facilitate not merely the subdivision of control processes in various biological conditions but also the comparative analysis of transcriptome variability between organisms and states, as exemplified in plant development and plant physiology studies (Alba et al., 2004). Also, cDNA microarray application to disease research, for example, in hematologic disorders like myelodysplastic syndromes (MDS), provides evidence of their promise for clinical use. By comparison of the expression patterns in neutrophils in MDS patients, researchers have made significant findings regarding the heterogeneity of gene regulation of this class of disorders. For instance, the application of cDNA microarrays has indicated the differential expression of RAB20 and ARG1 genes, which are involved in cell proliferation, as well as down-expression of cell survival genes , such as COX2. This research illustrates not just the complexity that is present in MDS but also the potential for identifying biomarker signatures that could aid diagnosis and treatment of patients (Pellagatti et al., 2004). Such findings illustrate the potential of cDNA microarrays to bridge the gap between clinical utility and basic research, elucidating the disease pathogenesis. The cDNA microarray promise is beyond its application for trivial profiling and as a robust platform for examining gene interactions and networks. It allows one to generate large amounts of data suitable for advanced bioinformatics analysis, enabling the discovery of regulatory networks and gene interactions. Most notably, cDNA microarray data integration with other omics technologies, such as proteomics and metabolomics, promotes a systems biology approach to studying biological processes. Such an integrated perspective is particularly necessary when characterizing complex traits, such as plant fruit development, where many genetic and environmental factors interact. Comparative genomics analysis of transcriptomic profiles across species further accentuates the comparative genomics point of view and allows for clarification of evolutionary relationships. With the ongoing advancement of cDNA microarrays, their integration into gene expression profiling paradigms will likely yield novel biological findings and therapeutic strategies in various areas of study (Alba et al., 2004).

5.3.2. Oligonucleotide Microarrays

The development of oligonucleotide microarrays has contributed in a major way to the study of gene expression profiling, offering a precious resource for researchers to study the transcriptome of numerous organisms. The microarrays facilitate high-throughput gene expression analysis through the use of short, single-stranded oligonucleotide probes that can hybridize to their corresponding mRNA targets. In contrast to spotted microarrays, in which probes are made before attachment, oligonucleotide microarrays use a method that enables direct printing of probes onto the surface of a solid, commonly glass or silicon. This advancement makes the process more reproducible and sensitive, and oligonucleotide microarrays hence make a significant contribution in research where accurate measurements of gene expression are most important. Second, the ability to tailor these arrays to specific genes of interest makes them maximally useful in a wide range of applications in genetics and molecular biology. Despite the advantages of oligonucleotide microarrays, researchers must consider the importance of appropriate normalization methods to ensure validation of their results. Normalization diminishes systematic technical variation that may hide biological information from gene expression data that is key in achieving meaningful comparisons among samples. Other normalization methods, such as loess and generalized Procrustes analysis, have been shown to significantly impact the statistical efficiency of these analyses. For instance, studies indicate that using methods like loess is capable of substantially reducing standard deviations while rendering detection of differential expression more sensitive, thus leading to more authentic conclusions about biological change (Meyer et al., 2012).

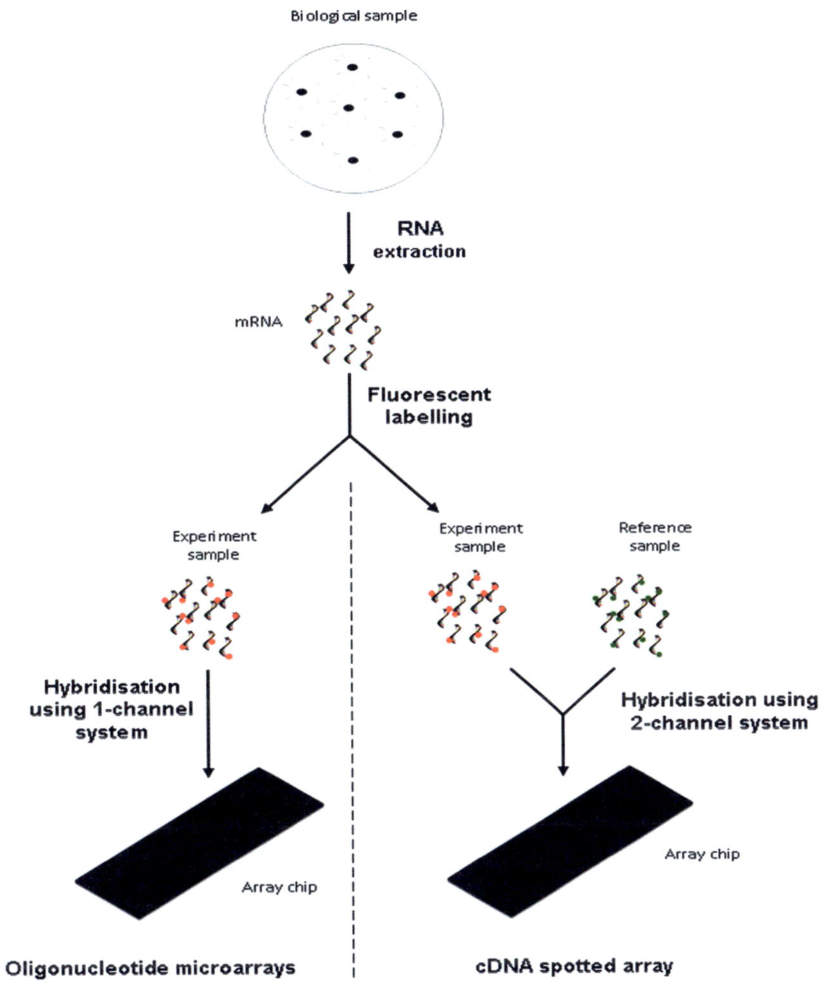

Figure 5.12. Oligonucleotide microarrays.

Source: https://www.researchgate.net/profile/Bichitrananda-Patra-2/publication/350008072/figure/fig3/AS:1000490619916291@1615546960970/The-microarray-experiments-Oligonucleotide-versus-cDNA-arrays.png.

All these attempts to further improve normalization techniques further increase oligonucleotide microarray capabilities, which render them an indispensable tool in today's genomic research.

Furthermore, the versatility of oligonucleotide microarrays to analyze gene expression in different environmental stresses further accentuates their applicability in cell biology and genetics research. By providing a detailed description of a cell's transcriptome, such microarrays enable scientists to ascertain how various stimuli or conditions affect gene expression at the genome level (Moreno & Pérez, 2016). This makes them an indispensable tool for studies that examine cellular reactions to extrinsic stimuli, where scientists can make connections between patterns of gene expression and biological functions. In spite of the emergence of a new generation of sequencing technologies as alternatives, the cost savings and versatility of oligonucleotide microarrays ensure they remain a worthwhile asset to gene expression profiling. Their ability to produce robust data with less pre-existing knowledge about the target organism highlights the ongoing applicability of microarrays to genomics (Figure 5.12).

5.3.3. SNP Microarrays

The advent of Single-nucleotide polymorphism (SNP) microarrays has revolutionized the genetic research environment, particularly in genomic variation and disease association studies. SNP microarrays leverage the capability of high-throughput technology to analyze thousands to millions of SNPs in the genome concurrently. This enables the detection of genetic markers associated with various diseases and traits, and this has been one of the significant contributions towards personalized medicine approaches. Because of their efficiency, these platforms allow not only the full profiling of genetic polymorphisms but also enhance our understanding of complex diseases that may be influenced by multiple genetic factors. The integration of SNP microarray information with other molecular profiling tools has opened the way towards further understanding the intricate relationship between genotype and phenotype and thus the development of targeted therapeutic strategies. Moreover, SNP microarray technical efficiency is enhanced through optimized hybridization conditions that minimize variability and maximize genotyping quality. Advances in probe design and the application of high fluid velocity during hybridization ensure reduced background noise and maximum signal intensity, a prerequisite to distinguish SNP variants. Studies have also shown that employing robust probes can reduce inter-experimental variation, which is necessary while comparing data from different studies. It is equally necessary to employ weaker probes that are specifically designed for detecting SNPs, since this enables better specificity in detecting minor genetic variations. These technological improvements show how ongoing improvements in microarray technology have a direct impact on the reproducibility and reliability of genotyping assays, thereby solidifying their status as an absolute tool of necessity within genomic medicine (Singh, 2013). The clinical use of SNP microarrays is most clearly achieved in oncology, where they are central platforms for uncovering the genetic basis of tumors. For instance, in ovarian cancer research, SNP microarrays have been employed for profiling some of the genetic alterations, including copy number alterations and gene expression alterations in chemosensitive and chemoresistant tumor tissues. Global profiling by scientists enables them to identify potential biomarkers for intrinsic resistance to treatment, thereby directing the treatment and improving the prognosis of the patient. The integration of SNP information with other genomic information, like miRNA and methylation signatures, also better explains the intricate biology of cancer, giving information on the pathways that manage tumor growth and treatment response. The inference of these findings is that SNP microarrays not just enhance our understanding of cancer but also pave the way for more personalized and effective therapeutic regimens (Koti et al., 2012).

5.4. Applications of Microarrays in Research

Microarray technology has revolutionized the field of genomics, particularly in the study of gene expression patterns. Through microarray technology, thousands of genes are measured at the transcriptome level simultaneously, which aids in the creation of a comprehensive understanding of cellular function and regulation. Microarrays find their main application in the categorization of cancer. For example, large-scale experiments have demonstrated microarrays' ability to discriminate among tumor subtypes based on gene expression profiles, which emphasizes their use in personalized medicine approaches. This precision in cancer diagnosis not only aids diagnosis but also directs the approach to treatment on the basis of individual patients, enhancing therapeutic outcome and reducing unnecessary interventions. Beyond cancer research, microarrays find applications in complex disease and biological process research.

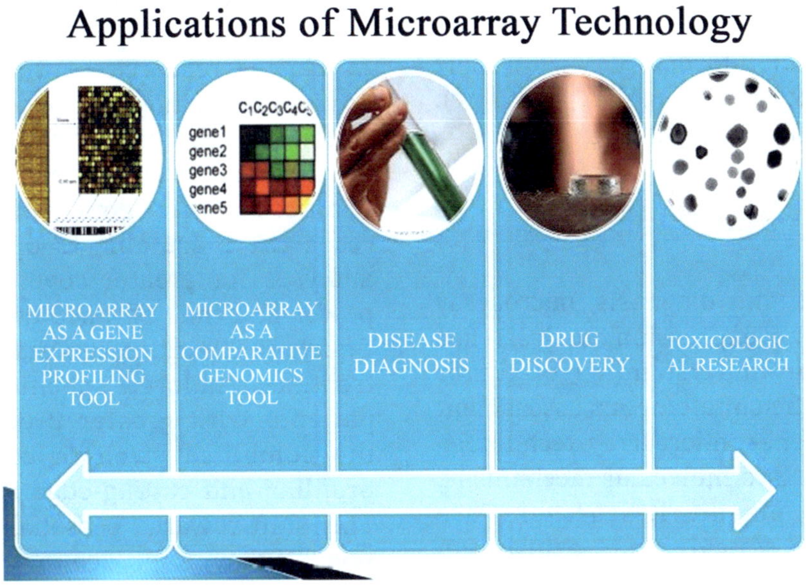

Figure 5.13. Applications of microarrays in research.

Source: https://i.pinimg.com/736x/74/c1/97/74c197af77daa9bfc4c42303c83c398f.jpg.

The ability to profile gene expression under different conditions or treatments allows researchers to identify potential biomarkers for diabetes, autoimmune diseases, and neurodegenerative conditions. Microarray technology also allows the study of interactions among genes as well as regulatory networks, allowing researchers to understand the pathophysiological mechanisms. The implication of this study extends beyond the identification of potential target therapies, in which particular genes responsible for the disease mechanism are studied in more detail. Microarrays, therefore, are an important tool in unraveling the complex link between genes and disease, leading the way towards new medical treatments. The Chinese Glioma Genome Atlas (CGGA) is a good example of combining microarrays with comprehensive genomic analysis. This platform accumulates large collections of genomic information, such as microarray data from almost 2000 glioma specimens, and offers researchers easy access to the necessary information for research purposes. By supplying extensive clinical information along with mRNA and DNA methylation profiles, CGGA overcomes accessibility barriers in functional genomics research. The interactive tools presented within the portal enable users to perform integrated analyses, including gene correlation and survival analysis among specific glioma subtypes. Such technologies highlight the broader impact of microarrays in scientific inquiry, facilitating collaborations and accelerating discoveries that drive increases in understanding tumor biology and potential treatment alternatives (Zhao et al., 2021). In addition, microarray data analysis helps to deal with high dimensionality and sparsity of gene information, highlighting the most significant genes to explore (Almugren & Alshamlan, 2019) (Figure 5.13).

5.4.1. Cancer Research and Diagnostics

In cancer research and diagnosis, microarray application to gene expression analysis has revolutionized our understanding of tumor biology. Through the simultaneous assessment of thousands of genes, microarray technology gives us an insight into molecular mechanisms of cancer development. Researchers are able to identify typical gene expression profiles that correlate with specific types of cancers, stages, or treatment outcomes. This throughput technology has made possible tumor classification, facilitation of stratification of patients by their prognostic signature and presumed response to treatment. The ongoing development and improvement of microarray technology platforms, such as the Affymetrix GeneChip, are evidence of a resolve to better diagnose and overall understanding of cancer biology in the context of genomics (Milchevskaya et al., 2017). These advances in microarray technology are matched by RNA sequencing data integration, which provides a more global view of gene expression. Many consortium projects , such as The Cancer Genome Atlas (TCGA) and the Genotype-Tissue Expression (GTEx) project, have yielded vast amounts of RNA sequencing data. This data can be mined to gain deeper knowledge of gene functions and their implications in cancer development. However, most existing expression analysis tools contain built-in shortcomings in addressing the unique needs of experimental biologists. The construction of platforms , such as GEPIA, with user-modifiable capabilities for differential expression analysis and patient survival analysis, facilitates the accessibility and usability of this enormous data and dissolves the gap between complex genomic findings and translational use in cancer diagnosis (Tang et al., 2017). As cancer research continues, the need for integration of microarrays and next-generation genomic technologies cannot be overstated. Through accurate probe set definition and project-specific gene annotation models, researchers are able to optimize microarray analyses for greater coverage and statistical power and thus advance the field of oncology. Oncology clinicians can diagnose and provide treatment tailored specifically to individual patients with greater precision by merging the combined strength of gene expression profiling and cutting-edge data analysis tools. This shift towards personalized medicine is a revolutionary approach that not only enhances therapeutic outcomes but also enhances the understanding of the intricate biology of cancer. As the field continues to advance, further collaboration between computational scientists and biomedicine researchers will have a critical role in unravelling the intricacy of cancer as well as enhancing diagnostic strategies.

5.4.2. Drug Discovery and Development

The face of drug discovery and development has been radically altered by the advent of microarray technology for the detailed profiling of gene expression. This new approach enables scientists to explore the intricate patterns of gene expression under a variety of conditions and thereby enables the identification of putative biomarkers for disease stratification as well as monitoring treatment responses. With microarrays, the transcriptomes of immune cells are analyzed, and researchers can detect differentially expressed genes that may influence drug efficacy and safety. This technology also allows direct sorting of immune cell subsets from whole blood, as recently shown, which provides a more precise snapshot of the biological factors present in patient populations. Therefore, the application of microarray data in the clinic is going to enhance the relative value of drug development programs by making the therapeutic intervention more specific to the individual's own genome (Letzkus et al., 2014). In addition to biomarker detection, microarray technology is also essential in solving the problem of individual variability in drug responses.

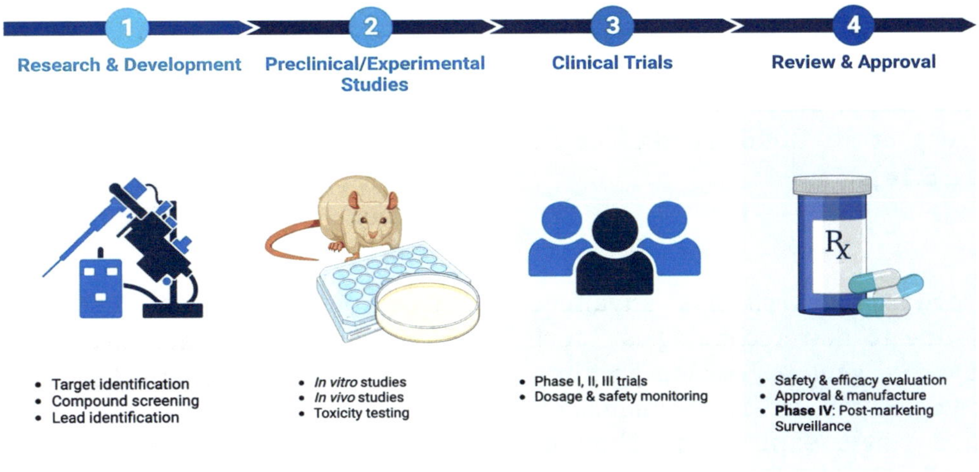

Figure 5.14. Drug discovery and development.

Source: https://pharmacologymentor.com/wp-content/uploads/2023/04/Drug-Discovery-and-Development.jpg.

Genetic variations, like the presence of cytochrome P-450 variants, can greatly influence the metabolism of patients to drugs, resulting in differences in effectiveness and tolerability. Through the use of the strength offered by microarrays, clinicians would be able to determine the genetic profile of patients, thus individualizing therapeutic regimens that respond to their individual requirements. Yet, as observed in the literature, the intrinsic complexity and presence of noise in high-throughput data require robust analysis methodologies. Emphasizing the importance of rigorous data processing, researchers suggest that the combination of gene expression profiling with model-based strategies using mathematical models can give reliable and faithful predictions of drug responses. This powerful synergy not only maximizes the drug discovery pipeline but also offsets the risks of adverse drug reactions (Herwig et al., 2006). The horizon of pharmaceutical research becomes increasingly intertwined with the principles of systems biology, a paradigm of systems thinking that redefines our understanding of biological systems. By merging the high-throughput capabilities of microarrays with the strategies of systems biology, scientists are able to study changes in gene expression within the context of entire biological pathways and expose intricate regulatory networks that govern cellular processes. This platform not only highlights prospective avenues that may be addressed during drug discovery but also enables the derivation of predictive models that can model treatment responses in individual patients. With increased advances in systems biology, scientists are increasingly enabled to investigate intricate interactions among genes, proteins, and the environment, ultimately achieving more effective and targeted treatments. These new methods have the potential to transform the drug discovery and development paradigm towards more data-informed and evidence-based clinical decision-making (Herwig et al., 2006; Letzkus et al., 2014) (Figure 5.14).

5.4.3. Study of Genetic Disorders

Genetic disorder research has advanced dramatically due to new technologies , such as microarrays and gene expression profiling. These technologies can screen for thousands of genes in a single experiment, showing patterns missed by traditional genetic studies. They are excellent tools for finding specific expressions of individual genes in individual disorders. For instance, by the detailed analysis of gene expression data, there are significant correlations that can be drawn between certain genetic markers and susceptibility to particular conditions.

As a result, integration of microarrays in genetic studies not only allows for enhanced comprehension of genetic conditions but also paves the way for more personalized medicine approaches with the prospect of treatments designed to fit individual genetic makeup, thereby ensuring maximum therapeutic efficacy. In the context of effective prediction of disease, the integration of machine learning algorithms with microarray data transforms the situation of genetic disorder research. Using advanced classifiers , such as Gaussian Naive Bayes and Decision Trees, scientists can identify influential gene sets involved in disease susceptibility. The method is based on feature selection, where major genes are ranked according to their statistical significance in disease incidence. This rigorous selection procedure reinforces the promise of microarrays not only in symptom detection but also in prognostic capacity. Furthermore, research demonstrates that consistent evaluation procedures and cross-validation methods can improve model quality, suggesting that strategic utilization of these algorithms is the key to revolutionary advancements in accurate prediction of genetic disorders and the design of preventive interventions, subverting conventional paradigms for diagnosis and treatment.

The hereditary basis of behavioral phenotypes, especially of anxiety disorders, also constitutes a significant area of research when it comes to studying genetic disorders. Selectively bred models , such as the bred High Responder (bHR) and bred Low Responder (bLR) rats, illustrate how genetically predisposed animals can express themselves in terms of certain behavioral phenotypes. By meta-analyzing microarray and RNA-Seq, researchers have identified discoveries about signature genes, such as Thyrotropin releasing hormone receptor (Trhr) and Uncoupling protein 2 (Ucp2), involved in mood control and energy metabolism. Results reflect not only the genetic complexity of behavior but also the practical implications of understanding human disorders. The research into microglial activation and the manner in which it is associated with neurodevelopment only continues to highlight the intricate interplay between genes and the environment in shaping response behavior, and hence the desire for research into the same to devise appropriate interventions for genetic disease (Verheijen & Sleegers, 2018; Venkata et al., 2024).

5.5. Advantages of Microarray Technology

Microarray technology offers profound advantages within the field of gene expression profiling, particularly with regard to enhancing the accuracy of disease diagnosis and treatment methods. Microarrays enable analysis of thousands of genes simultaneously, thus facilitating the possibility of developing a holistic view of gene expression profiles under different biological conditions. This is especially helpful for the identification of disease subtypes, as has been brought out by the development of gene expression profiles (GEPs) that can distinguish between aggressive lymphoma forms, like Burkitt Lymphoma and Diffuse Large B Cell Lymphoma. The application of GEP data has the potential to lead to maximally reclassified patients, tailored treatment approaches, and potentially better clinical outcomes, demonstrating the immediate effect microarray diagnostic capability has on therapeutic decision-making and patient care (Bouttell et al., 2023). Another shining advantage of microarray technology is the ability to analyze FFPE tissue samples, often the only remaining trace of biological material available for diagnostic testing. Conventional methods are limited by RNA degradation and modification during storage. The ability to recover and analyze gene expression using damaged samples is now provided by emerging genomic technologies, including the use of technologies like NanoString platforms. This technology not only widens the scope of microarrays but also broadens their application in the clinic, where scientists and clinicians can overcome sample quality restrictions. Therefore, microarray technology comes as a necessary piece of equipment for molecular studies, unlocking the door to knowledge regarding disease development and prognosis, especially when working with challenging sample types like FFPE (Manjunath et al., 2022). In addition to diagnostic and analytical benefits, microarray technology provides significant strengths in the context of high-throughput research environments. The capability for high-throughput analysis allows the study of gene expression across extensive conditions, resulting in greater speed in functional genomics. Comparative analysis via microarray analysis can be applied to unravel differential gene expression patterns between disease and health. This comparative power allows researchers to discover potential disease biomarkers, assess therapeutic targets, and uncover molecular mechanisms of pathologies. As such, microarray technology has become a critical tool in the arena of biomedical research, offering a platform for the thorough evaluation and manipulation of gene expression, through which our comprehension of complex biological systems is pushed further (Figure 5.15).

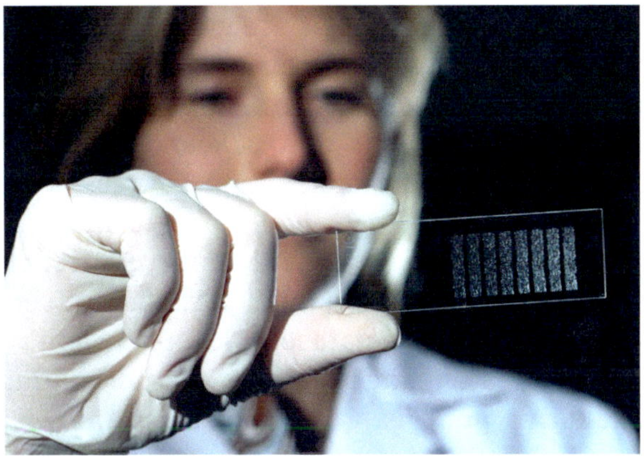

Figure 5.15. Advantages of microarray.

Source: https://cdn.britannica.com/40/262340-050-9FBD8959/Microarray-DNA-slide-genetics.jpg.

5.5.1. High-Throughput Capabilities

The emergence of high-throughput capability has revolutionized genomics science, particularly for microarrays and gene expression profiling. With these new technologies, researchers can study thousands of genes simultaneously, providing general insight into the complex regulatory networks operating in biological systems.

Utilizing these capabilities, researchers can effectively identify gene expression patterns associated with specific diseases and better understand cell responses to stimuli. This high-throughput approach minimizes the time and effort required to analyze specific genes and facilitates the rapid creation of strong datasets that can significantly enhance research outcomes. The ability to process high levels of data allowed discrimination among subtle variations in gene expression, which in turn accelerated diagnostic and treatment strategies for the combat of diseases, including parasitic diseases and cancers. With further development of bioinformatics, the integration of high-throughput data with computational models becomes progressively crucial. Next-generation sequencing and microarray technologies generate massive amounts of data, for which intelligent tools need to be used to make sense of it. Systems biology has been a crucial paradigm for which researchers can comprehend host-parasite interactions and cancer biology by combining multiple omics data sources. With the help of tools that enable one to map the intricate networks of interactions, researchers can identify patterns in data, perhaps not seen otherwise in huge datasets. High-throughput technologies enhance the potential to conduct exhaustive gene expression profile analyses, thus highlighting the multifunctional roles of genes in disease pathogenesis. The approach underscores the importance of transdisciplinary collaboration in realizing the complete potential of high-throughput technology in therapeutic research and personalized medicine. Clinical utility of high-throughput capacity extends beyond exploration into a significant contribution to personalized medicine development. As delimited in contemporary oncogenomics, the ability to analyze high-throughput gene expression information enables the stratification of cancer forms and the prediction of patient outcomes. The use of high-throughput methods enables the determination of individual biomarkers predicting therapeutic efficacy, thereby guiding clinical decision-making towards more tailored treatment protocols. Additionally, technological advancements in detection provide the greater sensitivity and resolution needed for the diagnosis and monitoring of various cancers. Most significantly, high-throughput capability not only enhances our understanding of disease pathogenesis but also allows for a rationale in the design of novel interventions that are adaptable to the unique genetic predisposition of the patient. This ability to translate genomic data into actionable clinical wisdom is the transformative power of high-throughput technology in modern medicine, with potential for novel innovations in patient care and management (Baianu, 2011; Jamshidi et al., 2015).

5.5.2. Comprehensive Gene Expression Profiling

Extensive gene expression profiling is an area that has radically transformed our understanding of the biological system, with the capacity to measure thousands of genes at the same time. Such high-dimensional analysis has a singular value in the clarification of the complex regulatory frameworks that control cell function and response to the environment. Microarray technology, as a foundation of gene expression profiling, facilitates scientists' ability to ask the entire transcriptome, which leads to knowing gene function, interaction, and expression dynamics. This is crucial for the discovery of disease biomarkers, understanding development processes, as well as the research of responses to environmental stressors. These in-depth profiles have provided the door through which targeted medicine is facilitated by referring to differential gene expression profiles that have the potential to guide therapeutic strategies, and thereby proving the necessity of standard methods of data analysis for sound conclusions in biology. Normalization methods are crucial to the accuracy of gene expression findings generated with the aid of microarrays. Successful normalization minimizes the effect of systematic technical variation, which is crucial if meaningful biological interpretation is to be derived from the data. Comparative evaluations on more recent methods of normalization were found to differ significantly in performance, and this influences the reliability of differential expression results. Techniques , such as loess, loessM, and generalized Procrustes analysis have proven to be superior options for buffering data against technical noise, offering improvements in sensitivity as well as inter-platform consistency of expression values. The ability to distinguish between actual biological changes and noise is imperative, especially in clinical practice, where precision is paramount.

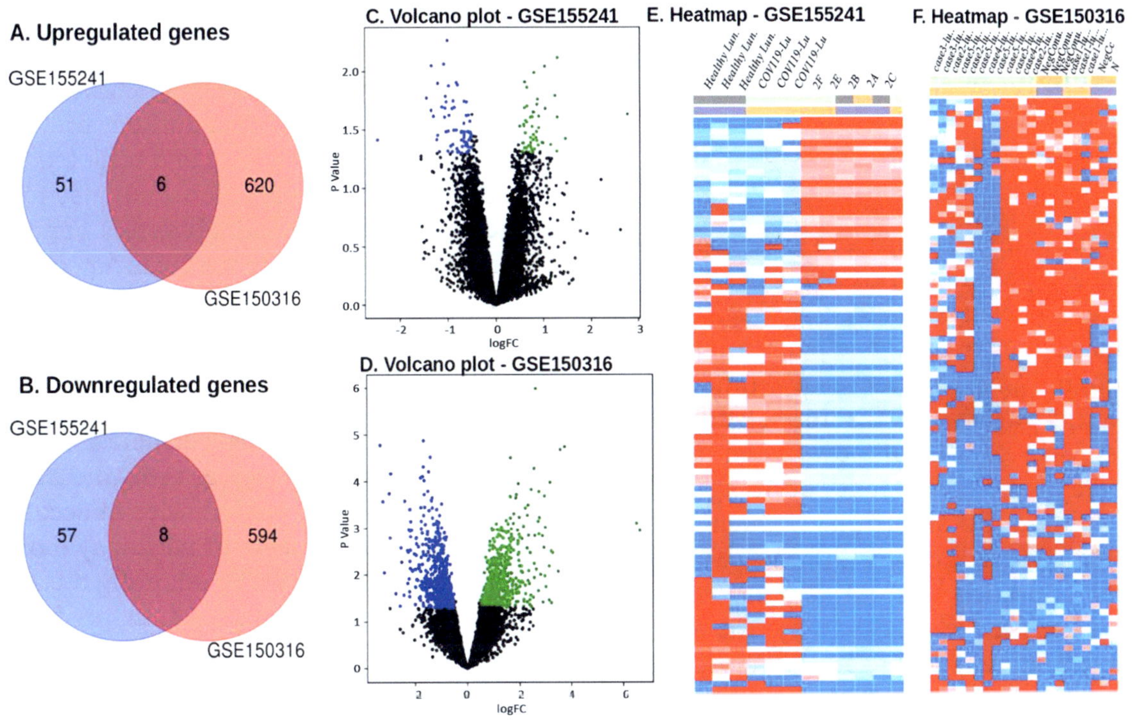

Figure 5.16. Computational gene expression profiling.

Source: https://external-content.duckduckgo.com/iu/?u= https%3A%2F%2Ftse4.mm.bing.net%2 Fth%2Fid%2FOIP.jBlGoIBnxK PL1T2hPF2hggHaE0%3Fr%3D0%26p id%3DApi&f=1&ipt= 9d300acb547be2feedffe4d53c44836 09eda7dd6421e463f81a3757d01b7de2b.

Thus, the judicious selection of normalization methods is an integral consideration in large-scale gene expression profiling for the guarantee of the integrity of results obtained from microarray experiments (Meyer et al., 2012). In addition to normalization, quantitative reverse transcription polymerase chain reaction (RT-qPCR) has also improved gene expression profiling capacity. The technology allows for the examination of specific mRNAs with great precision, even starting from extremely tiny sample inputs, making it a useful tool in studying molecular pathways in certain cellular settings. The combination of both microarray and RT-qPCR data enables a more comprehensive analysis that is appropriate for the identification and characterization of gene expression profiles between tissues or conditions. Notably, the employment of large-scale profiling techniques offers a deeper understanding of nephron heterogeneity and dominates the driving of diagnostic methodology for kidney diseases. Therefore, global gene expression profiling is not just a window onto basic biological processes but also a valuable resource for clinical diagnostics and drug development, an example of the potential resulting from concomitant advances in molecular biology (Cohen & Kretzler, 2002) (Figure 5.16).

5.5.3. Cost-Effectiveness Compared to Traditional Methods

The advent of microarrays and gene expression profiling is a paradigmatic era for personalized medicine, especially in cancer. Through the full-scale analysis of tumor gene expression, these technologies provide necessary information outside the purview of traditional diagnostic devices. One of the biggest advantages of microarrays is their cost-reducing ability when applied in situations , such as the treatment of breast cancer in India, where the standard approach to treatment is expensive and unwarranted chemotherapy. An analysis of cost-effectiveness based on a decision-analytic model revealed that gene expression profiling would identify approximately 40,000 patients annually who could safely avoid chemotherapy and therefore save its associated healthcare costs tied to overtreatment. This compelling evidence indicates that the use of gene expression profiling can yield substantial economic benefits along with enhanced patient outcomes through the application of specific therapies in response to individualized tumor profiles (Suresh et al., 2025). In contrast to the conventional treatment strategies that may rely heavily on blanket strategies of chemotherapy, gene expression profiling guarantees specificity because it selects merely those patients who will benefit from such measures. Such precision not only leads to enhanced healthcare outcomes but also decreases the economic burden on healthcare systems and patients in general. The study illustrated in the decision-analysis model proved a better cost-effectiveness, pointing out that the least costly gene expression test had an incremental cost-effectiveness ratio (ICER) that ranked it as a dominant strategy. On the contrary, traditional methods are of astronomical cost with no guarantee of improved prognostic accuracy or therapeutic benefit, necessitating a paradigm shift towards embracing newer and more efficient technologies in clinical practice (Suresh et al., 2025). In addition, the evolving culture of genetic profiling and targeted therapy is not for breast cancer alone, but also for other cancers like gastrointestinal cancers. For instance, with regard to late gastric cancer, biomarker profiling like that of vascular endothelial growth factor (VEGF-A) would delineate patients who would be suitable for anti-VEGF therapy, and thus tailor treatment protocols and potentially affect mortality rates. Nevertheless, the highly prohibitive cost of therapies using the traditional paradigm poses serious hurdles in accessibility and highlights the need for strikingly more cost-effective interventions. By adopting the strategic integration of gene expression profiling into treatment protocols, healthcare providers can optimize their treatments by making them wiser in how they use resources. This shift to cost-effective, personalized treatment modalities promises a sustainable healthcare model that is able to improve patient care without the excessive weight of cost constraints.

5.6. Limitations and Challenges

The application of microarrays for the profiling of gene expression in genomic science has several limitations and hindrances to achieving its full potential. The high dimensionality of the output data, for instance, can lead to overfitting when applying classical machine learning techniques. Classical methods struggle with the complex interactions between thousands of genes as they are not well equipped to handle high-dimensional vector spaces. As a result, it is difficult for scientists to extract useful biological information from the data since traditional methods of analysis will be unable to detect vital interactions necessary for the clarification of complex biological mechanisms. In an attempt to address this issue, scientists are now more inclined to explore quantum computing techniques, which ensure more computational power to manipulate and analyze high-scale gene expression data in a more effective manner (Akpinar et al., 2025). Another outstanding challenge of gene expression profiling is the technical limitations to determining functional gene expression signatures (FGES). While FGES are valuable sources of information as biomarkers for cancer diagnosis, their construction is marred with issues of background noise, gene cross-correlations, and the biological relevance of the resulting signatures. Not only is there variability within the gene expression measurement score measures themselves, but also within how scores correspond with clinical outcomes, as well. Additionally, the lack of standardization of FGES scores for testing can yield suboptimal and unstable results. More recently, these frailties have been met by proposals for validation pipelines utilizing a modified single-sample gene set enrichment analysis so that FGES quality can be ascertained in a more stringent and biologically sound way. This development gives emphasis to continuous improvement in techniques to increase the applicability of FGES in transcriptomic studies (Akpinar et al., 2025). Furthermore, interpretation of results from microarray studies remains a critical problem, particularly considering the vast complexity of biological systems. The integration of gene expression data with other layers of omics data, for instance, proteomics and metabolomics, remains a daunting task as researchers strive to construct global models of cellular pathways and disease. This is made even more difficult by biological variability that can obscure useful patterns in gene expression that are critical to therapeutic decision-making. Second, the threat of high false-positive rates in data sets characterizes the context of gene expression profiling and requires the application of strict criteria for result validation. Accordingly, improving the reproducibility and validity of results will be essential to advancing the science of microarray technology and increasing its application in clinical settings. Overcoming these various limitations is critical for releasing the maximum potential of gene expression profiling as a transformative technology for biomedical research and personalized medicine (Figure 5.17).

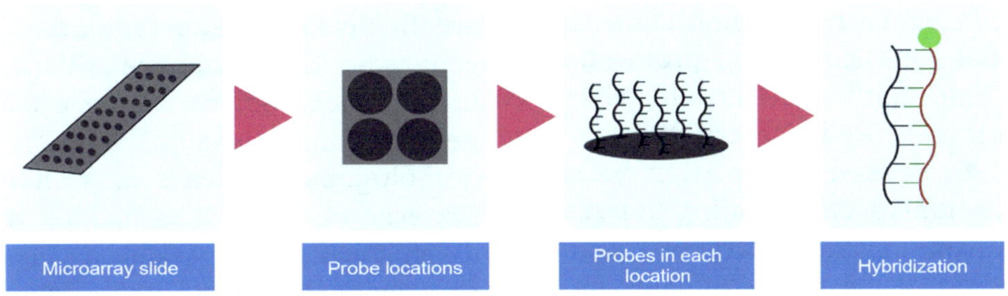

Figure 5.17. Limitations and challenges of gene expression microarray.

Source: https://geneticeducation.co.in/wp-content/uploads/2019/10/DNA-microarray.003-e1570163764401-768x266.jpeg.

5.6.1. Technical Limitations of Microarray Technology

Microarray technology, as significant as it has proved to be in advancing the science of gene expression profiling, is not without technical setbacks. The complexity of data interpretation is one of the greatest drawbacks of microarrays. The enormity of the output data from one microarray experiment commonly leads to problems in distinguishing true biological signal from noise. These are further enhanced by variations in background fluorescence, hybridization circumstances, and personal sample quality, all of which may introduce prejudice and affect the quality of the result. Additionally, statistical methods employed in handling microarray data can also give rise to misinterpretations, hence it is essential that researchers be cautious when concluding their findings. The intricacy involved in analyzing and mapping the data renders the technology both powerful and daunting, and for it to carry out meaningful analysis and interpretation, a strong support bioinformatics system must be in place (Shi, 2024). The second major disadvantage of microarray technology is the natural constraint of the number of probes available, which significantly affects its sensitivity and specificity. Microarrays interrogate RNA samples with pre-defined sequences and can thus miss new transcripts or splice forms not represented on the chip. Consequently, this limitation can lead to a partial gene expression profile and hide valuable information on the underlying biology of the investigated samples. Moreover, the challenge of cross-hybridization exists where there is non-specific binding between the probes and the unwanted targets, making data interpretation even more difficult. As a result, microarrays may provide a system for high-throughput examination of gene expression but may not effectively represent the dynamic and complicated image of gene activity seen in living organisms (Schwingen et al., 2020). Cost and accessibility also present significant barriers to the widespread use of microarray technology in research and clinical contexts. The expense of purchasing high-quality microarray chips, experimental hardware and reagents needed can be a significant cost factor, especially to small laboratory or limited-capital laboratories. In addition, the need for trained staff to drive the technology and interpret the resulting data introduces another level of cost and complexity. These financial limitations could limit the use of microarrays to well-funded research projects or major institutions, thus preventing the full potential of the technology from being used to fuel innovation among a wider scientific community. With the continued growth of the genomics industry, these cost and technical issues will need to be addressed to further improve the value and accessibility of microarray technology for gene expression profiling (Shi, 2024).

5.6.2. Data Interpretation Complexities

The interpretational complexity of data in the context of microarrays and gene expression profiling is great, largely because of the multi-dimensional nature of biological networks that are involved in gene regulation. Microarray-generated high-dimensional data tend to pose issues of noise and variability, which can hamper genuine biological signals. Moreover, genes in homologous pathways also share correlated patterns of expression, making it increasingly difficult to discern specialized gene contributions to specific biological processes. Without the application of appropriate statistical analysis and computational approaches, researchers can misread information and make wrong assumptions regarding gene function and interactions. Consequently, inclusion of advanced bioinformatics tools has become a prerequisite.

Tools like g:Profiler not only assist scientists in identifying enriched biological categories of gene lists, but also provide information for identifier conversion and ortholog mappings, thereby ensuring data interpretation transparency (Raudvere et al., 2019). Translation of genetic findings to functional gene insights in disease conditions like Alzheimer's disease provides further data interpretation complexities. Genetic correlations from microarray data generally point towards underlying pleiotropy in which single genes contribute to more than one phenotypic trait. This makes it hard to link genetic variation with disease mechanisms directly. Transcriptomic research, particularly for neurodegenerative disorders, has explained and confirmed genes of previously known risk and concurrently shown new associations. And yet, the physiological subtlety revealed by next-generation sequencing technologies once more underscores the challenge of converting genetic susceptibilities into meaningful biological understanding. By illustration in the pathways studied in Alzheimer's disease research, integrating transcriptomic with genetic information clarifies potential molecular mechanisms but underlines the continuing need for improved analytical methods to deal with this interpretational complexity (Verheijen & Sleegers, 2018). Furthermore, the concurrent application of gene expression information and interpretation presents additional layers of complexity that must be overcome by research scientists. Microarray and RNA sequencing techniques create vast quantities of data, yet their analysis and processing require competency in numerous bioinformatics strategies. Issues , such as batch effects, technical noise, and proper reference gene choice have the potential to impact outcome reliability significantly. Also, an understanding of differential expression results entails a nuanced understanding of the biological context with regard to the impact of regulatory elements as well as post-transcriptional regulation. Lacking an integrated approach that aligns genetic information with sound transcriptomic analysis, there is a danger of drawing wrong conclusions regarding gene function. Hence, ongoing advancements in computational methodology and bioinformatics strategies are necessary in transforming raw data to valuable biological interpretations, which guide subsequent investigations and therapeutic interventions in multifactorial disease (Raudvere et al., 2019).

5.6.3. Ethical Considerations in Gene Expression Studies

The field of ethical focus for gene expression research, particularly in microarrays and gene expression profiling, is full of moral issues that have to be scrutinized. Much as new technologies of molecular biology allow researchers to manipulate gene expression with increased accuracy, the attendant ethical implications of the practice become increasingly pertinent. For instance, the prospect of genetic engineering raises questions about the moral status of the involved organisms, most notably the case of embryonic stem cells derived from fertilized embryos. This has raised issues of concern for consent, the worth of potential life, and the importance of creating genetically altered organisms. Thus, the development of a moral code of conduct is essential to render research responsibly performed, with scientific progress in the right proportion weighed against societal values and ethical concerns. Shifting the focus of research to other sources for gene expression research, i.e., parthenogenetic embryonic stem cells, introduces another layer of ethical complexity. These stem cells derived from unfertilized oocytes sidestep some of the ethical concerns of standard embryonic stem cell research. But issues related to the treatment of human reproductive material, its patenting and ownership remain debatable among scientists. As advances in gene analysis, as disclosed in studies carried out by means of microarrays, demonstrate auspicious potential for understanding the behavior of genes, scientists must navigate through a complex web of ethical dilemmas. Use of genetically modified parthenogenetic stem cells, though ethically desirable, is associated with problems , such as growth retardation, further muddying the controversy over permissible means in gene expression studies (Kwak et al., 2011). Moreover, implications of gene profiling extend beyond laboratory procedure into broader societal ramifications, and thus, transparency and public engagement are critical. The public, policymakers, and researchers are among the stakeholders who must engage in discussions focused on resolving the ethical concerns of gene expression studies. Gene manipulation has implications that can be extensive, affecting not just an individual's life but also populations, such as in studies where the impact of gene expression alteration on disease is being measured. It is therefore important to create an inclusive discussion that harmonizes both the scientific promise of gene expression profiling and the ethical implications of its use. While researchers apply state-of-the-art methods , such as those relying on collaborative filtering to make predictions on gene expressions, they should also be aware of the ethical contexts generated by their findings and operate (Bayrak & Oğul, 2019) (Figure 5.18).

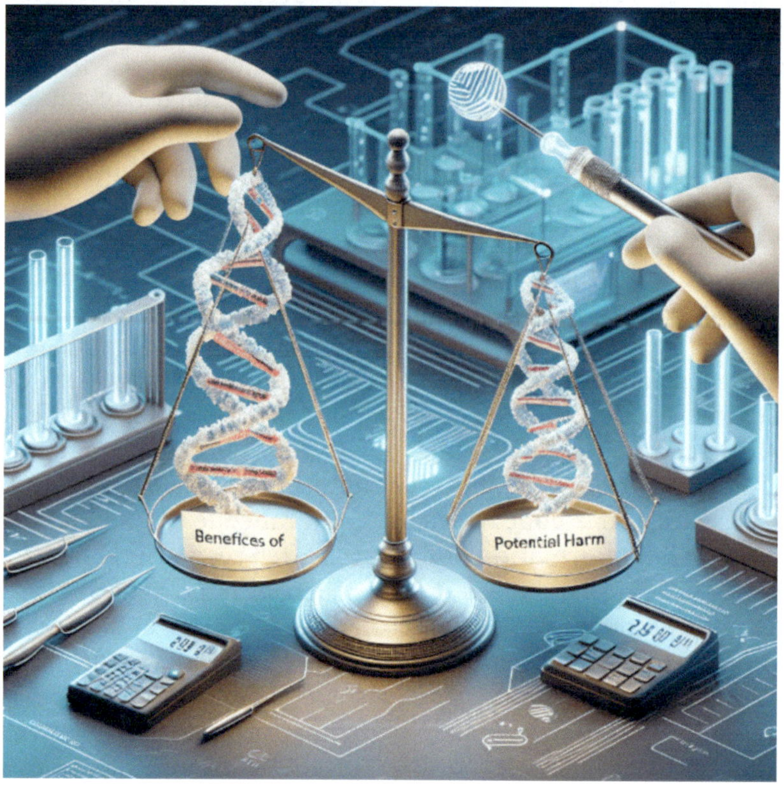

Figure 5.18. Ethical considerations in gene editing.

Source: https://healthindustrytrends.com/wp-content/uploads/2024/10/the-ethics-of-gene-editing-crispr-and-beyond-2.png.

SUMMARY

The study culmination of microarrays and gene expression profiling offers testament to the significance of these technologies in enhancing our understanding of cellular function and disease processes. By making it possible to examine thousands of genes simultaneously, microarrays have revolutionized the landscape of genomics, providing insight into transcriptional profiles with close associations with biological functions. This capability not only raises the finding of disease-related biomarkers but also the identification of potential therapeutic targets, unveiling the intricate pathways of different diseases. Increasing data output of such analysis, there is a significant evaluation of methodologies, including normalization techniques employed, in a bid to attain accuracy and reproducibility of findings. As mentioned in our review, the choice of normalization methods can have an important influence on the outcome of gene expression studies, and therefore necessitates standardization across microarray platforms. Loess and generalized Procrustes analysis are promising approaches for variability reduction and increasing inter-platform concordance. These developments highlight the importance of making the right analytical choices to yield dependable data that are reproducible in subsequent studies. Moreover, with the use of high computational capacities combined with experimental designs, researchers cannot only study gene expression but also study the functional relevance of such patterns in disease biology and therapeutic targeting, as the priorities of precision medicine would dictate in today's era. In general, the trajectory of microarray technology and its application in gene expression profiling reflects an active interplay between experimental and computational biology. Ongoing improvement in oligonucleotide design and in bioinformatics is required to optimize the accuracy of transcriptional assessments, as illustrated in current studies in the area. Together, experimental biologists and computational scientists combine to fortify the strength of genomic research, eventually leading to the development of revolutionary diagnostic and therapeutic interventions. With the advancing science, it is crucial that researchers remain adaptable and continue to make adjustments in their approach so that the promise of microarrays as a revolutionary gene expression analysis tool reaches its maximum potential in unraveling the complexity of life and disease (Adebiyi, 2006; Meyer et al., 2012).

The use of microarrays in gene expression profiling has revolutionized plant genetics research by providing the means of high-throughput transcriptomic change analysis. The use case of this impact, which is a milestone study, is the targeted chromosome engineering in *Arabidopsis thaliana*, which revealed surprising gene expression in spite of extreme chromosomal remodeling. The research demonstrated that phenotype and transcriptomic analysis of translocated lines exhibited little transcriptional influence, suggesting that gene expression control systems can tolerate very extensive genomic modifications (Akpinar et al., 2025). Based on the application of principal component analysis to verify morphological analysis, the research demonstrates the potential of microarray technologies in exposing underlying genomic resilience and plasticity in plant species. Moreover, these findings facilitate the application of gene expression profiling in answering how plants react to genetically engineered changes. Apart from structural genomic modifications, microarray studies also enable researchers to examine the effects of various transcription factors on plant development and stress responses. To begin with, the discovery of valine-glutamine (VQ) motif-proteins in mustard (*Brassica juncea*) highlights their vital role as transcriptional regulators. The current study identified 120 VQ genes and examined their expression patterns under cold stress, which resulted in numerous of these genes being differentially expressed across developmental stages and environmental conditions. These results support the complexity involved in gene regulatory networks because microarrays can be employed to determine functional associations among genes and their corresponding responses to abiotic and biotic stresses (Zheng et al., 2022). Thus, these findings demonstrate the potential for gene expression profiling to continue making contributions to crop improvement and resistance methods. Lastly, the general conclusions reached by means of gene expression profiling support the relevance of advanced methodology to plant genetics. The combined focus on both structural chromosomal mechanisms and dynamic gene expression responses demonstrates an integrated approach to the study of plant biology. Through microarray technology, researchers can unveil the cis-acting components that control transcription, thereby leading to a deeper understanding of gene function and interaction. The implications of such research are far-reaching, enhancing not only the basic knowledge of plant physiology but also offering avenues for applied agricultural innovations. Microarray-based techniques used in gene expression profiling will keep providing insightful information, influencing the direction of future research, and translating into sustainable development for long-lasting crop varieties.

A LOOK TO THE FUTURE

CHINESE GLIOMA GENOME ATLAS (CGGA)

The Chinese Glioma Genome Atlas (CGGA) represents a landmark effort in the field of cancer genomics, offering one of the most comprehensive and accessible repositories of multi-dimensional genomic data derived specifically from Chinese glioma patients. Gliomas, the most frequent and aggressive primary malignant brain tumors in adults, pose significant clinical challenges due to their heterogeneity, poor prognosis, and limited therapeutic options. Understanding the molecular underpinnings of these tumors is thus essential for advancing diagnostic, prognostic, and therapeutic research. CGGA was established to address this need by creating an expansive, systematically curated platform for functional genomic data that supports both basic research and clinical applications. Launched in 2012 and made publicly accessible in 2021, CGGA integrates diverse types of genomic and clinical information from nearly 2,000 glioma samples collected across multiple Chinese medical centers. The database includes whole-exome sequencing, mRNA sequencing and microarray, DNA methylation microarray, and microRNA microarray data, accompanied by detailed clinical annotations such as age, gender, WHO tumor grade, treatment status, and survival outcomes. This breadth of data empowers researchers to probe the complex genetic and epigenetic landscapes of glioma subtypes, facilitating new discoveries in tumor biology and patient stratification.

One of the core strengths of CGGA lies in its commitment to open access and ease of use. The platform provides user-friendly web tools enabling interactive exploration of mutation landscapes, gene expression patterns, methylation profiles, and survival analyses without requiring advanced computational expertise. These functionalities lower technical barriers for researchers worldwide, democratizing access to high-quality genomic data and fostering collaborative discovery.

Importantly, CGGA places a particular emphasis on recurrent gliomas and subtype analyses, areas often underrepresented in other major genomic resources. By including data on both primary and recurrent tumors, the database supports investigations into tumor progression, treatment resistance, and mechanisms of malignancy. The inclusion of multi-omics datasets further allows for integrative analyses that can reveal how genomic alterations interact with transcriptional and epigenetic changes to drive tumor behavior. Over the years, CGGA has become a cornerstone resource for the neuro-oncology community, contributing to numerous high-impact studies and facilitating advances in biomarker discovery, therapeutic target identification, and personalized medicine approaches. As genomic technologies and analytical methods continue to evolve, the ongoing expansion and refinement of CGGA will undoubtedly remain invaluable for unraveling the complexity of gliomas and improving outcomes for patients globally.

REFERENCES

1. Abstract 6538: Development and refinement of functional gene expression signatures as a computational tool for comprehensive characterization of transcriptomic data. (2023). *Cancer Research*. https://www.semanticscholar.org/paper/7e3811ad555cfe1173f024a407dc0463e04667a1 (accessed on 17th July 2025).
2. Adebiyi, E. F. (2006). Systems biology and the development of vaccines and drugs for malaria treatments. https://core.ac.uk/download/12356713.pdf (accessed on 17th July 2025).
3. Akpinar, E., Hangün, B., Oduncuoglu, M., Altun, O., Eyecioğlu, Ö., & Yalcin, Z. (2025). Quantum-enhanced classification of brain tumors using DNA microarray gene expression profiles. *ArXiv, abs/2505.02033*. https://www.semanticscholar.org/paper/8ab83b4ecbf01ba5cf529a43225a548083922738 (accessed on 17th July 2025).
4. Alba, R., Fei, Z., Payton, P., Liu, Y., Moore, S. L., Debbie, P., Cohn, J., et al. (2004). ESTs, cDNA microarrays, and gene expression profiling: Tools for dissecting plant physiology and development. *The Plant Journal, 39*, 697–714. https://doi.org/10.1111/j.1365-313x.2004.02178.x (accessed on 17th July 2025).
5. Almarzouki, H. Z. (2022). Deep-learning-based cancer profiles classification using gene expression data profile. *Journal of Healthcare Engineering, 2022*. https://www.semanticscholar.org/paper/00deec259516ae58c3290a7ea5e0cd1fc6ef90a6 (accessed on 17th July 2025).
6. Almugren, N., & Alshamlan, H. (2019). A survey on hybrid feature selection methods in microarray gene expression data for cancer classification. *IEEE Access, 7*, 78533–78548. https://doi.org/10.1109/access.2019.2922987 (accessed on 17th July 2025).
7. Balanu, I. C. (2011). Translational oncogenomic and human cancer interactome networks. https://core.ac.uk/download/pdf/290188.pdf (accessed on 17th July 2025).
8. Barrionuevo Moreno, I., & Del Espino Pérez, Á. (2016). Microarrays as a functional approach to the transcriptome. https://core.ac.uk/download/62908347.pdf (accessed on 17th July 2025).
9. Bayrak, T., & Oğul, H. (2019). A new approach for predicting the value of gene expression: Two-way collaborative filtering. *Current Bioinformatics*. https://www.semanticscholar.org/paper/7f1b275815e46fdd3585212e6ac62cd09396f125 (accessed on 17th July 2025).
10. Birt, I. A., Hagenauer, M., Clinton, S., Aydin, C., Blandino, P., Stead, J. D. H., Hilde, K. L., et al. (2019). A meta-analysis of hippocampal transcriptional profiling studies in a selectively-bred rat model provides converging evidence with genetic sequencing to implicate specific candidate genes and pathways in the liability for internalizing and externalizing psychiatric disorders. *bioRxiv*. https://www.semanticscholar.org/paper/5841037fec28869091cf4c46b927f9d7a2a8358b (accessed on 17th July 2025).
11. Bouttell, J., Hawkins, N., Masson, R., & Goodlad, J. R. (2023). OP79 gene expression profiling in the diagnosis of aggressive large B cell lymphoma: An early exploratory economic evaluation. *International Journal of Technology Assessment in Health Care, 39*, S21–S21. https://www.semanticscholar.org/paper/cb1027e1855699d3eeeb36c3ed36a70579d60224 (accessed on 17th July 2025).
12. Chu, C., Yao, C., Chang, Y. T., Chou, H., Chou, Y., Chen, K. H., Terng, H., et al. (2014). Gene expression profiling of colorectal tumors and normal mucosa by microarrays meta-analysis

using prediction analysis of microarray, artificial neural network, classification, and regression trees. *Disease Markers, 2014*. https://www.semanticscholar.org/paper/90c6cd3f99704e787288a6ddd0a9e3bc08ea9f16 (accessed on 17th July 2025).

13. Cohen, C. D., & Kretzler, M. (2002). Gene expression analysis in micro dissected renal tissue – current challenges and strategies. https://core.ac.uk/download/16432506.pdf (accessed on 17th July 2025).

14. Hassan, M., Awan, F. M., Naz, A., deAndrés-Galiana, E. J., Álvarez-Machancoses, Ó., Cernea, A., Fernández-Brillet, L., et al. (2022). Innovations in genomics and big data analytics for personalized medicine and health care: A review. *International Journal of Molecular Sciences, 23*, 4645–4645. https://doi.org/10.3390/ijms23094645 (accessed on 17th July 2025).

15. Helia, O., Matúšová, B., Havlová, K., Hýsková, A., Lyčka, M., Beying, N., Puchta, H., et al. (2025). Chromosome engineering points to the cis-acting mechanism of chromosome arm-specific telomere length setting and robustness of plant phenotype, chromatin structure and gene expression. *The Plant Journal, 121*. https://www.semanticscholar.org/paper/5430c799deddf734e57f71605a30cf5e16ca0d88 (accessed on 17th July 2025).

16. Herwig, R., & Lehrach, H. (2006). Expression profiling of drug response–from genes to pathways. *Dialogues in Clinical Neuroscience, 8*, 283–293. https://www.semanticscholar.org/paper/20679702d205f16e726b914451504f2462fc79f5 (accessed on 17th July 2025).

17. Hoffmann, K., Berger, H., Kulbe, H., Thillainadarasan, S., Mollenkopf, H. J., Żemojtel, T., Taube, E. T., et al. (2020). Stable expansion of high-grade serous ovarian cancer organoids requires a low-Wnt environment. *The EMBO Journal, 39*. https://doi.org/10.15252/embj.2019104013 (accessed on 17th July 2025).

18. Jamshidi, N., Lewis, N. E., Swann, J., Winzeler, E., et al. (2015). Systems analysis of host-parasite interactions. https://core.ac.uk/download/323077861.pdf (accessed on 17th July 2025).

19. Meyer, S. U., Kaiser, S., Wagner, C., Thirion, C., & Pfaffl, M. W. (2012). Profound effect of profiling platform and normalization strategy on detection of differentially expressed microRNAs--a comparative study. *PloS one*, *7*(6), e38946. https://doi.org/10.1371/journal.pone.0038946c(accessed on 17th July 2025).

20. Kim, S.-K., Qiao, G., Yoon, J., & Jang, I. (2015). Acute toxicity of cadmium on gene expression profiling of fleshy shrimp, *Fenneropenaeus chinensis* postlarvae using a cDNA microarray. *Journal of Environmental Sciences-China, 24*, 623–631. https://www.semanticscholar.org/paper/fe79dd4636174e41e6cbefeb7ae84b32f23c23de (accessed on 17th July 2025).

21. Koti, M., Vidal, R., Nuin, P. A. S., Haslehurst, A., Weberpals, J., Childs, T., Bryson, P., et al. (2012). Abstract 3645: Integrative molecular profiling in serous epithelial ovarian cancer for identification of biomarkers of chemoresistance. *Cancer Research, 72*, 3645–3645. https://www.semanticscholar.org/paper/7e01db6436b38cb1fd20faf1a2b345d1607bb9b8 (accessed on 17th July 2025).

22. Kulikov, E. P., Mertsalov, S. A., Shumskaya, E. I., & Piskunov, R. O. (2023). Expression Microarrays: Possibilities of Application in Clinical Oncology. *NAUKA MOLODYKH (Eruditio Juvenium), 11*(2), 229–240. https://doi.org/10.23888/hmj2023112229-240(accessed on 17th July 2025).

23. Kundaje, A., Meuleman, W., Ernst, J., Bilenky, M., Yen, A., Heravi-Moussavi, A., Kheradpour, P., et al. (2015). Integrative analysis of 111 reference human epigenomes. *Nature, 518*, 317–330. https://doi.org/10.1038/nature14248 (accessed on 17th July 2025).

24. Kwak, M., Hong, S., Yu, S. l., Sim, B. W., Seo, J. S., & Kang, J. (2011). Parthenogenetic embryonic stem cells with H19 siRNA-mediated knockdown as a potential resource for cell therapy. *International Journal of Molecular Medicine, 29*(2), 257–262. https://www.semanticscholar.org/paper/9deba1475464d9374831ac32b31697a952f54d73 (accessed on 17th July 2025).

25. Labonté, B., Suderman, M., Maussion, G., Navaro, L., Yerko, V., Mahar, I., Bureau, A., et al. (2012). Genome-wide epigenetic regulation by early-life trauma. *Archives of General Psychiatry, 69*. https://doi.org/10.1001/archgenpsychiatry.2011.2287 (accessed on 17th July 2025).

26. Lee, S.-T., Muench, M. O., Fomin, M. E., Xiao, J., Zhou, M., de Smith, A. J., Martín-Subero, J. I., et al. (2015). Epigenetic remodeling in B-cell acute lymphoblastic leukemia occurs in two tracks and employs embryonic stem cell-like signatures. *Nucleic Acids Research, 43*, 2590–2602. https://doi.org/10.1093/nar/gkv103 (accessed on 17th July 2025).

27. Letzkus, M., Luesink, E., Starck-Schwertz, S., Bigaud, M., Mirza, F., Hartmann, N., Gerstmayer, B., et al. (2014). Gene expression profiling of immunomagnetically separated cells directly from stabilized whole blood for multicenter clinical trials. *Clinical and Translational Medicine, 3*, 36–36. https://www.semanticscholar.org/paper/9f2d65922d071d5ec63ebaef8f3f24b770fe9989 (accessed on 17th July 2025).

28. Liao, J., Lu, X., Shao, X., Zhu, L., & Fan, X. (2020). Uncovering an organ's molecular architecture at single-cell resolution by spatially resolved transcriptomics. *Trends in Biotechnology, 39*, 43–58. https://doi.org/10.1016/j.tibtech.2020.05.006 (accessed on 17th July 2025).

29. Manjunath, H., Al Khulaifi, M., Sidahmed, H., Ammar, A., Vadakekolathu, J., Rutella, S., Al-Mohannadi, M., et al. (2022). Gene expression profiling of FFPE samples: A titration test. *Technology in Cancer Research & Treatment, 21*. https://www.semanticscholar.org/paper/35703dfd0ad70720b551a055d5bafac2f61a0a9c (accessed on 17th July 2025).

30. Milchevskaya, V., Tödt, G., & Gibson, T. (2017). A tool to build up-to-date gene annotations for Affymetrix microarrays. *3*, 38. https://www.semanticscholar.org/paper/b060257dd85c54b66c7753dc6dd43b52aa1fa02c (accessed on 17th July 2025).

31. Moretto, M., Sonego, P., Villaseñor-Altamirano, A. B., & Engelen, K. (2019). First step toward gene expression data integration: Transcriptomic data acquisition with COMMAND>_. *BMC Bioinformatics, 20*. https://www.semanticscholar.org/paper/2f75ee7e79131ebc539ba72f0ed47e16bc63ceb3 (accessed on 17th July 2025).

32. Nie, H. (2010). Genome-wide gene expression surveys and a transcriptome map in chicken. https://www.semanticscholar.org/paper/a0a24552ce06958a373408d09dc99f156591fcae (accessed on 17th July 2025).

33. Oh, E., Lee, J., Kim, H. S., Park, J. Y., Choi, S. Y., Choi, K. D., Kim, J. S., et al. (2023). Gene expression analysis in recurrent benign paroxysmal positional vertigo: A preliminary study. *Frontiers in Neurology, 14*. https://www.semanticscholar.org/paper/39ff7db09093d47993be16b4c1306a2d26ea6b07 (accessed on 17th July 2025).

34. Pellagatti, A., Esoof, N., Watkins, F., Langford, C. F., Vetrie, D., Campbell, L. J., Fidler, C., et al. (2004). Gene expression profiling in the myelodysplastic syndromes using cDNA microarray technology. *British Journal of Haematology, 125*, 576–583. https://doi.org/10.1111/j.1365-2141.2004.04958.x (accessed on 17th July 2025).

35. Raudvere, U., Kolberg, L., Kuzmin, I., Arak, T. V., Adler, P., Peterson, H., & Vilo, J. (2019). g: Profiler: A web server for functional enrichment analysis and conversions of gene lists

(2019 update). *Nucleic Acids Research, 47*, W191–W198. https://doi.org/10.1093/nar/gkz369 (accessed on 17th July 2025).

36. Ritchie, M. E., Phipson, B., Wu, D., Hu, Y., Law, C. W., Shi, W., & Smyth, G. K. (2015). *limma* powers differential expression analyses for RNA-sequencing and microarray studies. *Nucleic Acids Research, 43*, e47–e47. https://doi.org/10.1093/nar/gkv007 (accessed on 17th July 2025).
37. Sahoo, R., & Pradhan, R. (2023). Effectiveness of principal component analysis in functional mapping of gene expression profiles. *2023 International Conference on Recent Advances in Electrical, Electronics & Digital Healthcare Technologies (REEDCON)*. https://www.semanticscholar.org/paper/f27155087e968d5ed65062b7465211476b11733e (accessed on 17th July 2025).
38. Schwingen, J., Kaplan, M., & Kurschus, F. (2020). Review—Current concepts in inflammatory skin diseases evolved by transcriptome analysis: In-depth analysis of atopic dermatitis and psoriasis. *International Journal of Molecular Sciences, 21*. https://www.semanticscholar.org/paper/6ee59a0c354092ff8a56259ed0f47d759b3d1db2 (accessed on 17th July 2025).
39. Shi, C. (2024). DNA microarray technology principles and applications in genetic research. *Computer Life*. https://www.semanticscholar.org/paper/9b26de86de8c0d107e7b523850163489eaef3559 (accessed on 17th July 2025).
40. Singh, R. (2013). Signal oscillation is another reason for variability in microarray-based gene expression quantification. *PLoS ONE, 8*. https://www.semanticscholar.org/paper/39e45a103d29a8e823ff0bbf80dd0ee2da1d6d85 (accessed on 17th July 2025).
41. Srivastava, S., Srivastava, A. K., Suprasanna, P., & D'Souza, S. F. (2012). Identification and profiling of arsenic stress-induced microRNAs in *Brassica juncea*. *Journal of Experimental Botany, 64*, 303–315. https://doi.org/10.1093/jxb/ers333 (accessed on 17th July 2025).
42. Sukhamwang, A., Thananchai, H., Yodkeeree, S., Dejkriengkraikul, P., & Limpakan (Yamada), S. (2025). Abstract 5918: Vascular endothelial growth factor A (VEGF-A) gene expression profiling in Northern Thai gastric cancer patients and potential biomarker for anti-VEGF therapy selection. *Cancer Research*. https://www.semanticscholar.org/paper/d051b432904a444ccd789a4d7163217dde234cc9 (accessed on 17th July 2025).
43. Suresh, A. V. S., Singaraju, M., & Dadireddy, P. K. (2025). Cost-effectiveness analysis of gene expression profiling for breast cancer treatment decisions in India. *International Journal of Community Medicine and Public Health*. https://www.semanticscholar.org/paper/c0b8d48d945cba1b3d430f9d064bb417c178140e (accessed on 17th July 2025).
44. Syed, A. H., Abujabal, H., Ahmad, S., Malebary, S., & Alromema, N. (2024). Advances in inflammatory bowel disease diagnostics: Machine learning and genomic profiling reveal key biomarkers for early detection. *Diagnostics, 14*. https://www.semanticscholar.org/paper/017d30feecd3654909bd51ff19c7e7e54787f773 (accessed on 17th July 2025).
45. Tang, Z., Li, C., Kang, B., Gao, G., Li, C., & Zhang, Z. (2017). GEPIA: A web server for cancer and normal gene expression profiling and interactive analyses. *Nucleic Acids Research, 45*, W98–W102. https://www.semanticscholar.org/paper/231be65e77b73a3b1e554b19a8bde6bda751d488 (accessed on 17th July 2025).
46. Tirosh, I., Izar, B., Prakadan, S. M., Wadsworth, M. H., Treacy, D. J., Trombetta, J. J., Rotem, A., et al. (2016). Dissecting the multicellular ecosystem of metastatic melanoma by single-

cell RNA-seq. *Science, 352*, 189–196. https://doi.org/10.1126/science.aad0501 (accessed on 17th July 2025).

47. Venkata, N., Rama, A., Srikanth, G., Devendra, V., Haritha, D., & Krishna, D. L. (2024). Synergistic genomic profiling and predictive modeling for health outcome anticipation: A holistic strategy leveraging gene expression analysis. *2023 4th International Conference on Intelligent Technologies (CONIT)*. https://www.semanticscholar.org/paper/789f73733a7cfc92aab63d45963d581d16ec314c (accessed on 17th July 2025).

48. Verheijen, J., & Sleegers, K. (2018). Understanding Alzheimer disease at the interface between genetics and transcriptomics. *Trends in Genetics, 34*, 434–447. https://doi.org/10.1016/j.tig.2018.02.007 (accessed on 17th July 2025).

49. You, Y., Lai, X., Pan, Y., Zheng, H., Vera, J., Liu, S., Deng, S., et al. (2022). Artificial intelligence in cancer target identification and drug discovery. *Signal Transduction and Targeted Therapy, 7*. https://doi.org/10.1038/s41392-022-00994-0 (accessed on 17th July 2025).

50. Zarzar, M., Razak, E., Htike, Z., & Yusof, F. (2015). Prognosis of early cervical carcinoma using gene expression profiling. *Advanced Science Letters, 21*, 3485–3488. https://www.semanticscholar.org/paper/2d7bfe9d1095aea2366fd3cd56c3527a9573e649 (accessed on 17th July 2025).

51. Zhang, X., Jonassen, I., & Goksøyr, A. (2021). Machine learning approaches for biomarker discovery using gene expression data. *Bioinformatics*. https://www.semanticscholar.org/paper/66342b1031c06f44a2582ba1f22028d8885e1ca2 (accessed on 17th July 2025).

52. Zhao, Z., Zhang, K., Wang, Q., Li, G., Zeng, F., Zhang, Y., Wu, F., et al. (2021). Chinese Glioma Genome Atlas (CGGA): A comprehensive resource with functional genomic data from Chinese glioma patients. *Genomics Proteomics & Bioinformatics, 19*, 1–12. https://doi.org/10.1016/j.gpb.2020.10.005 (accessed on 17th July 2025).

53. Zheng, J., Li, H., Guo, Z., Zhuang, X., Huang, W., Mao, C., Feng, H., et al. (2022). Comprehensive identification and expression profiling of the VQ motif-containing gene family in *Brassica juncea*. *Biology, 11*. https://www.semanticscholar.org/paper/b4982e0b3fa3e036f958acffd9425acb6fdfccf5 (accessed on 17th July 2025).

54. Zhou, Y., Zhou, B., Pache, L., Chang, M. W., Khodabakhshi, A. H., Tanaseichuk, O., Benner, C., et al. (2019). Metascape provides a biologist-oriented resource for the analysis of systems-level datasets. *Nature Communications, 10*. https://doi.org/10.1038/s41467-019-09234-6 (accessed on 17th July 2025).

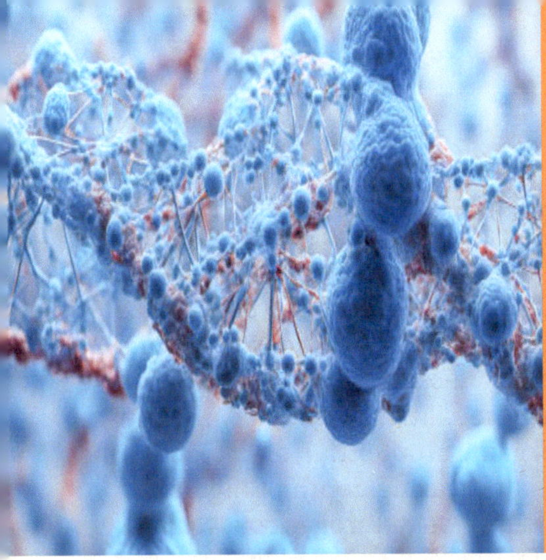

Chapter 6
MOLECULAR ONCOLOGY

Contents

Introduction

Molecular oncology is an essential interface between molecular biology and cancer research, which provides hints regarding the molecular and genetic processes of tumorigenesis. By exploring cellular and molecular alterations that are responsible for triggering cancer progression, scientists can identify specific biomarkers not just for better diagnoses but also to design therapeutic strategies. New knowledge regarding head and neck squamous cell carcinoma (HNSCC), for instance, emphasizes the central role of human papillomavirus (HPV) in tumor development, particularly in HPV-positive tumors. Such a distinction is very significant, since patients with HPV-positive HNSCC have better outcomes compared to their HPV-negative counterparts. Therefore, molecular oncology work is beyond mere genetic defects; it encompasses the intricate biological interactions that form the basis of tumor behavior and patient response and hence mandates integrated approaches to cancer research and treatment. Integration of molecular genetics into oncology has led to the application of personalized medicine, whose approach individualizes treatment protocols as a function of particular genetic patterns. For example, knowing about specific mutations in specific cancers can guide the selection of targeted therapy, with increased efficacy and fewer side effects. Synthetic lethality, where combined perturbation of two genes is lethal to the cell but individual perturbations are not, is a highly promising avenue for the discovery of new cancer drugs. Research in colorectal cancer has demonstrated that synthetic lethal approaches can exploit weaknesses in the setting of chromosomal deletions. This can be used to allow for the potential to engage genotype-specific treatments, thus advancing the aims of precision medicine and aligning treatment modalities with the inherent genetic architecture of tumors, which refers to the paradigm-breaking potential of molecular oncology in contemporary cancer therapy (Szyma et al., 2020). With increasing depth of molecular oncology, it becomes increasingly important in addressing the needs of heterogeneous cancer forms. This is through profound knowledge of tumor microenvironments, molecular pathways, and interactions with the immune system when designing effective interventions. This is particularly observed in cutting-edge research on how the molecular profile of a tumor affects its response to therapy, e.g., immunotherapy and chemoradiotherapy. For instance, the introduction of immune checkpoint inhibitors has revolutionized the therapy for recurrent or metastatic cancer , such as HNSCC, offering relief to patients who have few options now. The ongoing quest for the molecular biology of cancer is all ultimately directed to putting scientific discoveries into clinical practice, enhancing patient survival and quality of life by more effective, target-based therapies depending on individual tumor characteristics (Alyami et al., 2024) (Figure 6.1).

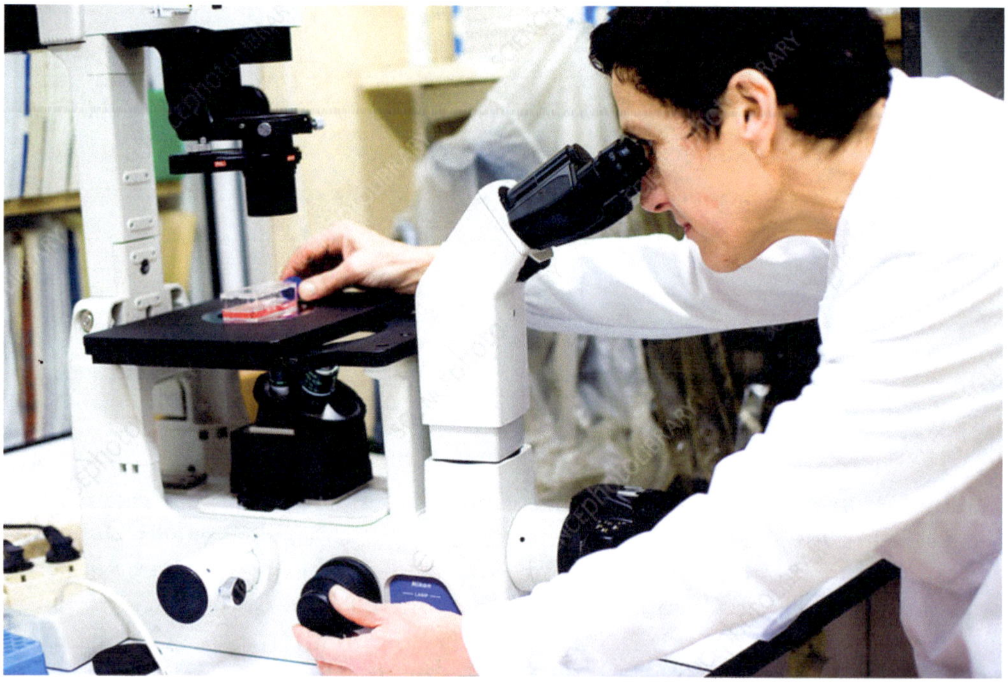

Figure 6.1. Molecular oncology.

Source: https://media.sciencephoto.com/image/c0326848/800wm/C0326848-Molecular_oncology.jpg.

Definition and Scope of Molecular Oncology

Molecular oncology is a specialty of cancer treatment and research encompassing the molecular and genetic events that occur in cancer initiation and progression. Molecular oncology integrates information from a wide variety of disciplines, ranging from molecular biology and genetics to biochemistry and pharmacology, to identify how cancer cells differ from normal cells at the molecular level. By identifying individual molecular alterations specific to different forms of cancer, researchers hope to develop targeted therapies with the potential to more effectively control or eradicate cancers. Molecular oncology thus encompasses both the identification of such biomolecular markers and their application to the development of new therapeutic approaches, ultimately enhancing the specificity of cancer therapy and minimizing patient morbidity. The scope of molecular oncology extends beyond merely understanding cancer biology; it also includes the application of personalized medicine strategies, which tailor therapy regimens based on unique genetic profiles. As illustrated in recent advances, correlation of specific genetic mutations and drug responsiveness has led to improved targeted therapies, enabling clinicians to choose the most efficacious regimens for their patients. Furthermore, ongoing research within molecular oncology is focused on explaining drug resistance mechanisms and developing means of overcoming them. This evolving knowledge is essential to address challenges posed by aggressive types of cancer, such as those outlined in the case of advanced metastatic breast cancer, where drug response may significantly vary between individuals (Fátima et al., 2018). Further, molecular oncology encourages the interdisciplinarity necessary to bypass the intricate nature of cancer. By combining genomics, bioinformatics, and drug discovery inputs, the discipline paves the door to novel, innovative clinical trials investigating new compounds and their combinations in the clinic. The overall concept is to translate bench science into effective clinical protocols that enhance survival without increasing side effects. Enhanced survival of advanced breast cancer, as recently noted, underscores the importance of such combined efforts. This combined approach, as mentioned in congresses and advisory reports, aims to maximize control of complex cancers and offers hope for enhanced long-term success for malignancy patients (Alyami et al., 2024) (Figure 6.2).

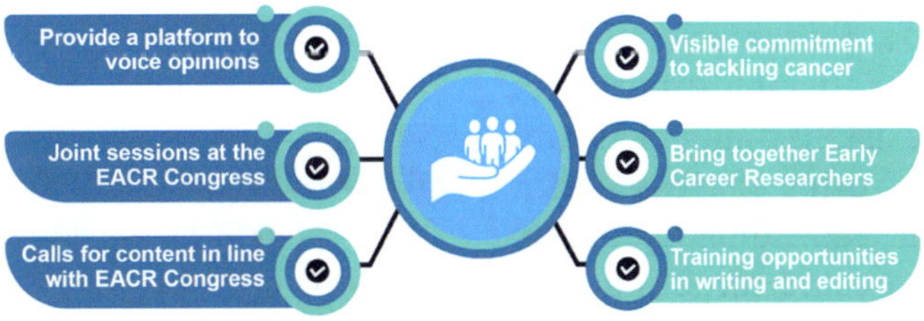

Figure 6.2. Scope of molecular oncology.

Source: https://febs.onlinelibrary.wiley.com/cms/asset/0ed6f9d8-3daa-456c-9d16-a0a3085461db/mol213445-toc-0001-m.jpg.

Historical Context and Evolution of the Field

The historical background of molecular oncology is inextricably linked with the process of developing our knowledge about cancer at the cellular and molecular levels. The subject gathered momentum in the early 20th century when scientists , such as Theodor Boveri put together the chromosomal theory of cancer. His research shed light on the role played by genetic factors in tumorigenesis, opening the door for subsequent research into the molecular origins of cancer. With advances in technology, particularly in DNA sequencing in the latter half of the 20th century, scientists began to find specific mutations that were associated with specific kinds of cancer and so initiated a shift towards more molecular-oriented research from traditional pathology. This advancement not only laid the groundwork for gene-specific treatments but also revolutionized the categorization and treatment of cancers, with its emphasis on personalized medicine for patient profiles. In the second half of the 20th century and early 21st century, an explosion of research into oncogenes and tumor suppressor genes propelled the discipline into new regions, laying bare the intricate genetic pathways to malignancies. Discovery of the role of the HER2 gene in breast cancer was a game-changer in this context, leading to the development of targeted therapy , such as trastuzumab. Further, discovery of the IDH gene mutations in glioblastomas was another demonstration of the pivotal role molecular diagnostics play in understanding the tumor biology, essential in guiding treatment. As has been noted in recent reviews, including consideration of IDH wildtype glioblastomas, the ongoing research into new therapies is crucial for the establishment of efficient treatments against these extremely resistant tumors (Alyami et al., 2024). These discoveries represented a tangible move away from traditional, cytotoxic therapies toward more specific targeting that attempted to interrupt specific molecular mechanisms. The molecular oncology history is also characterized by a growing recognition of the intricacies of dealing with cancer biology, particularly the interfaces between various cellular processes. New mechanisms of cell death , such as disulfidptosis, have emerged as major research areas in the field. Characterized by the accumulation of cystine in cancer cells due to the overexpression of specific transporters, this novel pathway demonstrates the dynamic nature of metabolic stress responses of tumor survival mechanisms (Chen et al., 2024). It is important to identify such regulatory pathways as they may serve as therapeutic targets, thus widening the treatment scope. As molecular oncology continues to develop, the issue will be how to apply these discoveries to clinically beneficial therapies. The integration of advanced techniques and greater insight into molecular interactions will be critical in reformulating treatment strategies and improving patient outcomes across a variety of malignancies.

Importance of Molecular Oncology in Cancer Research

The use of molecular oncology for the study of cancer cannot be overstated, particularly its potential to give a clearer picture of the genetic and molecular underpinnings of most cancers. By conducting studies on the molecular alterations that are accountable for cancer development and progression, researchers are capable of identifying the prospective biomarkers of early detection and prognosis. For instance, the study of prostate cancer yields useful information about the effects of molecular alterations on disease aggressiveness and patient prognosis. As has been documented, prostate cancer is the second most common neoplasm in men, and therefore, such studies are of immense value. It directs the need for more advanced diagnostic techniques, with new molecular targets being discovered as a result of research that investigates genetic mutations and tumorigenesis-related signaling pathways, thereby solidifying the groundbreaking role of molecular oncology in cancer therapeutic approaches as well as prevention measures (Rawla, 2019). Molecular oncology's role in making feasible advancements provides leeway far beyond personalized medicine, with individualized treatment approaches based on an individual's own genetic makeup. For example, understanding the mutations leading to specific cancers can lead to more effective targeted therapies compared to conventional therapies. This can be seen in prostate cancer, where gene profiling can guide treatment and improve outcomes for patients. Moreover, molecular oncology provides essential paradigms for the classification of subtypes of cancer based on molecular characteristics, enhancing the possibility of constructing clinical trials and performing epidemiologic studies guiding treatment protocols. The need for and value of sophisticated case definitions not only affect the effectiveness of treatment but also guide preventive intervention against cancer by outlining genetic vulnerability factors, underlining precision medicine's significance (Alyami et al., 2024). In addition, molecular oncology encourages interdisciplinary interaction, merging genetics, biochemistry, and clinical practice to advance cancer research and therapeutic paradigms. When scientists continue to unravel the intricate interactions among multiple molecular pathways, they are able to establish integrated models of cancer biology mirroring complexities in the real world. This integrated model is necessary to address cancer's multifaceted nature. It also underpins a more informed understanding of the way in which lifestyle and environmental influences meet genetic predispositions in the cause of cancer. Molecular oncology is thus a cornerstone for the progression of cancer research and, as such, is worth being up to date with for health professionals. With ongoing research aimed at uncovering emerging molecular targets and pathways, there is the hope of novel treatment modalities to continue expanding, which ultimately propels the fight against cancer (Rawla, 2019) (Figure 6.3).

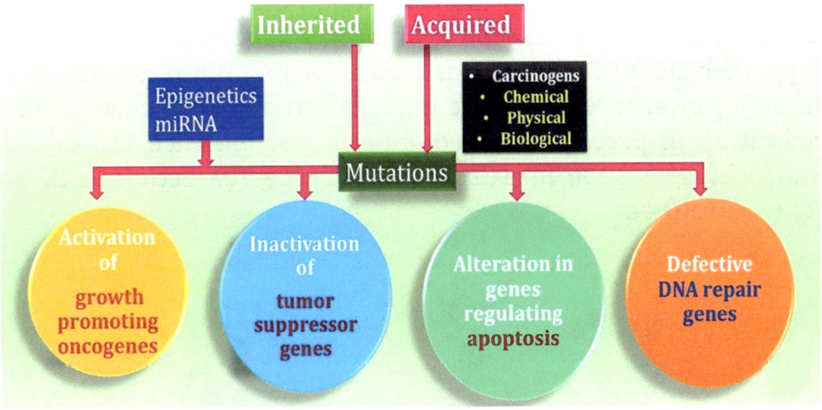

Figure 6.3. Importance of molecular oncology in cancer research.

Source: https://i.ytimg.com/vi/6IsVBHGhESw/maxresdefault.jpg.

6.1. Fundamental Concepts in Molecular Biology

The building blocks of molecular biology are basic processes , such as DNA replication, transcription, and translation, which map the flow of genetic information in a cell. Information regarding these processes is significant in molecular oncology because they are the processes through which genetic change can lead to the development of cancer. DNA is a blueprint to life, and alterations taking place during replication have far-reaching implications, with the potential of oncogene activation or inactivation of tumor suppressor genes. Furthermore, transcription and translation coordinate the synthesis of proteins that play crucial roles in cell growth and division. Any perturbation in these processes may lead to aberrant cell proliferation, a feature of cancer. Thus, an accurate comprehension of such elementary biological processes is not only important for general biological studies but also forms the pillars for therapeutic progress in oncology. Genomic changes arising due to mutations or epigenetic deregulations have a substantial impact on susceptibility to cancer as well as the progression of cancer. Molecular biology techniques , such as genome sequencing, have opened the way to the complexity of cancer genomes, revealing numerous mutations that can serve as biomarkers for treatment and diagnosis. Molecular oncology is founded on the concept of target treatment as a result of knowledge of these genetic alterations, which arose as the newest advancements in the discipline. For instance, next-generation sequencing makes it possible to precisely identify actionable genetic changes, guiding personalized treatment plans based on individual patient data. Integration of these genetic insights with cell-signaling pathways at the molecular level can optimize therapeutic gain while minimizing toxicities. It is therefore important to explain the relationship between genetic variations and their functional relevance in advancing the frontiers of precision medicine, a foundational principle of contemporary oncology treatment regimens. Understanding the molecular mechanisms of cancer not only guides current therapy but also enables the development of novel interventions for preventing and detecting early cancer. The study of key cell processes , such as apoptosis, cell cycle regulation, and DNA repair mechanisms, reveals vulnerabilities of cancer cells. The integration of molecular biology with emerging technologies like CRISPR and gene therapy opens the doors to new therapies aimed at the genetic defects of cancer. Furthermore, cancer research has come to better realize the importance of the tumor microenvironment in which the interaction between malignant and non-malignant cells can have a critical influence on disease evolution. By integrating the fundamental concepts of molecular biology with advanced methods and a proper understanding of cancer biology, researchers can develop powerful therapeutic models that not only cure established cancers but also target the eradication of precancerous conditions and enhance the overall effectiveness of cancer prevention measures, as seen in existing global research activities in precision medicine, such as Ryu (2023) (Figure 6.4).

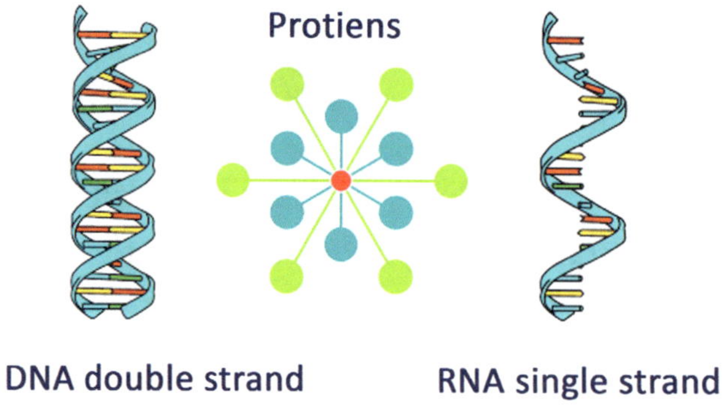

Figure 6.4. Fundamental concepts in molecular biology.

Source: https://blogger.googleusercontent.com/img/b/R29vZ2xl/AVvXsEj-YuKHpxN26oOedQQGkkvRtiy1PQ7QjbFbQIX9sGUwaiqVo_n9qEM9Z8HE4J2wcV7nA3NW6VaALnQGErDdTitSqIOVFyph_HEYWgjytoFV1gkXFHJKgHhMIUzcU-sijt-b5rVDZDVIeeDqTtosgGIextwjbyF-ZvG1nQ2Jk2Gziwf_7p-eB4Iof-tB/s640/The%20Basics%20of%20Molecular%20Biology%20Understanding%20the%20Fundamental%20Concepts.png.

6.1.1. DNA Structure and Function

The intricate structure of deoxyribonucleic acid (DNA) forms the foundation for its central role in biological functions, particularly cellular control and oncology. DNA is a double helix formed by two connected strands of nucleotides with a phosphate group, deoxyribose sugar, and nitrogenous bases (adenine, thymine, cytosine, and guanine). This organizational structure not only provides stability in the form of hydrogen bonding between complementary bases—cytosine with guanine and adenine with thymine—but also facilitates replication and transcription processes. Both processes are essential in the expression of genes and possible malignant transformations. In molecular oncology, it is necessary to understand this structure-function relationship because alterations in the integrity or mutations of DNA can lead to oncogenesis, where normal cells acquire the characteristics of cancer cells, thus promoting tumor growth and metastasis.

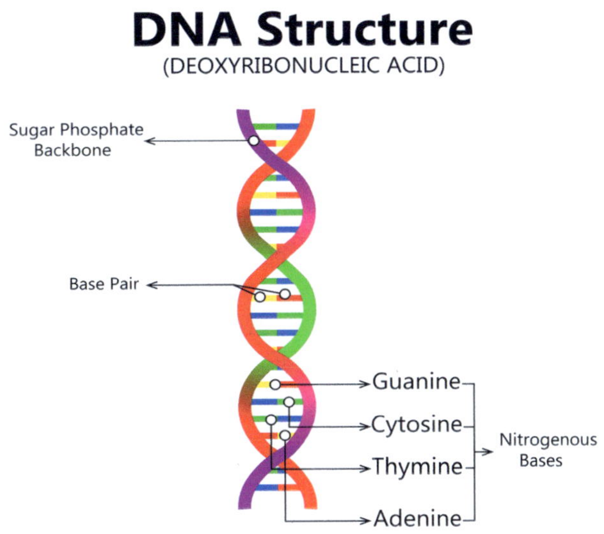

Figure 6.5. DNA structure and function.

Source: https://static.vecteezy.com/system/resources/previews/028/627/407/original/scientific-icon-spiral-of-dna-and-rna-an-illustration-of-the-differences-in-the-structure-of-the-dna-and-rna-molecules-image-poster-structure-rna-and-dna-vector.jpg.

The functional aspect of DNA has everything to do with its capacity for information storage and transmission to transmit genetic information that is critical for cellular function and the development of the organism. Genes, DNA molecules coding for specific proteins, direct the synthesis of these molecules, which are the structural components and functional units of cells. However, there may be various internal and external entities that result in mutation of DNA, ultimately disrupting the normal cell cycle and leading to aberrations , such as uncontrolled growth of cells. In molecular oncology, this is essential since the dysregulation of genes with specific functions in cell cycle control and apoptosis can cause cancer. Oncogene activation or silencing of tumor suppressor genes like p53, for example, may initiate a series of events for malignant transformation, highlighting the importance of genetic integrity to drive cellular homeostasis. Further, new developments in molecular science have enabled us to explore DNA at a never-before level, revealing cancer therapy possibilities. For instance, research on proteins involved in DNA repair mechanisms has revealed pathways that could be open to drug development. Brugia malayi-associated protein disulfide isomerase (PDI) is an example of structural dynamics that may be leveraged in targeted drug approaches across various biological systems, as its conformational behavior provides insights into enzyme function in cancer cell metabolism (Doharey et al., 2023). Also, the identification of riboflavin transporters and their overexpression in cancerous tumors presents the promise of exploiting their pathway as a form of targeted cancer therapy, demonstrating the potential of the intricate understanding of DNAs structure and functioning for new oncological treatments (Mariem et al., 2022) (Figure 6.5).

6.1.2. Gene Expression and Regulation

The intricate relationship between gene expression regulation and carcinogenesis lies at the core of molecular oncology. Gene expression is under significant regulation by a variety of internal and external influences, such as genetic mutations, epigenetic modifications, and environmental toxins. The impact of psychosocial influences on gene regulation, and the regulation of cancer survivors' genes in particular, is an especially important area of research. Research has indicated that psychosocial stressors can trigger biological processes leading to modulation of gene expression in tumor tissue and immune cells and affect disease outcome (Alyami et al., 2024). Such an intersection of gene expression and psychosocial risk factors is a reflection of the complexity of cancer biology and the necessity of an interdisciplinary approach to studying and treating cancer. Moreover, mounting evidence recognizes the role of specific genes in cancer initiation. For instance, the guanylate-binding protein 2 (GBP2) has been recognized as a significant driver for clear cell renal cell carcinoma (ccRCC). Studies indicated that GBP2 is often overexpressed in ccRCC and it is associated with adverse predictive outcomes. Its mechanism of action is through modulation of programmed death ligand 1 (PD-L1), hence having an effect on immune evasion of tumors as well as on immune cell infiltration (Ye et al., 2023). This indicates that gene expression not only supports tumor progression but also decides the tumor microenvironment, highlighting the role of using targeted therapeutic maneuvers with respect to these regulatory networks. An understanding of the regulation and expression of genes is crucial for new therapeutic approaches in cancer treatment. Such an understanding has bearing on new modes of treatment, such as immunotherapy, which attempt to tap into the body's own immune system as a way of combating cancer. Unveiling how the regulators of gene expression can contribute to the discovery of potential targets for therapeutic manipulation. For instance, modulating the expression of genes like GBP2 through interventions may increase the sensitivity of tumors to immunotherapeutic agents, ultimately resulting in improved patient outcomes. As molecular oncology evolves, further efforts at incorporating gene regulation studies into the clinic are required to improve the development of personalized medicine and increase survivorship in cancer patients.

6.1.3. Mutations and Their Role in Cancer Development

Mutations play a central part in cancer initiation, playing an important role in the tumorigenic process. These genetic mutations may happen at various levels, such as single nucleotide variation, insertions, deletions, and translocations at the chromosomal level. Certain mutations are inherited, thus being germline mutations, while others happen to an individual in their lifetime due to environmental factors, lifestyle, or random errors during DNA replication. Oncogene mutation causing enhanced cell proliferation and tumor suppressor gene mutation causing inhibition against unlimited proliferation can lead to uncontrolled growth of the cells and formation of tumor masses eventually. Understanding of these mutations not only explains how cancer develops, but it also helps in the creation of therapies targeting particular genetic mutations. The effect of some mutations on cancer is evidenced by the BRAF mutation in NSCLC. Approximately 4% of NSCLC patients carry BRAF mutations, the most relevant subgroup being the BRAF V600E, which occurs at approximately 2% incidence in the setting of advanced disease. The mutation enables abnormal activation of cell proliferation and survival signaling pathways, thus its oncogenic significance. Pursuant to the advent of targeted therapies , such as BRAF inhibitors, therapy for individuals affected by this mutation has become revolutionized, providing evidence for the clinical relevance of individualized therapy based on genetic screening. Moreover, guidelines of prominent cancer organizations now support routine diagnosis of BRAF mutations as a paradigm shift in oncologic practice that closes the gap between molecular defects and manageable therapy, resulting in better patient outcomes (Parisi et al., 2025). In breast cancer, several genetic factors contribute to the disease's multifactorial etiology, and germline mutations as well as single-nucleotide polymorphisms (SNPs) are of significant importance. Genome-wide association studies (GWAS) have been comprehensively examined to illustrate more than 180 polymorphic loci associated with breast cancer risk, illustrating the genetic etiology of its origin. The influence of well-established mutations, such as in BRCA1 and BRCA2, is, however, quite limited and occurs only in a minority of cases. These mutations, however, have profound implications for management at the clinical level and patient prognosis. The use of genetic marker analysis in breast cancer has elucidated the heterogeneity of the disease, indicating that the interaction of several modest-penetrance genes and the environment is necessary for the expression of individual risk profiles and the formulation of therapeutic plans (Pavlova et al., 2024) (Figure 6.6).

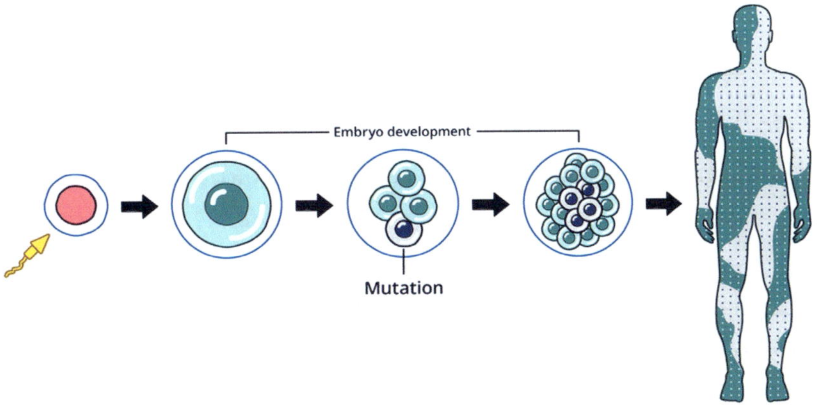

Figure 6.6. Mutations and their role in cancer development.

Source: https://www.cancer.gov/sites/g/files/xnrzdm211/files/styles/cgov_article/public/cgov_image/media_image/2022-04/OCPL-Cancer-Causing-Embryogenesis-Mutations.png?h=c7b81ad4&itok=klmGgc-r.

6.2. Cancer Genomics

The field of cancer genomics has revolutionized our understanding of oncogenesis by explaining the molecular mechanisms behind most cancers. By analyzing tumor genetic alterations, researchers can now identify specific mutations leading to the growth of cancers, drug resistance, and prognosis. For instance, in prostate cancer, high frequencies of pathogenic mutations in homologous recombination repair (HRR) genes have been observed and implicated in aggressive disease phenotypes. This realization has led to the creation of directed therapies that seek to exploit these genetic vulnerabilities. Furthermore, advances in genomic sequencing technology have made it possible to perform larger-scale tumor profiling, which has paved the way for individualized cancer treatment. Such precision medicine approaches specifically targeted are supposed to provide treatment based on one's genetic profiles, a drastic departure from the conventional one-size-fits-all approach in treating patients (González et al., 2025). Paragraph 10: Embedding genomic data within the clinic has tremendous implications, particularly with regard to improved diagnosis accuracy and therapeutic effectiveness.

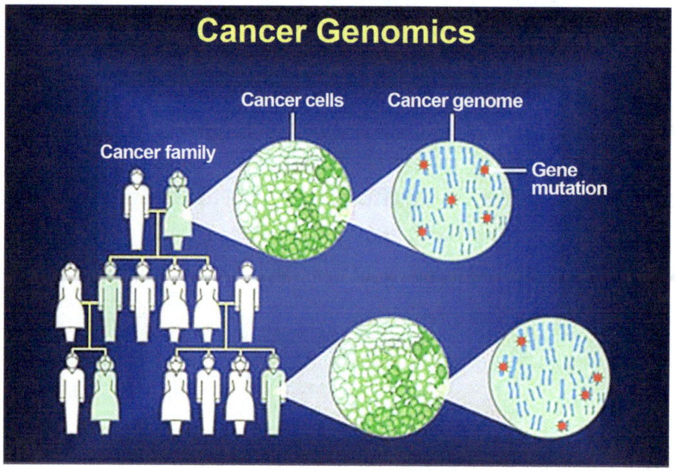

Figure 6.7. Cancer genomics.

Source: https://www.genome.gov/sites/default/files/genome-old/images/content/cancer_genomics.jpg.

The integration of genomic profiling with imaging modalities , such as PSMA-PET provides a richer picture of malignancy through combining anatomical, metabolic, and molecular attributes. For example, recent studies indicated that quantification of PSMA expression and genetic mutation status might be utilized to inform prognosis in metastatic prostate cancer. In other words, patients with pathogenic variants and high tumor volume by PSMA experienced poorer overall survival. This union of genomics information and molecular imaging not only assists in risk stratification of the patient but also aids the decision-making process towards treatment selection. As more and more oncologists embrace these new practices, the situation of cancer treatment continues to evolve with an emphasis on the significance of cancer genomics in aiding therapeutic outcomes (González et al., 2025). The emerging direction of cancer genomics is to advance predictive modeling to better enable us to predict disease progression and response to treatment. Through the use of sophisticated computational methods like machine learning and artificial intelligence, investigators hope to integrate complicated data sets that include genomic, clinical, and imaging data. Such models have the potential to uncover biomarkers with predictive metastatic behavior, alerting clinicians to patient prognosis and treatment. As would be expected from existing studies, combining genomic data with radiomics is set to deliver groundbreaking knowledge on tumor biology. Challenges remain, however, including keeping data variability and quality during model training. Resolving these issues in conjunction with advancing our understanding of the metastatic process is essential to the successful use of personalized strategies in oncology. Eventually, as methods become more advanced, predictive modeling will reimagine strategies for metastasis management (Figure 6.7).

6.2.1. Overview of Cancer Genomics and Its Significance

Cancer genomics represents a paradigm change in the molecular oncology science of discovering and characterizing genes that are involved in tumor development and growth. With the use of next-generation sequencing technologies, researchers can uncover a variety of genetic changes, including single nucleotide variants (SNVs), insertions and deletions (InDels), and copy number variations that are causative of malignancies. Identifying the genomic profile of tumors enables clinicians to personalize therapies based on the individual tumor profiles, significantly enhancing the effectiveness of therapy. For instance, in breast cancer, specific mutations , such as PIK3CA have been linked to resistance to treatment in neoadjuvant-treated patients. This highlights the potential of genomic data to serve as prognostic biomarkers and direct therapy, a shift away from conventional, shotgun approaches to more personalized, precision medicine strategies in oncology, thus paving the way for better patient outcomes (Paris et al., 2025). Aside from personalized treatment, the significance of cancer genomics is its central role in early detection and prevention (Paris et al., 2025). Genetic predisposition to specific cancers can be identified through broad-spectrum genomic screens, opening the door for early intervention with dramatic effects on survival. The development of genomic newborn screening for cancer predisposition syndromes (CPSs) highlights the potential for early detection. By defining germline mutations linked to increased cancer risk, healthcare systems can start surveillance and prophylactic treatments at birth, and in so doing, alter the course of disease progression. Moreover, introducing genomic data into public health programs also raises ethical concerns in terms of screening criteria and the confidentiality of patients. Extra vigilance is needed to balance the benefit of early detection against the dangers of worry and discrimination by individuals who are identified as being at genetic risk for cancer (Linga et al., 2024). With the emergence of cancer genomics, implications for research as well as clinical care are increasingly important. Integration of genomic data into clinical workflows necessitates collaboration among oncologists, geneticists, and data scientists to ensure that findings are effectively translated into actionable information. Furthermore, the continuous process of gene panel refinement employed in screenings needs to be adapted to changing scientific knowledge of cancer genetics for enhanced precision in risk evaluation of patients. As underpinned by new studies, identification of some mutations can lead to therapeutic paths of action, illustrating the interplay between genomics and treatment. The future of molecular oncology relies on the ability to employ genomic information to inform clinical decisions, thus maintaining the notion that a greater knowledge of cancer at the genetic level plays a critical role in advancing cancer therapy models and improving patient care (Paris et al., 2025).

6.2.2. Techniques Used in Genomic Analysis (e.g., Sequencing)

The landscape of molecular oncology has been profoundly changed with the use of advanced genomic analysis techniques, primarily sequencing technologies. Next-generation sequencing (NGS) is arguably one of the strongest methods that reflects this incomparable ability to achieve full insight into the genetic basis of cancer. With the ability to sequence millions of fragments of DNA simultaneously, NGS provides an extent of coverage and speed that previous approaches , such as Sanger sequencing, stand little chance of replicating. This capacity of throughput allows the identification of several genetic mutations and modifications, which are the cause of tumorigenesis, and the resultant development of knowledge in cancer biology.

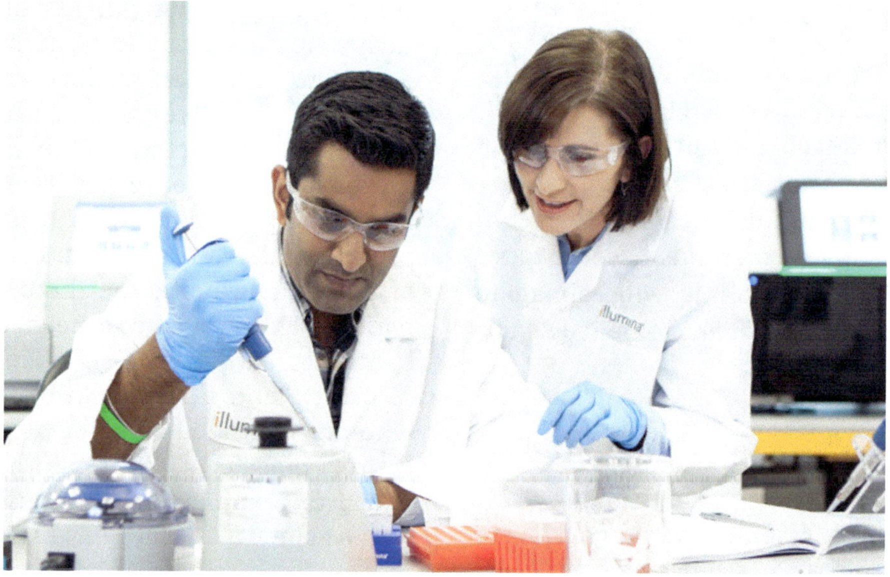

Figure 6.8. Techniques used in genomic analysis.

Source: https://assets.illumina.com/content/dam/illumina-marketing/images/techniques/scientists-lab-pipette-web-graphic.jpg.

The synergy of NGS with other molecular technologies, for example, polymerase chain reaction (PCR), enhances genomic data strength, thus providing greater specificity in identifying particular mutations and supporting clinical decision-making through tailoring treatment strategies, as demonstrated in recent studies on the effectiveness of genomic medicine in improving patient outcomes (Zuluaga et al., 2025). Apart from NGS, bioinformatics plays a crucial role in analyzing genomic data that significantly influences the interpretation of complex biological information. Development of platforms , such as the Open Navigator by Precision Oncology INformatics Technology (OnPOINT) attests to the potential of informatics solutions for precision oncology. These platforms enable genomic-clinical data integration to be automated such that clinicians can effectively match actionable molecular findings with suitable clinical trials (Botsis et al., 2025). The ability to systematically catalog genetic alterations and correlate them with FDA-approved medications or investigational treatments improves the ease with which to identify the best treatment options for patients. As patients present with variable mutations, such an informatics approach makes it such that every therapeutic option is not avoided, hence maximizing personalized medicine strategies, increasingly vital in the targeted treatment era. Lastly, the union of genomic sequencing technologies and bioinformatics not only hints at the promise of personalized medicine but also emphasizes the importance of ongoing research and innovation within the field. It is essential to consolidate multimodal sources of data, including variant registries and clinical databases, to facilitate the description of the clinical utility of genomic information (Botsis et al., 2025). With the evolving disciplines, putting effective solutions within reach, more so in the community, becomes exigent. Disparities in the utilization of these advanced techniques have the potential to curtail patient access to cutting-edge treatment. As evident in the most recent research evidence, the building of efficient platforms not only optimizes the engagement of patients in clinical trials but also enhances treatment outcomes as cancer therapy becomes personalized to unique genomic profiles (Zuluaga et al., 2025). Such breakthroughs pave the way for streamlined cancer management practices in pursuit of improved patient health and satisfaction (Figure 6.8).

6.2.3. Case Studies of Genomic Findings in Specific Cancers

The use of genomic analysis in cancer has provided significant advances in understanding individual cancers and their progression. For instance, the CAVE-2 GOIM trial is used for metastatic colorectal cancer (mCRC), where extensive genomic profiling (CGP) of ctDNA assists in the identification of actionable variants. Early observations are that a great majority of patients carry pathogenic variants within important genes , such as TP53 and APC, which are important markers for indicating the tumor behavior. The trial also revealed that around 31.4% of the patients carried RAS or BRAF mutations, which led to the identification of sophisticated resistance mechanisms to the therapies. These findings emphasize the role of genetic heterogeneity in cancer development, pointing to the necessity of patient-specific treatment strategies based on genomic information to optimize the prognosis of patients with mCRC (Napolitano et al., 2025). In pancreatic cancer, the genetic landscape is marked by vast heterogeneity and makes treatment routes more problematic. Evidence in extensive literature reviews has demonstrated that KRAS mutations are common, occurring in over 90% of malignant tumors in this category, and represent an obstinate challenge to treatment modalities. Pancreatic cancer is also often found not to harbor actionable mutations that molecular therapy can target, which represents a critical treatment deficit. Transcriptomic analyses have identified discordant tumor phenotypes, such as the squamous subtype, which are more resistant to conventional chemotherapy regimens and have poorer prognosis. This highlights the justification for employing a molecular-based strategy for the identification of subgroups of pancreatic cancer, targeting specific biomarkers, such as SMAD4 and TP53, which are treatment outcome-related (Ciulla & Luchini, 2024). The significance of cancer genomic findings extends far beyond the recognition of mutations; they carry implications for the creation of focused therapies with the promise of greater efficacy and lesser toxicity. As demonstrated in the cases of both mCRC and pancreatic carcinoma, genomic characterization not only assists in the elucidation of molecular underpinnings of tumor behavior but is useful for selection in favor of targeted therapeutic strategies. For example, in mCRC, actionable genomic alterations detected with CGP support personalized treatment regimens based on individual mutational profiles, while in pancreatic cancer, targeting the KRAS mutation remains a focal point for ongoing research. Finally, translation of genomic findings into clinical medicine practice holds important potential for treatment paradigm optimization, patient survival rate improvement, and molecular oncology establishment as a discipline (Ciulla & Luchini, 2024; Napolitano et al., 2025).

6.3. Molecular Mechanisms of Cancer

Understanding of molecular mechanisms associated with cancer has progressed substantially during the last few decades due to the discovery of oncogenes and tumor suppressor genes. One of the most studied of them is the TP53 gene that encodes the p53 protein, referred to as the guardian of the genome. p53 protein is a crucial transcription factor that controls numerous cellular responses by activating many target genes involved in cell cycle regulation, apoptosis, and maintenance of genomic stability. The mutation of TP53 causes the loss of its tumor-suppressing function and even triggers the activation of oncogenic properties in mutant proteins. As such, it is important to research the diverse mechanisms of the p53 signaling pathway and its role in cancer tumorigenesis for the development of targeted therapies in cancer that are able to effectively restore its activity in cancer cells (Wang et al., 2023).

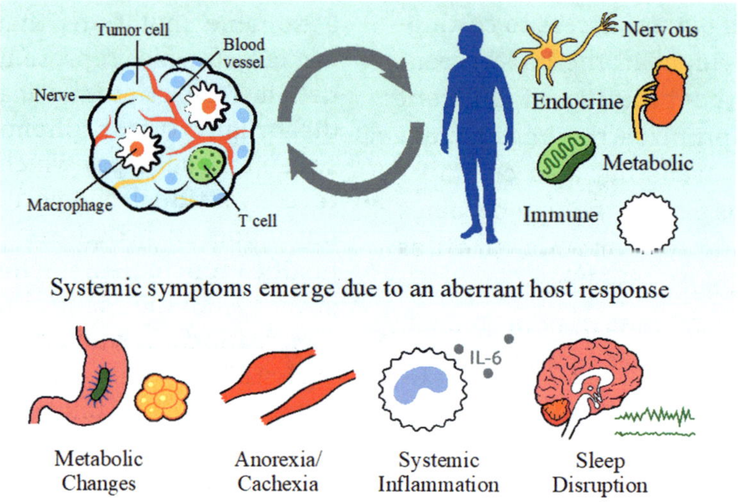

Figure 6.9. Molecular mechanisms of cancer.

Source: https://www.mdpi.com/ijms/ijms-20-02780/article_deploy/html/images/ijms-20-02780-g001.png.

In precision oncology, multi-omics methods have been an important approach to dissect the intricate molecular changes underlying tumorigenesis in cancer. These advanced approaches include genomics, transcriptomics, epigenomics, and more, to provide a holistic characterization of tumor biology. Multi-omics analysis not only enriches our understanding of fundamental processes in cancer but also illuminates treatment resistance and recurrence hazard. As these findings become increasingly implemented in practice, they emphasize the utility of personalized medicine and tailor-made treatment approaches. However, despite the potential of multi-omics, challenges to applying truly integrated analyses widely remain due to limitations in analytical infrastructure (Olivier et al., 2019). Addressing such challenges is crucial to advance the field and convert the discoveries into applications. Additionally, researching molecular processes in cancer transcends oncogenes and tumor suppressor genes to investigate multiple pathways involved in cellular metabolism and the tumor microenvironment. For instance, cross-talk between the cancer cells and their stromal cells can significantly influence the tumor's behavior and how it reacts to treatment. Exploring such interactions can reveal targets for therapy and methods that are mindful of the complexity of the tumor microenvironment. Ferroptosis, as well as autophagy regulators, have also been the target of interest because they are directly involved in the survival and growth of cancer cells when under stress. While the field of molecular oncology evolves, the research focus must more and more focus on deciphering these involved interactions and mechanisms to develop effective treatments that methodically break cancer's resilience (Wang et al., 2023) (Figure 6.9).

6.3.1. Oncogenes and Tumor Suppressor Genes

The roles of oncogenes and tumor suppressor genes are the focal point of cancer biology studies, often illustrated by their various functional mechanisms. Oncogenes are mutated forms of normal genes (proto-oncogenes) that promote cell growth and proliferation. Mutations in these genes, they can lead to overgrowth and proliferation of cells and thus tumorigenesis. Conversely, tumor suppressor genes are the guardians of the genome that hinder cell cycle growth and initiate apoptosis when there is DNA damage. Loss or inactivation of such safeguarding mechanisms could lead to excessive cell growth. This equilibrium between tumor suppressor genes and oncogenes is of utmost importance; shifting the balance on either side can initiate the cascade of events leading to cancer. Recognition of such dynamic interaction highlights the complexity of cancer and the need for focused treatments that can feasibly address aberrations in such significant genetic regulators. Advances in molecular oncology at an accelerated pace have revealed the intricate relationship between oncogenes and tumor suppressor genes, particularly in drug resistance development. The example of BRAF somatic mutations shows this overlap, with mutations of BRAF occurring frequently in various types of cancer, like melanoma and colorectal cancer. The study is that approximately 90% of BRAF mutations belong to the category of BRAFV600E mutations, which has a great impact on treatment and survival of the patient. Moreover, with the occurrence of co-occurring mutations in other oncogenes and tumor suppressor genes, the landscape of treatment options becomes difficult, and one solution may not prove sufficient. For instance, the interplay between BRAF mutations and secondary genomic alterations necessitates a multidirectional approach to treatment with targeted therapy coupled with immunotherapy. Thus, in-depth genomic profiling must be conducted to formulate effective treatment options tailored to individual patients, revealing insights into potential resistance pathways—often due to aberrant oncogenic signaling and impaired tumor suppressor gene function. The investigation of microRNAs, such as miR-192, further emphasizes the complexity of oncogenes and tumor suppressor genes in cancer biology. Chromosome 11q13.1's miR-192 is bidirectional in its activities as either a tumor suppressor or an oncogene, depending on the type of cancer. Dysregulation of miR-192 has been linked to the initiation of various malignancies, managing tumor dynamics through the regulation of gene expression and signal transduction pathways. This double role makes the process of miRNA-based therapeutics more complex because unraveling precisely how and why miR-192 works in a given situation is crucial to accessing its full potential. The fact that miR-192 is found everywhere in bodily fluids like serum and exosomes just highlights its potential as a non-invasive cancer prognosis and diagnosis biomarker. Lastly, it is important to possess a more differentiated understanding of oncogenes and tumor suppressor genes and their corresponding regulation mechanisms to drive personalized cancer medicine further, facilitating new detection strategies and treatments (Perfetto et al., 2025; Yang et al., 2025).

6.3.2. Pathways Involved in Cancer Progression (e.g., Signaling Pathways)

The intricate network of signal pathways involved in the process of cancer development is a key to understanding the molecular basis of most malignancies. The hub of this complex network is signaling pathways , such as PI3K/AKT/mTOR, RAS/RAF/ERK, and Wnt/β-catenin signaling cascades, which integrate cell processes , such as growth, survival, and proliferation. Abnormal regulation of these pathways is frequently observed in tumors, creating a disorderly cellular behavior. For instance, the PI3K/AKT/mTOR pathway is most commonly implicated in the maintenance of survival and growth in lung cancer, and the non-coding RNAs have a key function to play in their regulation.

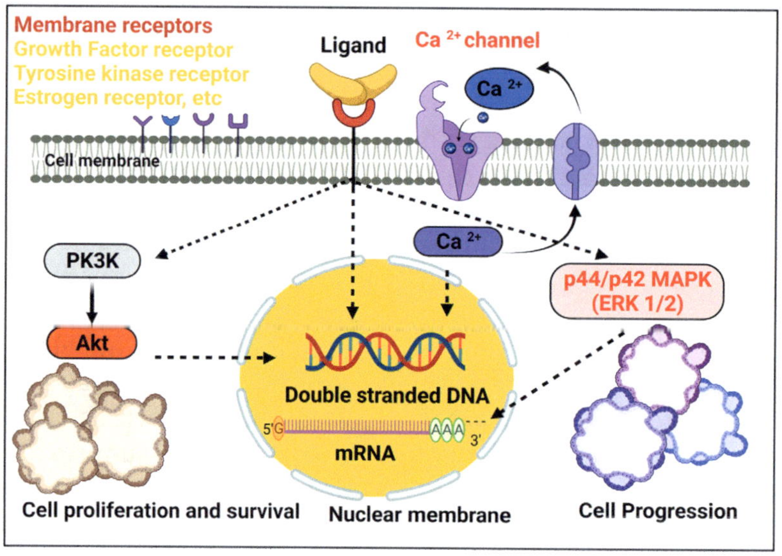

Figure 6.10. Pathways involved in cancer progression.

Source: https://www.researchgate.net/profile/Sumel_Ashique2/publication/360869858/figure/fig4/AS:1160944872882176@1653802235082/arious-signaling-pathways-involved-in-breast-cancer-proliferation-progression-and.png.

The involvement of these pathways in cancer transformation makes them candidates for possible therapy, aside from the existing treatment modalities highlighted in ongoing research. Understanding these signaling mechanisms is important to create more effective cancer therapies, aimed at reversing the specific changes taking place in cancer cells (Liu et al., 2023). In addition to well-established pathways, non-coding RNAs (ncRNAs) are also proving to be vital agents in cancer formation, regulating many signaling mechanisms. NcRNAs, including microRNAs, long non-coding RNAs, and circular RNAs, are of significant significance in modulating gene expression and thereby influencing cellular processes pivotal for tumorigenesis. For example, disturbance of the expression of specific miRNAs has been linked to the activation of oncogenic signaling pathways, thereby driving growth and development of lung cancer. These ncRNAs are found to have the capacity to modulate cancer processes by amplifying oncogenic signals or repressing tumor suppressor functions. With their roles in cancer biology increasingly understood, ncRNAs are also promising to act as both biomarkers and targets for therapy, transforming the landscape of cancer therapy and prompting the development of tailored approaches based on such molecular data (Liu et al., 2023). The CRC landscape also hints at the significance of signaling pathways in cancer development and resistance to therapy. Loss-of-function mutations of tumor suppressor gene and DNA repair genes often eliminate essential signaling cascades and promote malignancy. The clinical responses in CRC have traditionally augmented with chemotherapy and radiotherapy, but response to these treatments continues to vary due to the complexity of tumor biology. Understanding of the specific signaling pathways that drive CRC, such as Wnt and RAS pathways, makes the possibility of therapeutics that can overcome the limitations of conventional treatments possible. Through disclosure of the molecular signal that is implicated in CRC progression, researchers can design new therapies that specifically target these pathways, finally resulting in better patient outcomes and reduced disease progression (Figure 6.10).

6.3.3. The Role of the Tumor Microenvironment

The tumor microenvironment (TME) is a key notion in drug resistance and cancer biology. Not only does the TME consist of cancer cells, but also of an even more heterogeneous group of non-malignant cells , including immune cells, fibroblasts, and endothelial cells that interact with each other dynamically. These interactions can have significant influences on tumor growth, development, and metastasis. For instance, immune cells within the TME can suppress or enhance tumorigenesis depending on their phenotype and activation state. In this regard, manipulation of the TME has become an important area of study as it is susceptible to therapeutic manipulation with a view to optimizing patient outcomes, particularly combined with immunotherapies with a view to modulating immune checkpoint targets. Investment in the unmasking of the complexities of these interactions remains the hallmark of the landscape of treatment modalities in molecular oncology. Recent studies have mapped out the inherent heterogeneity of the TME in a tumor type-dependent and stage-dependent manner. Notably, the composition and function of the tumor microenvironments may determine therapeutic response and resistance. For instance, the results of recent studies have revealed that inter-individual differences in gut microbiome composition can influence the effectiveness of immunotherapies in patients with melanoma, with certain bacterial taxa being linked to responders and non-responders (Dimitriou et al., 2025). These findings explain the complex interaction between the biology of the tumor and the microbiome within the TME, and they highlight that modulation of the microbiome can enhance the therapeutic efficacy by creating a proper environment for immune stimulation. Thus, exploration of both the local and systemic features of the TME becomes essential to design innovative therapeutic strategies that can overcome resistance in numerous cancer types. Moreover, variations in the TME with aging introduce complexity, especially in the unique hematological malignancies , such as classical Hodgkin lymphoma (cHL). The unique biology of cHL, including the microenvironment rich in immune and stromal cells, underscores the importance of these factors in supporting malignant cells. Age-related variations in TME composition have been reported, with advancements in single-cell sequencing and spatial imaging technology having delivered critical information regarding variations in cellular interactions in younger versus older patients (Aoki et al., 2025). These variations can influence disease course and response to treatment, noting the need for age-specific treatment protocols. Understanding the variations of the TME in different populations not only assists in the identification of predictive markers but also provides access to tailor-made therapies that account for the distinct cellular environment in which tumors develop and progress.

6.4. Targeted Therapies in Oncology

Targeted therapies in cancer represent a paradigm shift in the management of cancer, focusing on molecular and genetic characteristics of cancer and not conventional practices targeting cells that are proliferating rapidly indiscriminately. This is a more tailored approach to treatment, where therapy is targeted at inhibiting certain pathways to drive the proliferation of cancer. The integration of advanced genetics, such as genomic sequencing and biomarker identification, has been significant in finding actionable mutations within the individual cancer. Individualized molecular signatures can be targeted by targeted therapies, making it possible to increase the efficacy of treatment while minimizing undesirable side effects.

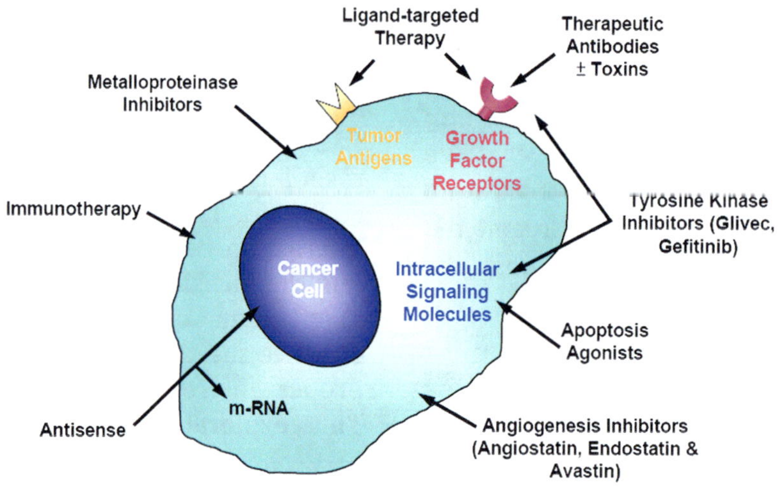

Figure 6.11. Targeted therapies in oncology.

Source: https://www.researchgate.net/profile/De-Kuan-Chang/publication/26576352/figure/fig3/AS:667716239237121@1536207365146/Targeted-therapy-refers-to-a-new.png.

As the discipline evolves and expands, an understanding of these molecular underpinnings is increasingly essential to optimize cancer care and outcomes in increasingly heterogeneous patient populations (Bhoyar & Chandu, 2025). Moreover, pharmacological science advancement and drug development have propelled the advancement and application of targeted therapies. Recent technological innovations in omics technologies, which systematically examine genetic, transcriptomic, proteomic, and metabolomic profiles, have significantly increased understanding of tumor biology. These advances enable clinicians to select treatments based on a patient's individualized molecular profile, thus raising the likelihood of successful treatment outcomes. In practice, the creation of molecular tumor boards demonstrates how multi-omics information can be used to guide clinical decisions, so that patients can be given the most promising treatments based on their individualized tumor characterization. Even with the advancements made, though, challenges persist in how to deliver these new treatments equitably and how to deal with the nuances of resistance mechanisms that can diminish their effects (Teleanu et al., 2025). Since targeted therapies continue to expand, their own critical analysis of value in patient stratification and treatment effectiveness is called for. Not all patients with actionable molecular alterations respond uniformly to targeted therapies, reflecting the complexities of drug response in relation to genetic background. In addition, as treatments become increasingly advanced, more interdisciplinary coordination among oncologists, geneticists, and data scientists will be needed to achieve a thorough understanding of tumor ecosystems. Challenging the efficacy of existing treatments using continuous clinical trials will also be essential for streamlining treatment approaches. The future of oncology is in realizing the full potential of targeted therapy and precision medicine, guiding the evolution of individualized models of treatment toward improved patient survival rates and outcomes overall (Bhoyar & Chandu, 2025; Teleanu et al., 2025) (Figure 6.11).

6.4.1. Definition and Examples of Targeted Therapies

Targeted medications are a characteristic of current oncological therapeutic policy, acting against specific molecular transformations of the neoplastic cells rather than against the broad group of cancer types. They inhibit routes responsible for tumor development and proliferation by impairing the activity of specific molecules, which play a crucial role in disease development. For instance, small-molecule inhibitors can engage a variety of different kinases, some of which participate in signaling pathway activation for cancer cell survival and proliferation. A case in point is the use of therapies against the AXL receptor, which has also been linked to aggressive tumor biology due to its roles in multiple tumor-promoting pathways, including enhanced cancer cell invasion, metastasis, and chemotherapy resistance. This particular targeting of molecular aberrancy not only maximizes the effectiveness of therapy but also minimizes the possibility of accidental harm to normal tissue, thereby reducing side effects inherent in traditional treatments. In the case of the particular example, targeted therapies have wide-ranging applications with various types of malignancies. One such example is the therapy of HER2-positive breast cancer with monoclonal antibodies that selectively target the HER2 receptor, blocking its growth signals and triggering apoptosis in cancer cells. Similarly, therapies for vascular endothelial growth factor (VEGF) target inhibiting angiogenesis, through which tumors form new blood vessels, thereby limiting cancer exposure to nutrients and oxygen. In hematologic malignancies, targeted therapies like imatinib that inhibit BCR-ABL fusion proteins in chronic myeloid leukemia are the clearest indication of the efficacy of individualized therapy in cancer management. Targeted therapy not only enhances the treatment outcome of patients but also sets the tone for developing individualized treatments based on the genetic composition of an individual's tumor, deviating from precision medicine in oncologic treatment. The complexity of tumor biology necessitates the continuous evolution of targeted treatments, particularly in the context of bypassing obstacles , such as therapeutic resistance. Tumor cells can resist initial therapy by evolving several mechanisms, such as activating alternate signaling pathways or through drug resistance mutations. For instance, studies have established that overexpression of AXL is involved in resistance to a large number of anticancer agents, highlighting the possibility of employing combination therapies that attack several routes simultaneously to increase efficacy and diminish the likelihood of relapse. The emerging interest in glioma treatment underlines the central role of glioma stem cells (GSCs) in tumor kinetic heterogeneity, underlining the need for new interventions that specifically target certain molecular pathways core to GSC activities. As ongoing research into molecular mechanisms of resistance deepens our insights, targeted therapies are the promise of transforming the practice of oncology due to their ability to change and respond to the intricate dynamics of tumor activity, as new research into GSCs and pathways aimed at maximizing clinical outcomes (Agosti et al., 2024; Yadav et al., 2025).

6.4.2. Mechanisms of Action of Targeted Drugs

The mechanisms of action of targeted drugs are a paradigm shift in oncological treatment regimens, emphasizing specificity over traditional regimens. They are designed to interfere with specific molecular targets that are involved in tumor development and progression, and their effectiveness is due to the ability to bind selectively to such targets without affecting normal cells in an adverse manner. For instance, small molecule inhibitors target specific signaling pathways, such as the EGFR or HER2 pathways, which are more active in cancer cells. By inhibiting these pathways, targeted therapy can close down critical processes , such as cell division and survival. Moreover, antibody-drug conjugates demonstrate a personalized strategy by delivering cytotoxic payloads to cancer cells directly, thereby minimizing collateral damage to normal tissues. Accordingly, the multifaceted mechanism of action of these agents plays an integral part in their optimization for maximal therapy with minimal toxicity and in transforming the oncological paradigm at its very core. To overcome the mysteries of dose optimization in the application of targeted therapies, there must be an in-depth understanding of their mechanisms of action. Unlike in conventional chemotherapy, with the maximum tolerated dose forming the principle that informs it, targeted drugs can deliver therapy at considerably lower doses. This shift in strategy is significant as it not only minimizes the risk of acute toxicity but also aligns with the most recent FDA recommendations favoring dose optimization as informed by molecular knowledge. Current literature recommends splitting such therapies into four distinct classes based on their mechanisms, e.g., small molecule targeted therapies and large molecule antagonists, each with its own set of dose optimization problems and solutions (Johnson et al., 2020).

For instance, while efficacy can be demonstrated in small molecules at sub-maximal doses, there may be a need to fine-tune efficacy and safety for large molecule antagonists to offer a therapeutic approach with a balance. Quantitative pharmacology and statistical modeling become a part of drug development to elucidate mechanisms of action for targeted therapies. Pharmacodynamic and pharmacokinetic data need to be combined to tailor dosing for the best patient effect with minimal undesired effects. Moreover, applying proof of activity as a gating criterion for dose escalation provides optimal decision-making on dose choice in early-phase clinical trials. This approach enhances the potential of achieving successful outcomes and also optimizes patient resource use, as discussed in framework papers on the classification of targeted drugs (Zhu et al., 2025). Essentially, understanding and optimizing the mechanisms of targeted treatments is key to enhancing molecular oncology to deliver more effective and personalized interventions tailored to the specific molecular characteristics of the individual tumor (Figure 6.12).

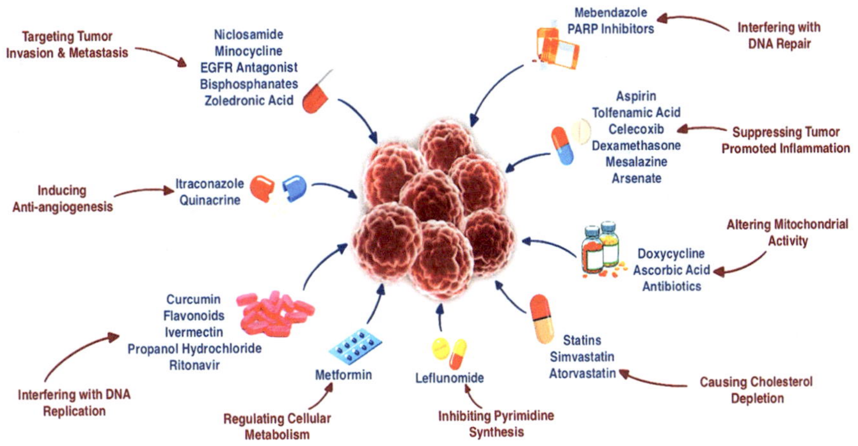

Figure 6.12. Mechanisms of action of targeted drugs: A fundamental shift in oncological treatment paradigms.

Source: https://www.researchgate.net/publication/361261794/figure/fig1/AS:11431281084277272@1663120441200/of-the-various-mechanisms-of-action-targeted-by-non-oncology-drugs-in-cancer-cells-making.png.

6.4.3. Challenges and Limitations of Targeted Therapies

The landscape of targeted therapies in molecular oncology is fraught with challenges that significantly deter their application to the clinic. Tumor heterogeneity is one of the central challenges that tumors with several changes in their genetics, which may occur within the same patient. This heterogeneity makes it challenging to define actionable targets, as therapy effective for one mutation will be ineffective for a comparable one present in the same cancer. In addition, the absence of uniform procedures for comprehensive genomic profiling deepens this problem, pointing out the inequity in access to sufficient molecular testing, especially in public healthcare systems. As documented in non-small cell lung cancer (NSCLC) studies, a significant number of patients are denied genomic testing by factors like inadequate facilities and awareness, ultimately affecting downstream treatment options and outcomes, as stated by Schneider et al. (2025). Further, the administration of targeted medications is challenging because the drugs face barriers in reaching tumors, particularly in the central nervous system (CNS). The blood-brain barrier limits the activity of numerous therapeutic agents, and tumor microenvironments may introduce further resistance to therapy. Such limitations call for novel drug delivery systems and sophisticated imaging modalities that can deliver treatments more effectively. For instance, advances in neuro-oncology in the recent past have evoked interest in window-of-opportunity trials, which provide the opportunity to assess drug effect within a real-time setting, providing important data for further refinement of treatment regimens. But considering the heterogeneity of tumors and microenvironments, as discussed by Geurts et al. (2025), only identifying a mutation won't do; drug development has to adopt tailor-made approaches to bypass these problems. Finally, the effectiveness of targeted therapies is also made difficult by the rapid evolution of resistance pathways within tumors. Over time, the cancer cells may even acquire mutations that render the previously effective treatments ineffective, creating a formidable challenge in the long-term survival of the patient. Such a process underscores the necessity of constant monitoring and treatment strategies that adapt to newly emerging mechanisms of resistance. In addition, the discovery of new experimental drugs for less common oncogenic drivers underlines the necessity of optimizing clinical trial designs to accommodate the diverse topographies of cancer biology. Its solution, apart from engaging the scientific community's united effort, requires a broader debate about healthcare policies to grant equal access to advances in precision oncology, as emphasized by Geurts et al. (2025).

6.5. Immunotherapy and Molecular Oncology

Immunotherapy has emerged as a leading technology in molecular oncology, particularly in the treatment of tumors with advanced mechanisms for immune evasion. This is due to the application of the body's own immune system to identify and destroy cancer cells, typically enhancing the efficacy of available treatments , such as chemotherapy and radiotherapy. With clarification of the molecular mechanisms of different cancers with advanced research tools, specific immunotherapeutic strategies are also being developed.

For instance, the immune microenvironment of head and neck squamous cell carcinoma (HNSCC) has been characterized with the help of omics technologies, which present interactions between tumor cells and immune elements in their vicinity. This information is crucial for the prediction of treatment response, treatment strategy optimization, and ultimately optimizing the survival of patients under the threat of in-built resistance to immunotherapy (Liu et al., 2025). Moreover, advances in comparative immuno-oncology have illuminated immune response complexity between different species, optimizing cancer treatment practice. By studying naturally occurring tumors in animals, scientists can compare and conclude about oncolytic virus (OV) mechanisms and their behavior in eliciting anti-tumor immunity. Such a comparison not only promotes deeper knowledge of how different animal immune systems tackle malignancies but also forms the groundwork for designing successful cancer treatments in the veterinary as well as human realms. Preclinical design in animal models has become an essential part of OV therapy assessment, providing a comprehensive evaluation of their efficacy and safety.

Multidisciplinary design bridges veterinary and human oncology gaps and, as such, refines translational research and imposes new treatment paradigms (Alkayyal, 2025). As immunotherapy continues to develop, integration of molecular oncology and bioinformatics will be key in shaping future paradigms of cancer treatment. Advances in genomic sequencing and data analysis will continue to enable better definitions of tumor heterogeneity, enabling clinicians to devise personalized therapies based on unique molecular profiles. By determining biomarkers associated with responses or resistance to treatment, scientists can develop new immunotherapeutic approaches, tailoring individual treatment regimens that hold the potential for improved effectiveness. Additionally, as our understanding of the tumor environment continues to grow, novel immunotherapy targets are being identified, revealing potential combination therapies that may synergize to positively affect patients. As the field of cancer treatment continues to evolve, the ongoing emphasis on both molecular characterization and targeted immunotherapy can potentially significantly impact the future of cancer treatment (Figure 6.13).

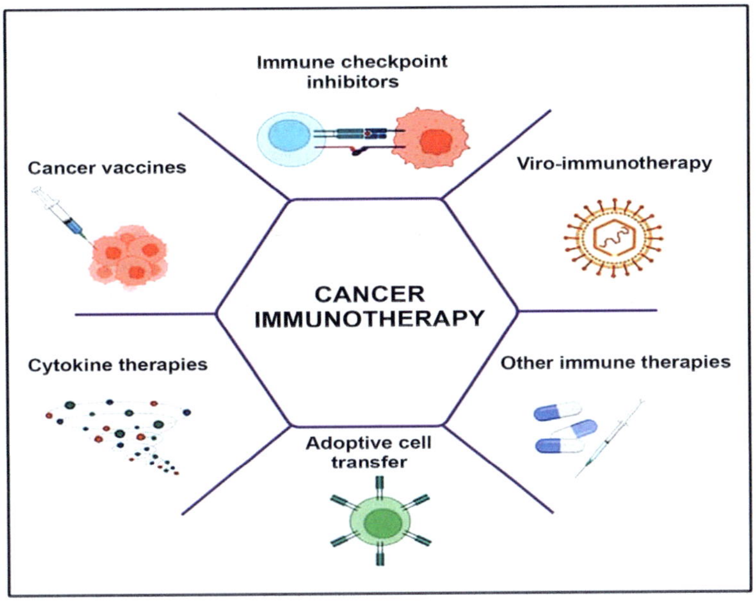

Figure 6.13. Immunotherapy and molecular oncology cancers.

Source: https://encyclopedia.pub/media/item/202305/6464751a703abcancers-15-02721-g004-550.jpg.

6.5.1. Overview of Immunotherapy Approaches

Immunotherapy is a revolutionary modality of molecular oncology that employs the intrinsic strength of the immune system against cancer. A number of approaches , such as checkpoint inhibitors, adoptive cell transfer, and monoclonal antibodies have gained more prominence in the clinic. Checkpoint inhibitors, in turn, target mechanisms that suppress immune responses, thus unleashing T-cells to recognize and destroy cancer cells. Therapies like pembrolizumab and nivolumab have proven highly effective in melanoma and lung cancer, with some patients responding with durable outcomes. However, not all patients respond to these drugs, which has stimulated research to find biomarkers that will predict sensitivity to immunotherapy. Understanding the molecular mechanisms involved in immunotherapy, including tumor antigen presentation, is critical to the design of optimal patient selection for these novel therapies and again underlies the requirement for an individualized strategy in oncology. Adoptive cell transfer (ACT) is another central immunotherapy strategy, whereby a patient's own T-cells are harvested, engineered or expanded *ex vivo*, and subsequently reinfused to fight the tumor. Chimeric antigen receptor (CAR) T-cell therapy is a renowned case, where T-cells are genetically modified to carry tumor antigen-binding receptors that enhance their specificity in targeting and destroying cancer cells (Ebru, 2022). The therapy has been extremely successful for hematological malignancies , such as acute lymphoblastic leukemia, but has been challenging to extend it to solid tumors due to the complexity of the tumor microenvironment. Despite these obstacles, advances in gene editing and next-generation CAR T-cell development mark a new frontier in personalized cancer treatment. Future study of the restriction and potential of ACTs will be essential in translating therapies into more broadly applicable treatments for a variety of cancer subtypes. The role of the tumor microenvironment (TME) in determining the efficacy of immunotherapy should not be overplayed. Composed of immune cells, extracellular matrix elements, and signaling molecules, TME can either enhance or suppress antitumor immunity. To illustrate, immunosuppressive cells , such as regulatory T-cells and myeloid-derived suppressor cells, can interfere with the functioning of therapeutic agents, resulting in the emergence of therapy resistance. Under these circumstances, combination strategies that integrate immunotherapy with other treatments, e.g., chemotherapy or targeted therapy, are being explored to overcome these obstacles. Further, emerging models , such as humanized mice provide robust platforms for the investigation of TME complexity and assessment of novel immunotherapeutic modalities more effectively. Investigation of the multi-factorial interaction of the TME and immune response is important in the augmentation of the build-up of even more effective immunotherapies that may yield improved outcomes for cancer patients (Chen et al., 2023; Li et al., 2024).

6.5.2. The Role of Biomarkers in Immunotherapy

The application of biomarkers in immunotherapy is a significant advance in the field of molecular oncology, particularly in the tailoring of cancer treatments to individual patients. Biomarkers are key markers that can ascertain the biological condition of tumors, and thus allow clinicians to determine which patients will be responsive to immunotherapy. For instance, the presence of specific immune checkpoints , such as PD-L1 expression, has been correlated with increased responses to checkpoint inhibitors, guiding treatments. This harmonization of treatment protocols with molecular prognostics optimizes the aggregate efficacy of immunotherapeutic interventions and minimizes unnecessary side effects. As science is progressing, it is essential to discover new biomarkers that not only determine the suitability of the patient for specific therapies but also elucidate the mechanisms of resistance towards the ultimate development of more targeted approaches in cancer therapy. Moreover, the role of metabolic biomarkers is becoming evident in the phenomenon of resistance to immunotherapy as well. Metabolic alterations in the tumor microenvironment can greatly detract from immune function and contribute to therapeutic failure. Upregulation of glycolysis and defective amino acid metabolism yield an immunosuppressive milieu that inhibits T-cell activation and function. Metabolite production, such as lactate, for example, can lead to the development of myeloid-derived suppressor cells and regulatory T cells, which inhibit effective antitumor immunity. Understanding these metabolic pathways has resulted in the identification of therapeutic strategies that have been found to target such changes, thereby enhancing the efficacy of immunotherapies. From metabolic biomarkers, scientists can develop enhanced strategies that are capable of reversing resistance mechanisms, thereby enhancing patient outcomes for immunotherapy (Shende et al., 2025). In case of cancers , such as glioblastoma, the application of biomarkers in guiding the treatment pathways is especially crucial due to the tumor's complex genetic makeup. Clinical trials on the efficacy of targeted therapies normally rely on specific molecular markers for patient stratification, which ensures the necessity of biomarker-guided treatment. But although genomically driven analysis can uncover potential by establishing lead indicators, the majority of clinical trials lack biomarker specifics in their study design. This lack of integration compromises the breadth of target therapies that can be provided to patients and represents a deficiency within the field of oncology that must be overcome. Expanding the use of molecular biomarkers can expand future clinical trial designs so that all the potential for personalized medicine is realized to successfully treat recurrent glioblastoma and other refractory cancers (van Opijnen et al., 2024) (Figure 6.14).

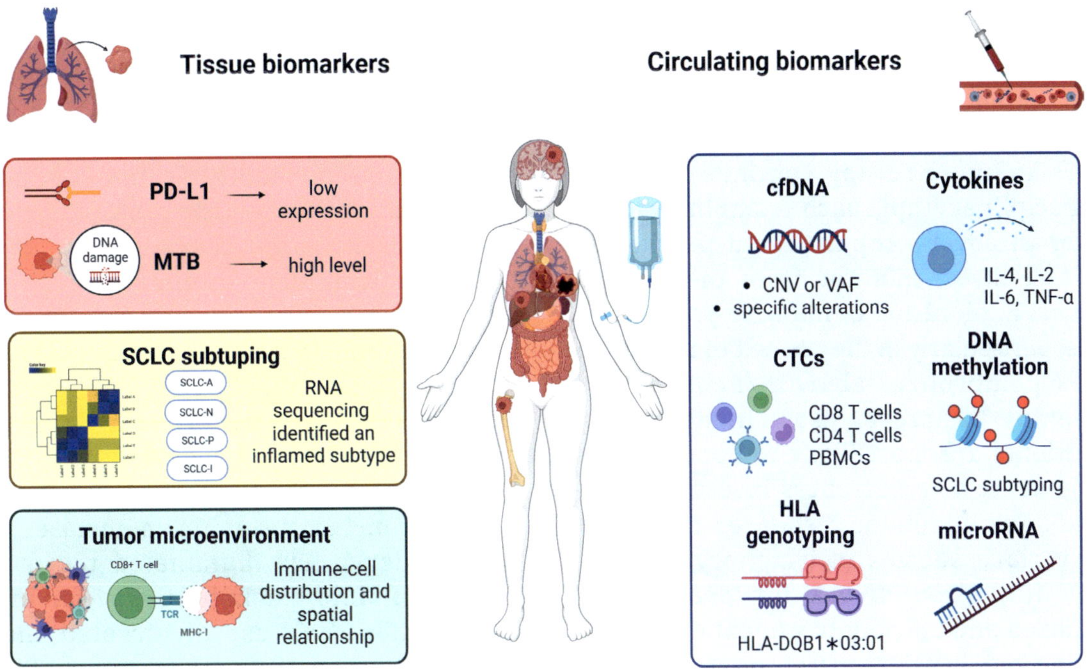

Figure 6.14. The role of biomarkers in immunotherapy.

Source: https://www.frontiersin.org/files/Articles/1308109/fimmu-15-1308109-HTML/image_m/fimmu-15-1308109-g001.jpg.

6.5.3. Success Stories and Ongoing Research in Immunotherapy

The field of immunotherapy has seen astounding expansion, and the beaconing success of combining checkpoint inhibitors with neoadjuvant chemotherapy in the case of triple-negative breast cancer (TNBC) is a case in point. The KEYNOTE-522 trial demonstrated that pembrolizumab, an anti-PD-1, combined with chemotherapy, dramatically increased the rate of pathological complete response (pCR) in early-stage TNBC patients. This landmark trial not only emphasized the potential of immunotherapy to enhance response to standard treatment but also formed the basis for the inclusion of immune-based strategies in treatment regimens. Continued investigation still strives to understand the immune dynamics in these responses, with studies showing that intratumoral infiltrating lymphocytes (iTILs) and Natural Killer (NK) cells are the major determinants of response to chemotherapy. This evolving landscape is filled with optimism regarding how we may engineer immune-related treatments to maximize overall patient gain in TNBC and elsewhere (Gasparini et al., 2024). Alongside these optimistic clinic results, the advent of patient-derived tumor organoids (PDTOs) is a paradigm shift in how researchers are approaching cancer immunotherapy. These organoids, which are cultured from patient tumor biopsies, accurately mimic the histological and molecular characteristics of primary tumors, providing a valuable model for preclinical studies. PDTOs not only facilitate better characterization of tumor behavior but also enable the identification of novel therapeutic targets and verification of immunotherapeutic agents. With the representative power of PDTOs, researchers are defining the way to personalized medicine, building on the success of immunotherapies to further improve efficacy and minimize side effects. However, there remain challenges in refining these models to address the omission of incorporating tumor microenvironment components within organoid cultures, which will also define the further progression of this vibrant field (Thorel et al., 2024). Immunotherapy continues to take a multidisciplinary approach, combining new biomarker discovery, sophisticated preclinical models, and direct monitoring of the patient in real time. Exploration of immune population dynamics, particularly in the context of therapies , such as pembrolizumab with neoadjuvant chemotherapy, has proven useful in identifying which patients are most likely to benefit from given regimens. As researchers investigate the processes behind immune responses, including roles of various subsets of lymphocytes, they are providing groundwork for even more individualized and efficient treatment protocols. By defining the interactions between immune cell profiles and treatment response, present treatments are looking to maximize and refine therapeutic techniques for TNBC and other cancers with the ultimate goal of maximizing the effectiveness of immunotherapy. With the continually evolving field of oncology, such holistic approaches have a lot of potential to further augment the patient's outcome and the future of cancer treatment (Gasparini et al., 2024; Thorel et al., 2024).

6.6. Future Directions in Molecular Oncology

The face of molecular oncology keeps changing with the advent of precision medicine, under which the treatment regimens are given top priority based on a patient's personalized genetic and molecular profile. With the progression of research, genomic sequencing and biomarker detection are now coming forward as important elements. Both these enable oncologists to identify genetic mutations that can enhance cancer growth and thus enable them to personalize therapy options. The role of artificial intelligence (AI) and machine learning (ML) cannot be overstated; they facilitate the analysis of large genomic datasets, improving diagnostic accuracy and treatment predictability. In the coming years, molecular oncology will be centered on creating personalized therapy that not only maximizes treatment but also minimizes side effects. This is a paradigm shift, and it is the promise of improved patient outcomes in oncology (Bhoyar & Chandu, 2025). New therapeutic approaches and targeted treatments are transforming the destiny of molecular oncology, particularly the treatment of complex diseases , such as melanoma brain metastases (MBM). New evidence has illuminated the molecular drivers of MBM, paving the way for improved intervention. The use of targeted therapies, along with immunotherapies and sophisticated treatments like stereotactic radiosurgery (SRS), has already proven to significantly improve survival in patients. However, additional studies are needed since current therapies will not be universally applicable due to the heterogeneity of the tumors. The future direction of MBM control will most likely be through a greater understanding of tumor biology and molecular signaling pathways that will enable clinicians to resort to an increasingly personalized treatment strategy that cares for patients as per their individual needs in detail. This will initiate a shift towards more personalized and effective care (Shrestha et al., 2025). As there are continuous developments in molecular oncology, gaps urgently have to be bridged through interdisciplinarity to drive innovative research and therapeutic strategies. Chemists, biologists, doctors, and data scientists must work with one another to establish new frontiers in cancer comprehension and therapy. Interdisciplinary research can accelerate the translation of laboratory advances to the clinic so that innovative methods become part of patient care with maximum speed. Furthermore, the development of comprehensive databases and biobanks will contribute importantly to the progression of research, facilitating the aggregation of large amounts of genetic as well as clinical data. These will be needed to support large-scale research that can validate the efficacy of new treatments, allowing for informed decisions in the planning of treatment. Lastly, this collaborative model is the most important factor in achieving the full potential of molecular oncology in the fight against the complexities of cancer treatment (Bhoyar & Chandu, 2025; Shrestha et al., 2025) (Figure 6.15).

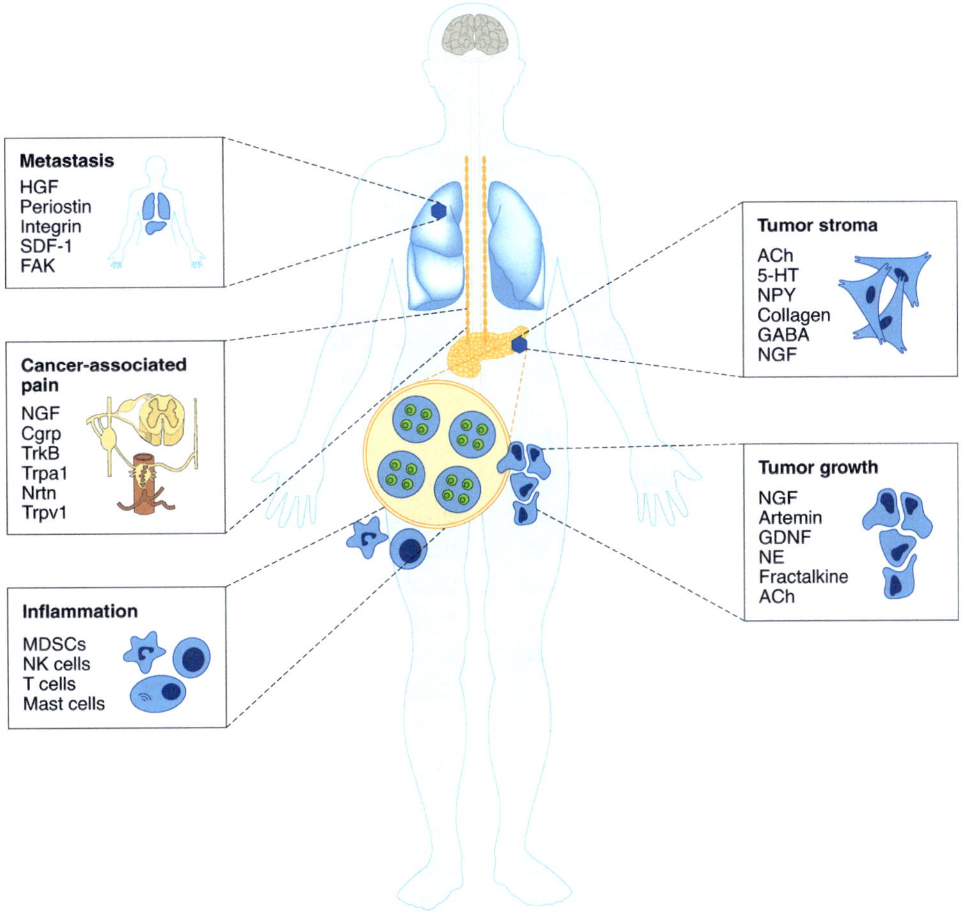

Figure 6.15. Future directions in molecular oncology.

Source: https://media.springernature.com/full/springer-static/image/art%3A10.1038%2Fs43018-020-00146-9/MediaObjects/43018_2020_146_Fig1_HTML.png.

6.6.1. Emerging Technologies and Their Potential Impact

The face of molecular oncology is rapidly evolving after the advent of new technologies that not only enhance our understanding of cancer biology but also advance treatment approaches. One such example is next-generation sequencing (NGS), which provides precise genomic data that reveals the complex and unique genomic alterations in every patient's cancer. This fresh approach demands a paradigm shift in the treatment protocols, from the traditional tissue-based therapy to biomarker-driven therapies tailored to the patient's genetic profile. As indicated in recent research,

NGS's ability to disentangle the complex genomic tapestry of cancers makes it possible the possibility of personalized medicine strategies that can substantially improve patient outcomes. The implications of such progress are vast, and they look towards the creation of accurately precise medicines that are based on the specific molecular etiology of cancer rather than merely its histology, thus optimizing the curative regimens (Nikanjam et al., 2025). Along with genomic science, progress within radiology is also increasingly becoming key to the field of molecular oncology. Advanced imaging modalities like MRI, PET, and CT have dramatically increased the promise of cancer detection, diagnosis, and treatment monitoring. These modalities give clinicians essential information on tumor behavior and biology, which are crucial to staging and treatment planning. Functional and molecular imaging also further expands clinicians' ability to understand the biology of tumors in an advanced manner. Furthermore, artificial intelligence (AI) is increasingly becoming an important instrument that can enhance radiological readings, improve diagnostic accuracy, and facilitate individualized treatment planning. According to recent literature, the integration of AI with hybrid imaging modalities may lead to dramatic enhancements in cancer management and thus render treatment increasingly personalized according to the patient profile, thus emphasizing the potential of these emerging technologies to transform oncological practice (Bakshi, 2024). The convergence of these technologies is a watershed moment for oncology research and practice, and it emphasizes the need for adaptive infrastructure within medical settings to facilitate personalized approaches. With molecular oncology embracing such innovations, there is still a challenge in ensuring equitable access to new treatments and technologies. For instance, tissue-agnostic clinical trial growth needs regulatory frameworks to be re-evaluated for effective streamlining of novel therapy method approval timelines based on unique molecular alterations rather than tumor types. Furthermore, decentralized studies hold the promise to improve access to underprivileged patients, addressing inequalities typically underlying cancer care. By emphasizing patient-centered strategies and applying real-world data, the practice can foster a framework that not only increases treatment options but also enhances clinical results within all demographic subgroups (Bakshi, 2024; Nikanjam et al., 2025).

6.6.2. Personalized Medicine and Its Implications

The paradigm shift to personalized medicine is a revolutionary approach in the field of molecular oncology, wherein cancer therapy becomes increasingly personalized to the genetic makeup of the patient. This is driven by the genomic revolution in technologies, namely Next-Generation Sequencing (NGS) and biomarker assessment, whereby scientists can uncover specific mutations that are amenable to being targeted by drugs. A combination of such technologies allows oncologists to move away from a uniform treatment approach towards more personalized and effective modalities. Personalized medicine, through the targeting of tumors' genetic and molecular profiles, aims not only to maximize therapeutic gain but also to prevent collateral side effects of conventional treatment and thereby improve overall patient benefit. These aspects point out the clinical and economic importance of this approach, which is critical in optimizing cancer care in the context of an escalating health problem (Ujjan et al., 2025). Personalized medicine must be economically evaluated to understand its effect on healthcare systems. Even though personalized treatments may be associated with higher upfront costs due to complicated testing and tailored treatment, research has shown they possess great potential to cause significant long-term benefits like high progression-free survival (PFS) and overall survival (OS) rates. For instance, research findings have shown that patients who are treated with personalized therapies often possess significantly higher survival benefits compared to patients who receive standard treatments. In particular, biomarker-driven therapies have proven more effective in patients with actionable gene mutations , such as EGFR and BRCA. This would imply that an investment in personalized medicine can ultimately yield higher quality-adjusted life years (QALYs), which would be a potentially cost-saving intervention in spite of initial economic expenditures (Ujjan et al., 2025). Accordingly, a comprehensive evaluation of tailored treatments must balance clinical and economic factors to inform health policy and open the door to patient access. The integration of artificial intelligence (AI) into personalized medicine adds to the value of individualized treatment in molecular oncology. AI is able to handle vast amounts of information from genomic profiling, identifying patterns that may not be obvious to other computational tools. By combining molecular profiling with artificial intelligence, physicians are able to make more accurate predictions of treatment outcome, facilitating further optimization of personalized treatments. For example, AI will be able to facilitate personalized radiation therapy planning by incorporating biological variation, thus resulting in better treatment outcomes and reduced toxicity. In addition, AI for real-time dose monitoring during radiotherapy can optimize patient safety and increase the quality of treatment planning. As these technologies are increasingly integrated into clinical practice, the role of personalized medicine in molecular oncology may change, initiating a new era of precision and agility in the treatment of cancer (Figure 6.16).

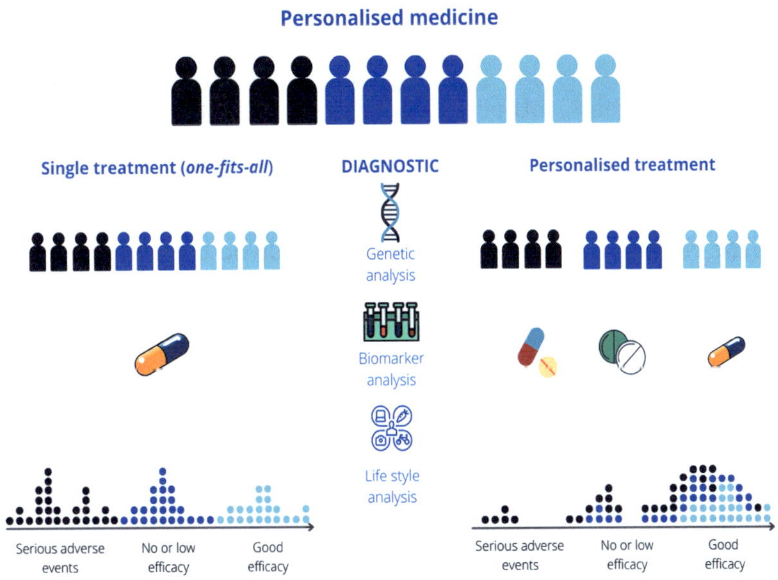

Figure 6.16. Personalized medicine and its implications.

Source: https://www.genosalut.com/wp-content/uploads/2022/05/Genosalut_Personalised_medicine-1024x683.png.

6.6.3. Ethical Considerations in Molecular Oncology Research

The expansion of molecular oncology research necessitates the serious consideration of the ethical concerns surrounding patient involvement and consent. Central to ethical conduct of research is the need for informed consent, which ensures the patient fully understands their inclusion in clinical trials. This includes awareness of potential risks, benefits, and the experimental condition of drugs being tested. Challenges are most evident among low health literacy groups, where comprehension of complex therapeutic regimens and research protocols can be challenging. Also, since molecular oncology often requires the harvesting of genetic material, researchers must navigate the terrain of genetic privacy and the eventual potential for misuse of genetic data. To offer robust protocols for confidentiality and ethical supervision is thus not only a legislative requirement, but an ethical requirement to foster confidence in patients and researchers alike in the rapidly evolving field of cancer therapy (Lopci et al., 2022). Equity of access to new therapies is an interesting ethical concern in molecular oncology research. With the advent of new treatments, inequalities in access can further widen health inequalities, particularly among vulnerable groups. They are typically associated with socioeconomic status, geography, and systemic healthcare inequalities. Ethical research must ensure maximum inclusivity by attempting to represent underrepresented groups in clinical trials, such that the findings generalize widely across populations. Moreover, researchers are faced with the challenge of espousing policies that facilitate fair access to new treatments. This requirement is more than individual studies; it calls for a collective commitment by the scientific community to build an environment where research leading to first-in-class oncology therapies can be made accessible to any patient, regardless of his or her situation or context. As such, this thrusts the virtue of justice in biomedical science (Young, 2020). In addition, the balance between scientific rigor and ethical stewardship poses an integral challenge in molecular oncology. The rapid evolution of potential treatments has a tendency to press research staff and clinicians into providing new treatments beyond their proven safety and efficacy. Therapeutic misconception, therefore, becomes likely whereby subjects are presupposed to believe that they are receiving tested treatment rather than experimental treatment. Such ethical consideration should include ongoing education of research participants and staff to counteract such a misconception, so that there is mutual understanding of clinical trials' experimental nature. In addition, strict post-trial monitoring of long-term effects and patient outcomes must be conducted to guide future practice and form ethical policy on patient protection and well-being. All concerned with molecular oncology research must therefore weigh innovation against moral principle, so that the pursuit of knowledge does not unjustifiably encroach upon patient welfare (Lopci et al., 2022).

SUMMARY

The comprehensive probe of molecular oncology has illuminated the sophisticated mechanisms of cancer biology and facilitated significant advances in therapeutic strategies. As the science unfolds, the single greatest conclusion is that the understanding of molecular signatures for various cancers not only enhances diagnostic precision but also facilitates treatment planning. This shift is evident in the bibliometric analysis of resistance to oral cancer drugs, as the shift from basic mechanisms to examining cancer stem cells and tumor microenvironments is part of a greater shift towards the integration of methods in oncology. These results highlight the importance of multi-disciplinary research within the scientific community, looking to apply learned knowledge towards meaningful clinical use, ultimately resulting in better patient care in oncology (Xu et al., 2025). Moreover, the application of machine learning to precision oncology is a milestone, but also hints at what lies in store in terms of challenges. While gigantic strides have been made in managing and analyzing data, especially in the instance of genomic profiling and digital pathology, clinical application of machine learning is limited. Researchers have pointed out many challenges, including the existence of data and those related to privacy and fairness. These must be addressed so that the full potential of machine learning to optimize treatment regimens and individualize patient care can be realized. As the field faces these challenges, the focus on building robust clinical guidelines and making technology an enabling tool and not a replacement for clinical expertise is more essential than ever before (Nittas et al., 2025). In summary, the future of molecular oncology hinges on overcoming existing obstacles while setting a teamwork culture for innovation. As continued research informs clinical practice and machine learning methods continue to improve, the possibility exists for creating more directed, effective cancer treatments. Ultimately, it will be the convergence of diverse research findings, such as drug resistance and machine learning potential, which will play a central role in defining effective treatment models. To convert these breakthroughs to the clinic effectively, ongoing conversation among clinicians, researchers, and ethical actors is essential, paving the way for a more responsive and agile oncology culture optimized for patient benefit and therapeutic efficacy.

Molecular oncology is a developing frontier in cancer treatment, in which the analysis of tumor-based genetic mutations is employed to guide specific treatments. It emphasizes precision medicine, whereby drugs are tailored to the patient's cancer's unique molecular profile. For instance, studies have shown that patients carrying specific genomic mutations—, such as those in the cyclin D-CDK4/6-INK4a-Rb pathway—may benefit from targeted inhibitors like palbociclib. Interestingly, in a pediatric patient trial of refractory tumors, while tolerable, no objective responses occurred, demonstrating both the potential and the limitation of such targeted therapies in such complex biological circumstances (Agosti et al., 2024). This goes to illustrate how there is always the need to explore molecular pathways further to maximize response rates and achieve improved outcomes in oncology. Expanded analysis of clinical trial design addresses the difficulty of cancer treatment assessment. Trials would have multiple endpoints, like primary and secondary measures, to establish efficacy over time. For instance, the trial of hypofractionated versus conventional radiation for prostate cancer illustrated the importance of long-term data, with a presentation of cumulative data that helps in disease-free survival rates. As results reach maturity, existing analyses can inform new clinical practice and research directions, such as improved biochemical failure management methods. Though both treatments were non-inferior for disease-free survival, biochemical recurrence and adverse event rates are an important area for future research (Lee et al.,

2024). Integrating complete trial results is critical for the optimization of therapeutic strategies in molecular oncology. Finally, the overlap of treatment results with molecular alterations demands a greater understanding of the biology of cancer development. The need for biomarkers in therapeutic selection reflects a growing trend towards personalized medicine, exemplified by the significant interest in actionable gene mutations in various cancers. For example, pilot trials with tumors harboring targeted genetic aberrations highlight the way certain therapies can take advantage of the distinct susceptibility of cancer cells and therefore increase the efficacy of treatment. However, the reported lack of significant responses in certain groups, such as those receiving palbociclib, raises questions about key issues regarding heterogeneity in tumor biology (Agosti et al., 2024). A grasp of these dynamics is needed to further molecular oncology and work on optimizing strategies exploiting genetic knowledge for more efficient patient-specific treatments.

A LOOK TO THE FUTURE:

GENOMIC SEQUENCING TECHNOLOGIES:

Genomic sequencing technologies have revolutionized the biological sciences, transforming how researchers decode the genetic information of organisms and how clinicians apply genetic insights in medicine. At its core, genomic sequencing refers to the laboratory process that determines the order of nucleotide bases in DNA or RNA molecules, thereby revealing the complete genetic blueprint of an organism. This process provides fundamental insights into genetic variation, function, evolution, and disease mechanisms, underpinning major advances in fields ranging from evolutionary biology and agriculture to personalized medicine and infectious disease surveillance. The history of genomic sequencing began with early methods such as the Maxam–Gilbert and Sanger sequencing techniques, with the Sanger method—based on chain-termination chemistry—dominating the field for nearly four decades after its development in 1977. While Sanger sequencing provided high-quality data for small-scale projects, its relatively low throughput and high cost limited its utility for whole-genome analyses. The advent of next-generation sequencing (NGS) in the early 2000s marked a dramatic turning point. These second-generation technologies use massively parallel sequencing to analyze millions of DNA fragments simultaneously, enabling large-scale projects such as whole-genome, exome, and transcriptome sequencing to be performed more rapidly, cost-effectively, and at higher throughput than ever before.

NGS platforms, including widely used sequencing-by-synthesis methods like those pioneered by Illumina, have expanded the scope of genomic research. They generate massive volumes of short-read sequence data that can be assembled and analyzed to detect genetic variants, gene expression levels, and even microbial populations in metagenomic samples. Despite these advances, short reads can make assembly of complex or repetitive genomic regions challenging, leading to the development of third-generation or long-read sequencing technologies. These platforms—such as Pacific Biosciences' single-molecule real-time (SMRT) sequencing and Oxford Nanopore Technologies—directly sequence individual DNA molecules without prior amplification, producing much longer reads that improve genome assembly and reveal structural variants.

Beyond these foundational methods, innovative approaches like linked-read sequencing and genome skimming continue to diversify the technological landscape, offering hybrid solutions that combine long-range context with high throughput and reduced sample requirements.

Today, genomic sequencing technologies are not just research tools but essential components of public health, clinical diagnostics, and precision medicine. They support rapid pathogen identification during outbreaks, enable genetic risk profiling for personalized treatments, and contribute to a deeper understanding of biological diversity and evolution. As sequencing costs continue to drop and analytical methods evolve, these technologies will remain central to future breakthroughs across science and medicine.

REFERENCES

1. Abbas, G. H., Khouri, E. R., Thaher, O., Taha, S., Vladimirov, M., Oviedo, R. J., Schmidt, J., et al. (2025). Predictive modeling for metastasis in oncology: Current methods and future directions. *Annals of Medicine and Surgery, 87*, 3489–3508. https://www.semanticscholar.org/paper/ddf0ef23d9ea741354a3f0d4d978f039582b30e6 (accessed on 17th July 2025).
2. Agosti, E., Antonietti, S., Ius, T., Fontanella, M., Zeppieri, M., & Panciani, P. (2024). Glioma stem cells as promoter of glioma progression: A systematic review of molecular pathways and targeted therapies. *International Journal of Molecular Sciences, 25*. https://www.semanticscholar.org/paper/15a85e605f55b9c1f91ff004830ccec505bfa08a (accessed on 17th July 2025).
3. Alkayyal, A. (2025). Insights from veterinary models for advancing oncolytic virotherapy through comparative oncology. *Frontiers in Molecular Biosciences, 12*. https://www.semanticscholar.org/paper/4b4fae0144dd6f936f4cf1410be41492219c09de (accessed on 17th July 2025).
4. Alyami, A. A., Alaqil, N. M., Alsulayyim, A. S. M., Al Yami, R. M. K., Salem, F. J. M., Al Hatailah, A. M. H., Al Zandan, S. A., et al. (2024). Comprehensive review of laboratory automation, quality control, and workforce adaptation. *Journal of Eco Humanism*. https://www.semanticscholar.org/paper/23b9d8d1d1bb86a22de2c37049b5ac58007775bf
5. Aoki, T., Wierzbicki, K., Sun, S., Steidl, C., & Giulino-Roth, L. (2025). Tumor-microenvironment and molecular biology of classic Hodgkin lymphoma in children, adolescents, and young adults. *Frontiers in Oncology, 15*. https://www.semanticscholar.org/paper/9bc7cfddd7261ce540d90d7d34dd9cef1ea146a5 (accessed on 17th July 2025).
6. Bakshi, I. (2024). From detection to therapy: The transformative power of radiology in oncology. *International Journal for Multidisciplinary Research*. https://www.semanticscholar.org/paper/cd08306eb7b2b8501923169b2120091517a70f80 (accessed on 17th July 2025).
7. Ben Mariem, O., Saporiti, S., Guerrini, U., Laurenzi, T., Palazzolo, L., Indiveri, C., Barile, M., et al. (2022). *In silico* investigation on structure–function relationship of members belonging to the human SLC52 transporter family. *Proteins: Structure, 91*, 619–633. https://www.semanticscholar.org/paper/e57d466d08746825670317cc69d9f1ad16f060ec (accessed on 17th July 2025).
8. Bhoyar, N. ., & Nirmal Chandu, H. . (2025). The future of precision medicine in personalized cancer treatment. *Journal of Neonatal Surgery, 14*(1S), 373–377. https://doi.org/10.52783/jns.v14.1551(accessed on 17th July 2025).
9. Botsis, T., Spiker, J., Kreimeyer, K., Jamali, A., Ziakas, I., Sherief, M., Fatteh, M., et al. (2025). OnPOINT: Development of an open navigator through precision oncology informatics technology to support precision oncology decisions and genotype-matched clinical trial enrollment. *Journal of Clinical Oncology*. https://www.semanticscholar.org/paper/429aa8baf9b5c4342903980d2f1a62ac3568b67f (accessed on 17th July 2025).
10. Cardoso, F., Senkus, E., Costa, A., Papadopoulos, E., Aapro, M., André, F., Harbeck, N., et al. (2018). 4th ESO–ESMO International Consensus Guidelines for Advanced Breast Cancer (ABC 4). *Annals of Oncology, 29*, 1634–1657. https://doi.org/10.1093/annonc/mdy192 (accessed on 17th July 2025).

11. Chen, A., Neuwirth, I., & Herndler-Brandstetter, D. (2023). Modeling the tumor microenvironment and cancer immunotherapy in next-generation humanized mice. *Cancers, 15*, 2989–2989. https://doi.org/10.3390/cancers15112989 (accessed on 17th July 2025).

12. Chen, J., Ma, B., Yang, Y., Wang, B., Hao, J., & Zhou, X. (2024). Disulfidptosis decoded: A journey through cell death mysteries, regulatory networks, disease paradigms and future directions. *Biomarker Research, 12*. https://doi.org/10.1186/s40364-024-00593-x (accessed on 17th July 2025).

13. Ciulla, C., & Luchini, C. (2024). Genomic determinants of biological aggressiveness and poor prognosis of pancreatic cancers: KRAS and beyond. *Expert Review of Molecular Diagnostics, 24*, 355–362. https://www.semanticscholar.org/paper/c1ca38bd60497c3d1abcd6370a27360c412525de (accessed on 17th July 2025).

14. Dharia, N., Zhu, J., Schroeder, A., Frank, S., Boetsch, C., Jamois, C., Kassir, N., et al. (2025). Abstract 2514: Refining oncology dose selection: A framework for tailored dose optimization in the era of targeted and immunotherapies. *Cancer Research*. https://www.semanticscholar.org/paper/c36767b207e0abb11e505641cc2ad806f878c80b (accessed on 17th July 2025).

15. Dimitriou, F., Damania, A. V., Nagarajan, P., Prabhakaran, S., Sahasrabhojane, P., Hoballah, Y., Mitra, D., et al. (2025). Delineating the role of the microbiome and tumor microenvironment interactions driving mucosal melanoma (MM) response and resistance to immune checkpoint inhibitor (ICI) treatment. *Journal of Clinical Oncology*. https://www.semanticscholar.org/paper/6434f690b30933205558d08d69d83951c8f9ef57 (accessed on 17th July 2025).

16. Doharey, P. K., Verma, P., Dubey, A., Singh, S., Kumar, M., Tripathi, T., Alonazi, M., et al. (2023). Biophysical and *in-silico* studies on the structure–function relationship of *Brugia malayi* protein disulfide isomerase. *Journal of Biomolecular Structure and Dynamics, 42*, 1533–1543. https://www.semanticscholar.org/paper/c763fabf5537242953717b08ea92faacb9be1bc0 (accessed on 17th July 2025).

17. Ebru, N. (2022). Therapeutic targeting of molecular pathways in colorectal cancer. *Experimental Oncology, 44*(1), 2–6. https://www.semanticscholar.org/paper/f93e0b23f161726732c83040c75c8b49207d9094 (accessed on 17th July 2025).

18. Gasparini, E., Ragazzi, M., Manzotti, G., Torricelli, F., Salviato, E., Bisagni, A., Zanetti, E., et al. (2024). Evaluation of the immune landscape associated with the efficacy of immunotherapy in patients with triple-negative breast cancer: Starlet study, synergy between research and clinical work. *Journal of Clinical Oncology*. https://www.semanticscholar.org/paper/a3987bff9782aaa71257a1947eab61f7ad6737c7 (accessed on 17th July 2025).

19. Gattu Linga, B., Mohammed, S. G., Farrell, T., Rifai, H., Al-Dewik, N. I., & Qoronfleh, M. W. (2024). Genomic newborn screening for pediatric cancer predisposition syndromes: A holistic approach. *Cancers, 16*. https://www.semanticscholar.org/paper/bab457f57d639416c359c885e633a733e789f474 (accessed on 17th July 2025).

20. Geurts, M., Blaquier, J., Wijnenga, M., Kamson, D. O., & de la Fuente, M. I. (2025). Incorporating targeted therapy into neuro-oncology practice. *American Society of Clinical Oncology Educational Book, 45*(3), e473324. https://www.semanticscholar.org/paper/9a4f8a801c82e399369524d2dc9d927d8e2b5015 (accessed on 17th July 2025).

21. González Rueda, S. D., García-Pérez, F., Sobrevilla-Moreno, N., Scavuzzo, A., Ramos-Ramírez, M., Soldevilla-Gallardo, I., Staufert-Gutiérrez, J., et al. (2025). Prognostic value of PSMA radio-

genomics in hormone sensitive synchronous metastatic prostate cancer. *Journal of Clinical Oncology*. https://www.semanticscholar.org/paper/8f5fe804416c37959f0eae37e1c3e5ad8bb017ad (accessed on 17th July 2025).

22. Johnson, D. E., Burtness, B., Leemans, C. R., Lui, V. W. Y., Bauman, J. E., & Grandis, J. R. (2020). Head and neck squamous cell carcinoma. *Nature Reviews Disease Primers, 6*. https://doi.org/10.1038/s41572-020-00224-3 (accessed on 17th July 2025).

23. Lee, W. R., Dignam, J. J., Amin, M., Bruner, D., Low, D., Swanson, G. P., Shah, A. B., et al. (2024). Long-term analysis of NRG Oncology RTOG 0415: A randomized Phase III noninferiority study comparing two fractionation schedules in patients with low-risk prostate cancer. *Journal of Clinical Oncology, 42*, 2377–2381. https://www.semanticscholar.org/paper/44f0f2adb31ddb2e16d95f7482d215b5fa7e6b2e (accessed on 17th July 2025).

24. Li, Y., Zhao, B., Peng, J., Tang, H., Wang, S., Peng, S., Ye, F., et al. (2024). Inhibition of NF-κB signaling unveils novel strategies to overcome drug resistance in cancers. *Drug Resistance Updates, 73*, 101042–101042. https://doi.org/10.1016/j.drup.2023.101042 (accessed on 17th July 2025).

25. Liu, X. H., Wang, G. R., Zhong, N. N., Wang, W. Y., Liu, B., Li, Z., & Bu, L. (2025). Multi-omics in immunotherapy research for HNSCC: Present situation and future perspectives. *NPJ Precision Oncology, 9*. https://www.semanticscholar.org/paper/912189c96adb11c46d52d489a82537e373b24448 (accessed on 17th July 2025).

26. Liu, Y., Ding, W., Wang, J., Ao, X., & Xue, J. (2023). Non-coding RNAs in lung cancer: Molecular mechanisms and clinical applications. *Frontiers in Oncology, 13*. https://www.semanticscholar.org/paper/ea501ab44d5a57b0c208c96545a26e7b83bc318a (accessed on 17th July 2025).

27. Lopci, E., Hicks, R., Dimitrakopoulou-Strauss, A., Dercle, L., Iravani, A., Seban, R., Sachpekidis, C., et al. (2022). Joint EANM/SNMMI/ANZSNM practice guidelines/procedure standards on recommended use of [18F]FDG PET/CT imaging during immunomodulatory treatments in patients with solid tumors version 1.0. *European Journal of Nuclear Medicine and Molecular Imaging, 49*, 2323–2341. https://www.semanticscholar.org/paper/b062e34802e78c69c42f97e6006cca9835667617 (accessed on 17th July 2025).

28. Lyon, A. R., López-Fernández, T., Couch, L. S., Asteggiano, R., Aznar, M. C., Bergler-Klein, J., Boriani, G., et al. (2022). 2022 ESC Guidelines on cardio-oncology developed in collaboration with the European Hematology Association (EHA), the European Society for Therapeutic Radiology and Oncology (ESTRO) and the International Cardio-Oncology Society (IC-OS). *European Heart Journal, 43*, 4229–4361. https://doi.org/10.1093/eurheartj/ehac244 (accessed on 17th July 2025).

29. Macy, M. E., Mody, R., Reid, J. M., Piao, J., Saguilig, L., Alonzo, T. A., Berg, S. L., et al. (2024). Palbociclib in solid tumor patients with genomic alterations in the cyclinD-cdk4/6-INK4a-Rb pathway: Results from National Cancer Institute-Children's Oncology Group Pediatric Molecular Analysis for Therapy Choice Trial Arm I (APEC1621I). *JCO Precision Oncology, 8*. https://www.semanticscholar.org/paper/4800adb5263b236dd43407bdc81d33dc679e59ae (accessed on 17th July 2025).

30. Napolitano, S., Boscolo Bielo, L., Martini, G., Pietrantonio, F., Pisconti, S., Sartore-Bianchi, A., Blasi, L., et al. (2025). The use of liquid biopsy comprehensive genomic profiling to identify the molecular landscape of patients with metastatic colorectal cancer who are candidates for anti-

EGFR rechallenge therapy: Findings from the CAVE-2 GOIM trial. *Journal of Clinical Oncology*. https://www.semanticscholar.org/paper/fe5ab7f0a0c3b5c1121bcc1fcfab50f1e963e84c (accessed on 17th July 2025).

31. Nikanjam, M., Kato, S., Allen, T., Sicklick, J., & Kurzrock, R. (2025). Novel clinical trial designs emerging from the molecular reclassification of cancer. *CA: A Cancer Journal for Clinicians, 75*, 243–267. https://www.semanticscholar.org/paper/ed31a3c6403c1b0469b4430cade90e86c2a9bb22 (accessed on 17th July 2025).

32. Nittas, V., Ormond, K., Vayena, E., & Blasimme, A. (2025). Realizing the promise of machine learning in precision oncology: Expert perspectives on opportunities and challenges. *BMC Cancer, 25*. https://www.semanticscholar.org/paper/5eeb4654f65bd7848865dfa20f586b24086b94a8 (accessed on 17th July 2025).

33. Olivier, M., Asmis, R., Hawkins, G. A., Howard, T. D., & Cox, L. A. (2019). The need for multi-omics biomarker signatures in precision medicine. *International Journal of Molecular Sciences, 20*, 4781–4781. https://doi.org/10.3390/ijms20194781 (accessed on 17th July 2025).

34. Paris, I., Minucci, A., Giaco', L., Generali, D., Nanni, S., D'Angelo, T., Pavese, F., et al. (2025). Abstract P2-05-28: High throughput analysis in HER2 positive locally advanced breast cancer (BC): pathological complete response (pCR) and mutational status. *Clinical Cancer Research*. https://www.semanticscholar.org/paper/d064eef09bb403d8c10f2dcbdba3334226aa425c (accessed on 17th July 2025).

35. Parisi, C., & Planchard, D. (2025). BRAF in non–small cell lung cancer: From molecular mechanisms to clinical practice. *Cancer, 131*. https://www.semanticscholar.org/paper/d6fcd0c03419d20104338cc08ea9e3897c3a0565 (accessed on 17th July 2025).

36. Pavlova, N. V., Dyomin, S. S., Churnosov, M., & Ponomarenko, I. (2024). A modern view of the role of genetic factors in the etiopathogenesis of breast cancer. *Advances in Molecular Oncology*. https://www.semanticscholar.org/paper/f5d8a3e4abab3013f99304 35ac123f46ef46a83e (accessed on 17th July 2025).

37. Perfetto, C., Aprile, M., Cataldi, S., Giovannetti, E., & Costa, V. (2025). Unraveling BRAF alterations: Molecular insights to circumvent therapeutic resistance across cancer types. *Cancer Drug Resistance, 8*. https://www.semanticscholar.org/paper/e7fa7f528d2835416489339d23ab2a839922e3b0 (accessed on 17th July 2025).

38. Rawla, P. (2019). Epidemiology of prostate cancer. *World Journal of Oncology, 10*, 63–89. https://doi.org/10.14740/wjon1191 (accessed on 17th July 2025).

39. Ryu, H. (2023). Latest trends in cancer clinical trials using genomics. *Journal of the Korean Medical Association*. https://www.semanticscholar.org/paper/039ac417b622424211122d28b444b91e816fc568 (accessed on 17th July 2025).

40. Schneider, L. P., Maselli-Schoueri, J. H., Gutierres Aguiar, B. de S., Aguiar, P. N., & del Giglio, A. (2025). Addressing challenges in the implementation of precision oncology: An in-depth examination of limitations and disparities in the treatment of non-small cell lung cancer in the Brazilian public healthcare system (SUS). *Global Public Health, 20*(1), 2450412. https://www.semanticscholar.org/paper/6f106973e200e81334740cc0eae336c7c3167af3 (accessed on 17th July 2025).

41. Shende, S., Rathored, J., & Budhbaware, T. (2025). Role of metabolic transformation in cancer immunotherapy resistance: Molecular mechanisms and therapeutic

implications. *Discover Oncology, 16*. https://www.semanticscholar.org/paper/b64eeb278b99586cbf5c093ca6e286539fc05bb2 (accessed on 17th July 2025).

42. Shi, C. (2024). Molecular biology and genetics research on schizophrenia. *International Journal of Public Health and Medical Research*. https://www.semanticscholar.org/paper/ba7cac65bbd358e51265373eda138542db86ecbc (accessed on 17th July 2025).

43. Shrestha, S., Cook, C. M., Parekh, J., & Mattei, J. (2025). A review on melanoma brain metastases. *Current Pharmaceutical Design*. https://www.semanticscholar.org/paper/67b8081a9354a781d7388de39d15b6d0a5a1b92d (accessed on 17th July 2025).

44. Song, T., & Li, H. (2024). Artificial intelligence plus molecular profiling for personalized radiotherapy: Questions 105–107 in the 150 most important questions in cancer research and clinical oncology series. *Visualized Cancer Medicine*. https://www.semanticscholar.org/paper/032fb70c8614dc84f019a0be57c566435513ea36 (accessed on 17th July 2025).

45. Szymańska, E., Nowak, P., Kolmus, K., Cybulska, M., Goryca, K., Derezińska-Wołek, E., Szumera-Ciećkiewicz, A., et al. (2020). Synthetic lethality between *VPS4A* and *VPS4B* triggers an inflammatory response in colorectal cancer. *EMBO Molecular Medicine, 12*. https://doi.org/10.15252/emmm.201910812 (accessed on 17th July 2025).

46. Teleanu, M. V., Schneider, A., Ball, C. R., Leber, M. F., Stange, C., Krieghoff-Henning, E., Beck, K., et al. (2025). Celebrating Ulrik Ringborg: Multi-omics-based patient stratification for precision cancer treatment. *Biomolecules, 15*. https://www.semanticscholar.org/paper/34bb56e81b6723ff1391cbd76f39dc890fe404df (accessed on 17th July 2025).

47. Thorel, L., Perréard, M., Florent, R., Divoux, J., Coffy, S., Vincent, A., Gaggioli, C., et al. (2024). Patient-derived tumor organoids: A new avenue for preclinical research and precision medicine in oncology. *Experimental & Molecular Medicine, 56*, 1531–1551. https://www.semanticscholar.org/paper/fb7e05616fa991e9d12dc12f365beb1cbbe27ebd (accessed on 17th July 2025).

48. Tonetti, M. S., Greenwell, H., & Kornman, K. S. (2018). Staging and grading of periodontitis: Framework and proposal of a new classification and case definition. *Journal of Periodontology, 89*. https://doi.org/10.1002/jper.18-0006 (accessed on 17th July 2025).

49. Ujjan, M. Y., Noureen, A., Aftab, L., Mercado Mercado, G., Haroon, M., Tahir, Z., Yaseen, M., et al. (2025). Evaluating the impact of personalized medicine on cancer treatment outcomes. *Journal of Medical & Health Sciences Review*. https://www.semanticscholar.org/paper/2f9ee3533489d87a8c2769caf8e94b50a1495621 (accessed on 17th July 2025).

50. van Opijnen, M. P., de Vos, F., Cuppen, E., Geurts, M., Maas, S., & Broekman, M. (2024). The role of molecular biomarkers in recurrent glioblastoma trials: An assessment of the current trial landscape of genome-driven oncology. *Medical Oncology (Northwood, London, England), 41*. https://www.semanticscholar.org/paper/25fb7cf82ab4593582080d2fad065d02251a7f90 (accessed on 17th July 2025).

51. Wang, H., Guo, M., Wei, H., & Chen, Y. (2023). Targeting p53 pathways: Mechanisms, structures and advances in therapy. *Signal Transduction and Targeted Therapy, 8*. https://doi.org/10.1038/s41392-023-01347-1 (accessed on 17th July 2025).

52. Wen, P. Y., Weller, M., Lee, E. Q., Alexander, B. M., Barnholtz-Sloan, J. S., Barthel, F. P., Batchelor, T. T., et al. (2020). Glioblastoma in adults: A Society for Neuro-Oncology (SNO) and European Society of Neuro-Oncology (EANO) consensus review on current management and future

directions. *Neuro-Oncology, 22,* 1073–1113. https://doi.org/10.1093/neuonc/noaa106 (accessed on 17th July 2025).

53. Xu, X., & Wang, Z. (2025). A two-decade bibliometric analysis of drug resistance in oral cancer research: Patterns, trends, and future directions. *Discover Oncology, 16.* https://www.semanticscholar.org/paper/0ab4e939ac17c905646b89fbed355a3f31f52a65 (accessed on 17th July 2025).

54. Yadav, M., Sharma, A., Patne, K., Tabasum, S., Suryavanshi, J., Rawat, L., Machaalani, M., et al. (2025). AXL signaling in cancer: From molecular insights to targeted therapies. *Signal Transduction and Targeted Therapy, 10.* https://www.semanticscholar.org/paper/5b11ca24c1c0d0861dfb253ed65e70dfc3b23d2f (accessed on 17th July 2025).

55. Yang, Y., Abdul Razak, S. R., Ismail, I. S., Ma, Y., & Yunus, M. A. (2025). Molecular mechanisms of miR-192 in cancer: A biomarker and therapeutic target. *Cancer Cell International, 25.* https://www.semanticscholar.org/paper/669c67378e55b4d7fe922c4b17615364e432b23d (accessed on 17th July 2025).

56. Ye, S., Li, S., Qin, L., Zheng, W., Liu, B., Li, X., Ren, Z., et al. (2023). GBP2 promotes clear cell renal cell carcinoma progression through immune infiltration and regulation of PDL1 expression via STAT1 signaling. *Oncology Reports, 49.* https://www.semanticscholar.org/paper/58962bc496c64a2231c4e8fd23d3d80333bab49e (accessed on 17th July 2025).

57. Young, G. (2020). Implications of the first FDA-approved anticoagulant in pediatrics: One ship has sailed but the next ones are at the dock–Highlight on [PBC-19-1346.R2]. https://www.semanticscholar.org/paper/3478533278fa2c5951845b5d16c88b9f28cd5078 (accessed on 17th July 2025).

58. Zebrack, B. J., Duan, F., Cole, S. W., Gareen, I. F., Prasad, P., Sicks, J. D., Cheung, C. K., et al. (2025). Social genomic mechanisms of health disparities among adolescent/young adult survivors of Hodgkin and non-Hodgkin lymphoma: ECOG-ACRIN EAQ211. *Journal of Clinical Oncology.* https://www.semanticscholar.org/paper/18bc7add672ee6e5d86a504672b9174421e89caf (accessed on 17th July 2025).

59. Zhu, J., Schroeder, A., Frank, S., Boetsch, C., Jamois, C., Kassir, N., Korfi, K., et al. (2025). Oncology dose optimization: Tailored approaches to different molecular classes. *Clinical Pharmacology and Therapeutics, 118,* 74–79. https://www.semanticscholar.org/paper/d7d1f33addef284fc505ca9e9f91f93762ba946f (accessed on 17th July 2025).

60. Zuluaga Zuluaga, M., Zuluaga, S., Ririe, A. K., Omana, N. J., Lizzy, N. C., & Kurniawaty, N. F. (2025). Molecular biology of cancer and new tools in oncology. *Journal of Medical & Health Sciences Review.* https://www.semanticscholar.org/paper/7504c8566a459436aca1443282d3b91fd8a63ab8 (accessed on 17th July 2025).

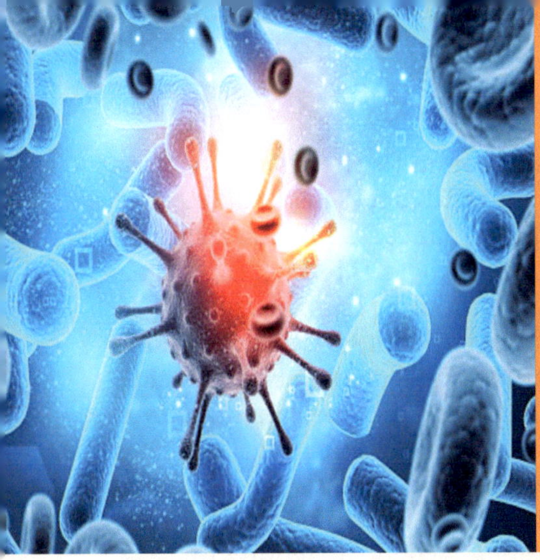

Chapter 7

MOLECULAR PATHOLOGY OF INFECTIOUS DISEASES

Contents

Introduction

The field of molecular pathology is inextricably linked to infectious diseases, outlining the complex processes through which pathogens cause disease at the cellular and molecular level. Knowledge of these mechanisms is crucial to the design of targeted therapy and prevention. By studying the molecular interactions between host and pathogen, scientists can identify the genetic and biochemical determinants that underlie susceptibility and progression to disease. For instance, antimicrobial resistance (AMR) has been a considerable problem in infectious disease management with far-reaching global health implications. Sophistication in AMR mechanisms, as this is currently understood in recent studies, necessitates an integrated conceptualization of gene mutations and how they affect the efficacy of cures (Donkin et al., 2022). Therefore, molecular pathology's inquiry offers invaluable data that are essential for fighting the wave of infectious diseases and ultimately reducing morbidity and mortality of such diseases. Additionally, host genetic factors' contribution offers a focal perspective in molecular pathology. The ABO blood group system, for instance, is found to affect susceptibility to many infections because of the presence of particular antigens on red blood cells. Studies have revealed that the different blood groups show different susceptibility to illnesses like tuberculosis, cholera, and even some cancers, complicating further the story of host-pathogen interaction (Abegaz, 2021). The phenotypic blood group variation has a strong impact on immune responses, pathogen attachment, and ultimate disease outcome. This association emphasizes the importance of looking at host genetics along with pathogen biology as a way of making personalized medicine approaches possible that can optimize the effectiveness of treatment and patient outcomes in infectious disease treatment. Lastly, an entire picture of the molecular pathology of infectious diseases needs to incorporate not just explanations of the distinct mechanisms alone but also address the interconnectedness of these factors within a greater biological context. Host genetics, microbial virulence factors, and environmental interactions control the pathogenesis of infectious disease. As reported in current studies, an understanding of these intricate interactions would provide the foundation for applying efficient public health interventions as well as therapy interventions (Abegaz, 2021; Donkin et al., 2022). Furthermore, understanding the molecular mechanisms of infection will guide future research directions, from vaccine production and the identification of new antimicrobial compounds. With the addition of molecular pathology proficiency, infectious disease studies can proceed to innovative solutions that counter the rising threats posed by pathogens in the more dynamic global health environment (Figure 7.1).

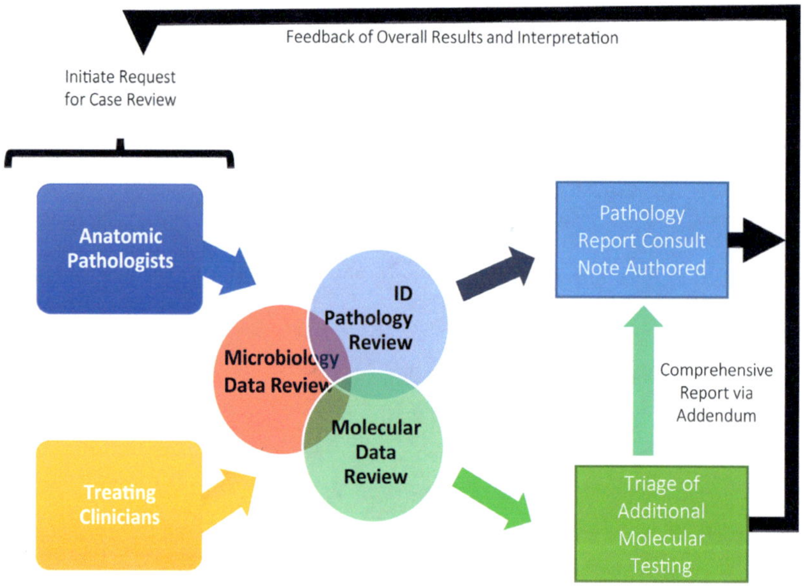

Figure 7.1. Molecular pathology of infectious diseases.

Source: https://www.modernpathology.org/cms/10.1016/j.modpat.2023.100168/asset/eb726e8f-b983-4fb5-9df9-1068b0f44501/main.assets/gr2_lrg.jpg.

Definition of Molecular Pathology

Molecular pathology is a unifying area within the field of biomedical science, serving as a bridge between pathology and molecular biology. The field focuses on the analysis of disease at the molecular level to report to clinicians and researchers the pathogenetic mechanisms that underlie pathological conditions. By studying genetic, epigenetic, and proteomic alterations in cells and tissues, molecular pathology demonstrates how infections interfere with normal cellular function. This information is not only essential for disease diagnosis but also for disease progression and treatment responsiveness prediction, thereby making it a cornerstone of precision medicine. Specifically in the instance of infectious diseases, where pathogens hijack host cellular machinery, understanding these molecular interactions can inform the modulation of targeted therapeutic strategies to target the root causes of disease rather than merely its symptoms. In searching for the dynamic interaction between molecular pathology and infectious diseases, scientists have begun to examine how changes in the host's molecular pathways induced by pathogens impact the immune response. For instance, circadian rhythm disruptions by infections have been emphasized as affecting immune function and pathogen susceptibility. The intricacy of the interaction between the circadian clock and immunomodulation underscores the intricacy of host-pathogen interaction. As evident in recent reviews, such disruptions not only affect immune cell function but also induce modifications in the host's inflammatory responses, which result in striking clinical effects. Such findings emphasize the need for the union of molecular findings with clinical presentations during infectious disease research to bring in new therapeutic approaches considering both molecular mechanisms and host response (Huang et al., 2023). Also, molecular pathology has essential functions in the diagnosis and treatment of some infectious diseases. Advances in technology within genomics, such as next-generation sequencing, have made it possible to identify unique molecular signatures of various pathogens. Such signatures can be applied in infection classification and facilitate the design of specific therapies. For instance, studies on genetic alterations within kinases for specific tumors, such as those caused by pathogens, provide useful knowledge about the molecular nature of such diseases. These findings not only establish targeted treatment methods but also enhance our understanding of the molecular determinants for disease progression. Lastly, application of molecular pathology in models of infectious disease shows the promise that knowledge of molecular mechanisms has in being transformed into better diagnosis, therapy, and outcome for patients within the complex setting of disease management (Donkin et al., 2022) (Figure 7.2).

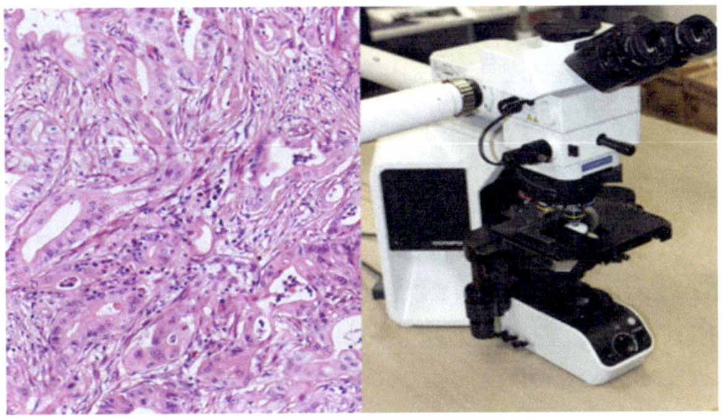

Figure 7.2. Molecular pathology .

Source: https://pod.ncc.go.jp/jp/ri/division/molecular_pathology/sub.png.

Importance of Studying Infectious Diseases

The relevance of learning infectious diseases is made apparent by the severe impact they have on public health and society as a whole. Over the past decades, outbreaks of infectious diseases have brought to the limelight loopholes in healthcare systems and the need for effective response mechanisms. The COVID-19 pandemic is a good example, showing how an infectious disease was able to upend global societal practices and economic frameworks. Understanding the molecular pathology of such diseases is not only crucial for vaccine development to be effective but also to create public health interventions that minimize their transmission. By exploring the manner in which pathogens work, researchers are able to identify potential targets for treatment that would otherwise pass them by, thereby maximizing health outcomes from epidemics and pandemics. This holistic comprehension is the basis for firm infectious disease training, one that is at the heart of today's health professionals who have to contend with new challenges. What is also taught by molecular pathology research is the intricate dynamics between infectious agents and host organisms. The study of virus-host interactions, such as the role of angiotensin-converting enzyme 2 (ACE2) in SARS-CoV-2 infections, is one instance of the relevance of such work. ACE2 has been found to be a primary virus receptor, and the understanding of this interaction has laid the foundation for potential therapeutic strategies, such as interventions involving human recombinant soluble ACE2 (hrsACE2) that are capable of efficiently inhibiting viral replication. Findings of this nature not only direct the treatment process but also enhance preventive measures to contain the effects of these diseases on populations. Ultimately, the rigorous scientific examination of such interactions forms a basis for knowledge essential to future medical science and public health advances. The applicability of infectious disease research extends far beyond immediate health effects to shape worldwide preparedness for possible future epidemics. Under conditions of increasing globalization, the risk of quick disease transmission rises. This knowledge allows us to put into place broad surveillance systems that can rapidly identify emerging threats. As past epidemics' history and today's impact of SARS-CoV-2 have demonstrated, a sound molecular foundation renders us better equipped to anticipate and counteract emerging viral threats. Preparedness strategies underpinned by thorough molecular pathology research not only strengthen individual and collective resilience but also serve as a global assurance against the inevitable emergence of new pathogens. By emphasizing the research of infectious diseases in the medical and scientific fields, we equip future generations with the tools and knowledge to effectively address current and emerging health emergencies.

7.1. Basics of Infectious Diseases

An understanding of the basics of infectious diseases is fundamental to their molecular pathology. Infectious diseases are caused by pathogenic agents, e.g., bacteria, viruses, fungi, and parasites, which infect the host, replicate, and disrupt normal physiological functions. Spread of the disease-producing agents may be due to various mechanisms, e.g., direct contact, air-borne transmission, and vector-borne transmission. The immune system battles these invaders through both innate and adaptive immunity mechanisms that identify and eliminate pathogens. Pathogens are constantly evolving, and this leads to challenges in the prevention and treatment , such as drug resistance. An understanding of these principles at their foundational level not only provides the basis for advanced research into molecular pathology but also highlights the necessity for public health programs in slowing the spread of infectious diseases and protecting community health. Molecular pathology is a dive into the nature of how pathogens work with host cells on the genetic and biochemical levels. This field examines the cell biology through which disease is caused by pathogens, those proteins and genes involved in pathogenesis. For instance, certain bacteria are capable of secreting exotoxins that disrupt cellular processes and enable tissue invasion. Viruses can also hijack host cell processes for replication and immune evasion. These encounters require a sophisticated understanding of biochemistry and molecular biology so that scientists can identify candidate therapeutic targets. With the continuous advancement in bringing together advanced technologies , such as genomics, proteomics, and bioinformatics, there is potential for paradigm-shifting understanding of disease processes and the development of novel treatment strategies (Qiu et al., 2023). This information is increasingly applicable in the fight against infectious diseases with the emergence of rapid mutations in many pathogens. Additionally, the introduction of artificial intelligence (AI) technologies has transformed the way infectious diseases are researched and managed, placing a premium on merging these innovations into infectious disease studies and molecular pathology. The ability of AIs to process large datasets has expanded diagnostics and individualized treatment approaches, overcoming major barriers in terms of cost and accessibility. With the application of machine learning and deep learning methodologies, disease outbreak prediction and identification of patterns in infections can be done with greater effectiveness by healthcare practitioners. The same technology can also facilitate enhanced vaccine discovery and therapeutic interventions with personalized genetic predispositions, resulting in enhanced healthcare interventions (Iqbal et al., 2023). But the rapid pace of AI technology advancement in the study of infectious diseases necessitates careful consideration of ethical principles, specifically data privacy and transparency of algorithms, to ensure that the benefits of integrating AI in healthcare come at no cost to patient rights or healthcare equity (Figure 7.3).

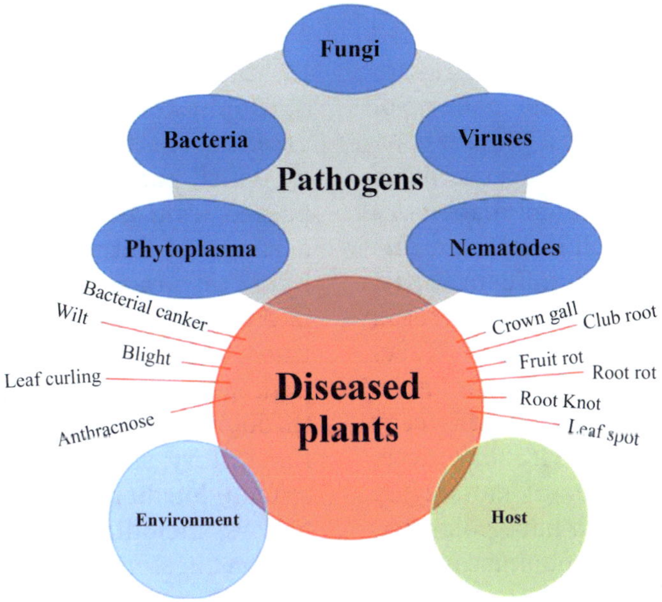

Figure 7.3. Understanding the basics of infectious diseases is vital to exploring their molecular pathology.

Source: https://www.researchgate.net/publication/338373529/figure/fig1/AS:843485842268161@1578114104097/Schematic-representation-of-plant-diseases-and-pathogens.png.

7.1.1. Types of Infectious Agents (Bacteria, Viruses, Fungi, Parasites)

In infectious illness, pathogenic agent classification plays a vital role in knowing their molecular pathology. Bacteria, which are one of the most common microorganisms, possess forms that vary and produce severe illnesses. They are single cells with unique special structures , such as cell walls, which separate them from eukaryotic cells. Whereas a majority of bacteria are neutral or beneficial, pathogenic strains can cause illness from a mild infection to a fatal disease like sepsis. The molecular mechanisms through which bacteria induce their pathogenic effect are typically specialized virulence factors, e.g., toxins that induce host tissue damage or invasion-facilitating enzymes. Second, the immune response to bacterial infections polarizes macrophages, and the latter can become a central element of the host's defense strategy, as has been elaborated in recent reviews of M1 and M2 macrophage phenotypes (Cerdeira & Brigagão, 2024). Viruses represent another significant category of infectious agents that possess the host cell dependence for their replication. In contrast to bacteria, viruses are acellular and are made up of genetic material wrapped inside a protein coat. Their pathogenicity is the result of mechanisms like the utilization of host cellular machinery for replication and causing cell death, and this will cause several diseases like influenza, HIV, and COVID-19. In molecular pathology, viruses are able to cause severe cytopathic effects and elicit host immune responses that make disease progression more complicated. Recent research has also indicated that viral infections have an effect on the behavior of monocytes and macrophages, and they can have polarized reactions that increase tissue inflammation and damage. The dynamic interaction between viral pathogens and the immune system demonstrates the complexity of treating viral infection in a clinical setting (Cerdeira & Brigagão, 2024). Fungi and parasites, being different in biology and pathology, play significant roles in the picture of infectious disease. Fungi account for a host of opportunistic infections, particularly among immunocompromised hosts, including species of Candida and Aspergillus. Pathogenicity among most such organisms is linked to their competence to evade the immune response of the host and form treatment-resistant biofilms. Parasites, which are comprised of , such as protozoa and helminths, possess intricate life cycles that involve more than one host. The pathogenic parasitic processes are mainly focused on nutrient competition and evasion of the immune system by the hosts. Notably, parasites' functions are not only limited to infection but also evoke significant alterations in the immunological setup of the host, leading to chronic disease and inflammation. Determination of the molecular interaction between such infectious pathogens and host responses is inevitable for successful treatment and diagnostic purposes.

7.1.2. Mechanisms of Infection and Transmission

In the understanding of the molecular pathophysiology of infectious diseases, it is essential to study the pathogenetic mechanisms by which pathogens infect their hosts and are passed from person to person. Pathogens use a range of entry portals, the most common being respiratory, gastrointestinal, and dermal pathways, which have a significant impact on transmission dynamics. For example, airborne pathogens like viruses can be easily transmitted through droplets in coughs or sneezes, making respiratory secretions a major factor in their spread. Furthermore, the pathogen's virulence factors, including surface proteins that assist with adhesion to host cells, are pivotal for developing infections. These mechanisms determine not only the initial infection but also the ability of the pathogens to avoid the host's immune response against them, thereby allowing them to thrive and survive within the host population. Antimicrobial resistance (AMR) in infection helps provide the context of how infection is spreading, as well as the implications. Certain species of bacteria, such as multi-drug-resistant bacteria, are especially relevant in medical practice and contribute to increased morbidity and mortality (Donkin et al., 2022). There were approximately 4.95 million deaths due to bacterial AMR in 2019, indicating the significant burden of resistance on public health (Donkin et al., 2022). Regarding transmission, resistant pathogens are transmitted more because they possess the ability to withstand treatment and thus are able to spread unchecked among populations. The association of these resistant strains with susceptible populations further magnifies prevailing health threats and requires a multi-pronged approach to epidemiological surveillance, efficient infection control, and namely, targeted therapeutic measures. The SARS-CoV-2 pandemic exemplifies the intricate mechanisms of viral transfer and the importance of an exhaustive comprehension of virus-host interaction. Coronaviruses like SARS-CoV-2 are primarily spread by respiratory droplets and have demonstrated the ability to transmit asymptomatically, rendering containment challenging (Lippi et al., 2020). The molecular mechanism of SARS-CoV-2 infection is typified by intricate virus-host interactions permitting the virus to hijack host cell machinery for replication. Investigation of these pathways not only reveals viral lifecycle vulnerabilities but also suggests areas of therapeutic targets for antiviral intervention. As research continues, better insight into such mechanisms will be important in developing vaccines and drugs that can effectively cut the transmission of zoonotic viruses in the future, emphasizing the role of molecular pathology in infectious disease regulation (Figure 7.4).

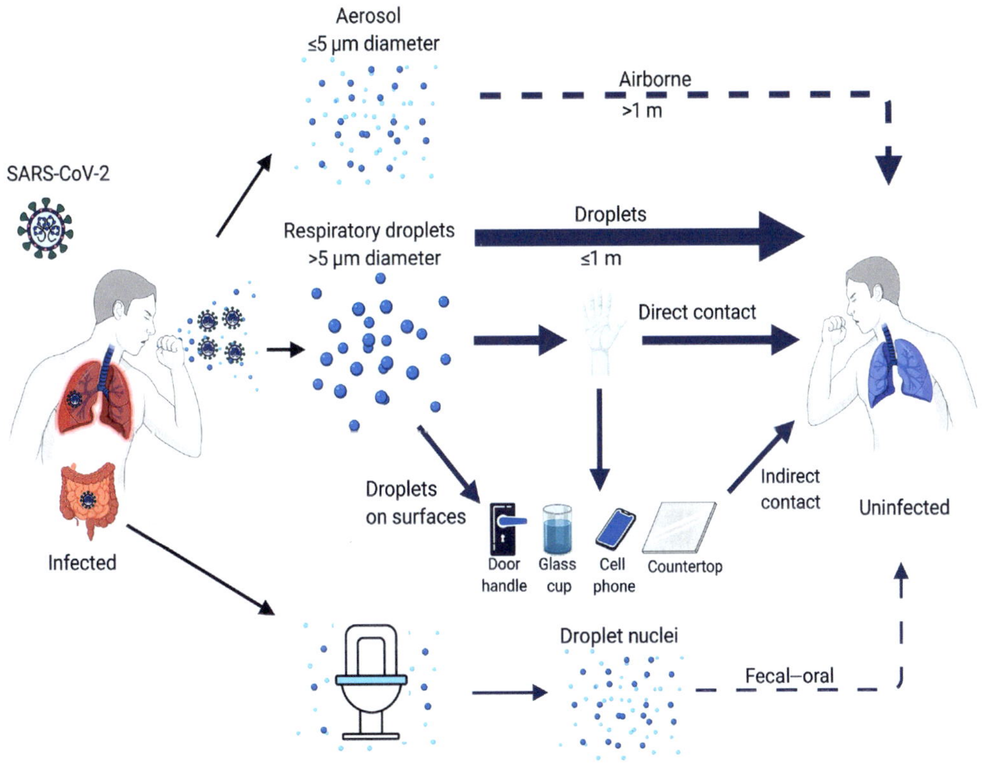

Figure 7.4. Mechanisms of infection and transmission in the molecular pathology of infectious diseases.

Source: https://www.cell.com/cms/attachment/212ae577-5665-40a3-97dc-ac8e99cde858/gr2_lrg.jpg.

7.1.3. Host Response to Infectious Agents

The host response to infectious pathogens is a multifaceted interaction of varied biological processes that are oriented towards identifying, combating, and destroying invading pathogens. In this case of infection, the innate immune system is the primary defense line, and it uses various cells, such as macrophages and neutrophils, which can identify and respond to the infection of pathogens. These immune cells release pro-inflammatory cytokines, initiating a fast inflammatory reaction that attracts more immune cells to the site of infection. This reaction, while crucial for containing infections, if not properly regulated, can also cause tissue damage. For instance, in human herpes virus 4 (HHV-4) caused infectious mononucleosis (IM), the proof is slowly building to associate it with autoimmune illness, demonstrating the complexity and potentially destructive nature of host reaction to certain infectious diseases (Naughton et al., 2024). Clarification of these dynamics is why certain people develop extreme disease symptoms and others are asymptomatic. The adaptive immune system then mounts a response, which is more specific and delayed but gives long-term immunity via memory T and B cells. APCs also present pathogen-derived antigens to T cells upon infection, which activate differentiated B cells to secrete antibodies against the pathogens. This antibody-mediated adaptive response is crucial for viral neutralization and marking infected cells for destruction. This adaptive response can be influenced by a range of factors, though, including the pathogen, the host's health and genotypic status, and previous immunity. Notably, the adaptive immune response in contagious infections , such as IM, can reveal vulnerabilities, as an abnormal immune response may potentially lead to inappropriate targeting of self-antigens and thus lay the groundwork for autoimmune diseases (Naughton et al., 2024). The implication of the results stresses the importance of understanding host-pathogen interactions at the molecular level. Most recently, progress in model studies has significantly advanced our understanding of the subtle host response to infection. Historically important traditional animal models, however, are generally not able to thoroughly simulate human disease. The pandemic of COVID-19 drove the development of *ex vivo* tissue challenge models, more relevant settings in which to explore immune response and host-pathogen interactions. These models allow researchers to examine the reaction of human tissues to various infectious pathogens and allow for the screening of potential therapies and vaccine targets. By comparing immune responses to various pathogens, like HIV-1 and SARS-CoV-2, scientists can identify common immunological pathways and therapeutic targets. Utilization of these new models not only avoids the limitation of classical approaches but also underscores the necessity to comprehend pathogen-specific immune responses, which is immensely helpful in creating effective interventions against infectious pathogens.

7.2. Molecular Techniques in Pathology

The insertion of molecular techniques into pathology has significantly transformed the landscape of diagnosing and understanding infectious diseases. These new technologies utilize genetic and molecular analysis to facilitate precise identification of pathogens, revealing their genetic composition and behavior. Techniques , such as the polymerase chain reaction (PCR) enable the amplification of pathogens' DNA or RNA to allow for detection of infection at much earlier stages than by conventional means. Particularly, real-time PCR is a prime technique for viral load measurement, which has implications for treatment and prognosis. Furthermore, next-generation sequencing (NGS) platforms facilitate high-resolution genomic typing of pathogenic agents, including sequence diversity, resistance profiles, and transmission dynamics. As a result, their combined application is not only a diagnostic innovation but also a milestone in the trajectory of personalized medicine in infectious disease management. To illustrate, in the case of emerging pathogens , such as SARS-CoV-2, molecular approaches have become a sine qua non to grasp the dynamics of disease development and presentation. Research has established that such technologies can identify the virus infection in various biological samples, like ocular fluids, thus revealing new routes of transmission that were underestimated earlier (Colavita et al., 2020). Such findings indicate the possibility of utilizing molecular techniques not only for diagnosis but even for surveillance in public health and control of outbreaks. The ability to evolve and implement molecular techniques quickly in response to an emerging pathogen signals their utility and key role in infectious disease management. For instance, the rapid isolation of SARS-CoV-2 from eye secretions in the COVID-19 pandemic shows that molecular pathology can be employed to guide specific health interventions and enhance our understanding of viral pathogenesis and infectivity at different tissue localizations. Also, the analysis of molecular mechanisms that are the roots of infectious diseases enhances therapeutic intervention as well as the construction of targeted interventions. By identifying specific genetic markers of virulence or resistance, it is easier for researchers to better individualize treatment regimens. Not only does this optimize therapeutic effect, but it also minimizes side effects that are attached to treatments of broader spectra. For instance, knowledge about the role of oxidative stress in gastrointestinal pathologies linked to infection is being utilized to identify potential antioxidant therapies (Vona et al., 2021). As molecular techniques continue to advance, they will continue to advance our knowledge of disease pathology, leading to increasingly effective prevention and therapeutic regimens. The move of molecular pathology from bench to bedside represents a paradigm shift and requires a culture of continuous research and innovation in the war against infectious diseases at the molecular level (Figure 7.5).

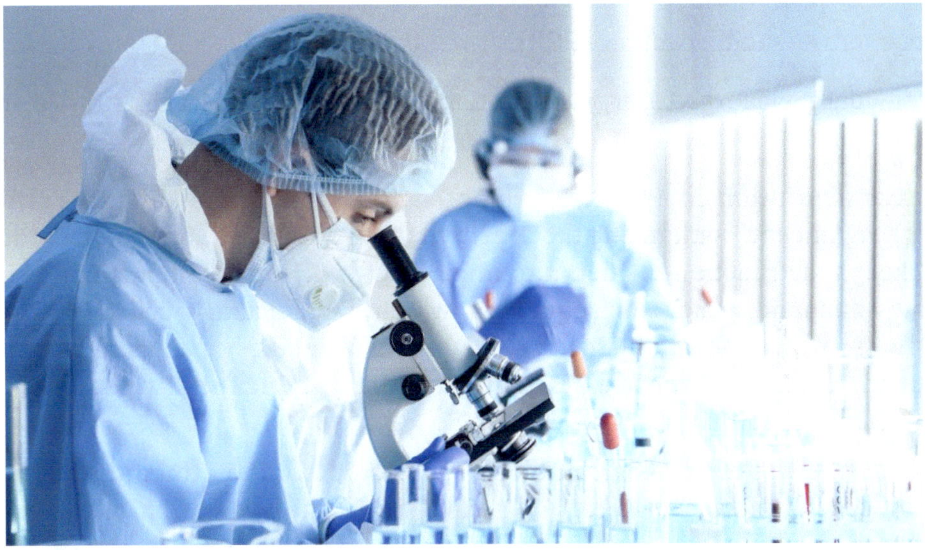

Figure 7.5. Molecular techniques in pathology.

Source: https://i.ytimg.com/vi/xIzV94bIerQ/maxresdefault.jpg.

7.2.1. Polymerase Chain Reaction (PCR)

The Polymerase Chain Reaction (PCR) is a milestone molecular technique in the infectious disease pathology paradigm. PCR enables the selective amplification of targeted DNA segments, and through this, it enables the quick detection of pathogens, allowing for the timely diagnosis and treatment. PCR has proven very valuable in the detection of a variety of infectious agents, from viral RNA to bacterial DNA, which proves its versatility. As exemplified in recent studies with prominent shrimp pathogens, such as the Infectious Myonecrosis Virus (IMNV), PCR's capability facilitates early pathogen detection critical to aquaculture disease management (Maharani & Sumsanto, 2024). PCR specificity and sensitivity equip physicians and scientists with precise information on whether pathogens exist, whether treatment procedures are effective, and overall public health interventions. These developments contribute to the broad vision for molecular pathology in clinical models of infectious disease, showing how technological innovation has a direct bearing on therapeutic and management treatments.

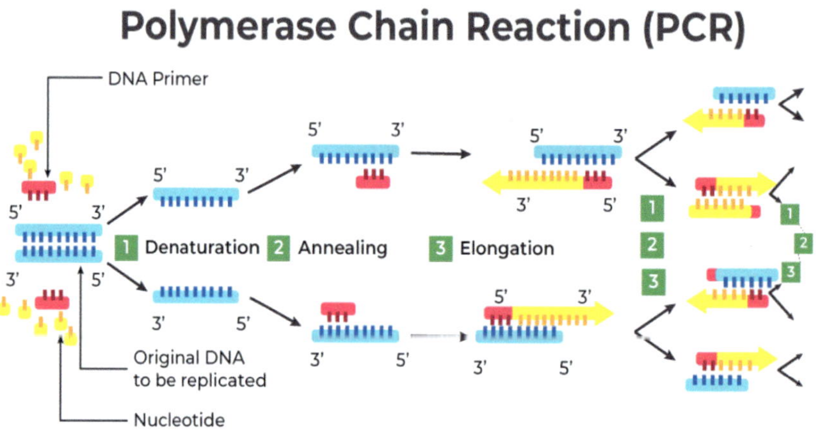

Figure 7.6. Polymerase chain reaction (PCR).

Source: https://media.geeksforgeeks.org/wp-content/uploads/20240122152308/Polymerase-chain-Reaction.png.

Technological innovation in PCR has prompted the evolution of Digital Polymerase Chain Reaction (dPCR), significantly enhancing the sensitivity and quantification of nucleic acids in clinical settings. dPCR keeps the reaction divided into millions of individual compartments, enhancing the detection of low-abundant pathogenic sequences, which is particularly crucial in the diagnosis of low-titer infections (Lauren et al., 2024). dPCR's precision makes it an excellent diagnostic and prognostic tool as it unravels constraints that accompany typical PCR methodologies, such as quantitative read-outs based on reaction efficiency.

Application of dPCR in molecular pathology enables doctors to attain absolute quantification of viral loads or genetic markers, thereby contributing to the evaluation of the disease process and response to treatment. As such, dPCR represents a paradigm shift in the case of monitoring and control of infectious disease, transforming classic diagnostic practice. The integration of PCR technologies in healthcare has completely transformed not just diagnostic microbiology but also the design of research and therapeutic approaches to infectious diseases. Enhanced PCR methods, ongoing, e.g., real-time PCR and multiplex systems, enable researchers to quantify and identify multiple pathogens simultaneously, a task previously hindered by the restrictions of past methods.

Engagement of such advances enables wide-scale epidemiological surveillance and prompt detection of outbreaks, both required in the prevention of infectious disease transmission. Besides, as has been evidenced by the practice of shrimp aquaculture, the application of PCR-based diagnostics makes it possible to optimize disease management practices in diverse settings (Maharani & Sumsanto, 2024). This convergence of molecular pathology and technology underscores the importance of advanced diagnostic techniques, ultimately translating into better health outcomes and informing public health policy in an era increasingly defined by the complexity of infectious disease control (Figure 7.6).

7.2.2. Next-Generation Sequencing (NGS)

The integration of Next-Generation Sequencing (NGS) technology in molecular pathology has transformed our perception of infectious diseases. Conventional diagnostic techniques tend to rely on culture methods or single-gene amplification, which can be tedious and narrow in outlook. In contrast, NGS allows for the concurrent sequencing of several nucleic acid fragments, yielding a broad panorama of the pathogen's genetic landscape.

This global strategy enhances our ability to identify known and emerging pathogens, characterize genetic mutations that bestow virulence, and understand the pathogen evolution dynamics and resistance mechanisms. Its quick evolution and adaptability make it imperative to employ the most recent technologies like NGS to match their evolution, making it a priceless instrument in today's diagnostics and infectious disease studies (Satam et al., 2023). In addition to making it easier to detect pathogens, NGS is also a valuable instrument for customizing the treatment schemes of infected patients. The more widely accepted idea of precision medicine extends to infectious diseases as well, where both the host and pathogen genomes are known to be required to determine efficacious therapeutic agents. Notably, NGS allows for the characterization of neoantigens—unique markers produced by tumor-specific mutations—which are capable of stimulating the immune response against cancer cells (Xie et al., 2023). Although extensively used in the context of oncology, the basic principles of neoantigen research can be adapted to create targeted immunotherapies against infectious disease pathogens, especially when standard treatments fail. Thus, the ability to apply NGS technology has the potential to provide more individualized treatment options based on patient and pathogen profiles. Besides, the applications of NGS extend beyond therapeutic and diagnostic clinical practice; they also extend to epidemiological surveillance as well as public health policy. The ability of NGS to quickly identify pathogen genomes enables a better understanding of transmission patterns during outbreaks, which is critical in stemming the spread successfully. By mapping transmission and spread-related genetic variants, public health officials are able to make more informed decisions regarding interventions and deployments of resources. Through the integration of NGS data with epidemiological models, researchers can forecast potential routes of outbreak, thereby enhancing readiness against new infectious diseases. Therefore, the impact of NGS on molecular pathology reaches far beyond the lab, enabling efforts that drive progress in public health outcomes as well as infectious disease prevention worldwide (Satam et al., 2023) (Figure 7.7).

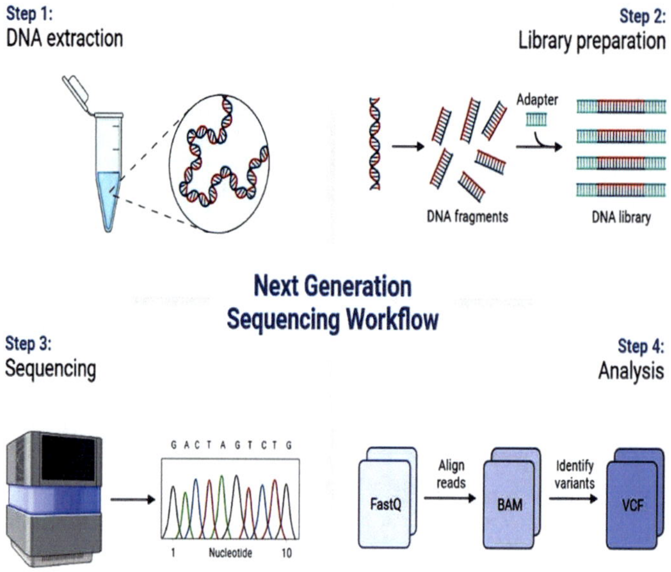

Figure 7.7. Next-generation sequencing (NGS).

Source: https://microbenotes.com/wp-content/uploads/2023/02/Next-Generation-Sequencing-NGS-1024x536.jpg.

7.2.3. In Situ Hybridization

In situ hybridization (ISH) represents a milestone technological advancement in molecular pathology, especially within the field of infectious disease. ISH allows for the localization of known nucleic acid sequences within tissue sections with precision, and it is irreplaceable in determining the presence and dynamics of pathogens at the cellular level. By employing labeled probes that hybridize to corresponding nucleic acids of interest, scientists can directly visualize the localization of the viral or bacterial genome in the context of tissue architecture. The spatial resolution is extremely beneficial in understanding the pathophysiology of disease since it illuminates the interaction dynamics between pathogens and host cells. ISH has enabled us to detect the virus in various pulmonary cell populations along the infection process and has enabled us to better interpret the pathogenic process (Ye et al., 2007). Apart from mere nucleic acid detection, ISH plays a key role in situating the morphological changes in the infected tissue into perspective. The combination of ISH with immunohistochemistry offers a twofold means of identifying both the existence of some pathogens and the host immune system reaction simultaneously. For instance, using ISH to identify SARS-CoV while conducting immunohistochemical analysis of immune cell markers, researchers can identify which immune cells are being used when infected. It helps to delineate the interaction between the pathogens and the host immune system, which is crucial in devising effective therapeutic interventions. As has been set out in pathologists' diagnostic capabilities, tools like ISH are precious in describing infectious pathogens and identifying the resultant histopathologic changes in tissue (Reller et al., 2001). More significantly, the worth of ISH goes beyond being a diagnostic tool to being that of prognosis as well as treatment monitoring. By determining the viral load and intracellular distribution of pathogens, ISH can advise clinicians on the likely course of disease and response to therapy. In chronic infections, the localization of the pathogen and dynamics of replication may be critical in determining the efficacy of antiviral drugs. With advancing molecular pathology, employing ISH becomes increasingly sophisticated, making it possible to track in real-time pathogen-pathogen interactions in tissue. Such ongoing development emphasizes the inclusion of advanced molecular techniques in routine diagnostic workup, which paves the way for improved understanding and control of infectious diseases and their related molecular processes (Ye et al., 2007; Reller et al., 2001).

7.3. Genetic Factors in Infectious Diseases

The pathogen is not the sole determinant of the dynamics of infectious diseases, as selectively host genetic determinants also modulate them. Genetic variation can create differential immune responses to identical infectious agents, leading to variations in disease severity among different hosts. Polymorphism in immune-related genes, for instance, can modulate cytokine production and hence the body's inflammatory response to infection. It is critical to learn about these genetic factors in molecular pathology because they can provide clues as to why certain populations are susceptible to certain diseases. Through such studies, researchers continue to de-mystify the genetic origins of infection and indicate why personalized treatment approaches are essential. These include taking into account an individual's genetic makeup for the purpose of enhancing curative benefits. Therefore, the genetics-infectious diseases interface is an important area of study that has practical application to public health as well as the practice of medicine. The relevance of genetics can also be seen when applied to the pathogens themselves, for the reason that they will change according to host genetic composition. The gene-for-gene relationship illustrates such interaction, wherein the presence of specific host resistance genes may be followed by the emergence of pathogenic counteradaptive responses. For example, viral mutations may arise to evade the immune response that is associated with specific human leukocyte antigen (HLA) types, pointing to a continuous evolutionary race between hosts and microbes.

This interaction needs to be studied in detail at the molecular level because particular genetic markers in both the host and the pathogen could guide more effective control measures for infectious diseases. Molecular pathology methodologies that include genetic analysis could, therefore, further illuminate infection processes in infectious diseases and lead to advancements in the development of vaccines and targeted therapies dependent on the population. Genetic predisposition plays a significant role in disease expression and development in autoimmune diseases , such as primary adrenal insufficiency. Notably, polymorphic markers of significant immune response genes have been associated with increased risks of some pathologies. For instance, research has pinpointed some genetic variants, such as IFNAR1 and IFNAR2 genes, as being predictive of primary adrenal insufficiency and highlighting the importance of genetic testing in the identification of at-risk individuals. The identification of such genetic associations makes for better diagnostic practices and informs personalized medicine strategies. Identification of susceptible populations based on genetic susceptibility allows medical practitioners to predict and intervene in complications more accurately, thereby maximizing patient outcomes. Thus, the integration of genetic factors into infectious disease studies emphasizes the necessity to explore molecular pathways for treatment as well as prevention, making molecular pathology of infectious diseases a more productive field (Figure 7.8).

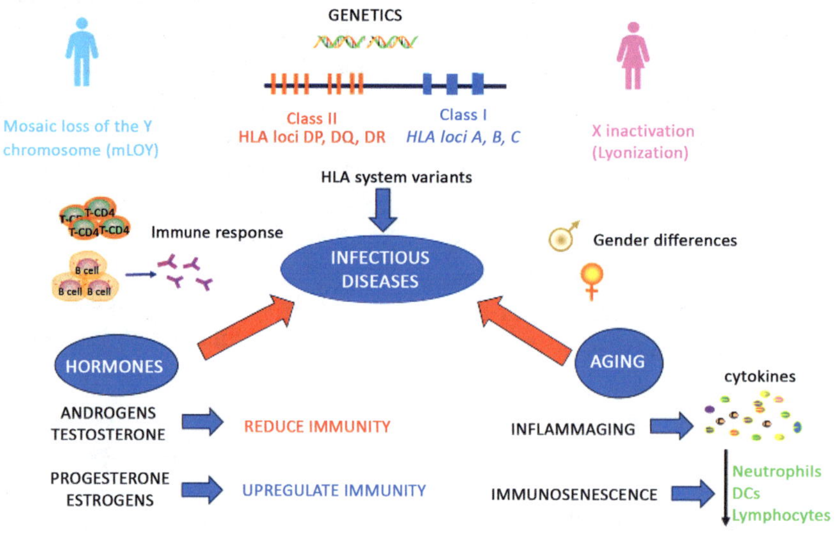

Figure 7.8. Genetic factors in infectious diseases.

Source: https://pub.mdpi-res.com/diseases/diseases-13-00179/article_deploy/html/images/diseases-13-00179-g001.png?1749536500.

7.3.1. Host Genetic Susceptibility

Identification of host genetic susceptibility is also at the core of molecular infectious disease pathology. Differences in genetic makeup from person to person play a significant role in how organisms respond to disease agents. For instance, variation in specific alleles may enable or disable immune function, thereby affecting the development of an infection. For malaria, research has indicated that genetic factors account for a large portion of the heritability of disease susceptibility among populations. This is attested by the identification of single-nucleotide polymorphisms (SNPs) associated with severe malaria, whereby certain CSMD1 gene variants are associated with increased risk, suggesting that there is a connection between severity of disease and genetic control (Damena et al., 2024). Host genetics-pathogen virulence interaction underlines the significance of an integrated perspective on such an interaction in the pathology of infectious disease. Apart from traditional infectious diseases, genetic susceptibility is also being examined in relation to emerging pathogens with wildlife reservoirs. As a case in point, studies on ophidiomycosis in snakes demonstrate how genetic variation can modulate the response to emerging fungal infections. Captive prairie rattlesnake trials infected with the pathogen Ophidiomyces ophidiicola demonstrated significant differences in gene expression based on tissue type and infection status. This gives credence to the position that host genetic factors are focal in determining infectious pathogen susceptibility and resistance, thereby dictating morbidity and mortality rates in wildlife populations (Mathur et al., 2023). Understanding these genetic responses can have a significant role in devising plans for conserving at-risk species against emerging pathogens, illustrating the central role of genetic variation in populations in nature. Lastly, understanding host genetic susceptibility not only aids understanding of individual and population response to infection but also can guide therapy. By recognizing the genetic factors that predispose an individual to serious disease, clinicians can tailor interventions more effectively. In infectious diseases like malaria, genetic risk factors play a role in offering the potential for developing personalized therapies that take into account variance among individuals. Moreover, the use of genomic data from different populations helps to account for environmental and evolutionary pressures shaping genetic susceptibility to infection. With emerging research, the integration of genetic data into the molecular pathogenesis of infectious diseases will be the panacea for combating these illnesses at a community and global level, which in turn will enhance public health interventions (Figure 7.9).

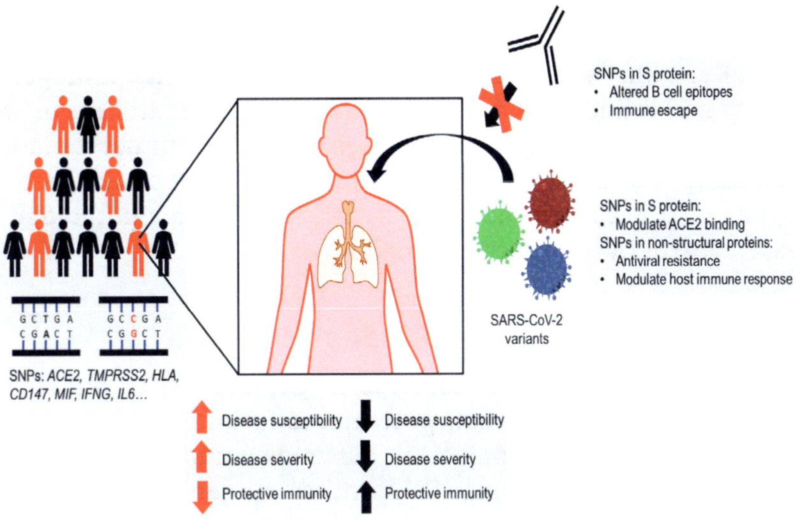

Figure 7.9. Host genetic susceptibility.

Source: https://onlinelibrary.wiley.com/cms/asset/d5dcd5cb-e4dc-4854-8e7a-25b1b7281960/imr12897-fig-0001-m.jpg.

7.3.2. Pathogen Genetic Variability

The genetic heterogeneity of the pathogen is of critical significance in the molecular pathology of infectious diseases and greatly impacts diagnosis, treatment, and epidemiology. Pathogens are found to be genetically very heterogeneous, and such heterogeneity is created by various parameters , including mutation rates, recombination, and host immune pressure selection. Such heterogeneity can potentially lead to changes in virulence and pathogenicity and hence influence disease outcome in infected hosts. The ability to detect and analyze genetic variation in pathogens underlies the comprehension of mechanisms for adaptation, transmission, and resistance to therapeutic intervention. Methods , such as polymerase chain reaction (PCR) and subsequent sequencing techniques have revolutionized diagnostic approaches by allowing scientists to select for unique genetic markers associated with pathogenicity and drug resistance, as uncovered in the advances outlined by Sperança et al. (2016). Furthermore, the importance of pathogen genetic variation extends beyond medicine to public health practices for the control and prevention of infectious diseases. As one example, understanding pathogen genome variations can provide insights into emerging strains that can present new challenges to the treatment and prevention of infectious diseases. This is especially exemplified in viral pathogens, whereby genetic variation can affect transmissibility as well as vaccine efficacy. An example of this is the work on the Infectious hypodermal and hematopoietic necrosis virus (IHHNV), where there was a lack of large-scale genetic variability within specific shrimp species. While the pathogen is of low impact, its potential to affect growth rates and productivity necessitates ongoing monitoring and examination of genetic variability (Feij et al., 2008). This points to the importance of constant innovation in molecular approaches to identify and monitor pathogen change with time. In addition to diagnostic and epidemiologic ends, information on genetic variation is valuable for the proper design of vaccines. Genetic variation within pathogens can complicate the development of vaccines since variations can lead to antigenic variation. The consequences of such diversity are significant, as it can interfere with the effectiveness of existing vaccines and necessitate continuous alteration of vaccine compositions to address new strains. Designing vaccines thus must consider genetic pathogen profiles to achieve optimal immunogenicity and reduce the risk of vaccine failure. Researchers using techniques , such as sequence analysis and fragment enzyme restriction can better understand the genetic makeup of the pathogens, opening doors for tailored vaccine policies (Sperança et al., 2016). Genetic variability of pathogens in this context not only benefits molecular pathology but also enhances the efficacy of disease control in all infectious pathogens.

7.3.3. Role of Plasmids and Mobile Genetic Elements

The role of plasmids and mobile genetic elements in the molecular pathogenesis of infectious disease increases with awareness due to their potential to facilitate the transfer of genes encoding antibiotic resistance between bacterial populations. Plasmids, small, often circular molecules of DNA, can replicate independently of chromosomal DNA and carry genes that confer useful traits, such as resistance to several antibiotics. These hereditary factors may be passed between bacteria to other bacteria by conjugation, transformation, or transduction, leading to the rapid dissemination of resistance characteristics in clinical and environmental environments. Therefore, the establishment of multi-drug resistant (MDR) strains poses a serious public health issue because it complicates treatment and increases morbidity and mortality rates of infectious diseases (Urban et al., 2022). Aside from that, mobile genetic elements like transposons and integrons are also crucial for the adaptation and evolution of bacterial pathogens. Transposons, or jumping genes, are elements that can insert into different genomic locations, thereby enabling the recombination of genetic material that increases the virulence and adaptability of bacterial populations. Integrons, on the other hand, are modules that are able to capture and express cassettes of genes, including genes for antibiotic resistance. This pooled gene system is a reservoir of resistance genes, which can easily spread by horizontal gene transfer in pathogenic and commensal bacteria and exacerbate the problem of infectious disease control. The mobilizable character of these elements necessitates rigorous monitoring and new means that can be adopted to combat antibiotic resistance (Berg et al., 2020). With the existing worldwide health pandemic caused by the emergence of antibiotic resistance, understanding the molecular activity of plasmids and mobile genetic elements is pivotal in the development of effective interventions. Their action on infectious diseases and the dissemination of resistance makes it important to study them more to describe the mechanisms underlying their action in various environments. In addition, this data can guide the discovery of new drugs and prevention measures that target these genetic elements, potentially reversing the course of the war against resistance. Hence, inter-disciplinary approaches between microbiology, genetics, and epidemiology are critical in designing comprehensive plans to combat the effects of MDR bacteria on human and animal health (Urban et al., 2022) (Figure 7.10).

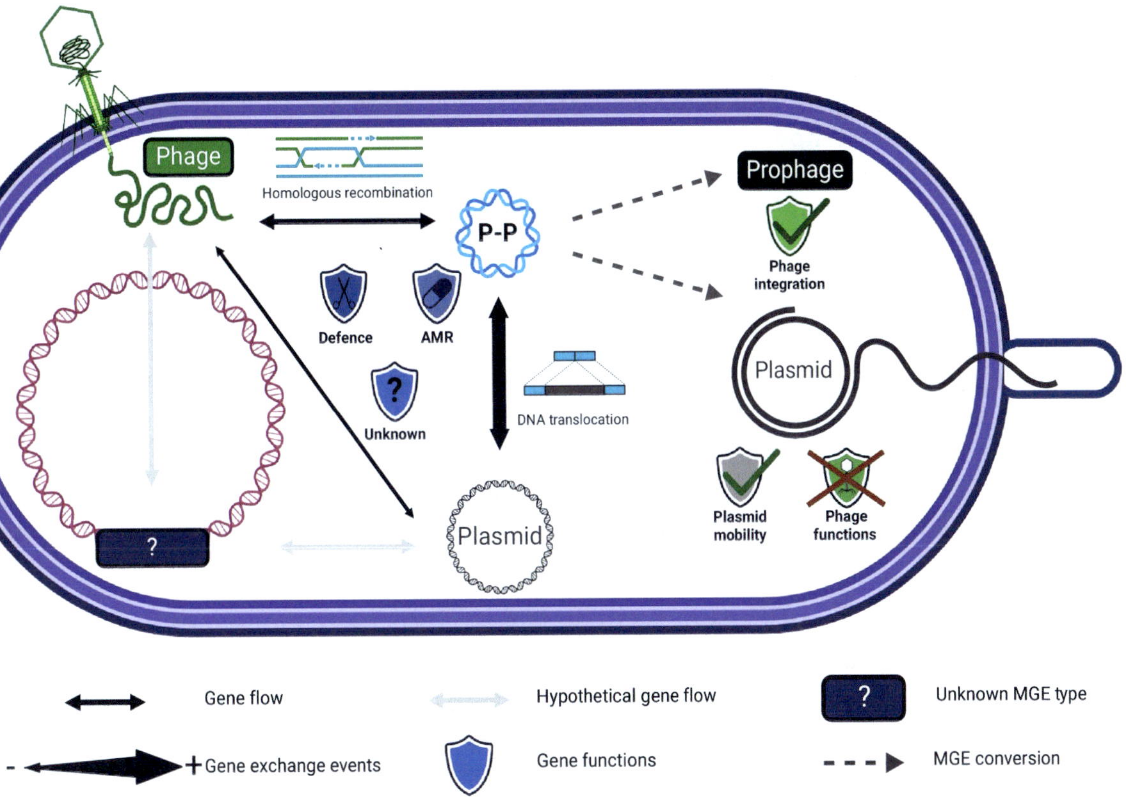

Figure 7.10. Role of plasmids and mobile genetic elements.

Source: https://www.cell.com/cms/attachment/40d9e225-8e99-44a1-8749-ae0e798125e0/gr1_lrg.jpg.

7.4. Pathogen–Host Interactions

Pathogen–host interactions should be understood for unraveling the complexities of infectious diseases. Pathogen–host interactions determine the infection dynamics, host immune response, and disease outcome, respectively. Pathogens employ various strategies to interfere with host defense, including antigen variation, immune suppression, and direct manipulation of host cells. Some pathogens, for instance, may secrete proteins that modulate host immune signaling pathways and facilitate their survival within the host environment. This subtle interaction between pathogenic virulence and host defense mechanisms is shaped by evolutionary pressures. Thus, the comprehension of these interactions not merely gives us an insight into the disease basis at the molecular level, but also gives us information about potential therapeutic strategies to enhance host resistance or target pathogenic processes directly. Breakthroughs in the past decade in molecular techniques have greatly enhanced our understanding of pathogen–host interactions, especially through the use of new diagnostic platforms. For example, next-generation sequencing and advanced PCR techniques allow scientists to identify and type pathogens to previously unattained levels of precision. In a typical study of the Galapagos sea lion, a multifilarial PCR test was developed, which reported the presence of *Dirofilaria immitis* and *Dirofilaria repens* among juveniles, which posed a gigantic danger of non-native pathogens. These strategies show how molecular diagnostics can be applied to inform conservation science and public health policy by providing essential information about the prevalence of pathogens and their relevance to the endemic species, highlighting the need to include molecular methods in infectious disease investigations (Malaguarnera & Cabrera-Pastor, 2024). Furthermore, the development of *ex vivo* tissue challenge models is a significant breakthrough in the study of host-pathogen interactions in a more human-relevant environment. Compared to conventional animal models, these new systems enable the specific study of immune responses to pathogens with the avoidance of some of the ethical and logistical issues related to *in vivo* studies. The COVID-19 pandemic dramatically increased the pace of adoption of such models, highlighting their use in viral pathogenesis studies and testing therapeutic interventions. With precise mimicry of human disease conditions, *ex vivo* models allow the study of molecular pathways involved in immune modulation to garner valuable insights into vaccine development and therapeutic targeting potential (Gordhan et al., 2023). Such developments not only advance knowledge regarding infectious disease pathogenesis but also pave the way for novel approaches towards disease prevention and treatment.

7.4.1. Mechanisms of Immune Evasion

The complexity of immune evasion mechanisms employed by pathogens forms an essential part of the molecular pathology of infectious disease. Pathogens have evolved different methodologies to counteract the host's immune mechanism, thereby ensuring that they can survive and grow despite the host's defenses. The mechanisms could be categorized as a group of different tactics , including antigenic variation, production of immune-modulating proteins, and recruitment of host cellular pathways. For instance, some viruses possess a high mutation rate, which enables them to rapidly modify their surface proteins and thereby escape being detected by antibodies and T-cells. This continuously changing nature complicates the development of effective vaccines and therapeutic interventions. Further, understanding such pathways is important in developing strategies for enhancing immune responses since current research focuses more and more on mimicking treatments that target specifically these evasive strategies with the aim of re-establishing immune function and effectively fighting infections (Sharma et al., 2024). Among the many studied pathogens, human cytomegalovirus (HCMV) stands as a paradigm example of immune evasion through superior molecular strategies. HCMV co-evolved with the host immune system and has specific genes , such as UL144 and UL141, that have significant roles in immune response modulation. UL144 is a herpesvirus entry mediator HVEM structural homologue, effectively transmitting inhibitory signals that limit the activity of T-cells. Meanwhile, UL141 is an analogue of the TIGIT immunoreceptor and has a significant role in evasion from natural killer (NK) cells. These mechanisms demonstrate not only the amazing flexibility of viruses like HCMV but also mirror the importance of glycosylation patterns of viral proteins, which aid in immune evasion by controlling ligand-binding interactions and enhancing the virus's stealth properties against the immune system (Nemčovičová et al., 2020). The potential of therapeutic intervention via manipulation of these immune evasion pathways cannot be overemphasized, particularly in the context of current advances noted with immunotherapy application. The achievement with the use of immune checkpoint blockade in oncology now offers an opportunity for generating similar approaches in treating infectious diseases. Blocking some of the checkpoints exploited by pathogens may enhance immune function and favor the elimination of chronic infections. For example, therapeutic targeting of UL144-dependent processes in HCMV may correct T-cell function, thereby increasing the host's ability to resist the virus. Overall, the intricate relationship between pathogens and host immunity underscores the necessity of understanding immunological processes better. This not only provides depth to the comprehension of the molecular disease pathology of infectious disease but also guides the development of new treatment strategies (Sharma et al., 2024) (Figure 7.11).

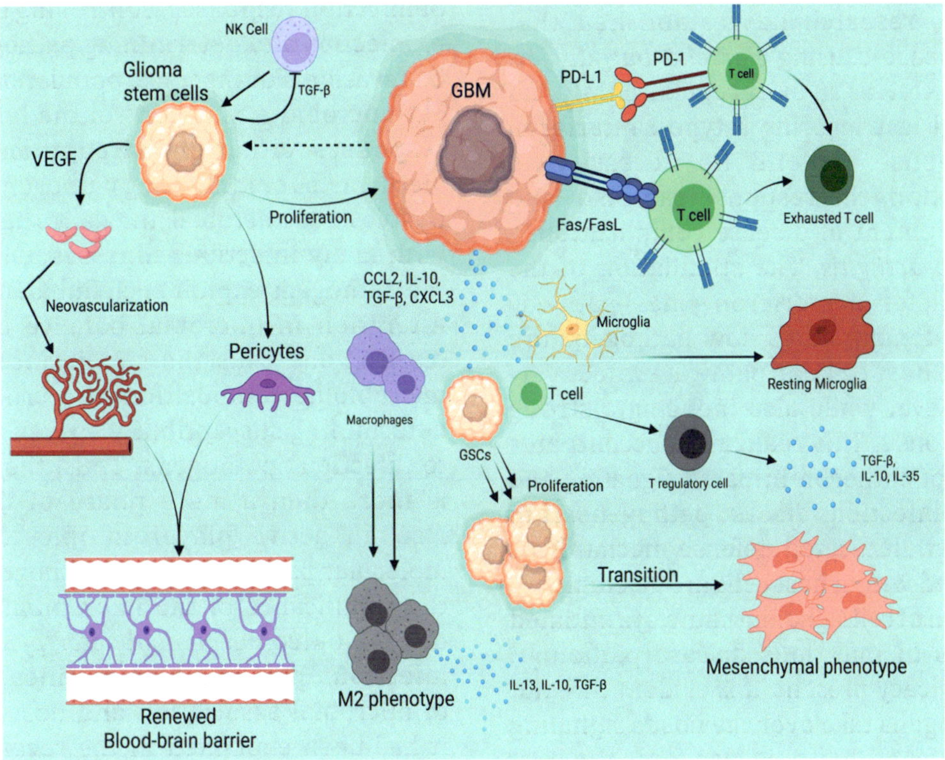

Figure 7.11. Mechanisms of immune evasion.

Source: https://www.researchgate.net/publication/361244037/figure/fig1/AS:1165971066757122@1655000573257/Visual-representation-of-the-immune-escape-mechanisms-of-glioblastoma-Utilizing-a.png.

7.4.2. Pathogen-Induced Cell Signaling Pathways

The engagement of host cell signaling pathways by pathogens is a critical aspect of infectious disease pathology. Pathogens employ diverse mechanisms for subverting host cell response through modulation of signaling pathways to facilitate their survival as well as replication in the host. Pathogen interactions usually elicit complex immune responses for their clearance. For example, host cell pattern recognition receptors (PRRs) can recognize pathogen-associated molecular patterns (PAMPs), which initiate cascade signaling that results in the production of a number of pro-inflammatory cytokines and chemokines. Immune activation plays a crucial role in the recruitment of immune cells to the site of infection, eventually enabling the host to generate a defensive response. Nevertheless, pathogens have evolved counter-strategies that can interfere with the signaling pathways so that they can bypass host immunity and be able to survive in the host, making the infectious disease-associated pathology more complex and challenging for treatment. One such mechanism by which pathogens can trigger host immune signaling is through the secretion of molecules , such as cyclic-di-adenosine monophosphate (c-di-AMP). For instance, research has established that the Lyme disease-causing *Borrelia burgdorferi* secretes c-di-AMP as an extracellular PAMP, and this is crucial in triggering a type-I interferon (IFN-I) response. Beyond its necessity to control infection, the response can also lead to the development of disease complications , such as *Lyme arthritis*. The stimulation of the STING (stimulator of interferon genes) pathway by c-di-AMP demonstrates how pathogens are able to hijack host cellular pathways effectively for their survival while also inducing a strong immune response. This realization accentuates the intricacy of pathogen-initiated signaling and its effects on infectious disease pathogenesis in general. The multifaceted defense mechanisms that are formed within host cells are an emphasis on the function of cell signaling pathways initiated by pathogens in infectious disease pathology. Given the intricacy present, it is evident that not only do pathogens take over the host's signaling to prevent defense, but they also force the host to initiate immunogenic mechanisms of cell death. These mechanisms, including apoptosis and pyroptosis, serve the purpose of killing infected cells and restricting pathogen growth. For example, the activation of these pathways by pathogens , such as *B. burgdorferi*, in response to stress, triggers a profound immune modulation. Information on the molecular processes that regulate such interactions gives hints towards therapeutic interventions. By defining the regulation mechanisms of these signaling pathways, scientists can develop intervention strategies that influence host immunity without undermining the severity of disease, promising a solution for future therapeutic interventions against infectious diseases (Li et al., 2024; Sharma et al., 2024).

7.4.3. Impact of Microbiome on Infectious Diseases

Interaction of human microbiome and infectious disease is a complex narrative that integrates host health and microbial dynamics. The microbiome is a significant immunoregulator of infection responses, controlling susceptibility to infection and determining pathogen behavior on invasion. For instance, population diversity in gut microbiota may control the host's immune responses either by strengthening defense mechanisms or facilitating pathogen colonization. Dysbiosis or microbial imbalance has been linked with many infectious illnesses, where some of the pathogens exploit such imbalances to infect. Alteration in microbial balance can augment disease, and thus the significance of defining microbiome composition as a crucial factor in determining susceptibility as well as resistance to infectious pathogens. Thus, the microbiome is more than a mere phase of infection but also an active player in infectious disease molecular pathology. Some pathogens exemplify the significance of the microbiome in shaping disease outcome. *Helicobacter pylori*, a proven infectious pathogen, exemplifies the overlap of microbial association and host wellness. As it has been explained in the recent consensus reports, not only is this infection linked to gastritis, but it also significantly alters the gut microbiota. Eradication of *H. pylori* infection has been hampered by increasing antibiotic resistance, encouraging reconsideration of therapeutic approaches. The *H. pylori*-gut microbiota interaction is a perfect example of how specific treatment regimens can manipulate microbial flora, potentially lowering the risk of developing complications like gastric cancer. Additionally, understanding these interactions would provide the potential for new therapies leveraging the microbiome to manage disease, proving the microbiome as both a facilitator of disease and a target for therapy, as identified by existing clinical guidelines (Malfertheiner et al., 2022). Additionally, the emerging science of the microbiome has implications for public health at large, namely its potential for disease prevention. Dysbiosis can cause higher inflammation and immune impairment, which contributes to higher susceptibility to a variety of infectious diseases like respiratory and gastrointestinal infections (Hou et al., 2022). Prevention can be considered through the facilitation of the balance of the microbiome by means of diet interventions and probiotics to enhance population immunity and resistance to pathogens. Also, recent findings suggest that microbiome modulation—through treatments , such as fecal microbiota transplantation—can provide new strategies for the treatment of recurrent infections and for the promotion of harmonious microbial communities. In this sense, the impact of the microbiome on infectious disease is vast, and its dual role as a disease pathology cause and as a therapeutic and prevention tool in molecular pathology is emphasized (Figure 7.12).

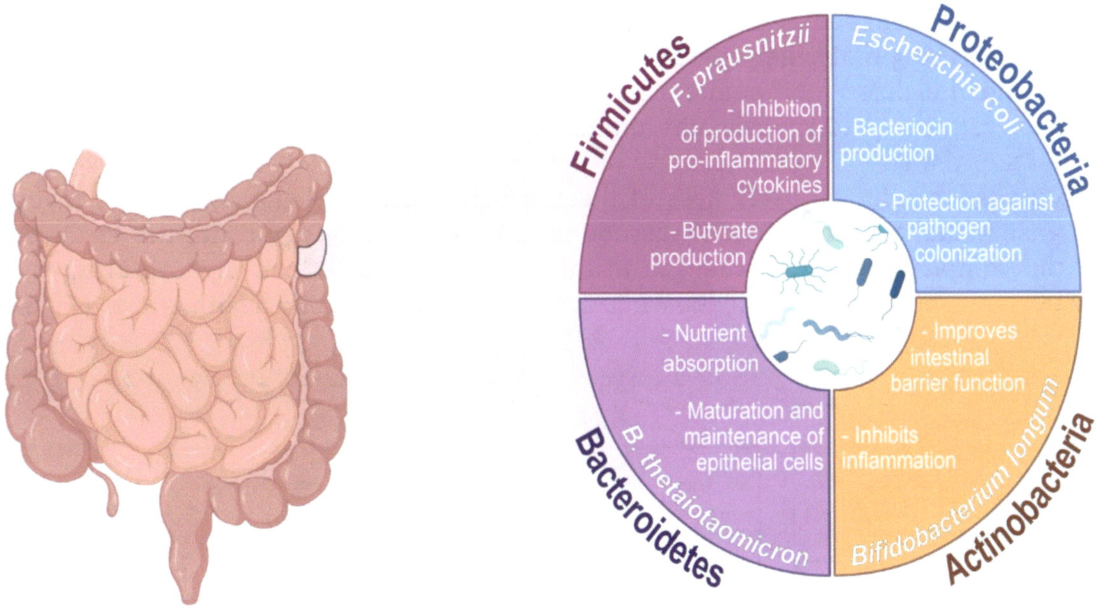

Figure 7.12. Impact of the human microbiome on infectious diseases.

Source: https://www.frontiersin.org/files/Articles/1098386/fmicb-14-1098386-HTML/image_m/fmicb-14-1098386-g001.jpg.

7.5. Diagnostic Advances in Molecular Pathology

The area of molecular pathology has experienced a great deal of advancement, particularly in the diagnosis of infectious diseases. Traditional microbiologic technique, including culture, can be hampered by the inability to culture fastidious pathogens or by previous antibiotic therapy effects, which can lead to suppression. Consequently, more effective molecular diagnostics , such as Universal Polymerase Chain Reaction (UPCR) testing, offer an improved approach that detects microbial nucleic acids in clinical samples regardless of the viability of the pathogen. Studies have proven that UPCR is an efficient tool to detect infections otherwise undetected by culture techniques, thereby bringing a revolutionary shift in pathogen diagnosis and treatment in complex infections. This has been vindicated by a study showing that antimicrobial therapy adjustment was directed by UPCR values and uncovering the potential of molecular techniques to inform clinical decision-making better than traditional techniques in isolation (Donkin et al., 2022). Apart from UPCR, novel imaging technologies , such as Atomic Force Microscopy (AFM) have also proven to be core tools in the molecular pathology of infectious diseases. AFM brings unparalleled resolution and sensitivity to bear, enabling researchers to study cellular and molecular changes that are associated with infectious processes. AFM can, for example, detect changes in cell morphology, adhesion properties, and mechanical compliance that typically mirror disease evolution. These parameters not only contribute to infection diagnosis but also to understanding the pathophysiological mechanisms involved in the onset and evolution of disease. In addition, AFM molecular characterization of the samples increases our understanding of the mechanisms through which the pathogens manipulate host cells, and thereby expanding the vistas of diagnosis as well as potential therapeutic avenues in infectious diseases (Kiio et al., 2020). With such diagnostic advances coming into existence, a path is made for personalized medicine in the management of infectious diseases. The ability to diagnose more specifically using molecular methods has significant implications in patient management as it allows for individualized therapeutic interventions based on the causative pathogens. Moreover, their inclusion can shorten diagnosis time, ultimately culminating in enhanced therapeutic outcomes while mitigating the risk of complications of delayed treatment. However, there are still studies needed to assess the clinical usefulness of these developments holistically. Further investigation will help ensure that the diagnostic landscape in molecular pathology continues to develop so it can face the complexities and challenges in infectious diseases effectively, capturing the subtle interplay between pathogens and hosts, while furthering overall public health efforts (Figure 7.13).

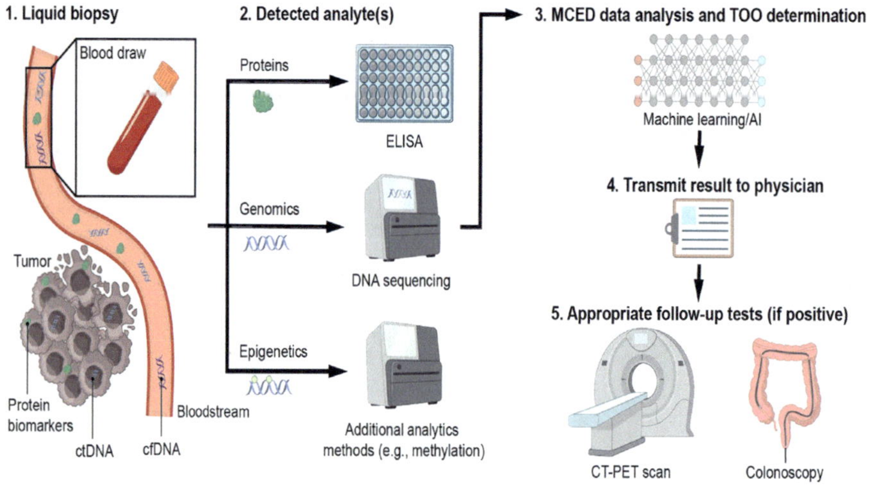

Figure 7.13. Diagnostic advances in molecular pathology.

Source: https://www.advancesinmolecularpathology.com/cms/10.1016/j.yamp.2023.07.007/asset/7f840040-2b44-43b4-b0e1-6054409b32ba/main.assets/gr1_lrg.jpg.

7.5.1. Biomarkers for Early Detection

Identification of biomarkers for the identification of infectious disease at an early time point is a valuable advance in molecular pathology because it allows timely intervention and improved patient outcome. Biomarkers are proteins, nucleic acids, or other molecules that signify infection by an infectious agent and aid in diagnosis of the disease at a moment when treatment can be optimally initiated. For instance, the use of specific protein biomarkers can enable the clinician to differentiate between bacterial or viral infections, thereby guiding appropriate therapeutic strategies. The integration of biomarkers in diagnostic procedures frequently employs advanced technologies, such as biosensors, capable of rapidly assaying biological samples with high sensitivity and specificity. By implementing such innovative methods, clinicians will be able to progress early infection identification, which stops the transmission of such infections and facilitates proper management of patient care (Zhang et al., 2025). Furthermore, biosensors have revolutionized the epidemiology of early infection detection. These devices are based on the identification and quantification of biomarkers associated with various pathogens, both viral and bacterial. Biosensor design has been enhanced with the development of biomechanical principles that enhance their performance regarding sensitivity and response time. Piezoelectric sensors, for instance, can transform mechanical interaction with biomolecules into quantifiable signals, hence allowing real-time infection analysis. The ease of use of such devices makes them excellent alternatives to traditional laboratory methods, which are time-consuming and costly. As pressure to provide instant diagnostics grows, sustained R&D of biosensor technology has the potential to plug critical gaps in current healthcare infrastructure, ultimately improving patient outcomes by facilitating timely therapeutic approaches (Zhang et al., 2025). In addition to traditional biomarkers, extracellular vesicles (EVs) are also being explored for their potential to be applied within early detection strategies for infectious diseases. EVs are nano-sized particles released from cells that have a set of molecular signatures of their parent cell state. Due to their low immunogenicity and ability to traverse biological barriers, their properties render them extremely desirable for non-invasive diagnostics. EV cargo alterations have been found to serve as markers of infectious disease and to elucidate aspects of disease progression and immune response. In addition, studies have demonstrated that EVs from various biological fluids have been found to yield valuable information on the detection of specific pathogens. Thus, the study of EVs as biomarkers offers not only promising avenues for early diagnosis but also a greater insight into infectious diseases' molecular pathology.

7.5.2. Role of Molecular Diagnostics in Personalized Medicine

Integration of molecular diagnostics into personalized medicine is a significant advancement in the management of infectious diseases because it enhances the precision with which patients can be diagnosed and treated. Molecular diagnostics utilize techniques , such as polymerase chain reaction (PCR) and DNA sequencing to detect specific pathogens and genetic susceptibility, allowing clinicians to diagnose infection early and select the optimal treatment approach. This individualization fosters improved patient outcomes by reducing the risk of ineffective therapy as well as curbing drug resistance development, which often complicates the treatment of infectious diseases. With the developing nature of personalized medicine, the reliance on molecular diagnostics will only increase and will be the backbone of modern medical practice in infectious disease management. Also, beyond detection, the application of molecular diagnostics is essential in monitoring the progression of disease as well as response to treatment. Through detecting certain biomarkers, doctors can gain insight into how individual patients could metabolize drugs or how their bodies respond to certain therapeutic regimens. This capacity not only allows for the improvement of existing treatment protocols but also aids in developing new therapies with the goal of targeting specific pathways of infectious disease. The entry of AI and machine learning technology will further refine these diagnostic tools, enabling more accurate predictions and personalized therapeutic strategies, a paradigm shift in infectious disease control. As molecular pathology advances, it is essential to address the challenge and promise of the ubiquitous application of molecular diagnostics in personalized medicine. While such technologies are impressive in their benefits, such as fast turnaround times and increased specificity, there are problems , such as the need for rigorous quality control and ethical considerations of genetic information. Moreover, the adoption of such diagnostic technologies can also be costly and thus pose access barriers, particularly in resource-limited settings. Based on recent reports, the convergence of molecular diagnostics into the clinic must be accompanied by widespread training of medical staff and adequate infrastructure for these technologies. It is only through such a collaborative effort that the potential of molecular diagnostics can be fully unleashed in the pursuit of personalized medicine for infectious diseases (Lutsiv, 2024; Vinayaka, 2024) (Figure 7.14).

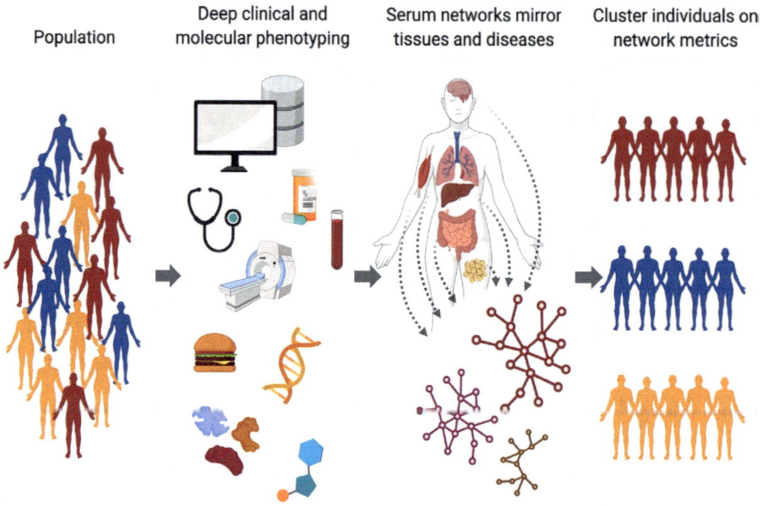

Figure 7.14. Role of molecular diagnostics in personalized medicine.

Source: https://www.cell.com/cms/10.1016/j.molmed.2020.09.003/asset/efcb8969-955f-4bb9-a38b-45b0ee56dd8c/main.assets/gr1_lrg.jpg.

7.5.3. Challenges in Implementing Molecular Diagnostics

The use of molecular diagnostics in infectious diseases presents several challenges that will undermine practical clinical uses. One major challenge is assay development and validation complexity. Molecular diagnostics, particularly those based on nucleic acid amplification techniques, require meticulous optimization for sensitivity and specificity. This involves issues like sample preparation, reagent selection, and complexities regarding the interpretation of results. Furthermore, maintaining high standards of quality control and assurance is paramount; the accuracy of molecular tests directly affects patient management decisions. As highlighted in recent literature, the need for fast and precise diagnostics has generated a spate of new testing technologies, but a number of them are challenged regarding their analytical performance and clinical utility, and thus, the need for sound validation procedures to bring about clinician and patient confidence (Kohale et al., 2023). In addition to technical issues, the financial burden of implementing molecular diagnostics cannot be overlooked. The cost of sophisticated equipment, reagents, and trained personnel often acts as a deterrent for general use, particularly in low-resource environments. The majority of healthcare environments are also unlikely to provide the requisite infrastructure to support complex molecular diagnostic platforms, resulting in health inequalities in access to cutting-edge testing technology. The COVID-19 pandemic highlighted these inequalities as laboratories encountered supply chain discontinuities and the high expense of nucleic acid amplification tests (Vona et al., 2021). Budget reductions can, therefore, decelerate innovation in how new molecular diagnostics are developed as research and development expenses become increasingly competitive. All these financial challenges must be addressed to make molecular diagnostics more accessible to various healthcare environments equitably. Lastly, the education of healthcare professionals in how to properly use and interpret molecular diagnostics is an ongoing challenge.

Although advances in molecular techniques will potentially improve disease identification and treatment, effective integration of the tools into practice requires extensive training and continuous professional education. Clinicians will not adequately understand test results, especially in complex cases where clinical data are important to interpretation. Misinterpretation of test results can have deleterious effects on patient care, as has been seen with the use of antibody testing during the early stages of the COVID-19 pandemic, which was marred by controversy regarding their accuracy and application (McLawhon & Fitzgerald, 2021). Therefore, emphasis on educational programs aimed at clinician knowledge development in molecular diagnostics is the need of the hour. These issues will be addressed in order for the full potential of molecular diagnostics in infectious diseases to be realized, leading to improved patient outcomes and decision-making.

7.6. Therapeutic Approaches

The modern therapeutic field of infectious illnesses is presently under threat increasingly by the development of antimicrobial resistance (AMR). Traditional anti-infectives, while still remaining fundamental treatment for most infections, are becoming less effective due to this decisive increase. Hence, researchers are turning towards several other modality alternatives that are capable of evading constraint by resistant pathogens. Of these, natural compounds have become of particular interest because of their availability and viability in biological activity. Among such a group of natural compounds, flavonoids, for instance, possess a lot of promise as antimicrobial drugs. Their diverse mechanisms of action—denaturing microbial membranes to interfering with nucleic acid synthesis—are a reflection of the potential they possess as adjunct therapeutic agents in combating infectious diseases. The discovery of such natural products could bring not just a new generation of defense but also inexpensive measures for poor-resource settings, thus broadening the armamentarium in treating infections (Ioannou & Baliou, 2024). A new therapeutic direction could include the application of high-multiplex tissue imaging (HMTI) techniques, significantly revolutionizing infectious diseases and other pathologies. Through the provision of detailed spatial and cellular information, HMTI enables researchers and clinicians to delineate complex tissue architecture, revealing distinct cellular interactions in the pathogen's microenvironment. Such are critical to understand pathogenesis, particularly for chronic infection and infectious diseases with a bearing on tumor biology. The use of cutting-edge computational technologies to interrogate this spatial data allows the identification of histopathologic biomarkers with associated disease outcomes, thus offering the potential to inform personalized therapeutic approaches. The incorporation of

HMTI technologies into clinical practice has the potential to ultimately drive personalized medicine approaches through the customization of treatment modalities according to the patient's pathology, improving the chances of effective interventions (Einhaus et al., 2023). As infectious diseases evolve, therapeutic research still remains absolutely essential. Beyond traditional pharmacological approaches, the necessity to incorporate emergent technologies , such as HMTI and the use of natural products like flavonoids is needed in the battle against the complicated challenges of resistant pathogens. Natural compounds possess a two-fold advantage: apart from exerting direct antimicrobial effects, their broad-range activity can be employed as prophylactic treatments against recurrent infections, e.g., in products , such as cranberry and D-mannose for urinary tract infections. The two-pronged strategy of applying both novel imaging methods and leveraging natural treatments can lead to more effective control strategies that can be adaptable to patient profiles. As research continues in this ever-evolving science, it is critical that these therapy strategies be supported by solid studies to guide efficacy, safety, and optimal use in practice (Ioannou & Baliou, 2024).

7.6.1. Antimicrobial Resistance and Its Implications

Antimicrobial resistance (AMR) is a severe issue in the infectious disease epidemic, directly affecting clinical outcomes and public health infrastructure worldwide. AMR is the process by which microorganisms acquire and develop the ability to resist once-effective treatments, thus rendering conventional treatments inappropriate. This effect does not result solely from gene mutations but is also directly affected by environmental and clinical practice, including the misuse and overuse of antibiotics. Therefore, infections caused by the resistant strains result in longer hospital stays, higher medical bills, and a greater mortality rate. The need to take action against AMR is underlined by health agencies, which cite it as a threat that will reverse decades of medical progress. A multifaceted approach, such as enhanced surveillance, judicious use of antibiotics, and innovation in new therapeutic technologies, will be required to fight AMR. In addition to patient health, AMR has broader economic and societal implications. Projections estimate that resistant infections are likely to result in an additional 10 million deaths annually by 2050 if the trend continues. The expensive nature of treating resistant infections tends to strain healthcare resources, diverting funds from other essential public health interventions. Furthermore, AMR is also poised to undermine the effectiveness of surgery and chemotherapy because the risk of infection is more and more insurmountable when prophylactic antibiotics that are otherwise effective become ineffective. The socio-economic impacts are profound, especially in low- and middle-income economies whose healthcare systems are already compromised. Solutions to combat AMR therefore, must address not only clinical innovation but also public health policy solutions that address socio-economic disparities that exacerbate the crisis. To effectively combat antimicrobial resistance, it is imperative to integrate modern technological advances in the monitoring and detection of pathogens. Notably, next-generation sequencing (NGS) has revolutionized infectious disease diagnosis by allowing rapid and accurate identification of resistant pathogens. The potential for DNA and RNA sequencing of many infectious pathogens offers greater insight into resistance mechanisms at the molecular level. The technique minimizes the limitations of traditional diagnostic techniques, making early and targeted interventions possible. Moreover, NGS reinforces epidemiologic surveillances, such as surveillance of infection outbreaks and resistance, which constitute key components in the fight against AMR. As the exposure to the impact of AMR continues, it will be essential to leverage technologies like NGS to create robust responses and counter the threat that resistant microorganisms pose, ultimately improving patient outcomes and public health impact (Gu et al., 2018) (Figure 7.15).

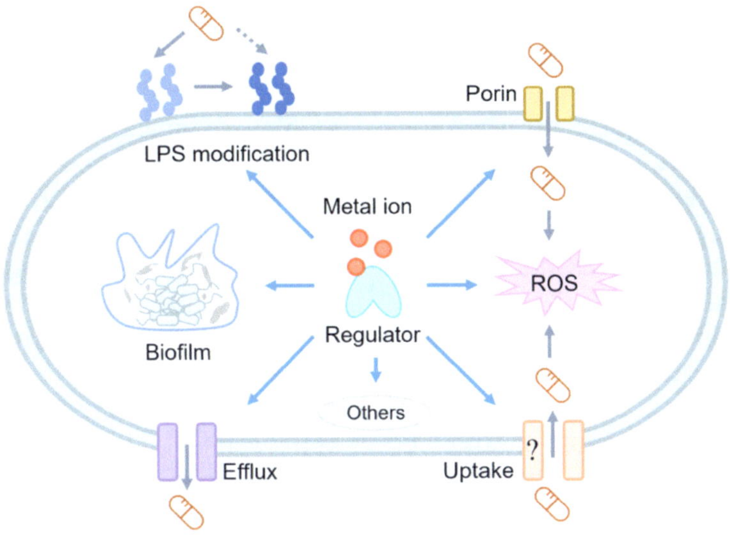

Figure 7.15. Antimicrobial resistance and its implications.

Source: https://enviromicro-journals.onlinelibrary.wiley.com/cms/asset/a4d11270-af04-478c-9990-38b30e6ec404/mbt214537-toc-0001-m.jpg.

7.6.2. Development of Targeted Therapies

The development of targeted therapies is a significant achievement in the molecular pathology of infectious diseases, representing a paradigm shift from the traditional treatment approaches toward more targeted interventions. This shift is most important in addressing the heterogeneous nature of infectious pathogens, with more than one mechanism of pathogenicity and unpredictable sensitivity to treatment. Targeted treatments attempt to identify specific molecular markers associated with infectious pathogens so that healthcare providers can align treatments with the unique biological characteristics of a pathogen. The integration of molecular pathology techniques, such as genomics and proteomics, streamlines the process of identifying these markers, thereby improving diagnostic accuracy and therapeutic efficacy. As per the literature, understanding the molecular mechanisms of infectious diseases is crucial for the development of effective treatment strategies that can reduce morbidity and mortality from infections (Sharma et al., 2024). Central to the success of targeted therapies is the concept of personalized medicine that emphasizes the role of individual patient parameters in therapeutic choice. Modern advances in molecular pathology have enabled clinicians to assess host factors, such as genetic variation and immune response, which play a significant role in an individual's susceptibility to infectious diseases. This specificity can lead to better treatment outcomes by ensuring that interventions are tailored not only to the pathogen but also to the host's individual biological circumstance. Furthermore, advancements in drug design, including monoclonal antibodies and small interfering RNA, more favorably enable the targeted disruption of single infection pathways with less off-target effects and adverse reaction risk. The ongoing development of such treatments underscores the importance of interdisciplinary collaboration during research as well as in clinical practice to optimize patient outcomes (Bauer et al., 2024). The future prognosis of targeted treatments in infectious diseases hinges on the continued refinement of our understanding of molecular pathogenesis. As research proceeds, new insight into alternative splicing and other post-transcriptional processes will likely provide further insight into how pathogens sidestep therapeutic targets. For instance, studies have revealed that splice variants of immunotherapeutic targets are capable of diminishing the therapeutic efficacy of such treatment modalities as monoclonal antibodies or CAR T-cell therapy. To overcome such challenges, it is important to thoroughly analyze splicing patterns and develop new strategies that consider such molecular variations. Ultimately, the integration of targeted therapy and molecular pathology will not only render treatment methods more specific but also encourage an even more active discussion between clinical research and basic applications in the control of infectious diseases (Sharma et al., 2024).

7.6.3. Vaccination Strategies and Molecular Vaccines

The experiments in vaccination strategy have taken inspiration from the fore at the forefront of addressing the molecular disease pathology of infectious diseases, particularly those that are caused by prominent bacterial pathogens. In the last few decades, conjugate vaccines have seen a massive change over the first-generation capsular polysaccharide vaccines, which largely developed T-independent immunity. This shift has resulted in vaccines that are able to induce good immunogenic responses, i.e., T-cell participation, which is so important in memory response and long-term antibody-producing cells. The availability of the Haemophilus influenzae type b (Hib) vaccine is a success story of this approach, demonstrating not only its efficacy in reducing morbidity and mortality from invasive disease but also its remarkable impact on herd immunity, as evidenced in populations where the vaccine has been implemented (Durando et al., 2015). Such developments highlight the important interaction between molecular understanding of pathogens and effective immunization strategies. Also, modern vaccination techniques have advanced as molecular techniques are employed, which allow more selective vaccine production methods. For instance, the molecular characterization of pathogens allows for the identification of targeted antigens that are capable of causing strong immunity. For the porcine reproductive and respiratory syndrome virus (PRRSV), extensive research into the virus's molecular biology has driven attempts to enhance vaccine efficacy with innovative approaches , such as reverse genetics and recombinant DNA technology (Archambault et al., 2014).

Beyond a focus on traditional vaccine preparations, these methods emphasize the application of heterologous viral antigens to generate strong neutralizing antibody responses. The problem is, however, that since PRRSV is highly genetically variable, this necessitates constant improvement and adaptation of the vaccine approach against rapidly evolving pathogens. Second, the convergence of immunological sciences and advanced biotechnological approaches is turning vaccination strategies into a multidisciplinary endeavor. The knowledge on immune system interaction with novel molecular vaccines indicates the intricate dynamics that control the efficacy of vaccination (Durando et al., 2015). Proof has been shown to establish that antigen conjugate vaccines elicit higher-affinity antibody responses with maturation and greater immunological memory. While analyzing these areas, scientists are also revealing not only the promise of existing vaccines but also the roadmap for developing new immunization technologies that can overcome emergent infectious diseases. Thus, the overall plan of immunization not only aims to combat current public health emergencies but also prepares to tackle future epidemics by establishing a foundation of scientific data and technology-based infrastructure required for effective immunization against various pathogens (Archambault et al., 2014) (Figure 7.16).

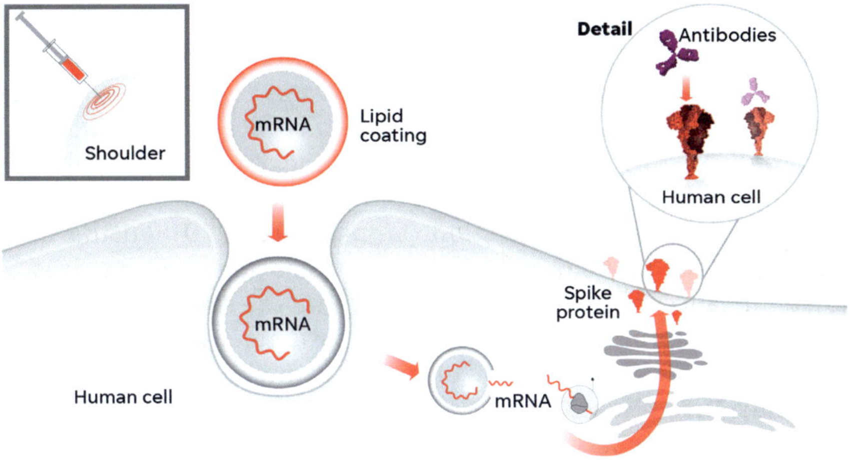

Figure 7.16. Vaccination strategies and molecular vaccines.

Source: https://www.gannett-cdn.com/presto/2021/01/22/USAT/92c43da6-bdb2-4b84-af13-2408258a0009-vaccine-all.png.

SUMMARY

In brief, the molecular pathology of infectious diseases offers a precious schema to understand the complicated interactions between pathogens and host responses. By such analysis, infectious diseases are better realized as not merely single events, but a continuum of biological reactions that evolve. For example, the SARS-CoV-2 or COVID-19 pandemic is one such phenomenon that demonstrates a multi-faceted progression at various stages , such as incubation, respiratory impairment, and pro-thrombotic events that culminate in recovery or death. As the characteristic pathogenic processes of SARS-CoV-2 demonstrate, the pathogenesis highlights divergent reactions of unique patients requiring idiosyncratic therapeutic input to address the characteristic biological derangements at the various phases of infection (Lippi et al., 2020). Furthermore, the molecular underpinnings of concomitant pathologies , such as Type 2 diabetes mellitus and periodontitis also illustrate the significance of molecular pathology in the treatment of infectious diseases. Identification of variously expressed genes between patients with these concomitant diseases is essential information for the development of targeted interventions as well as for diagnostic purposes. These conclusions validate that it is essential to have an integrated strategy, using molecular characterization to separate the interaction of more than one disease pathway. By elaborating on inflammation responses and the trafficking of immune cells in these co-morbidities, researchers can unveil a new generation of therapeutic targets, potentially able to improve patient outcomes significantly and support prevention strategies (Lippi et al., 2020). Lastly, the uses of molecular pathology transcend the realm of academic research to exert a significant influence on clinical practice. By establishing a better grasp of infectious disease biology, medical practitioners can facilitate individualized medicine approaches and improve early intervention processes. This integration of molecular data into infectious disease management not only enhances therapeutic outcomes but also circumvents potential complications due to misdiagnosis or delayed intervention. As the infectious disease world continues to evolve, responsiveness to these molecular nuances will be imperative to sustain public health and develop new solutions to address the increasing epidemic of infectious pathogens.

Molecular pathology of infectious diseases entails various sophisticated methodologies that significantly add to our information and grip on such diseases. The incorporation of molecular methods into traditional diagnosis is the most significant aspect of this field, allowing us to detect pathogens more specifically. For instance, next-generation sequencing (NGS) transformed how infectious disease diagnosis is carried out, making the way for the abandonment of traditional methods , such as culturing and serology. By enabling precise identification of pathogens at the genomic level, NGS enables more efficient surveillance and monitoring of infectious disease outbreaks, evidenced by its use during the COVID-19 pandemic to trace SARS-CoV-2 variants. This combination of molecular techniques with modern diagnostics has a very bright future in terms of improving patient outcomes and public health response to infection. The incorporation of molecular techniques into infectious disease pathology increases diagnostic effectiveness as well as streamlines treatment protocols. The introduction of precision medicine into this area emphasizes tailored approaches based on individual patient profiles, thereby increasing the outcome of treatment. Molecular testing supports the identification of individualized genetic markers associated with pathogens and host reaction, allowing for the timely formulation of targeted therapy. Nevertheless, although progress has been made, the bulk of the health systems continue to rely on conventional strategies. As has been set out, there is a wide gap in the application of bioinformatics towards infectious diseases, and this limits the research of molecular diagnostics. Filling the gap will entail investments in technological advancement as well as training in accordance with the need for more efficient analysis systems to support clinicians in the diagnostic process in infectious pathology. To realize the full promise of molecular pathology in infectious diseases, ongoing research and collaboration between hospitals are essential. As observed in Zambia, employment of new molecular techniques, such as digital pathology and molecular autopsy, can address certain key public health issues. Past research has shed light on priority areas of study that range from defining frequent causes of death to the development of cost-effective molecular approaches suitable for resource-constrained settings. Moreover, bioinformatics platforms delivered in the cloud, such as those used for precision medicine, are critical to advancing data analysis and usability. By adopting these technologies, the specialty has the opportunity to greatly advance infectious disease diagnosis and forensic pathology, eventually benefiting healthcare delivery systems. Strategic investment and collaboration in research will pave the way for evidence-based practice, improving the speed and accuracy of molecular pathology to help combat infectious diseases.

A LOOK TO THE FUTURE

LONG-TERM IMMUNITY:

Long-term immunity is a fundamental concept in immunology and public health, describing the sustained protection against specific pathogens that persists long after the initial exposure or vaccination. This enduring defensive capacity is essential for preventing reinfection and reducing disease severity, and it underpins key strategies in vaccine design, disease control, and global health policy. In contrast to short-term or passive immunity—which may disappear within weeks or months—long-term immunity involves biological processes that can last for years or even a lifetime, enabling the immune system to recognize and more effectively counter previously encountered pathogens. At the heart of long-term immunity is the adaptive immune system, a highly specific arm of host defense that evolves in response to infection or immunization. Upon first encountering a pathogen, the adaptive response mobilizes B and T lymphocytes that recognize specific antigens. Some of these activated cells differentiate into memory cells, which persist in the body long after the pathogen has been cleared. Memory B cells and memory T cells remain poised to respond quickly if the same pathogen reappears, producing antibodies and cell-mediated responses with greater speed and efficacy than during the initial infection.

Vaccination leverages this natural mechanism by exposing the immune system to harmless versions or components of a pathogen, stimulating memory cell formation without causing disease. This process forms the biological basis for many successful vaccination programs that have dramatically reduced or eliminated diseases such as measles and smallpox. An effective vaccine not only prevents acute infection but also establishes long-term immunological memory, offering protection that can extend across decades.

Although adaptive immunity is critical for durable protection, emerging research also highlights the role of **trained immunity** within the innate immune system. Trained immunity refers to a form of long-lasting functional adaptation in innate immune cells, such as monocytes and macrophages, which through epigenetic and metabolic changes exhibit enhanced responses upon subsequent challenges. While this form of immune memory is not antigen-specific in the traditional sense, it contributes to broader, prolonged readiness against pathogens.

The persistence and strength of long-term immunity can vary widely depending on the pathogen, host factors, and nature of exposure. Some diseases elicit immunity that is lifelong, while others—especially those caused by rapidly mutating viruses—may confer only transient protection or require booster immunizations to maintain immunity. Understanding these dynamics is critical for developing effective immunization schedules, anticipating disease resurgence, and shaping public health responses to emerging infectious threats. Ultimately, long-term immunity represents both a biological marvel and a central pillar of disease prevention strategies that safeguard global health.

REFERENCES

1. Abegaz, S. B. (2021). Human ABO blood groups and their associations with different diseases. *BioMed Research International, 2021*, 1–9. https://doi.org/10.1155/2021/6629060 (accessed on 17th July 2025).
2. Amgarten, D., Riyuzo, R., Dorlass, E., de Souza Reis, R., Rebello Pinho, J. R., Doi, A., & Fraga, A. M. (2024). Cloud-based bioinformatics platform for the analysis and diagnosis of infectious diseases. *São Paulo Medical Journal*. https://www.semanticscholar.org/paper/255b686a89004a2454313158c80228f1d0270f9e (accessed on 17th July 2025).
3. Archambault, D., Balasuriya, U., Rowland, R., Yang, H., & Yoo, D. (2014). Animal arterivirus infections. *BioMed Research International, 2014*. https://www.semanticscholar.org/paper/cb401ee25f19607600a610d49ff5ad2b2ebe8f81 (accessed on 17th July 2025).
4. Bauer, M., Schöbel, C. M., Wickenhauser, C., Seliger, B., & Jasinski-Bergner, S. (2024). Deciphering the role of alternative splicing in neoplastic diseases for immune-oncological therapies. *Frontiers in Immunology, 15*. https://www.semanticscholar.org/paper/b903fcc5d97bb638b227a8ad55252656bef4d825 (accessed on 17th July 2025).
5. Berg, G., Rybakova, D., Fischer, D., Cernava, T., Champomier Vergès, M. C., Charles, T. C., Chen, X., et al. (2020). Microbiome definition re-visited: Old concepts and new challenges. *Microbiome, 8*. https://doi.org/10.1186/s40168-020-00875-0 (accessed on 17th July 2025).
6. Cerdeira, C. D., & Brigagão, M. (2024). Targeting macrophage polarization in infectious diseases: M1/M2 functional profiles, immune signaling and microbial virulence factors. *Immunological Investigations, 53*, 1030–1091. https://www.semanticscholar.org/paper/8e41c55bcdc4d2bd1532ac1dff8987570e2acbdd (accessed on 17th July 2025).
7. Colavita, F., Lapa, D., Carletti, F., Lalle, E., Bordi, L., Marsella, P., Nicastri, E., et al. (2020). SARS-CoV-2 isolation from ocular secretions of a patient with COVID-19 in Italy with prolonged viral RNA detection. *Annals of Internal Medicine, 173*, 242–243. https://doi.org/10.7326/m20-1176 (accessed on 17th July 2025).
8. Corbi, S. C. T., de Vasconcellos, J. F., Bastos, A. S., Bussaneli, D. G., da Silva, B. R., dos Santos, R. A., Takahashi, C. S., et al. (2020). Circulating lymphocytes and monocytes transcriptomic analysis of patients with type 2 diabetes mellitus, dyslipidemia and periodontitis. *Scientific Reports, 10*. https://doi.org/10.1038/s41598-020-65042-9 (accessed on 17th July 2025).
9. Damena, D., Barry, A., Morrison, R., Gaoussou, S., Mahamar, A., Attaher, O., Issiaka, D., et al. (2024). A novel locus in *CSMD1* gene is associated with increased susceptibility to severe malaria in Malian children. *Frontiers in Genetics, 15*. https://www.semanticscholar.org/paper/787cd0d870c40e69f3619290a86e67c41c3480a0 (accessed on 17th July 2025).
10. Donkin, J., Emery, R. P., Polega, J., Behenna, C., Caulfield, A., & Simeunovic, G. (2022). 536. Evaluation of the clinical utility of universal polymerase chain reaction testing. *Open Forum Infectious Diseases, 9*. https://www.semanticscholar.org/paper/4ec008e765f34b4cd425f7d7f3ac15b869bda194 (accessed on 17th July 2025).
11. Durando, P., Faust, S., & Torres, A. (2015). Immunological features and clinical benefits of conjugate vaccines against bacteria. *Journal of Immunology Research, 2015*. https://www.semanticscholar.org/paper/2fe34bfee3d80af5d048721635fa9c3364f52f75 (accessed on 17th July 2025).

12. Einhaus, J., Rochwarger, A., Mattern, S., Gaudilliere, B. L., & Schürch, C. (2023). High-multiplex tissue imaging in routine pathology—are we there yet? *Virchows Archiv, 482*, 801–812. https://www.semanticscholar.org/paper/849340ea08ee05521ae77d484612548b25832e5a (accessed on 17th July 2025).

13. Feijó, R. G., Kamimura, M. T., de Oliveira, D. M., da Costa, R. B., Neto, M. F., Coêlho, M. G. L., & Maggioni, R. (2008). Avaliação da variabilidade genética do vírus da infecção hipodermal e necrose hematopoética (IHHNV) no camarão rosa, *Farfantepenaeus subtilis*, infectado experimentalmente. https://www.semanticscholar.org/paper/4a66b4217f2867dc96ee78d3b90ce5e8330c97f8 (accessed on 17th July 2025).

14. Gordhan, B., Liebenberg, D., Scarlatti, G., Herrera, C., Chiodi, F., Martinson, N., Fox, J., et al. (2023). *Ex vivo* challenges models for infectious diseases. *Critical Reviews in Microbiology, 50*, 785–804. https://www.semanticscholar.org/paper/c3c9a5615b328fc324f8f80647395118d9f76ec6 (accessed on 17th July 2025).

15. Gu, W., Miller, S., & Chiu, C. Y. (2018). Clinical metagenomic next-generation sequencing for pathogen detection. *Annual Review of Pathology: Mechanisms of Disease, 14*, 319–338. https://doi.org/10.1146/annurev-pathmechdis-012418-012751 (accessed on 17th July 2025).

16. Hou, K., Wu, Z. X., Chen, X. Y., Wang, J. Q., Zhang, D., Xiao, C., Zhu, D., et al. (2022). Microbiota in health and diseases. *Signal Transduction and Targeted Therapy, 7*. https://doi.org/10.1038/s41392-022-00974-4 (accessed on 17th July 2025).

17. Huang, H., Mehta, A., Kalmanovich, J., Anand, A., Bejarano, M. C., Garg, T., Khan, N., et al. (2023). Immunological and inflammatory effects of infectious diseases in circadian rhythm disruption and future therapeutic directions. *Molecular Biology Reports, 50*, 3739–3753. https://www.semanticscholar.org/paper/99dfe66b6e79c7c8bbe843b2ff365071bf8c7ad6 (accessed on 17th July 2025).

18. Ioannou, P., & Baliou, S. (2024). The molecular mechanisms and therapeutic potential of cranberry, D-mannose, and flavonoids against infectious diseases: The example of urinary tract infections. *Antibiotics, 13*. https://www.semanticscholar.org/paper/51e568c18b71d4fe9844028b71c4b42f87810e67 (accessed on 17th July 2025).

19. Iqbal, J., Jaimes, D., Makineni, P., Subramani, S., Hemaida, S., Thugu, T. R., Butt, A. N., et al. (2023). Reimagining healthcare: Unleashing the power of artificial intelligence in medicine. *Cureus*. https://doi.org/10.7759/cureus.44658 (accessed on 17th July 2025).

20. Kiio, T. M., & Park, S. (2020). Nano-scientific application of atomic force microscopy in pathology: From molecules to tissues. *International Journal of Medical Sciences, 17*, 844–858. https://www.semanticscholar.org/paper/6133d5b80cce90b14f43ff7a26713d307d527e55 (accessed on 17th July 2025).

21. Klubíčková, N., Dermawan, J., Mosaieby, E., Martínek, P., Vaněček, T., Hájková, V., Ptáková, N., et al. (2024). Comprehensive clinicopathological, molecular, and methylation analysis of mesenchymal tumors with NTRK and other kinase gene aberrations. *The Journal of Pathology, 263*. https://www.semanticscholar.org/paper/2f64dd7e4d79205060869432c84171bca58a3ba0 (accessed on 17th July 2025).

22. Knowles, S., Dennis, M., McElwain, A., Leis, E. M., & Richard, J. (2023). Pathology and infectious agents of unionid mussels: A primer for pathologists in disease surveillance and investigation

of mortality events. *Veterinary Pathology, 60*, 510–528. https://www.semanticscholar.org/paper/f5431df17afa785d98d6e3ff8938eef8e359f50d (accessed on 17th July 2025).

23. Kohale, M., Dhobale, A. V., Bankar, N. J., Noman, O., Hatgaonkar, K., & Mishra, V. H. (2023). Immunohistochemistry in pathology: A review. *Journal of Cellular Biotechnology, 9*, 131–138. https://www.semanticscholar.org/paper/370572f4a94c3243022134a5f07d752246650d8e (accessed on 17th July 2025).

24. Li, C., Qin, C., Wei, Y., & Shao, X. (2024). Interplays between host pattern-recognition receptors and pathogen ligands in immunogenic cell death. *Microbes & Immunity*. https://www.semanticscholar.org/paper/9d93fb891db4beb6c634860210896598067af2d4 (accessed on 17th July 2025).

25. Lippi, G., Sanchis-Gomar, F., & Henry, B. M. (2020). COVID-19: Unravelling the clinical progression of nature's virtually perfect biological weapon. *Annals of Translational Medicine, 8*, 693–693. https://doi.org/10.21037/atm-20-3989 (accessed on 17th July 2025).

26. Livingston, I. G., Gregory, T. M., Hawkins, E. C., Cave, A., Loyola, A., Vaden, S., Deresienski, D., et al. (2024). Molecular discovery of filarial nematode DNA in an endangered wild pinniped (*Galapagos sea lion, Zalophus wollebaeki*). *Ecology and Evolution, 14*. https://www.semanticscholar.org/paper/7df32408f06c05aa7c20fb2f5e2a69aff5af13c5 (accessed on 17th July 2025).

27. Locati, M., Curtale, G., & Mantovani, A. (2019). Diversity, mechanisms, and significance of macrophage plasticity. *Annual Review of Pathology: Mechanisms of Disease, 15*, 123–147. https://doi.org/10.1146/annurev-pathmechdis-012418-012718 (accessed on 17th July 2025).

28. Lutsiv, N. (2024). Molecular-biological methods of laboratory diagnostics. *Ukrainian Journal of Laboratory Medicine*. https://www.semanticscholar.org/paper/b23d88c3e4b71a568f8152c86915c0296af0d517 (accessed on 17th July 2025).

29. Maharani, D. S., & Sumsanto, M. (2024). PCR (Polymerase Chain Reaction) method as a detector of IMNV (infectious myonecrosis virus) disease in vaname shrimp (*Litopenaeus vannamei*). *Journal of Fish Health*. https://www.semanticscholar.org/paper/154194ebf7923af413aa08298c177dfa6ea4e097 (accessed on 17th July 2025).

30. Malaguarnera, M., & Cabrera-Pastor, A. (2024). Emerging role of extracellular vesicles as biomarkers in neurodegenerative diseases and their clinical and therapeutic potential in central nervous system pathologies. *International Journal of Molecular Sciences, 25*. https://www.semanticscholar.org/paper/3eb7861fc0ac1fb83620aec597246b90b6b2047c (accessed on 17th July 2025).

31. Malfertheiner, P., Mégraud, F., Rokkas, T., Gisbert, J. P., Liou, J. M., Schulz, C., Gasbarrini, A., et al. (2022). Management of *Helicobacter pylori* infection: The Maastricht VI/Florence consensus report. *Gut, 71*, 1724–1762. https://doi.org/10.1136/gutjnl-2022-327745 (accessed on 17th July 2025).

32. Mathur, S., Haynes, E., Allender, M., & Gibbs, H. L. (2023). Genetic mechanisms and biological processes underlying host response to ophidiomycosis (snake fungal disease) inferred from tissue-specific transcriptome analyses. *Molecular Ecology, 33*. https://www.semanticscholar.org/paper/285920e8f2ef48e95a83808d703106231d68c0da (accessed on 17th July 2025).

33. McLawhon, R., & Fitzgerald, R. (2021). SARS-CoV-2 serologic testing: Facts, fiction, and fallacies. *Clinical Chemistry*. https://www.semanticscholar.org/paper/95cde0663f90e43de550cb8677910e203325a792 (accessed on 17th July 2025).

34. Monteil, V., Kwon, H., Prado, P., Hagelkrüys, A., Wimmer, R., Ståhl, M., Leopoldi, A., et al. (2020). Inhibition of SARS-CoV-2 infections in engineered human tissues using clinical-grade soluble human ACE2. *Cell, 181*, 905–913.e7. https://doi.org/10.1016/j.cell.2020.04.004 (accessed on 17th July 2025).

35. Murray, C. J. L., Ikuta, K. S., Sharara, F., Swetschinski, L. R., Robles Aguilar, G., Gray, A. P., Han, C., et al. (2022). Global burden of bacterial antimicrobial resistance in 2019: A systematic analysis. *The Lancet, 399*, 629–655. https://doi.org/10.1016/s0140-6736(21)02724-0 (accessed on 17th July 2025).

36. Naughton, P., Enright, F., & Lucey, B. (2024). Infectious mononucleosis: New concepts in clinical presentation, epidemiology, and host response. *Current Opinion in Infectious Diseases, 37*, 157–163. https://www.semanticscholar.org/paper/54e2f2714d78458ce4b61926d94824 07c82fb41a (accessed on 17th July 2025).

37. Nemčovičová, I., Benko, M., Lenhartová, S., Kempová, V., & Nemčovič, M. (2020). New insights into the role of N-glycosylation involved in molecular immune checkpoint regulation by human cytomegalovirus glycoproteins with the implication in cancer therapy. *The Journal of Immunology*. https://www.semanticscholar.org/paper/a0ec7fa288e625802a8f7672cc242a826b3e868b (accessed on 17th July 2025).

38. Priya, R., Ye, M., Raghunanadanan, S., Liu, Q., Li, W., Yu, Q., Lou, Y., et al. (2024). *Borrelia burgdorferi* secretes c-di-AMP as an extracellular pathogen-associated molecular pattern to elicit type I interferon responses in mammalian hosts. *bioRxiv*. https://www.semanticscholar.org/paper/3096365ba908f7679849a546523a5abb31490deb (accessed on 17th July 2025).

39. Qiu, J., Li, L., Sun, J., Peng, J., Shi, P., Zhang, R., Dong, Y., et al. (2023). Large AI models in health informatics: Applications, challenges, and the future. *IEEE Journal of Biomedical and Health Informatics, 27*, 6074–6087. https://doi.org/10.1109/jbhi.2023.3316750 (accessed on 17th July 2025).

40. Rasskazova, N. D., Meremianina, E. A., Kalyuzhnaya, N. O., Abramova, N. D., Budanova, E., & Diakov, I. N. (2024). Association of polymorphic markers in innate immunity receptor genes with the risk of primary adrenal insufficiency. *Russian Journal of Immunology*. https://www.semanticscholar.org/paper/c569707c781004d704b19d0f6159a5d7e3b4affb (accessed on 17th July 2025).

41. Reller, L., Weinstein, M. P., Procop, G., & Wilson, M. L. (2001). Infectious disease pathology. *Clinical Infectious Diseases: An Official Publication of the Infectious Diseases Society of America, 32*(11), 1589–1601. https://www.semanticscholar.org/paper/8fb484a98d226b2868ad2fdac f8ced755a3c39dc (accessed on 17th July 2025).

42. Dr. Nishant Sharma, Dr. Shivam Vashisth, Dr. Varun Garg, Dr. Yogesh Kushwah, & Dr. Mustafa Khan. (2024). Understanding the Pathogenesis of Infectious Diseases: Insights from Pathology. *Universal Research Reports, 11*(4), 1–8. https://doi.org/10.36676/urr.v11.i4.1288(accessed on 17th July 2025).

43. Satam, H., Joshi, K., Mangrolia, U., Waghoo, S., Zaidi, G., Rawool, S., Thakare, R., et al. (2023). Next-generation sequencing technology: Current trends and advancements. *Biology, 12*, 997–997. https://doi.org/10.3390/biology12070997 (accessed on 17th July 2025).

44. Sperança, Márcia Aparecida, Rodrigo Buzinaro Suzuki, Aline Diniz Cabral, and Andreia Moreira dos Santos Carmo. 2016. 'Nucleic Acid-Based Diagnosis and Epidemiology of Infectious

Diseases'. Nucleic Acids - From Basic Aspects to Laboratory Tools. InTech. doi:10.5772/61965. (accessed on 17th July 2025).

45. Urban-Chmiel, R., Marek, A., Stępień–Pyśniak, D., Wieczorek, K., Dec, M., Nowaczek, A., & Osek, J. (2022). Antibiotic resistance in bacteria—A review. *Antibiotics, 11*, 1079–1079. https://doi.org/10.3390/antibiotics11081079 (accessed on 17th July 2025).

46. V'kovski, P., Kratzel, A., Steiner, S., Stalder, H., & Thiel, V. (2020). Coronavirus biology and replication: Implications for SARS-CoV-2. *Nature Reviews Microbiology, 19*, 155–170. https://doi.org/10.1038/s41579-020-00468-6 (accessed on 17th July 2025).

47. Vinayaka, A. M. (2024). Advancements in periodontal pathology: A systematic review and meta-analysis of molecular diagnostics, imaging techniques, regenerative therapies, and artificial intelligence. *Journal of Oral Medicine, Oral Surgery, Oral Pathology and Oral Radiology*. https://www.semanticscholar.org/paper/f6ac7cf3b86a29036f4ad25f222a794f268b6105 (accessed on 17th July 2025).

48. Vona, R., Pallotta, L., Cappelletti, M., Severi, C., & Matarrese, P. (2021). The impact of oxidative stress in human pathology: Focus on gastrointestinal disorders. *Antioxidants, 10*, 201–201. https://doi.org/10.3390/antiox10020201 (accessed on 17th July 2025).

49. Wainman, L. M., Sathyanarayana, S. H., & Lefferts, J. (2024). Applications of digital polymerase chain reaction (dPCR) in molecular and clinical testing. *The Journal of Applied Laboratory Medicine, 9*(1), 124–137. https://www.semanticscholar.org/paper/cc09f8bb5da8368e4413f860bec177719a6a561b (accessed on 17th July 2025).

50. Wezi, K., Mbawe, Z., Chisanga, A., Ellison, M., Frenshus, T., Zulu, H., Adutwum-Ofosu, K., et al. (2025). Forensic pathology research priorities for Zambia: Strengthening justice and public health through evidence-based practice. *International Journal of Research and Scientific Innovation*. https://www.semanticscholar.org/paper/9d98f1e748117ac7525cb8c3d1e4388a0af064a9 (accessed on 17th July 2025).

51. Xie, N., Shen, G., Gao, W., Huang, Z., Huang, C., & Fu, L. (2023). Neoantigens: Promising targets for cancer therapy. *Signal Transduction and Targeted Therapy, 8*. https://doi.org/10.1038/s41392-022-01270-x (accessed on 17th July 2025).

52. Ye, J., Zhang, B., Xu, J., Chang, Q., McNutt, M., Korteweg, C., Gong, E., et al. (2007). Molecular pathology in the lungs of severe acute respiratory syndrome patients. *The American Journal of Pathology, 170*, 538–545. https://www.semanticscholar.org/paper/aac7333bd2ea92f3faf915908bd815d7e6fc0499 (accessed on 17th July 2025).

53. Zhang, H., Xu, B., & Lai, N. S. (2025). Recent progress on the application of biosensors in biomechanics for the early detection of infectious diseases. *Molecular & Cellular Biomechanics*. https://www.semanticscholar.org/paper/9db4ae1b0e9327dfaafc341e44b2b443ac3823e5 (accessed on 17th July 2025).

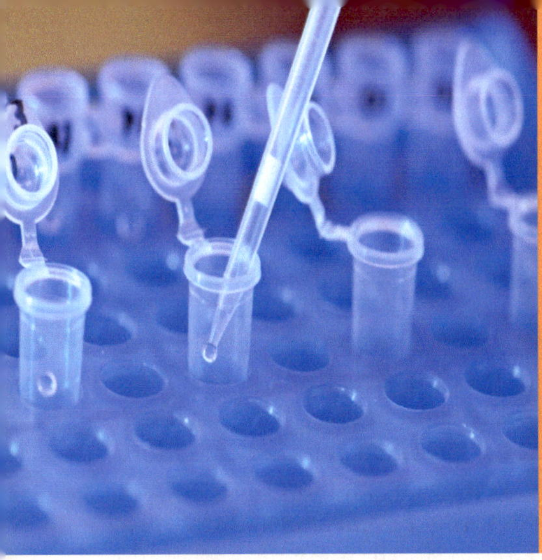

Chapter 8

INHERITED GENETIC DISORDERS

Contents

Introduction

Inherited genetic illnesses represent a wide category of human illness, having their beginning in the inherited genetic material in parent-to-child transmission. As a medical genetics subdiscipline, it examines how alterations in DNA could lead to phenotypic expressions of disease ranging from mildly ill to deathly sick states. These types of illnesses result from mutations in genes, which can be referred to as autosomal dominant, autosomal recessive, or sex-linked. Correct understanding of inherited genetic disorder spread is not just important for the patients themselves but for broader medical and social purposes, including genetic counseling and public health policy. As our understanding ever increases through genomic research developments, the importance of early diagnosis and intervention cannot be overstated. The rising prevalence of genetic disorders makes a serious need to perform an in-depth analysis of their etiology that would be the foundation of exploring potential therapeutic approaches. The pathogenesis of inherited genetic disorders is complex and typically both genetic and environmental in nature. Such interaction stresses the role of the human microbiota and other biological mechanisms able to influence the expression of genetic traits and vulnerabilities. Recent studies have investigated the deep impact of microbial diversity on health, indicating that the environment an individual is raised in, such as diet, can have powerful effects on gene expression and even the triggering of particular disorders. For instance, factors that impact microbiota composition during early life, including antibiotics use or mode of birth, may have the potential to shape conditions linked with genetic predispositions. Understanding these interactions is essential in addressing inherited disorders holistically in a way to best react to cure and preventive programs. The interaction of genetics and environment remains rich with future promise for therapies and interventions. Advances in cutting-edge technologies, particularly genomics and bioinformatics, have revolutionized research on inherited genetic disorders, providing researchers with new tools to unravel intricate genetic information. The advent of whole-genome sequencing has made it possible to identify not only monogenic diseases but also multifactorial conditions caused by the interaction of a number of genes. This can lead to more precise diagnoses and better insight into disease mechanisms, paving the way for personalized medicine. Further, the integration of artificial intelligence in data analysis helps identify new drug targets and biomarkers for disease early detection. With research ongoing to elucidate the genetic cause of various diseases, the hope for the development of new treatments and preventive strategies grows. The interface of genetics, technology, and clinical practice will certainly be the route to tremendous progress in the treatment of inherited genetic conditions, ultimately leading to improved patient outcomes and quality of life (Figure 8.1).

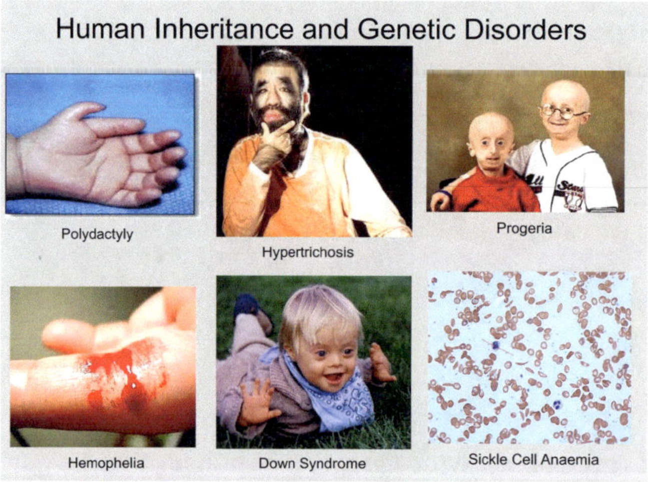

Figure 8.1. Inherited genetic disorders are human ailments.

Source: https://image.slidesharecdn.com/04-09-11ppt-humaninheritancegeneticdisorders-120507235837-phpapp02/75/Human-Inheritance-Genetic-Disorders-1-2048.jpg.

Definition of Inherited Genetic Disorders

Inherited genetic diseases happen as a result of a mutation in genes transmitted over generations of families. These diseases happen as a result of alterations in the DNA sequence of particular genes, which could lead to various health issues. The mode of inheritance of these diseases can be divided into types, including autosomal dominant, autosomal recessive, X-linked, and mitochondrial inheritance. Autosomal dominant disorders, for instance, Huntington's disease, require only a single copy of the gene causing the disease from one diseased parent to result in expression of the disease. Autosomal recessive disorders, for instance, cystic fibrosis, require two copies of the causative gene for the patient to manifest symptoms. The diversity of patterned inheritance demonstrates the complex relationship between genetics and the phenotypic expression of the disease. The impact of inherited genetic disorders extends beyond the individual's health, profoundly affecting families and communities. Patients with these disorders can undergo not only physical handicap but also psychological issues and social distress. These disorders have an enormous economic impact due to the long-term care and specialist treatment they might require. Besides the direct health implications, families may also experience psychological distress as they go through the diagnostic process, treatment, and potential genetic counseling in future families. Furthermore, the reality of inherited genetic disorders may strain relationships within the family, thereby justifying the social support systems in supporting the affected families. Consequently, it is imperative to understand these intricate dynamics in a bid to develop effective interventions that address not only the medical but also the psychological and social aspects of inheriting genetic disorders. Recent advances in genetic research have provided an entryway to improved identification and understanding of inherited genetic disorders. Impressive techniques , such as next-generation sequencing have revolutionized the exploration of genetic variation and, most notably, enabled researchers to uncover novel correlations among specific genes and genetic disorders. For example, the establishment of strong gene-disease associations has been a cornerstone of understanding disorders with complex inheritance, including familial hypercholesterolemia and hereditary cancer syndromes. Recently, the field of genetics has also recognized the significance of structural variants and copy number variations in triggering such disorders. As highlighted in research, the integration of advanced genomic methods into clinical practice can enhance the accuracy of diagnosis and facilitate the identification of new therapies in patients with inherited genetic disorders (Iuliano & Paduano, 2024). By combining scientific innovation with clinical practice, the ongoing research work attempts to improve results and quality of life for patients and families with these challenging conditions.

Importance of Understanding Genetic Inheritance

A detailed understanding of genetic inheritance is important in the determination of the mechanisms of inherited genetic diseases. Inheritance rules provide hints about the way traits and possible diseases may be passed down from generation to generation. By examining genetic inheritance, scientists and doctors can determine which genes are responsible for specific disorders, thus facilitating more accurate diagnoses and personalized treatment methods. This information is particularly relevant in the treatment of genetic diseases like retinitis pigmentosa, where certain mutations can lead to typical phenotypic expressions. With this knowledge, clinicians can provide informed genetic counseling to permit families to understand the risks and implications of inherited disease and treatments that can mitigate the impact of such disorders on the afflicted as well as their relatives. Moreover, explaining the complexities of genetic inheritance is pivotal for the development of effective therapeutic approaches in hereditary diseases. With progressing research, geneticists are unraveling many variants causing diseases that contribute to a myriad of conditions, from as severe a disease as retinitis pigmentosa, with over 80 genes identified until now. Such genetic details are the foundation for new treatment approaches, from gene therapy to tailor-made medicine, taking individual genetic backgrounds into account. With the evolving therapeutic environment, understanding the intricacies of the role of genetic variation in influencing health can underpin the design of more precise interventions, with the value of improving patients' quality of life. This encapsulates the significance of genetic inheritance as a subject of research, not merely an academic endeavor, but as a precursor to the healthcare advancements of tomorrow.

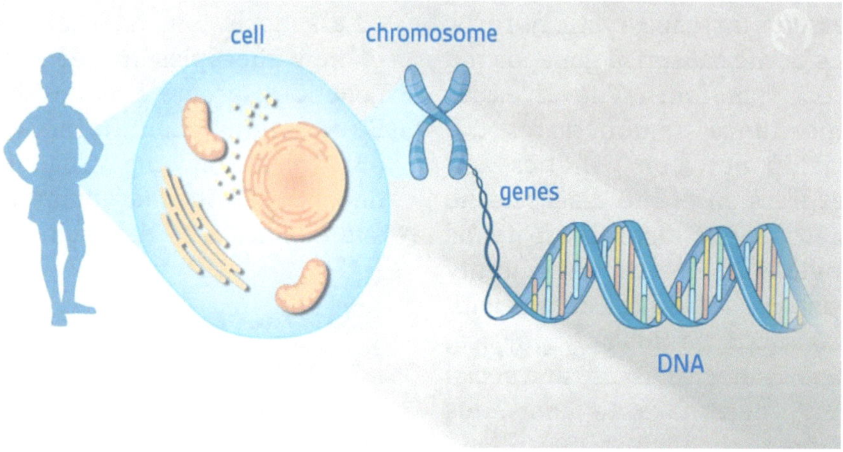

Figure 8.2. Importance of understanding genetic inheritance.

Source: https://i.ytimg.com/vi/50za3OPqe6k/maxresdefault.jpg.

Furthermore, genetic inheritance awareness facilitates preventive management of illness in high-risk groups. Being aware of the genetic susceptibility makes individuals capable of making appropriate life choices and of undergoing regular screening to identify potential disorders early. Where disorders like retinitis pigmentosa come into play, it makes it easier for individuals to receive timely interventions that will stop disease progression or alleviate symptoms. Genetic counseling is also a significant factor in such cases, as it educates people about what family planning measures are possible for them, including prenatal diagnosis and assisted reproduction techniques. Proactiveness not only enables people but also frees them from the emotional and financial burdens of having to cope with inherited ailments. Therefore, the knowledge of genetic inheritance significance is a vital element in creating public health strategies to reduce the prevalence and impact of inherited genetic illnesses (Figure 8.2).

8.1. Types of Inherited Genetic Disorders

Inherited genetic disorders are typically classified into three broad groups: single-gene disorders, chromosomal disorders, and multifactorial disorders. Single-gene or Mendelian disorders result from mutations in one gene and exhibit characteristic patterns of inheritance, such as autosomal dominant, autosomal recessive, or X-linked inheritance. Cystic fibrosis, sickle cell anemia, and Huntington's disease illustrate. Such conditions may have different phenotypes and are diagnosable by genetic tests with options for individualized medical treatment. Furthermore, the reliability of the prediction of their pattern of inheritance makes it possible to offer genetic counseling to affected families, with provision for anticipatory health surveillance and reproduction. Chromosomal disorders, on the other hand, occur due to chromosome number or structure aberrations. These abnormalities are brought about by non-disjunction during the cell division process and can result in the conditions of Down syndrome, Turner syndrome, and Klinefelter syndrome. The impact of these abnormalities can be catastrophic, disrupting growth and causing a myriad of medical issues. Individuals with chromosomal abnormalities are likely to need multidisciplinary care geared towards the integration of their unique medical and educational needs. Medical practitioners must recognize these syndromes so that they can offer sufficient support to both the individuals and their families. There are three crucial groups, with multifactorial disorders having etiologies that result from a combination of genetic and environmental factors. Single-gene and chromosomal disorders do not lead to simplistic models of inheritance, but these disorders lead to complicated interactions between different genes and environmental influences. They include heart disease, diabetes, and cancer. In nations like Saudi Arabia, congenital blood disorders , such as thalassemias and hemoglobinopathies highlight the importance of genetic diseases influenced by both environmental and genetic factors, underscoring the role of public health interventions specifically aimed at controlling these conditions. Limited knowledge on these disorders can prevent effective management interventions, which demonstrates the importance of educational interventions that boost the level of knowledge and awareness among affected populations (Alruwaily, 2025) (Figure 8.3).

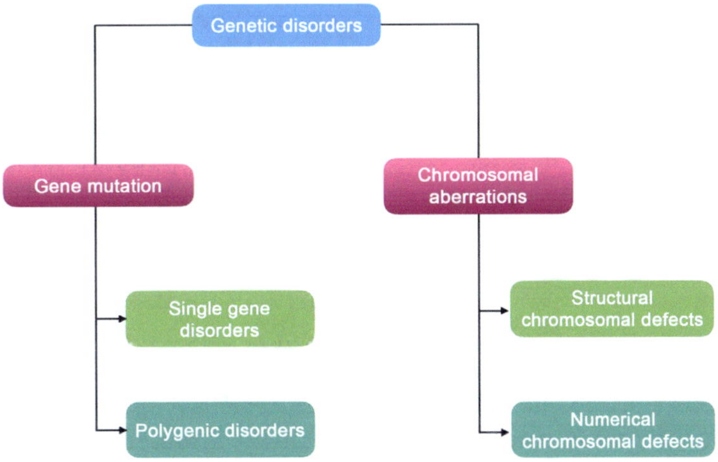

Figure 8.3. Types of inherited genetic disorders.

Source: https://geneticeducation.co.in/wp-content/uploads/2020/03/genetic-disorders.001-e1583144181972.jpeg.

8.1.1. Autosomal Dominant Disorders

Classification and definition of autosomal dominant diseases have progressed so far, but yet they are still complex since they are heterogeneous. Autosomal dominant disorders arise if only one copy of a faulty gene is sufficient to cause the disease, and thus the inheritance patterns play particularly significant roles. The clinical manifestations and signs may vary significantly even among those with the same familial defect. The heterogeneity of these diseases makes diagnosis and treatment challenging. A good example would be inherited retinal diseases (IRDs), wherein some amino acid substitutions in protein domains cause variable phenotypic presentation among disease-affected individuals. While researchers struggle to unravel the complexities of such disorders, computational resources for variant classification arise, and therefore, the necessity of improved diagnostic methods in the clinic (Iuliano & Paduano). Understanding pathogenic mechanisms of autosomal dominant disorders also enables the development of targeted therapeutics. The development in the identification of causative genes has a tremendous effect on the treatment approach, targeting the individual genetic susceptibility of persons afflicted with the condition. In autosomal dominant epilepsy with auditory characteristics, for example, the discovery of a new variant in the LGI1 gene not only provides genetic confirmation of the disease but also improves the efficacy of treatments. These patients may be given individually tailored anti-seizure medications that revolutionize their quality of life. This indicates the importance of genetic testing as a prerequisite for the correct diagnosis and management of autosomal dominant disorders, thereby demonstrating the profound impact of genetic data on clinical practice (Moloney et al., 2022). In addition, the application of multi-classifier methods is a promising direction for the detection of pathogenic variants in patients with autosomal dominant diseases. The success of tools applied to measure variant pathogenicity, such as that of MutScore and BayesDel in the evaluation of IRD variants, demonstrates collective endeavor in genetics and bioinformatics. These resources facilitate improved classification and diagnosis, most critically enabling the identification of novel, uncharacterized variants. As the complexity of genetic disease is conquered, these resources not only facilitate our abilities to understand such conditions but also pave the way for additional precision medicine, giving hope to patients and families with inherited genetic diseases. With advancements in technology and greater knowledge of the genetic processes, there is a future ahead with improved interventions and diagnostics as the norm (Iuliano & Paduano, 2024).

8.1.2. Autosomal Recessive Disorders

The mechanism of autosomal recessive diseases is a significant area of study in inherited genetic disorders, pointing to a significant characteristic of human genetics. In the conditions of this disorder, two copies of a mutated gene need to be present, such that the individual displays the disorder, most commonly when both parents have the gene mutation. This mode of inheritance is most relevant in consanguineous communities, where the possibility of two carriers being mated together is higher, hence the risk of affected offspring due to autosomal recessive disorders is higher. These disorders consist of a high range of phenotypes, and hence, while some patients have an extremely severe clinical presentation, others do not have any clinical presentation, which is reflective of the range of complexity in genotype-phenotype correlation in such diseases (Reuter et al., 2017). The autosomal recessive disorders' genetic heterogeneity is reason enough for the need for specific diagnostic techniques to identify affected individuals at an early age. The majority of autosomal recessive disorders are brought about by mutations in essential genes that play critical roles within several biochemical pathways. For instance, disorders , such as cystic fibrosis, Tay-Sachs disease, and phenylketonuria are brought about by specific gene mutations that hinder normal cell functions. In cystic fibrosis, mutations of the CFTR gene disrupt chloride ion transport and cause severe respiratory and gastrointestinal disease. Tay-Sachs disease, caused by mutation of the HEXA gene, also causes progressive nerve cell degeneration and eventual premature death.

The phenotypic effects of such diseases illustrate the necessity of the impaired pathways and the significant clinical effects that mutations can have. Also, autosomal recessive conditions can require full genetic counseling, especially in such families having a written history of such conditions, promoting informed reproductive choices and likely intervention steps (Parenti et al., 2020). Genetic screening and diagnostic methods have advanced significantly, greatly enhancing the identification and management of autosomal recessive conditions. Next-generation sequencing technologies, particularly whole-exome sequencing, have facilitated the ability to detect disease-inducing mutations in affected patients, even in multisystem diseases with multiple genetic contributors. Research has indicated a high rate of diagnostic yield in consanguineous pedigrees, as in research that detected putatively pathogenic variants in a large proportion of such pedigrees (Reuter et al., 2017). Furthermore, the identification of novel candidate genes through exome sequencing is a significant step towards the elucidation of the genetic basis of these conditions. Not only do these developments facilitate early diagnosis but also open up avenues for targeted therapy and personal therapy, which can reverse patient outcomes for autosomal recessive disorders, validating that there should be more research in this dynamic field of genetics (Parenti et al., 2020) (Figure 8.4).

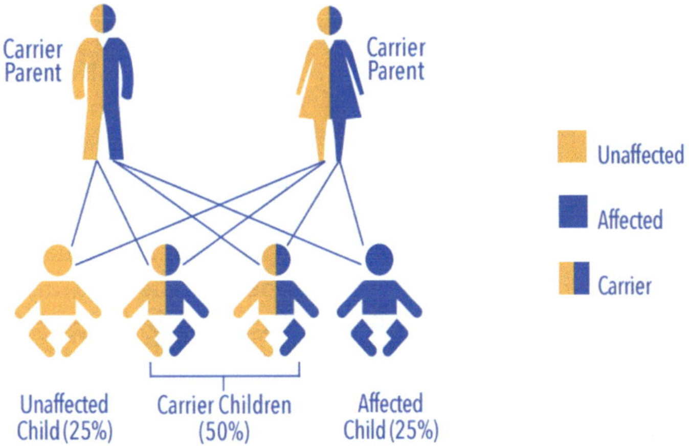

Figure 8.4. Autosomal recessive disorders.

Source: https://www.researchgate.net/profile/Shahin-Asadi/publication/345120487/figure/fig4/AS:952801547022337@1604176999131/Schematic-of-the-autosomal-recessive-inherited-pattern-followed-by-Schindler-syndrome.jpg.

8.1.3. X-Linked Disorders

X-linked disorders represent a significant group of inherited genetic disorders, which are predominantly encountered among males as they possess only a single X chromosome. These disorders are a result of X chromosome mutations and can be expressed in a variety of phenotypes. One well-known example is X-linked ichthyosis due to a hemizygous deletion of the STS gene. This condition is typically linked with severe dryness and scaling of the skin, reflecting the gene's significant role in lipid metabolism. Variability in the mutations with X-linked ichthyosis in other populations, for example, in the Republic of North Ossetia–Alania, has been described by researchers representing different ethnic groups, indicating a complex pattern of genes. The foregoing results emphasize the need for thorough genetic research for the diagnosis of X-linked disorders, especially among genetically diverse populations (Vasilyeva et al., 2023). The molecular diagnosis of X-linked disorders extends beyond ichthyosis as a gradient of genetic disorders manifested through various physiological dysfunctions. For instance, X-linked hypophosphatemia (XLH) involves mutations in the PHEX gene that result in phosphate wasting and skeletal deformities. The pathogenesis of XLH has a serious effect on individuals, whereby it is difficult for them to manage their body growth and general health. There might be an aggregation of genetic defects in certain families, particularly in situations where there is intense consanguinity, and diseases , such as spondyloepiphyseal dysplasia (SED) and XLH might co-exist. Studies that highlight such co-morbidities increase our degree of knowledge about the genetic interaction and the probability for concomitant expressions in impacted families, underlining the complexity of genetic inheritance (Ma et al., 2023). Implications of X-linked illness are not limited to clinical presentation but have profound implications for family planning and genetic counseling. Understanding the pattern of inheritance and the potential for carriers among unaffected female relatives is essential. Genetic counseling plays an important role in preparing affected families with knowledge regarding the inheritance of X-linked disorders to their offspring, especially males who are more at risk. Moreover, advancements in next-generation sequencing technologies have revolutionized the identification of pathogenic variants responsible for these disorders, which can now result in earlier diagnosis and targeted treatment modalities. With developments in the area of genetics, the inclusion of patient education and molecular diagnostics is necessary in facing challenges posed by X-linked disorders from the viewpoint of inherited genetic disorders in general (Ma et al., 2023; Vasilyeva et al., 2023).

8.2. Mechanisms of Inheritance

The mechanisms of inheritance are crucial in research on inherited genetic diseases, which show how traits and diseases are transmitted from one generation to another. Priority among them is Mendelian patterns of inheritance that encompass autosomal dominant, autosomal recessive, and X-linked. Autosomal dominant conditions arise when a lone copy of the gene for the disease results in the phenotype, such as in Huntington's disease. However, autosomal recessive illnesses, such as cystic fibrosis, stipulate that both alleles must carry the mutation for the disease to be manifested. In addition, X-linked illnesses, primarily seen in males, are the result of X chromosome mutations, which add yet another level of genetic trait inheritance complexity. Knowledge of these patterns is fundamental in genetic counseling and the calculation of the likelihood of disease expression in the next generation. In molecular genetics, the findings in techniques , such as CRISPR–Cas9 gene editing are revolutionizing our concept of inheritance mechanisms and their role in inherited diseases. Accurate delivery of a specific DNA sequence, CRISPR–Cas9 promises to treat the cause of a large number of genetic disorders by correcting a specific mutation at its source. This precision not only highlights the interface of inherited genetics and disease but also indicates a revolutionary direction toward tailoring treatments. CRISPR–Cas9's capability to restore normal gene function is symptomatic of the dynamism of inherited genetics in that it reverses the strictures of Mendelian patterns and becomes at ease with the complexity of epigenetic modifications. However, it is important to advance this technology with caution, given the ethical issues and long-term implications in germline editing (Kolanu, 2024). Clinical manifestations of genetic diseases inherited from generation to generation have a tendency to illustrate the intricate interaction of inheritance patterns, while some diseases display the nuances of gene expression and repeat expansions. Myotonic dystrophy type 1 (DM1), for instance, exhibits an interesting pattern of inheritance in relation to CTG repeat enlargements that correlate with the severity of the disease. Not only does the disease exhibit autosomal dominant inheritance, but it also has a characteristic known as anticipation, in which successive generations have increasing manifestations. The results of research in various populations indicate the multifaceted nature of DM1, with paternal age and maternal transmission playing a significant role in disease progression (Ionova et al., 2024). The results emphasize the importance of knowing multiple mechanisms of genetic inheritance as they have considerable implications for treating the disease and the future of genetics as a field (Figure 8.5).

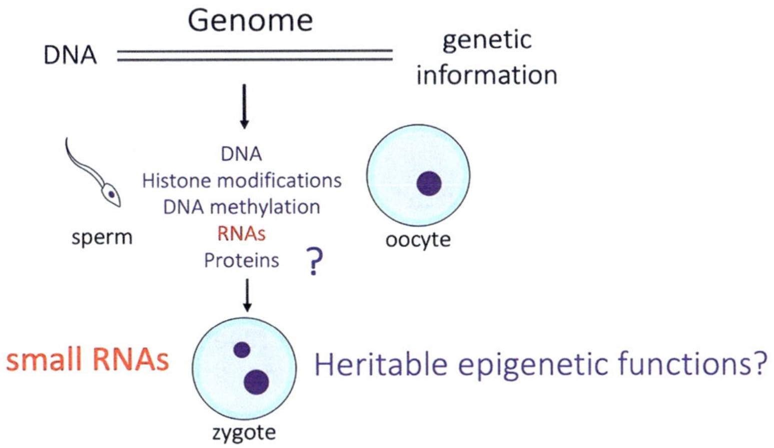

Figure 8.5. Mechanisms of inheritance in genetic disorders.

Source: https://research.pasteur.fr/wp-content/uploads/2015/08/research_pasteur-enmechanisms-of-epigenetic-inheritancefrmecanismes-de-lheredite-epigenetique-pasteur-web-1.jpg.

8.2.1. Mendelian Inheritance Patterns

Mendelian inheritance patterns form the foundation for understanding how genetic traits are inherited from parents to offspring. They are credited to Gregor Mendel, the first to ever conduct experiments on pea plants in an effort to understand the laws of inheritance, laws were formulated on how alleles sort out and organize. The two primary Mendelian inheritance patterns include autosomal dominant and autosomal recessive traits. In autosomal dominant illnesses, for instance, Huntington's disease, having one single copy of the mutant allele suffices to get the illness, thereby allowing the trait to be manifested in all the generations. Conversely, autosomal recessive disorders, such as cystic fibrosis, involve two alleles of the disease allele so that the disease might only be expressed if the individual has two copies of the allele, and this quite frequently leaves carriers themselves unaffected but passing on the condition to their offspring. Mendelian inheritance patterns are particularly relevant in the context of inherited genetic disorders. Identifying these patterns allows clinicians and genetic counselors to predict the likelihood of an individual to pass or inherit a genetic disorder. Genetic testing has increased information regarding such disorders, such as hereditary cardiomyopathies, where specific mutations can be traced through family generations. In this regard, the Mendelian inheritance contribution is particularly underscored by its participation in family aggregation of disease, where relatives can have common genetic defects for the same health outcome. This consistency in genetics mandates a higher premium on early diagnosis and starting personalized treatment regimens with the goal to advance patient results, especially when intervention earlier would terminate high-level expressions of such inherited conditions (Garoia et al., 2025). Further, the recognition of the individual Mendelian patterns may provide more precise biological and therapeutic understanding in the field of genetics. For instance, research on the genetic etiology of anxiety disorders and their relationship to major depression has pushed innovative therapies by identifying individual genetic markers. With data provided through studies , such as the UK Biobank, researchers can study genetic variances associated with disorder-specific polygenic risk scores, leading to evidence-based practice in the clinic (Tesfaye et al., 2024). This precision in genetic testing not only allows for the identification of those at risk, but also creates the opportunity for the ability to provide personalized medicine, treatments individually tailored to the subject's specific genetic predisposition. Hence, Mendelian inheritance patterns remain at the forefront of informing both theory and practice in the management of inherited genetic disorders, ultimately leading to research into more efficient therapeutic interventions.

8.2.2. Role of Mutations in Genetic Disorders

The impact of mutations on genetic disease is enormous, playing a vital role in the pathogenesis of inherited conditions. Various kinds of mutations exist, including point mutations, deletions, and duplications, responsible for diverse clinical presentations. For instance, neurodevelopmental disorders (NDDs) tend to develop because of typical mutations disrupting vital neurodevelopmental processes. These disorders, characterized by intellectual disabilities and behavioral disturbances, illustrate how one mutation in a susceptible gene can have wide-ranging effects on intellectual and emotional development. The genetic heterogeneity of the mutations renders correlations between genotype and phenotype challenging to determine, making the understanding of these disorders a formidable but critical endeavor. An elaborate examination of the mutations provides significant insight into diagnostic and treatment strategies that are important to patient management and improved quality of life in affected individuals. Furthermore, the concept of mutational load—a term applied to the aggregate burden of genetic variants—provides greater understanding of the complexities of inherited conditions. Experiments have revealed that common and rare genetic variants are both involved in the risk of NDDs, and because mutations can interact with each other in intricate ways to influence phenotypic outputs, the relationship between them is potentially complicated by interactions involving genetic and environmental factors, particularly in multifactorial diseases where symptom expression depends on the co-occurrence of additional mutations or environmental stimuli. For example, the two-hit model proposes that a germline mutation must first arise and establish a predisposition to disease, and that follow-up somatic mutations would lead to the expression of the disorder. Now that such models have been recognized, scientists can understand how the occurrence of mutations overall influences the severity and expression of genetic disorders and consequently impacts potential intervention and treatment protocols. Epigenetic modifications also play a crucial role in deciding the phenotypic outcomes of genetic disorders, suggesting a two-level interaction of genes and epigenetics. Epigenetic modifications , such as DNA methylation and histone modification, possess the potential to modify gene expression without altering the underlying DNA structure and thus introduce complexity to hereditary genetic disorders. These differences may be influenced by environmental factors, diet, and even toxic exposures, as the interactive dynamics between genetic predispositions and epigenetic modifications with regard to disease expression reflect. The interaction between epigenetic modifications and genetic mutations highlights the relevance of a multidimensional investigation of inherited disorders. Identification of both genetic and epigenetic components helps us to understand better how inherited disease is generated and maintained across generations, thereby providing an opportunity for targeted therapies and precision medicine approaches that acknowledge this multifaceted interaction (Parenti et al., 2020; Ionova et al., 2024) (Figure 8.6).

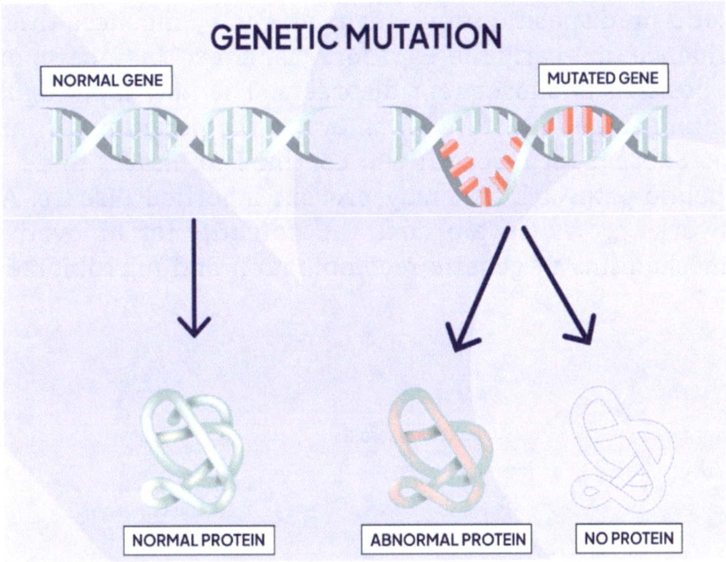

Figure 8.6. Role of mutations in genetic disorders.

Source: https://www.health.com/thmb/7UPmUcOC32y23cEXnKKjbbDzOjk=/1500x0/filters:no_upscale():max_bytes(150000):strip_icc()/Health-Genetic-Mutation-background-light-purple-a6ad7969c03e4780ae174b4c9f705c0c.jpg.

8.2.3. Genetic Recombination and Its Effects

Genetic recombination is at the heart of genetic variation and diversity, which is fundamental to evolution and adaptation. Recombination occurs during meiosis when there is the exchange of genetic material between homologous chromosomes, resulting in new combinations of alleles in gametes. Recombination is at the heart of the passing of traits that influence phenotypes that may be beneficial, neutral, or detrimental. However, this process also gives rise to inherited genetic disorders. Aberrations in recombination can lead to the erroneous distribution of genetic material to give rise to diseases , such as Down syndrome, where there is an extra complete chromosome as a result of nondisjunction processes during meiosis. The relationship between disease expression and genetic recombination underscores how this critical biological process can contribute both to increased genetic diversity and pathological effects. Moreover, the influence of genetic recombination extends beyond the immediate implications of genetic diversity; they have extensive impacts on gene therapy and targeted medicine. Advances in gene therapy have leveraged the pathways of recombination to correct genetic defects underlying inherited diseases. This approach aims to target particular genes through the utilization of viral vectors to deliver corrective codes into patient cells. An example is the recent innovation of viral vector-mediated therapy, which has been successful in correcting monogenic diseases—those caused by mutations within a single gene. Difficulties still persist, such as the potential for unwanted effects like insertional mutagenesis, induced by the corrective gene interfering with other important genes. Therefore, the understanding of genetic recombination is not an academic exercise; it plays a critical role in developing effective and safe treatments for inherited genetic illnesses (Bulcha et al., 2021). As research on genetic recombination is ongoing, its application towards overall genetic health and disease advancement becomes more relevant. The influence of microbiotas, more specifically via the gut-brain axis, offers a model for how genetic predisposition and environmental influences interact to create health outcomes. There is evidence that early life exposure can affect the microbiome and thereby gene expression and predisposition to subsequent disorders. The new field highlights the interaction among genetics, environment, and health with an eye to the potential for microbial interventions to reverse genetic risk. Subsequent research will continue to dissect these interactions, possibly leading to new therapeutic pathways that may prevent inherited disease. As our understanding of these complex networks grows, so too does the potential for innovative new methods that leverage the natural mechanisms of genetic recombination and microbiome interactions (Bulcha et al., 2021) (Figure 8.7).

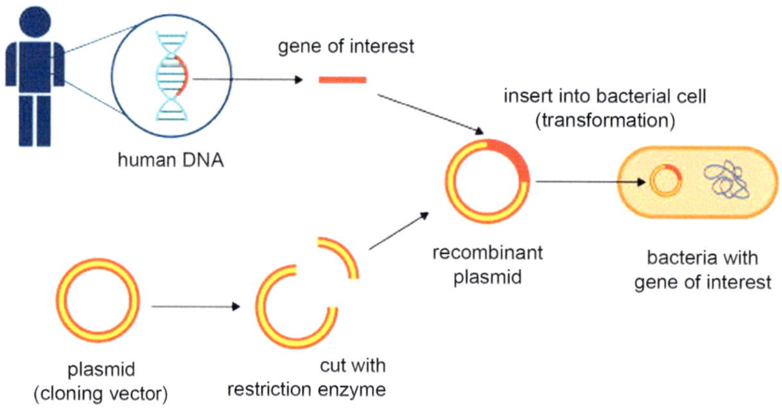

Figure 8.7. Genetic recombination and its effects.

Source: https://media.istockphoto.com/vectors/biological-diagram-explain-concept-of-recombinant-dna-production-from-vector-id1371723283?k=20&m=1371723283&s=612x612&w=0&h=MDlc60S9TCdaZzNN0jW6a2B9UF0i04QlBUKeIMJkNHE=

8.3. Common Inherited Genetic Disorders

Inherited genetic conditions constitute a considerable area of interest in human health, characterized by mutations in parentally inherited genes in their offspring. The conditions manifest themselves in varied presentations directed to different organ systems of the body and producing different clinical manifestations. A specific case in point is congenital disorders of glycosylation (CDGs), which arise from glycosylation process abnormalities. The heterogeneity of CDGs includes over 160 various types, and each of them manifests varied severity and symptoms. The diagnostic process in individuals who might be suffering from such disorders is also ridden with complications, as the conventional diagnostic tests may not yield immediate results. The position of genetic counselors is also significant in this case since they assist affected families in managing medical uncertainty, which includes issues of inheritance patterns, family planning, and coping with the condition, finally managing the emotional and psychological impact of the diagnosis (Weixel et al., 2024). Mucocutaneous bleeding disorders are another important group of inherited genetic disorders that affect the quality of life for affected individuals. Diseases , such as von Willebrand disease (VWD) and hereditary hemorrhagic telangiectasia (HHT) also cause excessive bleeding events that are serious and life-altering. The underlying biology for these diseases, although less well known than for more commonly diagnosed conditions , such as hemophilia, is not as well elucidated. Detection of diseases causing excessive mucocutaneous bleeding in a few patients takes years, with all the suffering and limbo illness that can create. The complex diagnostic process of such disorders makes the medical professionals overlook noted symptoms in instances where standard tests fail to show a cause. The gap needs to be closed because increased understanding and targeted research may lead to improved diagnostic and therapeutic treatment in patients (Sidonio et al., 2023). Growing knowledge of inherited genetic disorders emphasizes the importance of ongoing research and advances in genetic sciences. Effective management of such conditions is founded on an intensive knowledge of their genetic basis, including the characterization of pathogenic variants leading to disease phenotypes. Engagement of communities and cross-disciplinary collaboration among investigators, clinicians, and patients are significant to responding to priorities in research that have immediate effects on individuals with inherited conditions. For example, the establishment of a National Research Blueprint for Inherited Bleeding Disorders conveys a collective endeavor in focusing research on discovering useful therapies and improving patient care. With the genetic disorder paradigm evolving further, future developments in genetic testing, counseling, and therapeutic modalities will be instrumental in maximizing patient outcomes and quality of life for patients with inherited genetic disorders (Sidonio et al., 2023).

8.3.1. Cystic Fibrosis (CF)

Cystic fibrosis (CF) is a group of inherited diseases transmitted through generations because of the production of thick, sticky mucus that causes damage to many organs, especially the lungs and intestines. Cystic fibrosis is caused by a mutation of the CFTR gene that encodes for a protein responsible for the regulation of salt and water movement in and out of cells. The defective CFTR protein leads to abnormal ion movement that causes the characteristic mucus accumulation, plugging airways and creating an environment conducive to bacterial infection. The commonality of CF renders it important to study various inherited genetic diseases since it signifies how a mutation in one gene can have profound and dramatic consequences for health, emphasizing the need for accurate therapeutic interventions and enhanced research into the disease's molecular basis. The symptoms and manifestations of cystic fibrosis vary widely due to something referred to as variable expressivity, which is both genetically and environmentally caused. The individual with CF may or may not have long-standing respiratory disease, pancreatic deficiency, and malnutrition, among other manifestations. This variation complicates diagnosis and treatment, revealing the interaction between a person's genetic makeup and external influences. It has been proven in research that environmental factors also have a significant part to play in the decision of the severity and progression of CF, as they are capable of affecting the genetic flaws to make symptoms worse or better (Schmitthenner et al., 2025). This compels us to adopt a holistic approach involving both lifestyle and genetic factors to improve patient outcomes. Treatment interventions for cystic fibrosis have come a long way since their initiation, and instead of targeting the actual genetic mutation, they are now aimed at controlling symptoms and avoiding complications. Present interventions include airway clearance measures, inhaled drugs, and pancreatic enzyme supplementation, which together are designed to control respiratory and gastrointestinal symptoms. A new and revolutionary treatment approach has recently been witnessed with CFTR modulator therapies that are specifically designed to target the defect caused by the CFTR mutations. Nonetheless, further research is required to completely comprehend the extensive gene-environment interactions that influence disease presentation and therapy response (Schmitthenner et al., 2025). By utilizing knowledge gained from genetic modeling along with clinical expertise, researchers can develop more personalized treatment plans that reflect the genetic as well as the environmental heterogeneity of cystic fibrosis and eventually enhance patients' quality of life affected by this genetic disease (Figure 8.8).

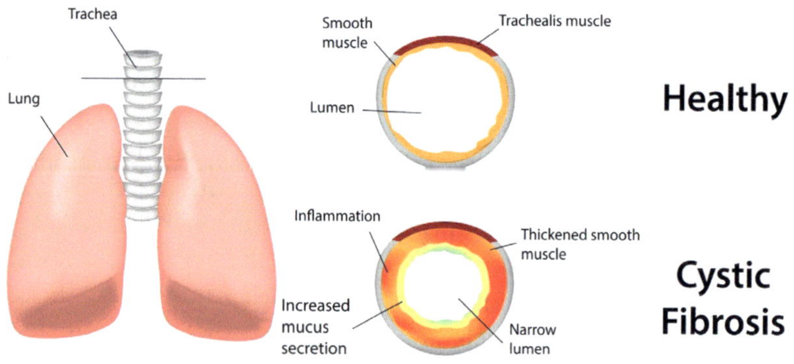

Figure 8.8. Cystic fibrosis (CF).

Source: https://image.shutterstock.com/shutterstock/photos/328687007/display_1500/stock-photo-cystic-fibrosis-328687007.jpg

8.3.2. Sickle Cell Anemia

Sickle cell anemia, the most highly studied of all the inherited genetic disorders, results from a mutation at the HBB gene on chromosome 11. The mutation causes one amino acid substitution in the beta-globin chain of hemoglobin to form sickle hemoglobin (HbS) from normal hemoglobin A. Under conditions of low oxygen tension, HbS polymerizes and induces the red blood cell to deform into a sickle shape. These mutated cells have a decreased lifespan and often result in chronic hemolytic anemia. The clinical manifestations of sickle cell anemia can be extremely variable, from episodic pain as a result of vaso-occlusive crises to acute chest syndrome, highlighting the complexity of the disorder and the need for exhaustive management plans that address both the acute complications and the long-term care (Shirani Asl & Tamaddon, 2025). The etiology of sickle cell anemia is intimately related to its mode of inheritance, defined as an autosomal recessive disorder. This means that two copies of the mutant gene from both parents are required for the patient to express the disease phenotype. Symptomless carriers or those who possess a single copy of the HBB mutation are typically asymptomatic but have a protective benefit against malaria. This differential pressure has increased the prevalence of sickle cell trait in malaria-endemic regions, which is one of the best examples of natural selection in human genetics. The global pattern of sickle cell disease demonstrates its impact not only on the wellness of individuals but also on public health systems, which are compelled to accommodate affected individuals with access to genetic counseling and new treatment modalities. Sickle cell anemia research and treatment developments have moved steadily forward, but there are great challenges. Advances , such as hydroxyurea, which causes fetal hemoglobin production, have been helpful to many patients. Gene therapy is paradigmatically promising as a cure, with correction of the genetic lesion or induction of normally beneficial fetal hemoglobin production. All these treatments must be balanced, however, with attention to ethical issues, inequities in access, and long-term evidence of efficacy. Besides, multidisciplinary sickle cell anemia management, incorporating hematology, genetics, and population education, is critical to enhance the management of the disease. Ongoing research is crucial to understand the biological mechanisms related to sickle cell anemia and develop better treatments to improve the quality of life of the affected (Shirani & Tamaddon).

8.3.3. Huntington's Disease (HD)

Huntington's disease (HD) is characteristic of the complexity of inherited genetic illness. Characterized by progressive neuronal loss, HD is caused by a longer-than-normal CAG repeat in the HTT gene on chromosome 4. The genetic defect leads to the production of a mutant form of huntingtin protein that is toxic to neurons in the brain, notably damaging areas responsible for movement and thought. Patients typically begin to manifest symptoms in mid-adulthood, which include chorea, psychiatric symptoms, and mental deterioration. Such impacts not only create health problems for the patient but also generate a massive emotional and social burden on family and caregivers, who must endure the devastating impact of this disorder as it escalates into appreciable disability and resultant premature death. The molecular pathophysiology of Huntington's disease is to illustrate an unprecedented interaction between genetic mutation and cellular failure. One of the most characteristic aspects of HD is the role of oxidative stress in neurodegeneration. Hyperproduction of ROS after mitochondrial damage has been thought to be an etiologically important component of HD pathogenesis. Mitochondria, instrumental in the production of ATP and metabolic activity, are impaired in the case of HD patients, further augmenting oxidative stress and susceptibility of the neurons. As Singh et al. (2019) suggest, oxidative stress has the potential to induce cellular damage, affecting macromolecules , such as DNA, lipids, and proteins, resulting in necrosis or apoptosis. This understanding of the biochemical changes that occur with HD illustrates the value placed upon comprehending oxidative processes involved in the pathogenesis of neurodegenerative disorders and emphasizes the necessity of therapeutic interventions to address oxidative damage. Genetic counseling is a crucial factor in treating Huntington's disease, especially in those at risk based on family history. Because HD is an autosomal dominant disorder, there is a 50% chance that an affected individual will pass the mutation on to the next generation. The complexities of testing, interpretation of results, and psychosocial consequences require careful genetic counseling on clinical and family histories. Genetic counselors guide individuals and families to make informed choices in risk awareness, selecting proper tests, and coping with the emotional effects of potential results. As the technology of genetic testing advances, Kelly (2013) outlines how genetic counselors are extending their approach, moving beyond the standard to provide more extensive genomic counseling. This is necessary for guaranteeing families and patients receive personalized, supportive care as they live with, or are at risk of, Huntington's disease (Figure 8.9).

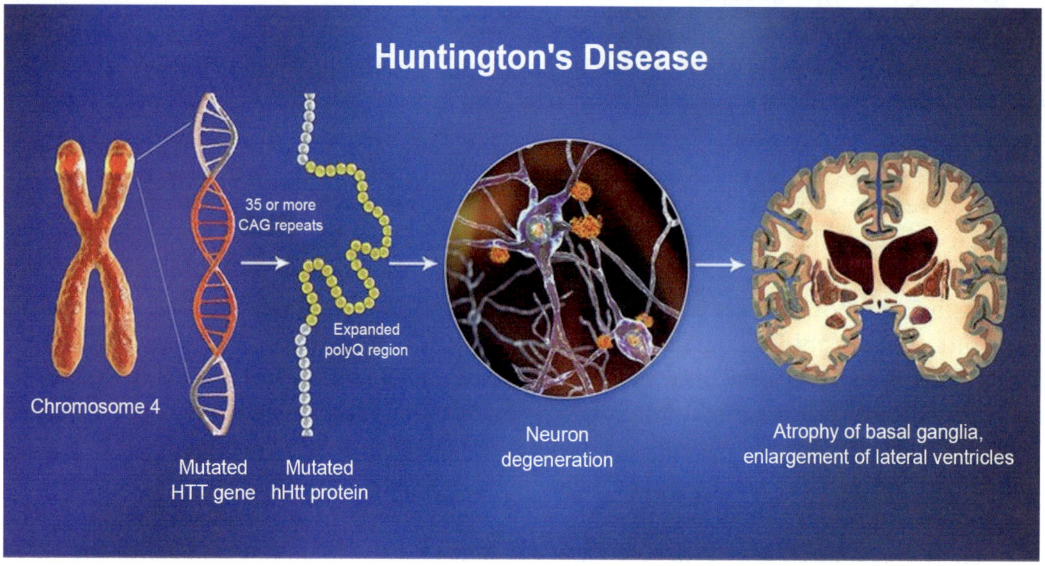

Figure 8.9. Huntington's disease (HD).

Source: https://www.fcneurology.net/wp-content/uploads/2022/07/Huntington's-disease-diagram.jpg.

8.4. Diagnosis of Inherited Genetic Disorders

Diagnosis of inherited genetic disorders has made great progress, thanks to advancing technology and an enhanced understanding of human genetics. Clinically, diagnosis previously relied heavily on family history and phenotypic presentation, which tended to be confusing because symptoms were similar between different disorders. The technology of advanced genetic testing methods, such as whole exome sequencing, has changed the diagnostic process by allowing for the identification of exact genetic mutations that cause inherited diseases. This is particularly significant because inherited diseases tend to manifest in different ways, most of the time making diagnosis complicated. With more advanced testing methods, physicians can now provide more personalized treatment options, greatly improving care for patients. Thus, the advent of genetic testing into routine clinical practice underscores its pivotal role in the successful diagnosis of inherited genetic disorders. A multidisciplinary approach has emerged as pivotal to increasing the accuracy and efficiency with which inherited genetic disorders are diagnosed. The paradigm bridges conventional practice, such as peripheral blood smear analysis for hematological disorders, with cutting-edge molecular approaches involving next-generation sequencing (NGS). For instance, in neonatal red cell disorders, accurate diagnosis of conditions like G6PD deficiency or hereditary spherocytosis is made possible through the integration of morphological examination and biochemical examination with genetic examination. Such advanced practices not only enhance the identification of a specific genetic mutation but also make it possible to perform early interventions that could effectively influence a patient's quality of life. With constant clinical practices modifying and embracing, the collaborative efforts of hematologists, geneticists, and clinical biochemists are likely to revolutionize the diagnostic landscape for inherited disorders. Recent studies have highlighted the relevance of new genetic testing approaches for diagnosing inherited kidney diseases (IKDs), demonstrating the broader picture for inherited genetic disorders. Current diagnostic paradigms highlight the important role of precise genetic identification, given that IKDs account for a significant proportion of childhood renal failure. Enhanced genetic testing has made it possible for clinicians to categorize these disorders by specific genetic abnormality and mode of presentation. Moreover, the call for early intervention strategies holds true in these developments since early diagnosis can effectively limit long-term morbidity of IKDs. New therapeutic modalities , such as gene therapy and organoids, not only promise improved outcomes of treatment but also underscore the dynamic interplay between therapy and diagnosis in the case of genetic disorders. Combined, these advances offer the possibility of a future where precision diagnosis and personalized medicine converge to enhance patient management in genetic health.

8.4.1. Genetic Testing Methods

Genetic testing methods have become indispensable in the diagnosis of hereditary genetic illnesses, providing a variety of mechanisms ranging from traditional methods to highly advanced molecular ones. While peripheral blood smear analysis has been a long-standing traditional routine diagnosing mechanism, particularly for the study of red blood cell morphology, its shortcomings necessitate the inclusion of more sophisticated techniques. The diagnosis of enzymatic deficiency and hemoglobinopathies, for instance, is considerably aided by biochemical tests, though in most instances these can be supplemented with genetic tests for confirmation. By using morphology together with biochemistry, clinicians can arrive at a better understanding of an inherited disease and thereby enhance patient management and therapeutic possibilities. Use of multidisciplinary diagnosis is also necessary owing to the fact that most genetic diseases are complex, with their phenotypic presentation being better utilized with multidisciplinary evaluation, with proper comprehension of the causative genetic mutation (Asl et al., 2025). Next-generation sequencing (NGS) is a revolutionary technological advancement in genetic testing, particularly for patients with hereditary genetic diseases. By enabling whole-exome sequencing (WES), NGS provides a compelling tool to identify pathogenic variants in the coding regions of the genome. Not only is it cost-effective, but it is also effective in its method, as it allows for complete analysis that can uncover the underlying genetic etiology of disorders that are not detected by routine tests. Despite its advantages, the NGS procedure is technologically complicated and often subject to variability in data interpretation, which can affect the results of diagnosis. This complexity makes it necessary for universal data analysis methods and laboratory guidelines to ensure reliability and uniformity of the output. Laboratory design, laboratory protocols, and quality control recommendations suggest practices that illustrate the imperative need for stringency in implementing WES in the diagnosis of genetic disease (Medical Genetics Branch of Chinese Medical Association, 2025). The implications of accurate genetic testing methods extend beyond diagnosis; they determine the very nature of therapeutic intervention and disease management of inherited genetic diseases. Early diagnosis through advanced testing technologies allows intervention to occur at the earliest time, from preventive strategies, tailored treatment plans, or even gene therapy in a few cases. As the genetic test continues to evolve, its integration into clinical practice not only facilitates better patient management but also helps bring about improved pathophysiological insight into most genetic diseases. In addition, emerging technologies and advanced test technologies promise increased diagnostic accuracy, which is needed to design targeted therapies. Consistent with this, encouraging collaboration between geneticists, clinicians, and laboratory professionals is essential for maximizing the potential of new testing technologies for the treatment of inherited genetic disorders (Figure 8.10).

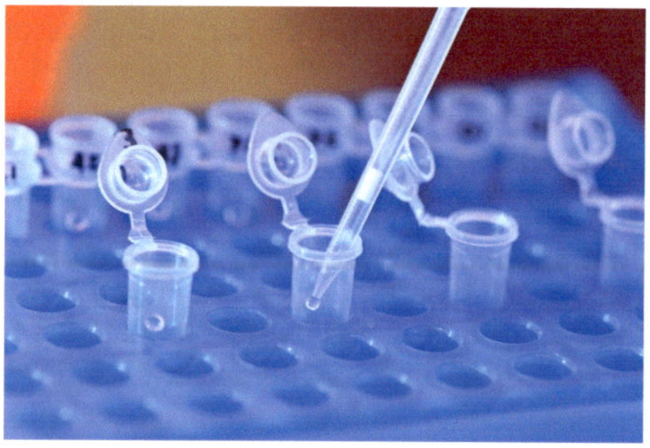

Figure 8.10. Genetic testing methods.

Source: https://www.esneft.nhs.uk/wp-content/uploads/2022/06/genetic-testing.jpeg.

8.4.2. Role of Family History in Diagnosis

The role of family history in the diagnosis of inherited genetic disorders cannot be overemphasized since it forms a preliminary critical element for interpretation of the risk and potential expression of genetic conditions in individuals. Detailed family history allows clinicians to identify patterns of inheritance, differentiate between relationships of various disorders, and determine the probability of offspring becoming affected. For instance, presence in multiple relatives of a specific condition may suggest an autosomal dominant mode, and therefore, testing and potential intervention recommendations are made differently. In addition, familial clustering of conditions typically informs recommendations for genetic counseling and screening practice, enabling providers to strategically target high-risk individuals for testing and improve outcome predictions and individualized management strategies. With advances in technology in genetic testing, the inclusion of family history in clinical assessment remains vital for determining the best course of diagnostic testing and family risk assessment. Variable expressivity and incomplete penetrance of genetic disorders also make it crucial to have comprehensive family histories. If a genetic mutation exists, it may present differently in family members, rendering it challenging to diagnose. For example, a single pathogenic variant might result in divergent presentations of a disorder among siblings, thus being a challenge to the diagnostic precision with a solitary sighting of an index case. Family histories uncover such nuances, which not only lead to the detection of at-risk individuals but also promote detailed information on how environmental factors and accompanying genetic defects can modulate the phenotypic spectrum of inherited diseases. As more recent evidence shows, interactions between several genes can modify the expressivity of inherited disorders, so that systematization of family history becomes increasingly important in clinical practice of genetic diagnosis, so as to continue refining prognostic information as well as patient management, thereby enabling more risk-stratified assessment. Also, the more individualized use of medicine being sought through genetic testing emphasizes the value of family history for risk stratification. Modern genetics is extending from single-gene testing to whole-exome and whole-genome sequencing tools that allow for the analysis of complex, multi-gene diseases in families with previous testing that has been uninformative. Research has shown that familial clustering of genetic disease frequently is accompanied by shared environmental exposures and genetic predispositions—highlighting a key aspect of patient management. Through the identification of common patterns that exist in family histories, health care providers can use this information to direct targeted interventions and preventive measures, especially in those disorders with oligogenic inheritance, as outlined in most cardiovascular diseases. This integrated approach not only ensures earlier and more accurate diagnoses but also allows for the embracing of preventive strategies aimed at risk reduction—a testament to the strength of family history in deconstructing inherited genetic conditions (Parenti et al., 2020; Wilde et al., 2022).

8.4.3. Advances in Prenatal Screening

The advancement of prenatal screening technologies is a significant achievement in the early detection of inherited genetic diseases. Of particular interest, non-invasive prenatal testing (NIPT) has revolutionized clinicians' assessment of the risk for chromosomal abnormalities in the growing fetus. The latest iteration, NIPT2.0, utilizes high-throughput sequencing to provide an accurate approach to identifying fetal chromosomal aneuploidies, microdeletion/microduplication syndromes, and dominantly inherited monogenic disorders. This new technology surpasses the limitations of older techniques with improved detection and accuracy, particularly for complex genetic diseases that would never have been possible before. Such improvements in prenatal screening techniques make it possible to intervene early and make decisions by potential parents, pointing to the clinical significance of incorporating cutting-edge genetic testing into prenatal care strategies (Reproductive Health Branch of China Maternal and Child Health Association, 2024). Besides, clinical application of NIPT2.0 needs careful consideration of how it will be used in practice. In conferences where experts come together to develop consensus best practice, a number of considerations are realized concerning its use, including the identification of the target diseases, choosing candidate populations, and offering sufficient pre- and post-test genetic counseling. Implementing standard protocols can help to actualize the potential benefits of this novel technology while alleviating the problems associated with its adoption, such as interpretation of findings and psychological impact on pregnant couples. Emphasis on quality control and outlining the boundaries of the tests are crucial aspects in developing a responsibly implemented prenatal genetic testing policy. With adherence to professional guidelines, medical practitioners can be certain that NIPT2.0 is used responsibly and ethically, ultimately leading to improved healthcare for mother and child (Reproductive Health Branch of China Maternal and Child Health Association, 2024). Beyond identifying chromosomal abnormalities, prenatal screening addresses such conditions as sickle cell disease. Being one of the most common inherited blood disorders globally, sickle cell disease is extremely dangerous to patients. Recent prenatal diagnostic methods make early detection possible and provide valuable information regarding the genetic mutations that cause the disease. Additionally, the technologies enable medical professionals to forecast disease severity and complications, thus enhancing treatment strategies for the affected families. Concurrently, the development of gene-editing technology and alternative treatments, including stem cell transplantation, illustrates the ongoing efforts at managing and mitigating the impacts of sickle cell disease. Together, these advances in genetic science and prenatal diagnosis not only assist families in making informed reproductive choices but also set the stage for new therapies with the promise to alter the course of these genetic diseases (Figure 8.11).

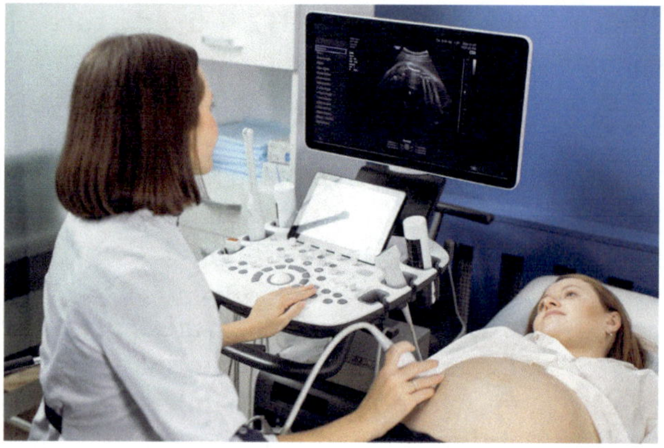

Figure 8.11. Advances in prenatal screening.

Source: https://www.whmcenter.com/wp-content/uploads/2024/07/AdobeStock_407329436-Large.jpeg.

8.5. Treatment Options

The management of inherited genetic diseases is usually complicated and multilayered, particularly with the diversity and complexity that defines such conditions. Management can range from symptomatic relief to targeted therapy that aims to repair the genetic mutations underlying the disorder. To illustrate, conditions , such as Charcot-Marie-Tooth (CMT) have driven a great amount of genetics research, and this has made it possible to identify the key mutations that are responsible for the disorder. This understanding allows for the development of personalized therapies that can alter the course of the disease by directly repairing the specific genetic flaws found in the patients (Caruso et al., 2020). Significantly, this shift towards personalized medicine allows for personalized therapies based on the genetic makeup of the individual to enhance therapeutic efficacy and minimize side effects. In the case of liver diseases, i.e., hepatocellular carcinoma (HCC), the therapy schemes are becoming more sophisticated. Given that HCC is diagnosed at a late stage, therapeutic programs are usually bound by tumor heterogeneity and resistance to conventional treatments. Multikinase inhibitors and immune checkpoint inhibitors are some of the approved drugs currently, but these therapies have overall low survival benefits (Caruso et al., 2020). The challenge is one of understanding both the tumor microenvironment and the molecular determinants of resistance, so as to infer that a more nuanced approach is needed. Ongoing research into tumor genetics and personalized treatment protocols has the potential to lead to improved outcomes but assumes innovative preclinical models reflecting the complexity of HCC pathology. Innovative treatment approaches for other inherited genetic disorders serve to identify the potential of gene therapy and RNA-based treatments. These technologies attempt to repair or compensate for genetic defects in their onset. For example, the development of CRISPR technology is making gene editing precise, with the potential for treating diseases that currently have no acceptable treatment. Tackling the disease-causing mutations head-on, such as some forms of CMT, there is hope for disease modification rather than symptomatic management (Morena et al., 2019). In addition, gene therapy is also potentially key to diseases like HCC, where alterations in genes are identified and scientists come up with a designed therapeutic intervention that could significantly enhance patient survival. Lastly, as genetics advances further, novel treatments for inherited conditions are increasingly a reality, with the potential to enhance control and outcome.

8.5.1. Gene Therapy

Gene therapy is one of the most promising approaches to combat inherited genetic disorders, aiming at the root genetic mutation responsible for these diseases. Traditional medical treatments mainly address symptoms and not the source of the disease, leading to persistent patient morbidity and suffering. Gene therapy aims to repair or replace defective genes with a potential treatment for conditions like cystic fibrosis, hemophilia, and some hereditary eye disorders. Emerging developments have brought to the forefront the capabilities of non-viral delivery systems, which are capable of overcoming the limitations of traditional viral vectors. Emerging methodologies, including liposomes and nanoparticles, enhance the safety profile and specificity of gene deliveries, a feature critical in conditions where targeted intervention is needed to prevent complications and improve therapeutic outcomes (Jony et al., 2025). Application of gene therapy is most groundbreaking in genetic retinal diseases (IRDs), which are more likely to lead to blindness or vision loss due to specific genetic mutations. Traditional treatment approaches have been met with moderate success in these complex disorders, and new solutions were called for.

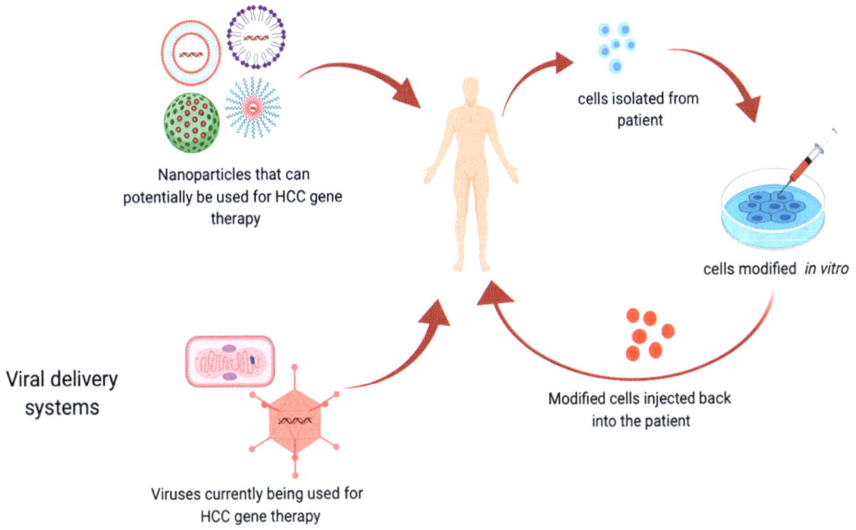

Figure 8.12. Gene therapy.

Source: https://st.adda247.com/https://www.studyiq.com/articles/wp-content/uploads/2022/12/15163620/Gene-Therapy.jpg.

A new burst of clinical trials in applying gene therapy to treat IRDs is a reflection of an increasing realization of the potential. Treatments for diseases , such as Leber congenital amaurosis and retinitis pigmentosa demonstrate the promise of gene therapy in restoring partial or full vision by directly delivering functional copies of genes into retinal cells. By circumventing the drawbacks introduced by traditional treatments, including immunogenicity and delivery precision, gene therapy is an oasis of hope for patients with IRDs. The future of such an approach seems bright with ongoing studies deciphering the complexities of these disorders to create a model for therapy interventions (Umair, 2024). Additionally, the greater significance of gene therapy moves into personalized medicine, where treatments are targeted on the basis of the individual's unique genetic profile. This paradigm shift emphasizes a more individualized approach in the management of inherited genetic disorders, so precise interventions can lead to better patient outcomes. Aside from the correction of genetic defects, gene therapy can also be utilized to enhance genetic resistance against certain diseases, which can potentially lead to preventive treatments. With continuing research progress, ethical concerns and accessibility of care need to be a priority to bring the advantages of gene therapy to the world's multi-faceted population. Possibilities provided through individualized gene therapy use are an enormous step towards unraveling genetics and disease management, and the therapeutic future of genetic disorders will be revolutionized while opening new heights to modern medicine (Jony et al., 2025) (Figure 8.12).

8.5.2. Symptomatic Treatment Approaches

Symptomatic management protocols serve as a vital component of the treatment of inherited genetic diseases, particularly when curative therapies are yet to be developed. For many conditions, such as Perry disease (PeD), where the genetic mutations dictate the course of the disorders, symptom relief is a priority in improving the quality of life for patients. PeD is such a typical example in this regard, as it is accompanied by Parkinsonism, psychiatric impairment, and other debilitating effects of TDP-43 protein aggregates within the brain. Treatment for symptomatic relief targets the disease symptoms without interfering with the genetic cause, via means , such as pharmacological interventions targeting neurochemical pathways. Researchers have theorized that several potential targets for therapy, including monoamine oxidase B (MAO-B) and serotonin receptors, may form the cornerstone for the generation of effective symptomatic treatments of neurodegenerative conditions like PeD (Gajda et al., 2024). Inherited metabolic epilepsies (IMEs) also illustrate the necessity for symptomatic treatment modalities in the context of genetic diseases. IMEs, being an idiopathic epilepsy with heterogeneous metabolic dysfunctions, demonstrate the difficulty in developing targeted treatments due to their rarity and heterogeneity. Therapeutic measures in the majority of cases are dominated by symptom control by the use of antiepileptic drugs and supportive therapy and not the correction of the metabolic disorders per se. However, progress in molecular genetics has assisted in raising awareness of the pathomechanisms of IMEs and inspired the development of new diagnostic methods and treatment strategies. Current advances suggest that nutritional therapy, vitamin replacement, and other supportive therapies may confer a considerable benefit in managing symptoms from these metabolic disorders, which could lead to future targeted treatments (Latzer et al., 2024). Although symptomatic treatments are required for the management of inherited genetic disorders, they act optimally variably depending on the specific condition and its specific presentations. For instance, in PeD, symptomatic treatments may reverse the neurodegenerative presentation, allowing for overall improvement in the well-being of patients. Therapeutic interventions for IMEs remain more heterogeneous, involving an array of methods from dietetic modifications to potential enzyme and gene therapies. With advancing studies, the focus will even more be on not only improving symptom control but also designing more focused and efficient therapy regimens targeting the molecular underpinnings of such genetic diseases. Ultimately, the fact that genetic studies are ongoing is poised to bear upon future strategies, balancing symptom relief against getting closer to complete therapeutic solutions to inherited genetic disorders (Latzer et al., 2024).

8.5.3. Importance of Early Intervention

The significance of early intervention for inherited genetic diseases cannot be overstressed, as early intervention has the potential to significantly alter the life course of those affected. Newborn screening programs highlight the key role of early diagnosis in preventing the adverse effects of congenital genetic and metabolic disorders. For instance, research on Fars Province, Iran, approximated an inherited metabolic disorder (IMD) birth prevalence of 1:1000, encompassing major conditions , such as phenylalanine metabolism disorders and fatty acid oxidation disorders (Salarian et al., 2025). With early detection of such disorders before their onset in terms of signs and symptoms, healthcare workers are able to implement pertinent interventions, which reduce morbidity and accompanying health complications. In addition, the ability to screen and treat these disorders early offers windows of ongoing care and treatment, further raising the necessity of these screening programs to better increase long-term outcomes for such populations.

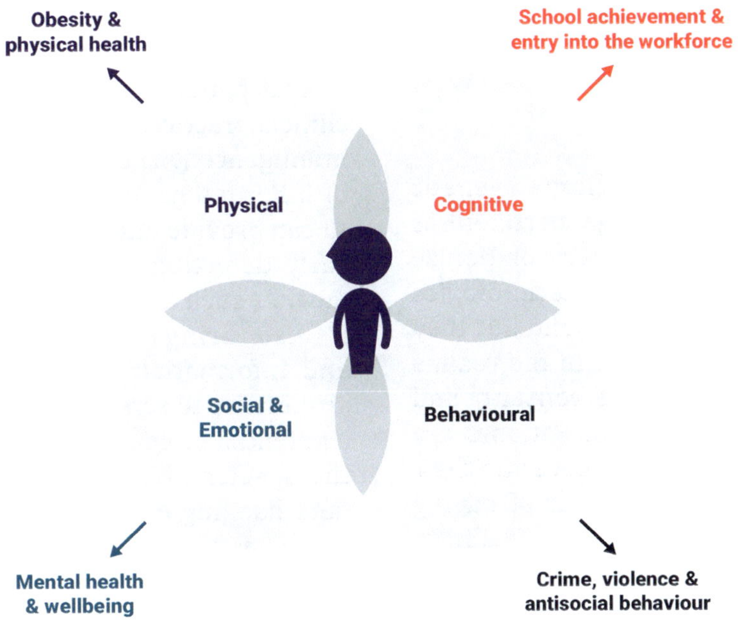

Figure 8.13. Importance of early intervention.

Source: https://www.eif.org.uk/files/image/about/mtc-four-domains.png.

Beyond individual health outcomes, early intervention is also positive for overall public health outcomes. Newborn screening aligns with the intent to reduce the healthcare costs of untreated genetic disorders. With successful screening programs, the onset of disorders that require a great deal of medical intervention can be prevented, therefore limiting the burden on families and healthcare systems (Kannoth & George, 2024). For such families who get early diagnosis, there is an opportunity for prevention, diet modification, or medication to be introduced successfully. Communities benefit from fewer cases of severe disability, leading to a more effective society overall. Therefore, economic justification for early intervention is not only in short-term healthcare cost savings, but also in promoting healthier, more capable future generations. Moreover, increasing awareness of inherited genetic disease and the importance of early intervention can potentially result in more beneficial overall societal opinions regarding genetic health. Educating parents, health practitioners, and communities about conditions , such as vitamin-dependent genetic disorders emphasizes the need for keen screening and timely treatment for enhancing quality of life (Kannoth & George, 2024). Through extensive education efforts, individuals are rendered empowered to seek early genetic testing in the event that there is an existing family history of the same disorders. Public education campaigns can contribute to enhancing participation in screening programs, thus leading to increased early detection rates. These concerted efforts enable understanding of proactive healthcare strategies as being imperative not only for individual health but also for population health improvement, driving towards a societal movement to value preventive interventions in healthcare (Figure 8.13).

8.6. Ethical Considerations

Ethical concerns surrounding inherited genetic disease are becoming increasingly pertinent as genetic testing and biotechnologies revolutionize the healthcare landscape. These technologies offer greater diagnosis and treatment, but they pose significant moral dilemmas in the realms of patient autonomy, informed consent, and the potential for discrimination. Patients are faced with the complexities of discovering their genetic vulnerabilities, often in fear of having this knowledge. Therefore, the responsibility of healthcare providers is heavier, with the obligation to make sure the patients understand the implications of genetic testing completely. Misconceptions rooted in genetic illiteracy have the potential to hinder well-informed decision-making, calling for individualized education interventions to facilitate patients and families in their genetic testing and counseling choices (Alruwaily, 2025). An even-handed reaction to ethics of genetic disorders, thus, must target open communication and equitable access to means, in an attempt to foster an informed population of patients. Healthcare providers play a role in caring for ethical matters relating to inherited genetic disorders. Physicians must attempt to walk the thin line between delivering potential benefit and patient confidentiality and autonomy. As noted in recent studies, there are experiential knowledge gaps in understanding the genetic etiology of disorders among patients and caregivers that might lead to misinterpretation of the utility of genetic testing (Alruwaily, 2025). Concerns for healthcare providers also address implications for disclosing genetic information, particularly in relation to familial effects and risk of genetic discrimination. Ethical education and principles are required to prepare health professionals to deal with the delicate aspect of genetic test results and the potential implications of revealing such details to patients and families. This indicates the requirement of a serious ethics course in the medical sector so that patient well-being is the top priority in clinical practice. New technologies like artificial intelligence (AI) complicate the ethical context of inherited genetic disorders even further. As AI can provide unprecedented advantages in the early detection and diagnosis of ailments via means , such as facial recognition technologies, it also brings along questions of privacy and information security. The possibility for authorities to screen massive databases creates a potential threat of government overreach, with the specter of the misuse of sensitive genetic data hanging over it. This is a scenario where there has to be a robust framework to play on the rights of human beings and robust fences around leaks and discrimination. The balance of innovation and moral accountability is the ideal, as integration of AI into genetic health has to be preceded by preventive measures towards protecting patients' interests. In navigating this crossroads of technology and ethics, stakeholders need to develop a healthcare environment that holds individual privacy in high esteem even as it leverages the visionary potential of genetic discoveries.

8.6.1. Genetic Privacy and Discrimination

The arrival of genetic testing has revolutionized the field of medicine, particularly in the diagnosis and management of inherited genetic disorders. Despite this being a significant advancement, it is accompanied by actual and serious concerns of genetic privacy and discrimination. Genetic information are in their nature, private and sensitive and reveals predisposition to a variety of illnesses, which may then be abused by employers, insurers, and even family members. Fear of genetic discrimination may discourage individuals from having potentially lifesaving tests, thereby hindering public health efforts to detect and treat inherited diseases. Without robust legal protection for genetic data, patients are open to the threat of job loss or exorbitant health insurance rates, creating a concerning paradox in which information about genetic danger imposes social expenses rather than enhanced health, as noted in the treatment of ethical issues in behavioral genetics (Tofiloski, 2025).

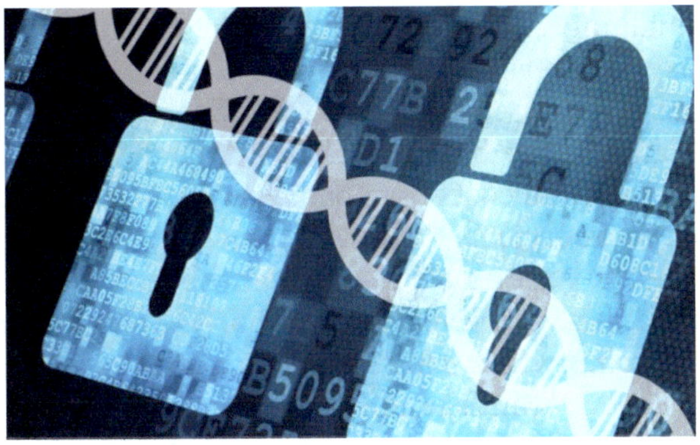

Figure 8.14. Genetic privacy and discrimination.

Source: https://external-content.duckduckgo.com/iu/?u=https%3A%2F%2Fgeneticliteracyproject.org%2Fwp-content%2Fuploads%2Felementor%2Fthumbs%2Fprivacy-pe4uw8hgsoyd9eery5ry9ysz8kv65ye8y31zbf1nns.jpg&f=1&nofb=1&ipt=b217e7cc87d4c7449e167dd3f66525e22ad6b15321e7bcbc5a613dfa54d93de6.

Moreover, the ethical ramifications of genetic screening extend beyond individual privacy to social implications. With more advanced genetic studies, the threat of stigmatization based on genetic vulnerability also grows. Patients carrying clearly identifiable genetic markers for illnesses , such as Huntington's disease or certain cancers can become socially ostracized or discriminated against, not only by insurers or employers but also among their communities. The potential for genetic profiling to aggregate existing biases and inequalities in society raises concern about the proper ethical standards under which genetic research and its applications exist. Overcoming such concerns requires collaborative efforts to ensure transparency, inclusivity, and respect for individuals' autonomy in genetic research, as outlined in the comprehensive literature review of behavioral genetics and molecular psychiatry (Tofiloski, 2025). Further, arguments surrounding genetic privacy also overlap with broader arguments surrounding informed consent and the moral use of genetic information. As molecular markers become more and more a part of disease diagnosis and treatment of genetic disease, it is necessary to have guidelines in place that protect individuals against genetic discrimination. This means having policies that limit access to genetic information and manage it so that it is not abused, but necessary research is enabled. Complications within the interpretation of genetic information provide another level of complication to this setting, as misinterpretation has the ability to feed into occurrences of discrimination. Ultimately, the aim must be a fine line between the potential of genetic findings and the necessity for individual rights, paving the way for an eventual future where genetic testing is used to create more understanding and health equity and less discrimination (Figure 8.14).

8.6.2. Implications of Genetic Testing

The applicability of genetic testing, particularly in relation to inherited genetic disease, goes beyond straightforward diagnosis and impacts all aspects of familial and societal function. Testing may identify carriers of autosomal recessive and X-linked disease, providing useful information for potential parents. Advances in genetic screening technology, such as the CarrierTest, permit the detection of multiple genes at once for mutations. This combined strategy allows one to understand their genetic susceptibility, thereby impacting reproductive decisions. It also enhances preconception care by , including numerous risk tests as part of an effective assessment, which ultimately identifies the health of generations to come. Genetic testing, by facilitating these critical evaluations to be made, plays a significant role in the lifetime disease trajectory of an individual, ensuring that decisions are made through concrete genetic evidence (Diblík et al., 2022).

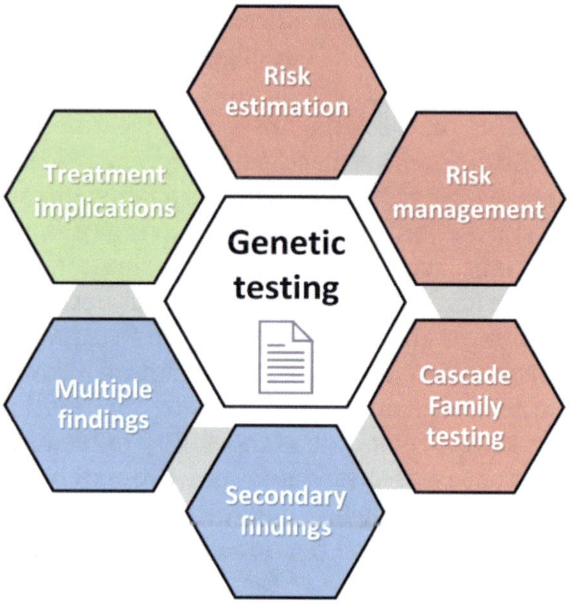

Figure 8.15. Implications of genetic testing.

Source: https://www.preprints.org/img/dyn_abstract_figures/2021/05/f4c067daf16fcfeec855a843effdaabf/preprints-42714-graphical.v1.jpg.

Secondly, the moral implications of genetic testing must be taken into account. The rate of progress in genetic technology has prompted an immediate need to avoid the abuse of genetic information, potentially leading to employment or insurance discrimination. Lesch–Nyhan syndrome illustrates such complexities and indicates the large challenges presented by families in coping with genetic diseases. An earlier diagnosis through genetic testing has the potential to inform families with information, thus allowing them to make evidence-based choices regarding care and interventions. However, the decisions accompany emotional struggles and ethical dilemmas regarding the amount of treatment and management methods. The implications of genetic testing extend into the ethical sphere, demanding intense debate about patient rights, autonomy, and the ethics of genetic interventions (Zhang et al., 2022). Furthermore, genetic testing holds significant public health policy and resource allocation implications. As screening technology increases and becomes more common, population detection of genetic disorders could lead to increased demands for healthcare provision for managing such conditions. Policymakers will have to determine how genetic screening should be included in existing healthcare systems, balancing the benefits of early diagnosis with the potential costs of subsequent treatment and support services. Moreover, data gathered using massive genetic screening can be utilized for public health prevention and early intervention programs, which can reduce the health care load of genetic conditions. Lastly, the implications of genetic tests have core considerations of population and individual health that need a holistic response to its ethical, clinical, and policy dimensions (Diblík et al., 2022) (Figure 8.15).

8.6.3. Ethical Dilemmas in Gene Editing

The ethical dilemma of gene editing, and the use thereof with reference to inherited genetic disease in particular, raises profound questions about the scientist's responsibility and that of society at large. Germline gene editing, i.e., altering genes in human embryos, acquires not just touted medical advances but has significant ethical undertones as well. While advances in tools , such as CRISPR-Cas9 have given rise to optimism regarding the eradication of genetic diseases, they also bring controversy regarding the implications of "playing God." As debated in deliberations of the European Society of Human

Reproduction and Embryology, there is a balance between the hope that gene editing will bring and ethics in its application. The complexities ushered in by legislative laws and social values require ongoing debate to determine whether the future of gene editing is worthwhile for the ethical effects it has on society (De Wert et al., 2018).

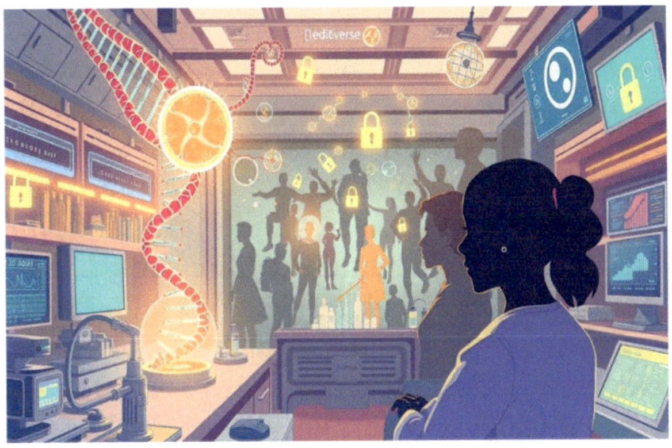

Figure 8.16. Ethical dilemmas in gene editing.

Source: https://editverse.com/wp-content/uploads/2024/09/Gene-Editing-Ethics-CRISPR-scaled.jpg.

The case of He Jiankui's gene-edited twins serves as a prominent example of the functional complexities and ethical challenges associated with gene editing technologies. Advocates of such innovations argue that they could prevent the onset of severe genetic disorders, ensuring that gene editing not only would put an end to human suffering but also improve overall well-being. But there are dozens of counterarguments and they revolve around the risk of unintended genetic alterations and the potential genealogy of off-target mutations with irreversible impacts on future generations. This incident has prompted self-reflection in the scientific community regarding standards of safety and efficacy, necessitating a re-evaluation of the regulatory principles under which human germline editing is performed. The controversy highlights the fine line between innovation and moral responsibility, with the quest to eliminate genetic diseases raising questions on the potential for unforeseen consequences that could make the human condition more complex (Bolton et al., 2024). Furthermore, the socio-economic ramifications of gene editing technology introduce another layer into the ethical equation. As gene editing becomes more accessible, there is fear that it will expand existing health disparities. Wealthier segments of society will have privileged access to these technologies, creating a gap between those with the means to alter their genetic destiny and the rest of society. This innovation presents deep ethical concerns over equity, justice, and the potential for a new genetic elite. Society is confronted with whether gene editing should be allowed to remain an elite privilege or opened up for all, and the issue brings an imperative for equitable access to medical advancements. As the conversation around inherited gene disorders and gene editing continues to advance, it is crucial to apply ethical considerations to policies and procedures that govern these cutting-edge technologies so that the pursuit of health gain does not result in social conflict (De Wert et al., 2018) (Figure 8.16).

SUMMARY

In summarizing the presentation of inherited genetic disorders, it is important to note the serious effect such diseases have on the patient and society at large. Genetic diseases , such as thalassemia and inherited ocular diseases manifest themselves in several manifestations that can have a profound impact on the quality of life. These disorders are diagnosed and treated through an interdisciplinary approach involving genetics, clinical medicine, and patient education. Furthermore, the psychological and emotional burdens endured by affected families are indicative of the need to be able to offer thorough support mechanisms. With this knowledge of these disorders at a molecular level, researchers and doctors can take strides toward designing specific treatments that might end the effects of these disorders or even cure them in others. Advances in technology in genetic testing procedures have revolutionized the study of inherited genetic diseases, allowing more accurate and reliable diagnoses. Next-generation sequencing (NGS) has been a central among such advances, allowing detection of numerous genetic variants associated with disorders like inherited retinal diseases. Apart from its advantage in diagnostic improvement, this also allows the formulation of new treatment approaches through personalized medicine. Research demonstrating the utility of gene therapy for thalassemia and other diseases points toward the revolutionary possibilities of genetic research in the practice of medicine. With advances in our understanding of the genetic basis of such conditions, application of new diagnostic methods and treatment strategies will only reshape patient management in the years to come. Moreover, the ethical consequences of genetically acquired diseases should not be overlooked. With new technology providing further insight into genetic predisposition, privacy, consent, and the emotional impact of genetic information come to the forefront. Gene therapy poses questions about access and the equitable distribution of treatment across populations. It is important that the medical profession continue to debate the ethical issues of genetic intervention for benefits to be received by all segments of society. Ultimately, a thorough understanding of heritable genetic disorders, along with their biological, social, and ethical considerations, will guide the way towards improved measures for management and more beneficial results for afflicted individuals and families, emphasizing the realization of both scientific advancement and compassionate care.

An understanding of inherited genetic disorders requires a critical evaluation of their clinical and genetic subtleties. A crucial aspect of this understanding is the recognition of genetic associations among diseases. For instance, studies have identified strong genetic correlations between kidney stone disease (KSD) and other gastrointestinal ailments, as evidence of the multifaceted interaction of genetics among different organ systems. By analyzing large genome-wide association studies, researchers discovered that diseases , such as irritable bowel syndrome and Crohn's disease shared the same genetic architecture as KSD, as evidenced by positive genetic correlations and pleiotropic single-nucleotide polymorphisms that underlie both sets of diseases. This intricate genetic association suggests a shared mechanism of pathophysiology that can be employed to inform future therapeutic approaches and prevention strategies, thereby emphasizing the place of thorough approaches in the treatment of these diseases (Wang et al., 2025). Another prominent feature in the context of inherited genetic disorders is the ongoing evolution of diagnostic and therapeutic approaches. In pediatric patients, particularly, inherited kidney diseases (IKDs) present complex issues requiring innovative solutions. With the introduction of genetic testing technologies , such as whole exome sequencing, diagnostic practice has changed to permit precise detection of over 150 genetic defects that lead to IKDs. This detail in the diagnostic techniques is of importance as not only does it enhance the accuracy of disease categorization, but also allows for early intervention, which can be vital for significantly improved patient outcomes. Further, classification of IKDs based on genetic defects and clinical manifestations assists in further comprehension of their diverse presentations and mechanisms, ultimately towards more precise and effective management plans for the involved individuals (Wang et al., 2024). The convergence of new therapies , such as gene therapy and organoids, also better showcases the potential for revolutionary advancements in the therapy of inherited genetic disorders. The potential of gene therapy for previously untreatable diseases has the potential to transform the therapeutic landscape, offering hope to patients with debilitating genetic diseases. Organoid technology, allowing for the creation of patient-specific models of tissue, has the potential for personalized medicine, enabling clinicians to tailor treatment based on a patient's genetic blueprint. As these novel treatments are developed and refined, ongoing research and clinical trials must be used to test their effectiveness and safety. These innovations not only increase the knowledge about genetic diseases inherited in an autosomal dominant manner but also lay the groundwork for more effective, personalized therapy that may substantially improve the quality of life of patients with such challenging diseases (Wang et al., 2024).

A LOOK TO THE FUTURE:

NEW TREATMENT MODALITIES:

In recent years, the landscape of medical treatment has undergone a profound transformation as new treatment modalities expand the possibilities for preventing, managing, and curing disease. Traditionally, therapeutic approaches relied heavily on broad categories such as surgery, pharmacotherapy, radiation, and supportive care; however, advances in molecular biology, genomics, immunology, and engineering are ushering in a new era of innovative modalities that transcend conventional paradigms. These emerging treatments offer highly targeted mechanisms of action, often tailored to individual patient biology, and hold the promise of addressing unmet medical needs in fields ranging from oncology and genetic disorders to infectious disease and chronic conditions. At the forefront of these innovations are biological and precision therapies, which include modalities such as antibody–drug conjugates, bispecific antibodies, and engineered proteins and peptides. Antibody-drug conjugates combine the selectivity of antibodies with potent cytotoxic agents, enabling direct targeting of cancer cells while minimizing systemic toxicity. Bispecific antibodies, designed to bind two distinct antigens simultaneously, further enhance therapeutic precision by engaging multiple disease-relevant pathways. Engineered peptides and proteins continue to expand functional diversity through improved stability and specificity in binding, broadening their utility across therapeutic areas. Cell and gene therapies represent a particularly transformative class of modalities. Chimeric antigen receptor (CAR) T-cell therapies harness a patient's own immune system by genetically modifying T cells to recognize and eliminate cancer cells, and variants such as CAR-NK and CAR-M cells are now entering clinical development. Similarly, gene editing technologies like CRISPR/Cas systems enable precise correction of disease-causing mutations, exemplified by recent clinical success in sickle cell disease and beta-thalassemia, offering potential one-time curative treatments. Other promising approaches include nucleic acid-based therapies, such as RNA interference and antisense oligonucleotides, which modulate gene expression to treat underlying causes of disease, and oncolytic viruses that exploit engineered viral agents to selectively destroy tumor tissue. New delivery systems, including nanoparticles and novel vectors, are expanding the reach of these therapies by improving stability and cellular uptake. Beyond biologics, biophysical modalities such as sonodynamic therapy and electroporation-enhanced treatments are emerging as innovative non-pharmacologic strategies to enhance efficacy and reduce invasiveness. Collectively, these new treatment modalities reflect a broader shift toward precision and personalized medicine, where treatments are increasingly tailored to the genetic, molecular, and clinical features of individual patients. While challenges remain—such as ensuring safety, equity of access, and sustainable cost—these advancements underscore a paradigm shift in therapeutic development that promises deeper biological insight and improved patient outcomes across diverse diseases.

REFERENCES

1. Ali, S., Mumtaz, S., Shakir, H. A., Khan, M. A., Tahir, H. M., Mumtaz, S., Mughal, T. A., et al. (2021). Current status of beta-thalassemia and its treatment strategies. *Molecular Genetics & Genomic Medicine, 9*. https://doi.org/10.1002/mgg3.1788 (accessed on 17th July 2025).
2. Alruwaily, B. K. Q. (2025). Comprehension of premarital screening and genetic disorders. *International Journal of Medical Science and Clinical Research Studies*. https://www.semanticscholar.org/paper/e4904d60908a8887947da831eb9865c8bf1b56cc (accessed on 17th July 2025).
3. American Diabetes Association. (2018). Classification and diagnosis of diabetes: *Standards of medical care in diabetes—2019. Diabetes Care, 42*, S13–S28. https://doi.org/10.2337/dc19-s002 (accessed on 17th July 2025).
4. Assiri, K. A., Alrasis, M. S., Mashlawi, A. I., Alayda, M. H., & Aljndbai, A. M. (2024). Role of molecular markers in identifying genetic disorders. *International Journal of Community Medicine and Public Health*. https://www.semanticscholar.org/paper/97e39be19bbc4b6479474c9448f01062b1acae6a (accessed on 17th July 2025).
5. Bao, E. L., Cheng, A., & Sankaran, V. G. (2019). The genetics of human hematopoiesis and its disruption in disease. *EMBO Molecular Medicine, 11*. https://doi.org/10.15252/emmm.201910316 (accessed on 17th July 2025).
6. Bolton, A. (2024). The future of human germline genome editing: Analyzing He Jiankui's experiment. https://core.ac.uk/download/640869304.pdf (accessed on 17th July 2025).
7. Brock, D. C., Wang, M., Hussain, H. M., Rauch, D. E., Marra, M., Pennesi, M., Yang, P., et al. (2024). Comparative analysis of *in-silico* tools in identifying pathogenic variants in dominant inherited retinal diseases. *Human Molecular Genetics*. https://www.semanticscholar.org/paper/b84e7b3348f064963812ae09bbc5f3ed9b09a12a (accessed on 17th July 2025).
8. Bulcha, J., Wang, Y., Ma, H., Tai, P. W. L., & Gao, G. (2021). Viral vector platforms within the gene therapy landscape. *Signal Transduction and Targeted Therapy, 6*. https://doi.org/10.1038/s41392-021-00487-6 (accessed on 17th July 2025).
9. Caruso, S., O'Brien, D. R., Cleary, S. P., Roberts, L. R., & Zucman-Rossi, J. (2020). Genetics of hepatocellular carcinoma: Approaches to explore molecular diversity. *Hepatology, 73*, 14–26. https://doi.org/10.1002/hep.31394 (accessed on 17th July 2025).
10. De Wert, G., Heindryckx, B., Pennings, G., Clarke, A., Eichenlaub-Ritter, U., van El, C. G., Forzano, F., Goddijn, M., Howard, H. C., Radojkovic, D., Rial-Sebbag, E., Dondorp, W., Tarlatzis, B. C., Cornel, M. C., & European Society of Human Genetics and the European Society of Human Reproduction and Embryology (2018). Responsible innovation in human germline gene editing: Background document to the recommendations of ESHG and ESHRE. *European journal of human genetics : EJHG, 26*(4), 450–470. https://doi.org/10.1038/s41431-017-0077-z(accessed on 17th July 2025).
11. Cryan, J. F., O'Riordan, K. J., Cowan, C. S. M., Sandhu, K. V., Bastiaanssen, T. F. S., Boehme, M., Codagnone, M. G., et al. (2019). The microbiota–gut–brain axis. *Physiological Reviews, 99*, 1877–2013. https://doi.org/10.1152/physrev.00018.2018 (accessed on 17th July 2025).
12. Diblík, J., Jarošová, R., Bittóová, M., Zembol, F., Dohnalová, L., Vilímová, Z., Soldatova, I., et al. (2022). O-146 Extended carrier testing of inherited disorders for reproductive risk

assessment in preconception care. *Human Reproduction*. https://www.semanticscholar.org/paper/287b9a9ba280405fc12dce506a062371a42722c8 (accessed on 17th July 2025).

13. ElSayed, N. A., Aleppo, G., Aroda, V. R., Bannuru, R. R., Brown, F. M., Bruemmer, D., Collins, B. S., et al. (2022). Classification and diagnosis of diabetes: *Standards of care in diabetes—2023. Diabetes Care, 46*, S19–S40. https://doi.org/10.2337/dc23-s002 (accessed on 17th July 2025).

14. Gajda, Z., Hawrylak, M., Handzlik, J., & Kuder, K. J. (2024). Perry disease: Current outlook and advances in drug discovery approach to symptomatic treatment. *International Journal of Molecular Sciences, 25*. https://www.semanticscholar.org/paper/f815da888859b80c1b97badaa7e5e35ae8403e6a (accessed on 17th July 2025).

15. Garoia, F., Capovilla, T., Reginato, A., Rubbo, F., Paldino, A., Pio Loco detto Gava, C., Bassetto, G., et al. (2025). Genetic testing in cardiomyopathies: Updates and future perspectives. *Journal of Cardiovascular Medicine*. https://www.semanticscholar.org/paper/049217ae1592b1a997f4110219612ac63279ff46 (accessed on 17th July 2025).

16. Gerard, J. P., Tan, A. H., Lim, S. Y., Ahmad-Annuar, A., Schee, J., & Gopalan, N. (2025). Genetic testing for Parkinson's disease in an underrepresented population: Knowledge, attitudes, and ethical considerations from a Malaysian perspective. *Journal of Genetic Counseling, 34*. https://www.semanticscholar.org/paper/db0081f2d172b1b221def775822b5fcbdf2e5cde (accessed on 17th July 2025).

17. Hagău, A. C., Iurian, D., Pop, M., Șus, I., Șuteu, C., Dunareanu, A. S., & Muntean, I. (2025). Arrhythmogenic cardiomyopathy in children: Case series and review of the literature. *Journal of Cardiovascular Emergencies, 11*, 36–42. https://www.semanticscholar.org/paper/b355497d3e63921907c73365d381f1204465c9a7 (accessed on 17th July 2025).

18. Ionova, S., Murtazina, A., Marakhonov, A., Shchagina, O., Ryadninskaya, N., Tebleva, I. S., Kadyshev, V., et al. (2024). The study of the inheritance mechanisms of myotonic dystrophy type 1 (DM1) in families from the Republic of North Ossetia-Alania. *International Journal of Molecular Sciences, 25*. https://www.semanticscholar.org/paper/5082022253a55697542bb5afb51a32a6ea7e01e5 (accessed on 17th July 2025).

19. Iuliano, R., & Paduano, F. (2024). Editorial on the Special Issue "Genetic and Molecular Basis of Inherited Disorders". *Genes, 15*. https://www.semanticscholar.org/paper/f990e2ab9395b7326ef636a4db7fdb1eb0b23b21 (accessed on 17th July 2025).

20. Jespersgaard, C., Fang, M., Bertelsen, M., Dang, X., Jensen, H., Chen, Y., Bech, N., et al. (2019). Molecular genetic analysis using targeted NGS analysis of 677 individuals with retinal dystrophy. *Scientific Reports, 9*. https://doi.org/10.1038/s41598-018-38007-2 (accessed on 17th July 2025).

21. Johnson, D. E., Burtness, B., Leemans, C. R., Lui, V. W. Y., Bauman, J. E., & Grandis, J. R. (2020). Head and neck squamous cell carcinoma. *Nature Reviews Disease Primers, 6*. https://doi.org/10.1038/s41572-020-00224-3 (accessed on 17th July 2025).

22. Jony, M. J., Joshi, A., Dash, A. K., & Shukla, S. (2025). Non-viral delivery systems to transport nucleic acids for inherited retinal disorders. *Pharmaceuticals, 18*. https://www.semanticscholar.org/paper/9f0676d6332f85e800822fc8a60cb4a28a79d1ca (accessed on 17th July 2025).

23. Kannnoth, A., & George, S. (2024). Vitamin-dependent genetic disorders of childhood: A comprehensive review. *International Journal of Advanced Research in Medicine*. https://www.semanticscholar.org/paper/f7bb912463619e1408db7fd2c42cba1eb32869cb (accessed on 17th July 2025).

24. Kolanu, N. D. (2024). CRISPR–Cas9 gene editing: Curing genetic diseases by inherited epigenetic modifications. *Global Medical Genetics, 11*, 113–122. https://www.semanticscholar.org/paper/78d72b039aedbb2dc73612f94139b0562e9703fb (accessed on 17th July 2025).

25. Kováč, P., Jackuliak, P., Bražinová, A., Varga, I., Aláč, M., Smatana, M., Lovich, D., et al. (2024). Artificial intelligence-driven facial image analysis for the early detection of rare diseases: Legal, ethical, forensic, and cybersecurity considerations. *AI*. https://www.semanticscholar.org/paper/48b479a78ec64873f6078910115f3812c2a5ebf3 (accessed on 17th July 2025).

26. Langerscheidt, F., Wied, T., Al Kabbani, M. A., van Eimeren, T., Wunderlich, G., & Zempel, H. (2024). Genetic forms of tauopathies: Inherited causes and implications of Alzheimer's disease-like TAU pathology in primary and secondary tauopathies. *Journal of Neurology, 271*, 2992–3018. https://www.semanticscholar.org/paper/8592fc291d81b2be420b967d34522607aa741a30 (accessed on 17th July 2025).

27. Latzer, I. T., & Pearl, P. L. (2024). Inherited metabolic epilepsies—Established diseases, new approaches. *Epilepsia Open*. https://www.semanticscholar.org/paper/57ee3a621549b53cd9962ce97e84235e60c6c3c3 (accessed on 17th July 2025).

28. Ma, J., Zhang, Y., Ding, X., Liang, Z., Yang, C., Deng, Z., He, H., et al. (2023). Co-occurrence of spondyloepiphyseal dysplasia and X-linked hypophosphatemia in a three-generation Chinese family. *Calcified Tissue International, 113*, 266–275. https://www.semanticscholar.org/paper/6a08473308735824a551bed39253f65ef9052f2c (accessed on 17th July 2025).

29. Medical Genetics Branch of Chinese Medical Association, Birth Defects and Molecular Genetics Branch of Chinese Preventive Medicine Association, Clinical Genetics Professional Committee of Shanghai Medical Association, Molecular Diagnosis Branch of Shanghai Medical Association, Bao, Y., Fan, Y., Su, M., et al. (2025). [Expert consensus on the standardized application of whole exome sequencing technology in diagnosis of genetic disorders]. *Zhonghua Yi Xue Yi Chuan Xue Za Zhi = Chinese Journal of Medical Genetics, 42*(1), 1–11. https://www.semanticscholar.org/paper/8e4daa190cac343067aa03ee38b6bf4105e448a7 (accessed on 17th July 2025).

30. Moloney, P., McHugh, J., O'Byrne, J., Llamas, Y., Lynch, T., & McGovern, E. (2022). Ictal aphasia in LGI1-related autosomal dominant epilepsy with auditory features. *Practical Neurology, 22*, 317–320. https://www.semanticscholar.org/paper/0aa8fbef1838e8c58d42a5c562dcff8e15f28cd9 (accessed on 17th July 2025).

31. Morena, J., Gupta, A., & Hoyle, J. C. (2019). Charcot-Marie-Tooth: From molecules to therapy. *International Journal of Molecular Sciences, 20*, 3419–3419. https://doi.org/10.3390/ijms20143419 (accessed on 17th July 2025).

32. Ormond, K. E. (2013). From genetic counseling to "genomic counseling". *Molecular Genetics & Genomic Medicine, 1*, 189–193. https://doi.org/10.1002/mgg3.45 (accessed on 17th July 2025).

33. Parenti, I., Rabaneda, L. G., Schoen, H., & Novarino, G. (2020). Neurodevelopmental disorders: From genetics to functional pathways. *Trends in Neurosciences, 43*, 608–621. https://doi.org/10.1016/j.tins.2020.05.004 (accessed on 17th July 2025).

34. Reproductive Health Branch of China Maternal and Child Health Association, Xu, C. M., Yin, C., Yin, A., Liu, S., Jiang, Y., Luo, Q., et al. (2024). [Expert consensus on the clinical application strategy of NIPT2.0, a new-generation non-invasive prenatal screening technology]. *Zhonghua Yi Xue Yi Chuan Xue Za Zhi = Chinese Journal of Medical Genetics, 41*(10), 1155–1163. https://

www.semanticscholar.org/paper/a1aeea4af3d11679e1b502ab2ab02008a74182f0 (accessed on 17th July 2025).

35. Reuter, M. S., Tawamie, H., Buchert, R., Gebril, O. H., Froukh, T., Thiel, C. T., Uebe, S., et al. (2017). Diagnostic yield and novel candidate genes by exome sequencing in 152 consanguineous families with neurodevelopmental disorders. *JAMA Psychiatry, 74*, 293–293. https://doi.org/10.1001/jamapsychiatry.2016.3798 (accessed on 17th July 2025).

36. Salarian, L., Ilkhanipoor, H., Amirhakimi, A., Afshar, Z., Nahid, S., Moradi Ardekani, F., Rahimi, N., et al. (2025). Epidemiology of inherited metabolic disorders in newborn screening: Insights from three years of experience in Southern Iran. *Orphanet Journal of Rare Diseases, 20*. https://www.semanticscholar.org/paper/6fb15439bbdf5b4b38e2ce3a8de0a57947fd5cf5 (accessed on 17th July 2025).

37. Shirani Asl, V., & Tamaddon, G. (2025). Red blood cell disorders in newborns: Bridging traditional and modern diagnostics. *Fetal and Pediatric Pathology*. https://www.semanticscholar.org/paper/3b367bd4e5a17980d48cd3f3daeb50c88086e23a (accessed on 17th July 2025).

38. Sidonio, R., Bryant, P. C., Di Paola, J., Hale, S. A., Heiman, M., Horowitz, G. S., Humphrey, C., et al. (2023). Building the foundation for a community-generated national research blueprint for inherited bleeding disorders: Research priorities for mucocutaneous bleeding disorders. *Expert Review of Hematology, 16*, 39–54. https://www.semanticscholar.org/paper/b54a729b63ef3d21292a95d0f4dd40fc69dd3209 (accessed on 17th July 2025).

39. Singh, A., Kukreti, R., Saso, L., & Kukreti, S. (2019). Oxidative stress: A key modulator in neurodegenerative diseases. *Molecules, 24*, 1583–1583. https://doi.org/10.3390/molecules24081583 (accessed on 17th July 2025).

40. Tebbi, C. (2022). Sickle cell disease: A review. *Hemato*. https://www.semanticscholar.org/paper/66ebae003acf1930b7be65139ef059cf50cec5ce (accessed on 17th July 2025).

41. Tesfaye, M., Shadrin, A., Parker, N., Jahołkowski, P., Parekh, P., Kutrolli, G., Birkenæs, V., et al. (2024). Comorbidity alters the genetic relationship between anxiety disorders and major depression. *medRxiv*. https://www.semanticscholar.org/paper/ecc8ccae0c5294eed8c7dc5249fc8aba168d0c49 (accessed on 17th July 2025).

42. Tofiloski, S. (2025). Navigating the ethical landscape of molecular psychiatry and behavioral genetics. *Contemporary Research Analysis Journal*. https://www.semanticscholar.org/paper/b9b377d9a77f8b0ff781e7ae6321e344add80a9c (accessed on 17th July 2025).

43. Tukker, A. M., Royal, C., Bowman, A. B., & McAllister, K. A. (2021). The impact of environmental factors on monogenic Mendelian diseases. *Toxicological Sciences, 181*, 3–12. https://doi.org/10.1093/toxsci/kfab022 (accessed on 17th July 2025).

44. Umair, M. (2024). Gene therapy for rare genetic disorders: Transformative progress, challenges, and future prospects. *Journal of Biochemical and Clinical Genetics*. https://www.semanticscholar.org/paper/74c3bf3cffead4762f7c3afda70aa7a831e830b5 (accessed on 17th July 2025).

45. Vasilyeva, T., Marakhonov, A., Tebieva, I. S., Kadyshev, V., Borovikov, A., Markova, Z. G., Chukhrova, A. L., et al. (2023). Genetic heterogeneity of X-linked ichthyosis in the Republic of North Ossetia–Alania, case series report. *International Journal of Molecular Sciences, 24*. https://www.semanticscholar.org/paper/26e6e59fc2452fb85a7377b3360b19bf25501682 (accessed on 17th July 2025).

46. Verbakel, S. K., van Huet, R. A. C., Boon, C. J. F., den Hollander, A. I., Collin, R. W. J., Klaver, C. C. W., Hoyng, C. B., et al. (2018). Non-syndromic retinitis pigmentosa. *Progress in Retinal and Eye Research, 66*, 157–186. https://doi.org/10.1016/j.preteyeres.2018.03.005 (accessed on 17th July 2025).

47. Wang, G., Liao, M., Tan, D., Chen, X., Chao, R., Zhu, Y., Li, P., et al. (2024). Advances in diagnosis and treatment of inherited kidney diseases in children. *Kidney Diseases, 10*, 558–572. https://www.semanticscholar.org/paper/4b92baa742f87b89335bd8827cb5c459d44a6a40 (accessed on 17th July 2025).

48. Wang, Y., Zhao, Z., Wang, R., & Hu, X. (2025). Genetic links between gastrointestinal disorders and kidney stone disease. *Kidney360, 6*, 616–626. https://www.semanticscholar.org/paper/2f9a55cf5ba639b482fd7332b3cc477b20adc646 (accessed on 17th July 2025).

49. Weixel, T., Wolfe, L. A., & Macnamara, E. F. (2024). Genetic counseling for congenital disorders of glycosylation (CDG). *Journal of Genetic Counseling, 33*, 1358–1364. https://www.semanticscholar.org/paper/7ee1ae3fa373f6e4fb50ad2dbdda87c6ce97b660 (accessed on 17th July 2025).

50. Wilde, A. A. M., Semsarian, C., Márquez, M. F., Sepehri Shamloo, A., Ackerman, M. J., Ashley, E. A., Sternick, E. B., et al. (2022). European Heart Rhythm Association (EHRA)/Heart Rhythm Society (HRS)/Asia Pacific Heart Rhythm Society (APHRS)/Latin American Heart Rhythm Society (LAHRS) expert consensus statement on the state of genetic testing for cardiac diseases. *Heart Rhythm, 19*, e1–e60. https://doi.org/10.1016/j.hrthm.2022.03.1225 (accessed on 17th July 2025).

51. Xavier, M. J., Roman, S. D., Aitken, R. J., & Nixon, B. (2019). Transgenerational inheritance: How impacts to the epigenetic and genetic information of parents affect offspring health. *Human Reproduction Update, 25*, 519–541. https://doi.org/10.1093/humupd/dmz017 (accessed on 17th July 2025).

52. Zeppenfeld, K., Tfelt-Hansen, J., Riva, M., Winkel, B. G., Behr, E. R., Blom, N. A., Charron, P., et al. (2022). 2022 ESC guidelines for the management of patients with ventricular arrhythmias and the prevention of sudden cardiac death. *European Heart Journal, 43*, 3997–4126. https://doi.org/10.1093/eurheartj/ehac262 (accessed on 17th July 2025).

53. Zhang, T., Briere, J. M., Leeman, K. T., Wojcik, M., & Agrawal, P. (2022). Ethical implications of early genetic diagnosis in an infant with Lesch–Nyhan syndrome. *Journal of Genetic Counseling, 31*, 1434–1437. https://www.semanticscholar.org/paper/a183f766e94a1dcf1d38f66739de2c3a6e45ef96 (accessed on 17th July 2025).

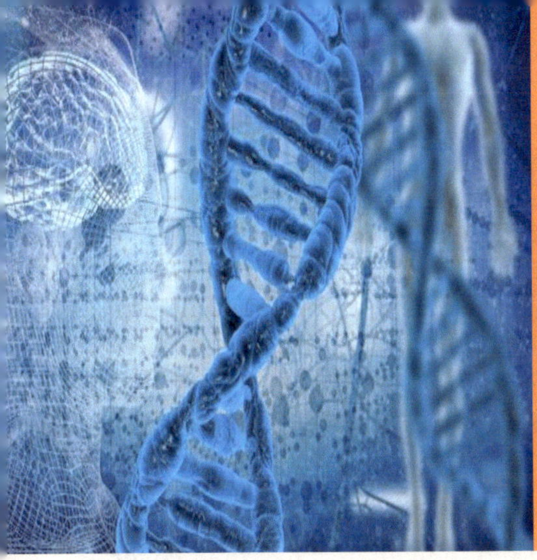

Chapter 9

EPIGENETICS AND DISEASE

Contents

Introduction

Understanding the complex interaction between the environmental and genetic components is crucial when examining the disease onset mechanisms. Epigenetics, or heritable changes in gene expression independent of alterations in the sequence of DNA, has emerged as an important area of interest in clinical investigations. By examining how nongenetic factors, such as lifestyle, diet, and environmental exposures, influence gene expression, researchers obtain information on new aspects of disease susceptibility and heterogeneity. This is particularly noted in conditions like Wilson-Konovalov disease (WKD), a genetic disorder exhibiting vast phenotypic diversity despite sharing an identical genotype among affected populations. The intersection of epigenetic alterations with intrinsic genetic vulnerabilities emphasizes the complexity of pathologies, suggesting that the understanding of such interactions is essential to further therapeutic interventions and preventive measures in disease treatment (Komarova et al., 2025). Moreover, the heterogeneity of metabolic health among obese subjects mirrors the significance of epigenetic regulation in cardiometabolic disease. Research has revealed that despite the prevalence of obesity as a significant risk factor for conditions , such as diabetes and hypertension, some proportion of obese individuals are metabolically healthy. This is because of differences in inflammation and resolution of inflammation, which may be underpinned by epigenetic alterations. Based on studies that categorize people in terms of metabolic health, there can be great variability in systemic inflammation levels and immune response, which illuminate how epigenetic mechanisms result in health outcomes during obesity. By delineating these pathways, not just our knowledge of disease is enhanced, but so is clinical practice and public health policy (Tavajoh et al., 2025). In essence, the study of epigenetics provides a valuable window into the investigation of most diseases, and indeed most significantly those with complex presentations from a mix of genetic and environmental influences. The heterogeneity in diseases like WKD and in individuals who are obese highlights the potential that epigenetics has to uncover significant information regarding disease mechanisms. Future research into the pathways whereby epigenetic changes drive gene expression and disease onset will be essential for the development of personalized medicine interventions, allowing health care providers to tailor interventions according to an individual's unique genetic and epigenetic profile. As the field matures, not only does it hold the promise of expanding our understanding of previously known diseases, but it also enables novel diagnostic and therapeutic approaches in the realm of epigenetics and disease (Figure 9.1).

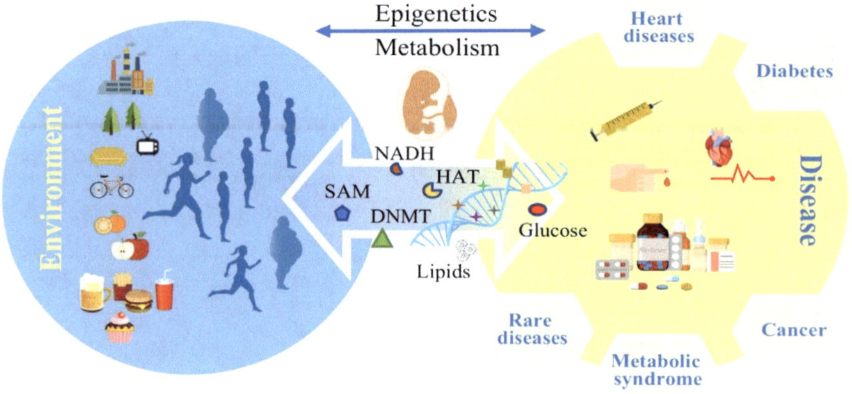

Figure 9.1. Epigenetics and disease.

Source: https://www.frontiersin.org/files/Articles/410886/fgene-09-00361-HTML-r2/image_m/fgene-09-00361-g001.jpg.

Definition of Epigenetics

Epigenetics is a fascinating intersection of genetics and the environment, effectively rewriting our understanding of heredity and gene expression. Epigenetics, by definition, is the stable and heritable adjustment of gene function that occurs in the absence of changes to the underlying DNA sequence. Such modifications, which can be initiated by environmental signals , such as diet, lifestyle, and poisons, ultimately determine which genes are activated or suppressed. The two major mechanisms of this complex regulatory system are DNA methylation and histone modification. DNA methylation involves the addition of methyl groups to cytosine bases within CpG dinucleotides, and it has the capacity to inhibit gene transcription. Meanwhile, histone modifications—through mechanisms , including methylation, acetylation, and phosphorylation—can alter chromatin accessibility and thus influence gene expression. The intricacy of such processes gives a dynamic stage from which the capacity of external factors to elicit phenotypically demonstrable change can be understood. Subsequent research repeatedly emphasizes the contribution epigenetics makes to disease conditions, most significantly metabolic and autoimmune disease. Epigenetic alterations have been called upon, for instance, in malignancies in which deranged patterns of DNA methylation have the capability to silence tumor suppressor genes or to activate oncogenes and thus foster malignancy. Furthermore, autoimmune diseases tend to have epigenetically dysregulated regulation, in which environmental signals can trigger dysregulated immune reactions via epigenetic means. Epigenetics is not merely the domain of disease, however, but also of therapeutic promise, since targeted epigenetic therapy can correct gene expression profiles during disease. This intricate interaction between epigenetics and disease underscores the necessity of further research into how epigenetic pathways are utilized for targeted therapeutic measures and prevention. Recent reviews attest to the evidence that diet- and bioactive compound-modulated genetic regulation is of promising interest for therapeutic intervention for the control of diseases involving epigenetic dysregulation. For example, the evidence indicates that certain natural compounds can modulate mitochondrial activity and alter epigenetic status, thereby influencing molecular networks necessary for cellular homeostasis. In metabolic dysfunction-associated steatotic fatty liver disease (MASLD), for example, dietary and lifestyle interventions are starting to be regarded as highly significant therapeutic interventions. Epigenetic modifications, like DNA methylation alterations and regulation of non-coding RNA, can play major roles in MASLD and disorder pathogenesis as well as treatment. These findings emphasize improved knowledge on how nutritional interventions can induce desirable epigenetic changes, leading to preventative medicine strategies and therapeutic innovations within the new epigenetics field (Caputo et al., 2023).

Importance of Studying Epigenetics in Relation to Disease

Epigenetics has increasingly been highlighted in research to uncover the basic mechanisms of many diseases. One of the key areas is the impact of environmental influences on gene expression, which is mostly controlled by epigenetic modifications. These include DNA methylation and histone acetylation, which control gene activity without directly altering the DNA sequence itself. This would mean that environmental factors like diet, stress, and exposure to toxins can lead to epigenome alterations that make one vulnerable to diseases. For instance, the consumption of short-chain fatty acids (SCFAs) in diets has been associated with epigenetic imprinting that is protective against inflammatory diseases, demonstrating how diets can significantly affect disease susceptibility through epigenetics (Fulton et al., 2021). Therefore, knowing these mechanisms could provide insights into prevention, resulting in personalized healthcare interventions that take into consideration the unique epigenetic makeup of individuals. Studying epigenetics is also a vital key in identifying complex diseases like cancer, wherein epigenetic modifications result in aberrant gene expression patterns. Tumors often have specific epigenetic signatures that distinguish them from normal tissues and could serve as biomarkers for diagnosis and prognosis in most instances. Moreover, epigenetic modification-guided therapeutic interventions, such as the use of histone deacetylase inhibitors, are also hopeful anticancer therapies. The ability to reverse deleterious epigenetic changes is the key to restoring normal gene function, and this opens up a novel therapeutic avenue (Gausman & Langer, 2020). The new treatment approach highlights the need to translate epigenetic research into practice, to expand our understanding of disease biology and treatment efficacy. Lastly, public health is the field impacted by the implications of epigenetic studies, specifically in addressing health disparities by socioeconomic status. The epigenome is sensitive to several environmental factors and lifestyle influences, which reinforce health disparities. Public health interventions can be developed from examination of these correlations and thereby reverse the adverse effects of socio-economic and environmental exposure on health outcomes. For example, interventions in favor of healthier lifestyles or dieting can significantly affect gene expression in chronic disease. For this reason, studying epigenetics offers an effective model for describing how genetics, environment, and lifestyle interact in causation and prevention of disease, resulting in improved health solutions and policy within diverse populations (Gausman & Langer, 2020; Fulton et al., 2021).

9.1. Basics of Epigenetics

The epigenetics concept is a paradigm change in the understanding of gene regulation and expression, which shows that the genome is not fixed but dynamic in reaction to internal and external stimuli. The epigenetic processes, such as DNA methylation, histone modification, and RNA interference, broadly modulate gene expression without changing the underlying DNA sequence. These processes direct sophisticated biological processes, such as cell differentiation, development, and reaction to the environment. In pathology, abnormal epigenetic alterations can lead to cancer and tumorigenesis. For example, it has been demonstrated that HDACs are significantly overexpressed in various cancers, which provides support for the tumor growth environment through the repression of apoptosis and cell cycle controlling genes (James et al., 2020). Therefore, knowledge of the basics of epigenetics enlightens us on the pathways that might be pivotal in both the onset and progression of diseases. Furthermore, knowledge of the basics of epigenetics is imperative for unveiling the mysteries surrounding cancer initiation and drug resistance. Epigenetic alterations may lead to cellular characteristics that are tumor cell-favorable in terms of survival and growth, as demonstrated in hematologic malignancies , such as acute lymphoblastic leukemia (ALL).

In such a case, the bone marrow niche plays a critical role in facilitating chemoresistance, a unifying hindrance to effective treatment. Literature has indicated that the interaction of leukemic cells with the environment of the bone marrow might lead to cell-protective strategies aiding survival within chemotherapy regimens (Quagliano et al., 2020). Of particular note, targeted epigenetic therapies have proven to be promising avenues of overcoming these adaptations. By modulation of epigenetic markers, cancer cells can become sensitized to chemotherapy, thereby enhancing treatment effectiveness and patient response. Aside from its use in cancer, the concepts of epigenetics are seen in other diseases, including neurodegenerative and metabolic syndromes. These diseases have generally been shown to possess altered epigenetic signatures, which could be due to a combination of genetic and environmental determinants , such as diet, stress, and exposure to toxins. For instance, epigenetic modulation of DNA methylation and histone marks has been implicated in diseases like Alzheimer's disease, where these modifications could regulate cognitive impairment by influencing neuronal survival and function. The discovery of the role of epigenetics in such diseases not only enhances our understanding of their etiology but also presents novel therapeutic options due to the reversible nature of epigenetic modifications. With continued research, the condition of epigenetics will only enhance preventive measures and treatments in the various branches of medicine (Figure 9.2).

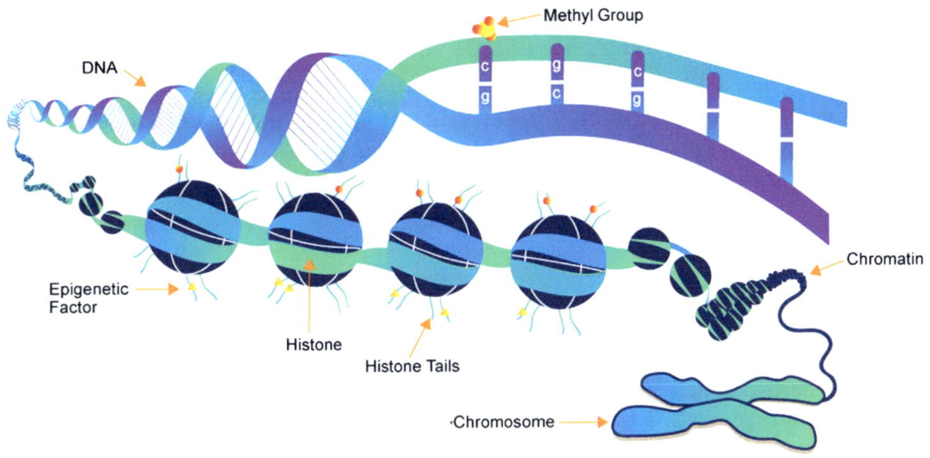

Figure 9.2. Basics of epigenetics.

Source: https://www.whatisepigenetics.com/wp-content/uploads/2013/07/dna-chromatin-histone.jpg.

9.1.1. Mechanisms of Epigenetic Regulation

The epigenetic mechanisms of regulation are significant in the control of gene expression without altering the actual DNA sequence. Of most significance among them are DNA methylation, histone modification, and non-coding RNAs. DNA methylation involves the addition of a methyl group to the cytosine residues, often to CpG dinucleotides, and this can lead to transcriptional gene silencing. On the other hand, histone modifications , such as acetylation and methylation relax or condense the chromatin structure, with an ultimate impact on entry to the transcription machinery. Moreover, non-coding RNAs, namely microRNAs and long non-coding RNAs, are also paramount actors in post-transcriptional regulation via messenger RNA degradation or chromatin dynamic regulation. Cumulatively, these mechanisms constitute a sophisticated system of regulation that is deeply interwoven with the pathology of numerous diseases and ultimately controls cellular behavior and identity. Pathological ramifications of deranged epigenetic control have been reported in various diseases, including neurodegenerative diseases and muscular dystrophies. Alzheimer's disease (AD), for instance, has shown a remarkable association with mitochondrial malfunction, which is complemented by the breakdown of epigenetic mechanisms. Evidence indicates that agents like alpha-lipoic acid (α-LA) are endowed with protective roles via the induction of mitochondrial biogenesis and control of inflammatory responses; significantly, α-LA also exhibits epigenetic controlling mechanisms by influencing the expression of inflammatory-related genes like COX-2 and TNF-α. This dual action is meant to emphasize the utility of targeting epigenetic pathways as therapeutic interventions aimed at halting or even reversing the course of diseases like AD. These newer approaches promise to transform disease control and offer new hope for more effective interventions. Facioscapulohumeral muscular dystrophy (FSHD) is a particularly intriguing example of how epigenetic regulation can directly contribute to the emergence of disease. FSHD entails dysregulation by ectopic expression of the DUX4 gene, which disrupts normal muscle function. This occurs when the rearrangement of chromatin leads to the inappropriate expression of this gene, thereby triggering a pathogenic cascade that manifests in muscle pathology. By understanding the specific chromatin regulators involved in FSHD, scientists can selectively target these factors to normalize patterns of gene expression and reverse disease effects. The studies on FSHD not only underscore the importance of localized epigenetic mechanisms but also define new avenues for therapeutic development. Moving towards therapies by the eyes of epigenetic modification may open doors to targeted therapies aimed at correcting the underlying causes of genetic expression modifications, leading to improved patient outcomes (Figure 9.3).

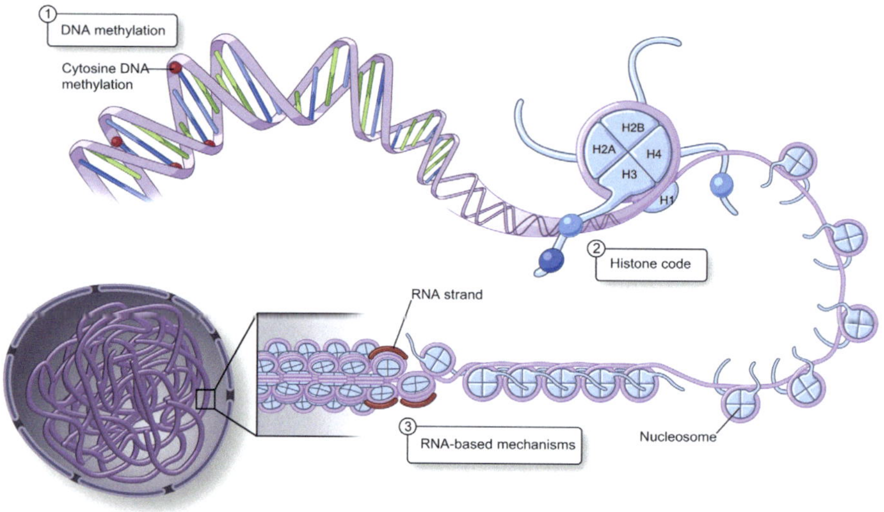

Figure 9.3. Mechanisms of epigenetic regulation.

Source: https://www.researchgate.net/profile/Charles-Matouk/publication/43299038/figure/fig1/AS:601788541579264@1520488977260/Three-fundamental-mechanisms-of-epigenetic-gene-regulation-Epigenetic-mechanisms-of-gene.png.

9.1.2. Role of DNA Methylation

DNA methylation is a key epigenetic regulatory mechanism that influences gene expression without altering the underlying DNA sequence. The alteration is typically in cytosine residues in CpG dinucleotides and is a critical mechanism in genomic imprinting, transcriptional silencing, and chromatin remodeling. As an epigenetic marker, DNA methylation is integral to numerous biological processes, such as the regulation of inflammation and immune response. The disease-DNA methylation connection has come to the forefront, particularly for chronic inflammatory diseases, where dysregulation of the methylation pattern can speed up the disease process. For example, in the case of systemic low-grade inflammation, the discovery of differential DNA methylation sites associated with biomarkers , such as C-reactive protein (CRP) bears consequences for understanding pathogenetic mechanisms and therapeutic approaches, evidence for a deep connection between methylation and chronic disease (Katu, 2024). Intensified investigation of DNA methylation indicates that it is involved in various pathological conditions, especially those affecting oral health diseases , such as periodontal and peri-implant diseases. The dysregulation of methylation in inflammatory response genes has been linked to variations in the susceptibility and severity of disease.

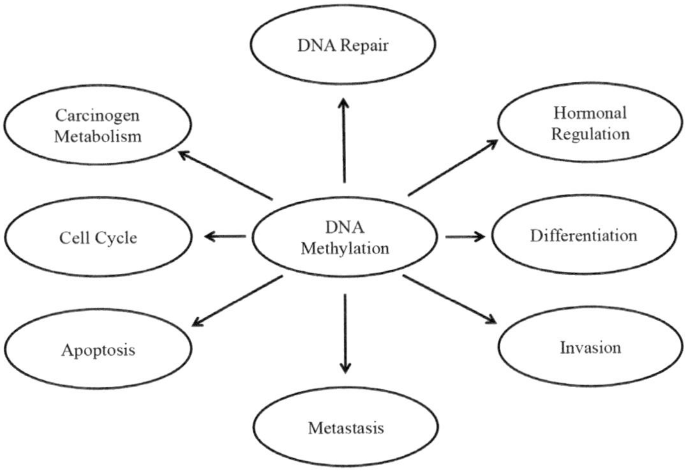

Figure 9.4. Role of DNA methylation.

Source: https://www.researchgate.net/profile/Eric-Buckles-2/publication/224871549/figure/fig2/AS:393839203373059@1470909991284/Fig-2-Schematic-diagram-of-involvement-of-DNA-methylation-in-different-cellular.png.

In periodontitis, for instance, increased levels of certain methylation enzymes correlate with the severity of the disease, influencing the production of pro-inflammatory cytokines and the initial-line immune response to microbial injury. In addition, studies delineate the role of DNA methylation in regulating innate immune response genes, again showing its complex interaction with inflammatory pathways like the toll-like receptor signal pathway. This has emphasized the importance of acquiring such knowledge in comprehending the molecular processes to develop targeted treatments and preventive strategies in oral diseases (Larsson et al., 2024). Interestingly, advancements in research on methylation dynamics extend beyond the DNA because emerging evidence has emphasized the role of RNA methylation as well. In diseases like periodontitis and peri-implantitis, RNA methylation pattern modifications have been linked to immune response modulation and inflammation. For instance, methylation modifications , such as N6-methyladenosine (m6A) have been shown to regulate gene expression as well as inflammatory cytokine production. These findings push the pursuit of a more combined concept of molecular states of disease and interactive functions of DNA and RNA methylation in directing pathophysiological states. By interrogating these epigenetic networks, researchers can continue to reveal mechanisms that result in disease and even inform novel therapeutic pathways that leverage these insights for improved patient outcomes (Larsson et al., 2024) (Figure 9.4).

9.1.3. Influence of Histone Modification

The role of histone modification in gene expression is the leading area of study in epigenetics and disease mechanisms, and in this respect, histones, the protein subunits around which DNA winds, are amenable to a variety of post-translational modifications, i.e., acetylation, methylation, and phosphorylation. Each of these modifications has a significant impact on chromatin structure and gene accessibility, thus controlling transcriptional activity. Emerging research has elucidated how aberrant patterns of histone modifications lead to dysregulated gene expression implicated in most diseases, more so neurodegenerative diseases like Alzheimer's disease (AD). Notably, studies have demonstrated that some modifications of histones are associated with the expression of genes related to neuronal function and synaptic plasticity, important processes whose disruption might underlie AD pathology (De Plano et al., 2024). Therefore, understanding the role of histone modifications sheds light on the molecular mechanisms of disease development and can result in new therapies. Histone modifications are not only biomarkers of disease progression but also potential targets for therapy.

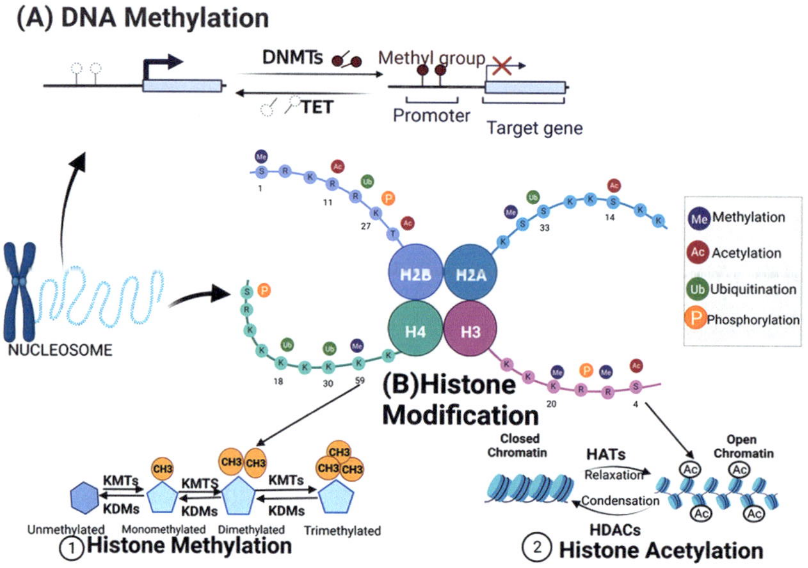

Figure 9.5. Influence of histone modification.

Source: https://www.researchgate.net/publication/362300155/figure/fig1/AS:11431281097640882@1668655865883/The-mechanism-of-DNA-methylation-and-histone-modification-in-detail-ADNA-Methylation.png.

In cardiovascular diseases, hypertension in particular, histone modifications proved to be key regulatory processes that regulate blood pressure regulation and vascular homeostasis. Dysregulation in histone acetylation and methylation patterns is most closely linked with essential hypertension pathophysiology. The research identifies that such alterations can affect the expression of genes involved in crucial pathways, like the renin-angiotensin system, a significant blood pressure regulator (Karabaeva et al., 2024). With the unwinding of such complex interactions by researchers, the hope is growing that manipulation of histone modifications can create new avenues to treat high blood pressure, especially in comorbid diseases like type 2 diabetes mellitus, where the susceptibility to coronary artery disease is heightened. The dynamic relationship between histone modifications and the environment once again points towards the pivotal role of epigenetics in disease and health. Environmental determinants , such as diet, stress, and exposure to toxins could lead to histone mark alteration, which would eventually impact disease susceptibility and advancement. For example, certain nutrients in food have been reported to regulate histone acetylation, enhancing or inhibiting gene expression involved in disease conditions like obesity and related complications. Consequently, histone modification research offers a profound understanding of the two-way interaction between genes and the environment, with emphasis on epigenetic determinants of disease etiologies. With more research, de-mystifying these interactions will not only produce increased understanding of disease mechanisms but also inform the development of targeted treatment approaches that account for individual epigenetic signatures and environmental responses to modifications (Figure 9.5).

9.2. Epigenetics and Cancer

The intricate association between epigenetics and cancer is evidenced by the presence of abnormal gene expression patterns during tumorigenesis. Epigenetic modifications like DNA methylation and histone alterations are important in regulating gene function without altering the underlying DNA sequence. For instance, in colorectal cancer (CRC), development from benign polyps to malignant tumors is coupled with intricate genetic and epigenetic changes that encompass the cancer's development. Exosome involvement, small vesicles implicated in intercellular communication, has been a significant focal point. Exosomes transport molecular cargoes that determine cancer biology, particularly metastasis, where they convey factors that control tumor behavior. This convergence of exosomal dynamics and epigenetics accentuates the complexity of CRC advancement and suggests therapies employing these pathways in the battle against malignancy (Rani, 2025). Following the elucidation of roles for exosomes in CRC, additional research into other epigenetic pathways should be pursued. Histone modification, particularly that which is performed by SET domain bifurcated 1 (SETDB1), is a major paradigm in the meeting of epigenomics and cancer. SETDB1 is a lysine histone methyltransferase, and it mediates the methylation of histone 3 lysine 9 and leads to the repression of transcription of essential genes. Overexpression and inappropriate activation of SETDB1 are linked to unfavorable prognosis in most cancers, including HCC. This connection demonstrates the feasibility of targeting such epigenetic modifiers in the development of effective immunotherapeutic strategies. By understanding the molecular mechanisms through which SETDB1 influences tumorigenesis and immune evasion, researchers can identify novel therapeutic approaches aimed at reversing these epigenetic alterations (Zhang et al., 2024). The reciprocal interplay between cancer and epigenetic alterations represents not only a sophisticated understanding of tumor biology but also the potential for novel forms of therapy. As science continues to evolve, the detection of particular epigenetic markers will improve early diagnosis and prognosis for numerous cancers. Furthermore, the application of epigenetic therapy can normalize gene expression profiles in the tumor and reverse or halt cancer progression. Identification of ceramide-dependent exosomal cargoes and their function in CRC is only one part of the intricate web that relates epigenetics to cancer. Application of such findings will be a key factor in uncovering novel therapeutic avenues that bridge biological understanding to the clinical setting. Lastly, the inclusion of epigenetics in diversifying cancer treatments is of monumental potential in maximizing patient benefits and fighting malignant disorders' multi-factorial challenges (Rani, 2025; Zhang et al., 2024) (Figure 9.6).

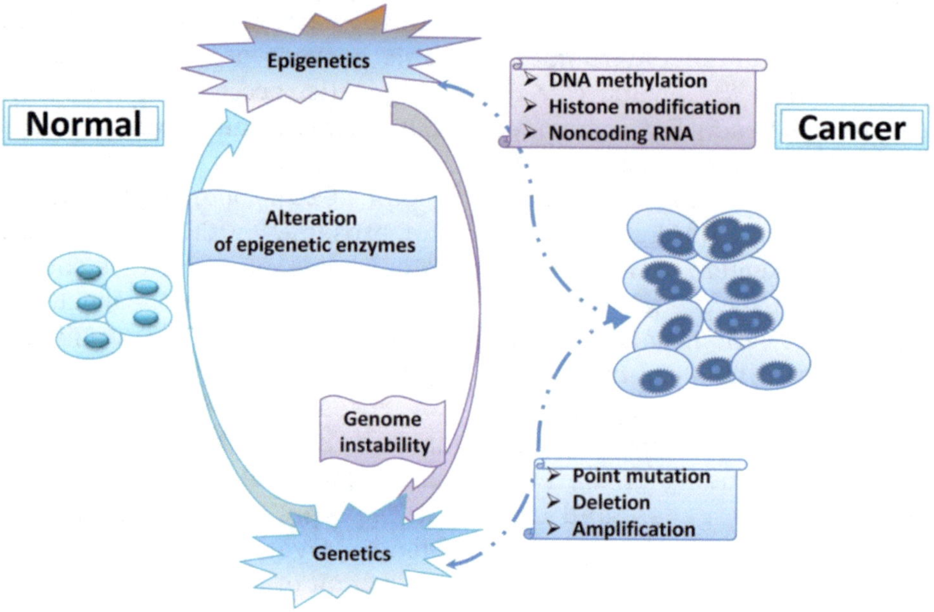

Figure 9.6. Epigenetics and cancer.

Source: https://www.spandidos-publications.com/article_images/or/31/2/OR-31-02-0523-g02.jpg.

9.2.1. Epigenetic Changes in Tumorigenesis

The intricate interaction between tumorigenesis and epigenetic changes has recently gained significant attention, with an understanding of how these changes affect tumorigenesis. DNA methylation, one of the most significant epigenetic changes, is the addition of methyl groups to the cytosine residues in DNA and can have a significant effect on gene expression. Global DNA methylation pattern alteration has been linked to deregulating cellular pathways for carcinogenic changes. Notably, advances in DNA methylation profiling, including single-cell analysis and ultra-long read sequencing technologies, have enabled the establishment of a more precise understanding of these epigenetic changes in various cancers and thus highlight their essential contribution to tumorigenesis and cancer progression (Skvortsova et al., 2019). By the elucidation of methylation landscape between normal and cancerous cells, scientists are able to identify particular genes that can be candidate biomarkers for pre-diagnosis and therapeutic targets. Moreover, the role of histone modification in carcinogenesis complements existing knowledge about the dynamics of DNA methylation. Histones, the protein cores around which DNA is wrapped, undergo many modifications that activate or repress transcription. One such important player in this line of work is histone methyltransferase EZH2, whose involvement in repression of transcription via trimethylation of histone 3 lysine 27 (H3K27) has been established. Overexpression of EZH2 in ovarian cancer, for example, is a widespread phenomenon leading to global silencing of tumor suppressor genes and the ensuing aggressiveness of the disease. With its pivotal role in the epigenetic machine, EZH2 became a promising target for treatment, and several small-molecule inhibitors are currently in clinical trials to reverse the epigenetic derangements that underlie cancer growth (Jones et al., 2018). Such focus on therapeutic interventions underscores the significance of defining epigenetic modifications in combating cancer. Identifying epigenetic alterations in tumorigenesis not only sheds light on cancer biology but also opens up avenues for new treatment strategies. With ongoing investigation, the possibility of utilizing epigenetic alterations as diagnostic and prognostic markers is increasingly becoming a reality. The dynamic nature of these changes means that they must be reversible, and it is hoped that therapeutic intervention may result in a correction towards normal gene expression patterns within tumors. With broad studies on the epigenetic patterns of various cancers, the mechanisms of resistance against commonly used therapies, researchers are identifying novel targets for intervention. The ultimate goal will be a better understanding of the epigenetic changes in tumorigenesis, which will enhance the specificity of cancer therapy, resulting in more targeted and individualized therapy protocols with the potential to improve patient outcomes and survival rates along the continuum of cancer (Figure 9.7).

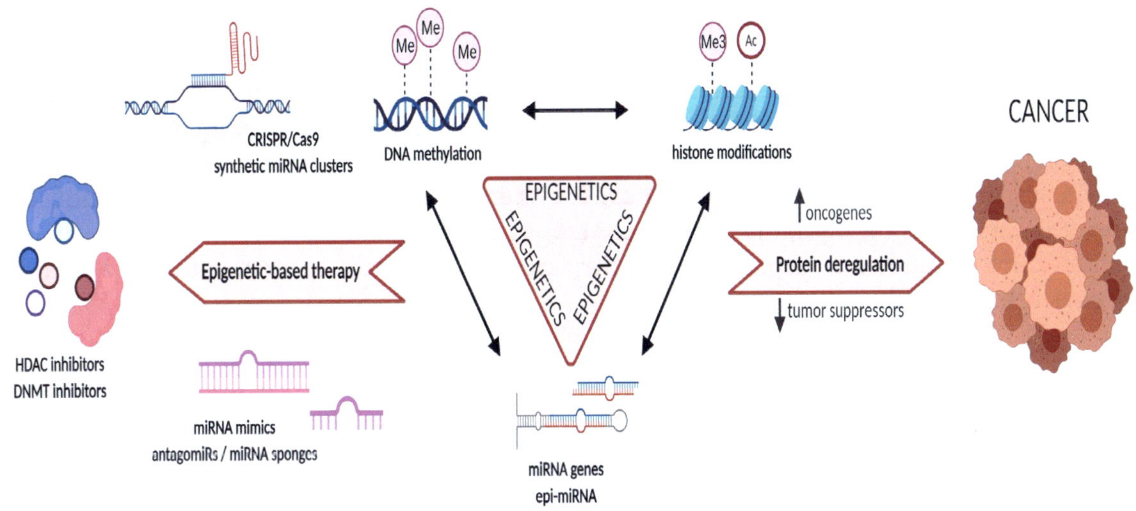

Figure 9.7. Epigenetic changes in tumorigenesis.

Source: https://pub.mdpi-res.com/cancers/cancers-13-01333/article_deploy/html/images/cancers-13-01333-ag.png?1616068590.

9.2.2. Role of Epigenetics in Cancer Progression

The convergence of carcinogenesis and epigenetics has emerged as a primary area of research, revealing the mechanisms by which heritable epigenetic alterations contribute to cancer development and metastasis. Unlike genetic mutations that alter the code of DNA, epigenetic modifications—, such as DNA methylation and histone modifications—regulate gene function without altering the underlying DNA sequence. These alterations can be induced by the cellular microenvironment, lifestyle, and environmental stimuli, creating a dynamic landscape in which normal cell function can become deregulated. For instance, hypermethylation of tumor suppressor genes can silence their activity to allow uncontrolled cell growth. Understanding these alterations is important to an understanding of the mechanisms driving cancer development and could pave the way for novel therapies aimed at specifically addressing these epigenetic modifications. Other than regulating genes directly, epigenetics is also essential in the broader scheme of cell signaling pathways, influencing the way cancer cells will respond to stimulation. MicroRNA function, small non-coding RNAs that have a function in post-transcriptional regulation, is often regulated by epigenetic elements, which affect cell growth, differentiation, and apoptosis. By these routes, epigenetic modifications can not only impart the intrinsic characteristics of cancer cells but also shape their behaviors in interacting with the surrounding tumor microenvironment. This reciprocal talk can further enhance cancer development by promoting angiogenesis, invasion, and immune evasion. Hence, treatments focusing on the reversal of epigenetic modifications are gaining attention as they hold the promise of restoring normal cellular function and suppressing tumor development. The potential for the use of epigenetic alterations as cancer diagnostic and prognostic biomarkers is an exciting new frontier in oncology. Epigenetic alterations can be detected in readily available bodily fluids, such as blood or urine, and thereby enable non-invasive cancer screening methods. Such biomarkers would provide crucial information regarding the presence and development of cancer and aid in earlier intervention and individualized therapeutic regimens. Moreover, the advent of epigenetic drugs that aim to reestablish regular epigenetic patterns offers possible avenues for the struggle against refractory cancer phenotypes. From the alignment of epigenetics and disease, or more specifically, cancer, researchers are able to conceptualize new approaches to maximize patient efficacy and stimulate innovation in cancer therapy models. Specifically, as is noted in the literature, the detection of anomalies in the control of epigenesis may reveal previously unknown pathways of carcinogenesis and provide an entry point for targeted interventions (Amina, 2024; Nicheperovich et al., 2025) (Figure 9.8).

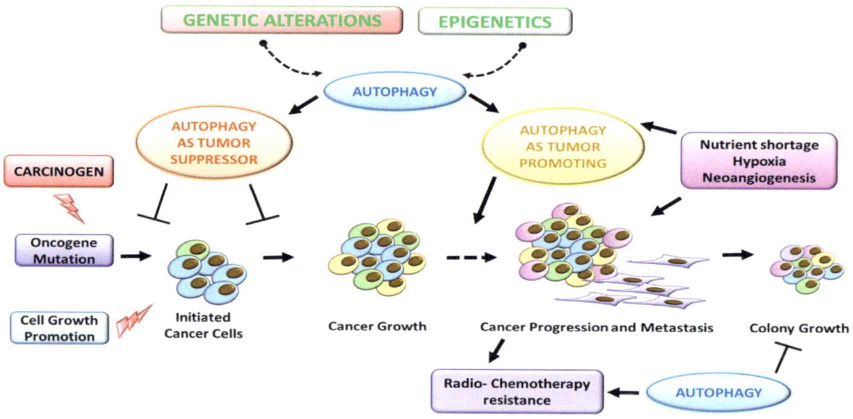

Figure 9.8. Epigenetics in cancer progression.

Source: https://www.researchgate.net/publication/360809469/figure/fig7/AS:1159223450845184@1653391816010/Dual-role-of-autophagy-in-cancer-progression-Involvement-of-epigenetic-mechanism-on.jpg.

9.2.3. Potential for Epigenetic Therapies in Oncology

The study of epigenetic therapies in cancer is a paradigm-shifting promise that aligns with the modern face of oncology. Epigenetics are heritable gene expression alterations that do not involve a modification of the DNA sequence but rather occur through mechanisms , such as DNA methylation and histone modification. These epigenetic modifications play an important role in tumoral growth and tumor progression because they can induce the activation of oncogenes or the repression of tumor suppressor genes. The reversibility of these epigenetic alterations under treatment propels the emergence of targeted treatment, which enhances the ability to target the unique molecular characteristics of cancers.

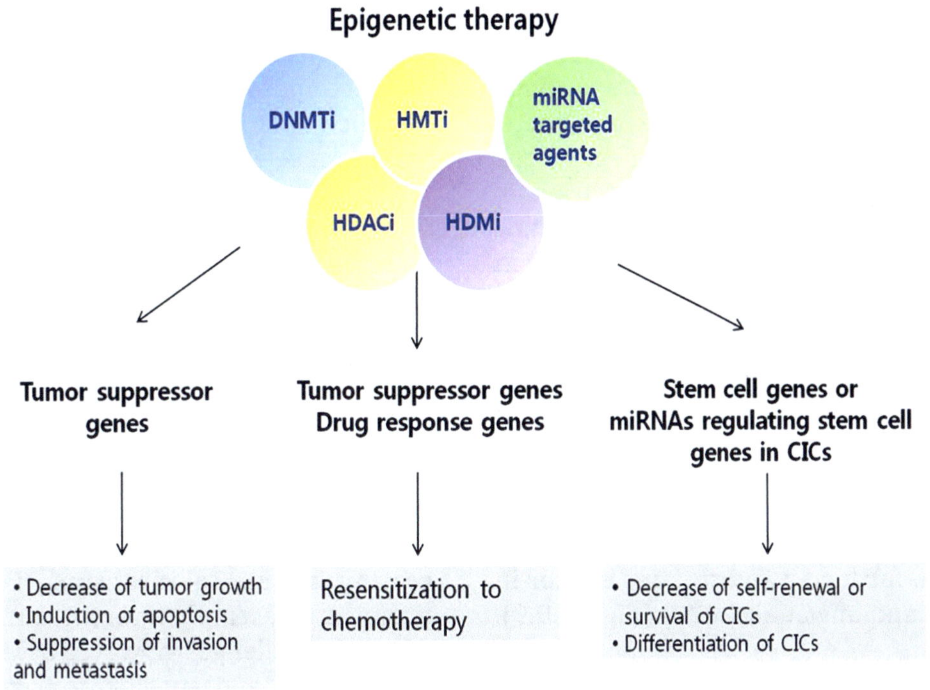

Figure 9.9. Epigenetic therapies in oncology.

Source: https://www.mdpi.com/ijms/ijms-12-00983/article_deploy/html/images/ijms-12-00983f2-1024.png.

The common role of epigenetic marks as cancer prognosis biomarkers and therapeutic targets underscores their significance in harmonizing personalized medicine approaches in oncology (Takahashi et al., 2024). Recent advances in the understanding of immune mechanisms, especially trained immunity, have opened up new possibilities for epigenetic therapy to be applied in cancer therapy. Trained immunity is elicited through epigenetic reprogramming of innate immune cells to enable them to mount better responses upon encountering pathogens or tumor cells. In the tumor microenvironment (TME), epigenetic modulation could enhance the therapeutic efficacy of immune checkpoint inhibitors and gene-engineered T cells. This is because it has the potential to generate an inflammatory milieu, enhance cytotoxic T cell populations, and reverse immunosuppression—

factors which directly lead to therapeutic outcome. Moreover, the knowledge of how various microorganisms and vaccines generate tumoricidal activity through trained immunity suggests the necessity of further investigation into the integration of these mechanisms with epigenetic strategies to treat cancer (Takahashi et al., 2024). Epigenetic therapy has become increasingly prevalent in clinical use with the approval of numerous small-molecule inhibitors of single epigenetic enzymes. Histone deacetylase inhibitors and DNA methyltransferase inhibitors have also shown therapeutic effects in the treatment of a wide variety of cancers, proving the ability to reverse disease-causing epigenetic modifications. Clinical applications of epigenetic drugs extend beyond the direct inhibition of tumor expansion but are also being increasingly included in combination therapies to augment the strength of proven treatments. Furthermore, ongoing research in detecting other epigenetic markers and their modulation using new methods provides a dynamic future prospect in cancer therapy. With increasing depth of understanding of epigenetic landscapes, the potential for novel therapeutic strategies based on epigenetics continues to expand, outlining a new paradigm for facing and treating cancer in the future (Zhanqiang et al., 2023) (Figure 9.9).

9.3. Epigenetics in Neurological Disorders

Epigenetics is important in our knowledge of diseases of the nervous system, providing information regarding the intricate biological processes that lie behind conditions like Alzheimer's disease and glioma. As more research is carried out in this area, it becomes clear that environmental influences, lifestyle options, genetics, and various factors interact with each other in complex manners to change gene expression without a change to the DNA sequence itself. This holds particularly for neurological diseases, where epigenetic alterations , such as DNA methylation and histone modification, can potentially influence disease pathology and course. The potential for therapy of epigenetic treatments, especially in conditions using cutting-edge technologies like CRISPR interference, provides promising new options for treatment and management of such diseases, with hopeful targeted therapies that can be employed to prevent symptoms or reverse disease progression. New advances in understanding the epigenetic context of neurological diseases emphasize the need for effective approaches to cope with the complexity of such disorders. For instance, CRISPR interference employs RNA-guided inhibited Cas proteins in the regulation of gene expression without causing double-strand breaks and hence less secondary genetic alterations. The approach has been said to be successful at the preclinical level, especially when it targets crucial genes that underlie the pathogenesis of Alzheimer's, such as APP, and gliomas by regulation of MGMT and TERT expression. Notably, these interventions function to correct disease-causing epigenetic changes, thus placing particular therapeutic potential on epigenetic editing as an intervention. Bringing such promising research into the clinic is open to daunting challenges, however, at least in delivery mechanisms and specificity across the blood-brain barrier. Public interest and perception in brain health also reflect the mounting realization of the interconnection between epigenetics and neurological disease. One interesting survey showed that, while the interviewees were aware of lifestyle effects on brain function, they were less aware of socioeconomic determinants that also play a significant role in the development of these diseases. Out of the polled group, a high level of connection was perceived between Alzheimer's disease and the significance of maintaining brain fitness through various stages of life. Notably, women and individuals with higher educational achievements placed more emphasis on determinants of brain health. These results require concerted public health activity aimed at generating awareness and promoting behaviors that can lower neurologic disease risk. The integration of such knowledge with novel epigenetic studies would potentially be able to inform future disease prevention and disease management approaches, thus contributing to the general body of knowledge about brain health and disease (Budin-Ljøsne et al., 2022; Lu, 2024) (Figure 9.10).

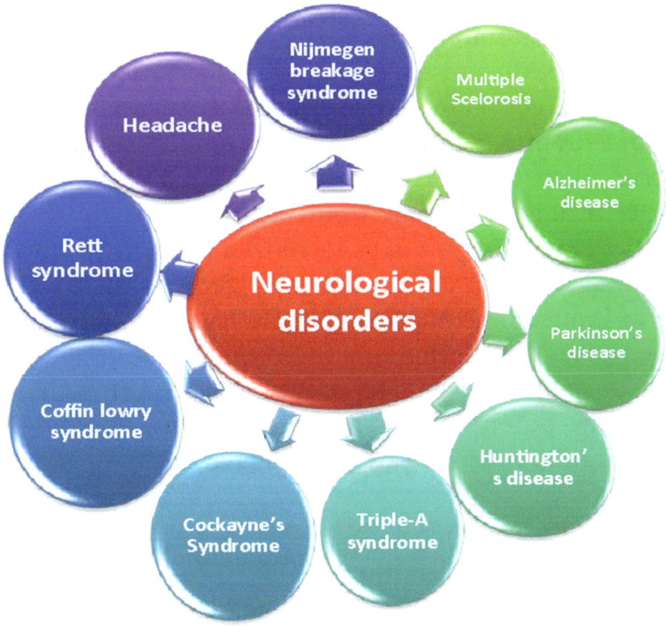

Figure 9.10. Neurological disorders.

Source: https://www.semanticscholar.org/paper/Epigenetic-and-Therapeutic-Analysis-of-various-Tripathy/e77fa511765189135078df33dadf76969be6617b/figure/0.

9.3.1. Impact of Epigenetics on Brain Development

The function of epigenetics in brain development is an important one, as it influences a number of biological processes that are fundamental to neurogenesis and cognitive functions. Epigenetic mechanisms like DNA methylation and histone modification regulate gene expression based on genetic predispositions and environmental factors. During critical phases of brain development, epigenetic modifications direct the development of neurons and synapses and ultimately influence cognitive processes , such as learning and memory. Neuronal early development is most epigenetically sensitive to modification, an effect that is caused by nutritional processes; for instance, folate should be consumed during pregnancy to prevent neural tube defects, an indication of the importance of good maternal nutrition in the establishment of epigenetic marks that control embryonic brain development. This information provides a complex interaction between internal and external genetic topography, with the possibility for lifelong effects related to neurological illness and cognitive ability. What is known suggests that certain substances utilized in metabolic pathways have a profound effect on brain development through epigenetic processes. For example, methylation is crucial in cell replication as well as gene expression, which is subservient to neural function. The availability of methyl donor compounds, e.g., S-adenosylmethionine, directly influences the effectiveness of such epigenetic alterations. Disruptions in these processes, such as those involved with folate deficiency, can result in aberrant neural development and are a factor in some neurological disorders. In addition, novel evidence points towards dietary influences, such as short-chain fatty acids (SCFAs) produced by gut microbiome fermentation of diet-derived fiber, playing a role in modifying brain development via epigenetic reprogramming. SCFAs have been demonstrated to modulate histone acetylation and consequent gene expression, hence being an integral part of the complex dance of neurodevelopmental processes. This emphasizes the pervasive regulatory network that is responsible for brain maturation by both genetic and epigenetic influences. The epigenetic modifications have consequences beyond typical brain development, extending to mental health and neurodevelopmental illness. Aberrant patterns of DNA methylation and histone modification have been implicated in such illnesses as autism spectrum disorders (ASD) as well as schizophrenia. Both conditions are likely to appear during times of critical development of the brain when epigenetic marks are established, thus early-life intervention becomes a potential to reorient disease trajectories. Investigating this association reveals to us that the interaction between genetic susceptibility and environmental stimuli has the potential to induce maladaptive epigenetic alteration. This information provides a window of opportunity for potential therapeutic interventions reversing epigenetic dysregulation to promote normal brain development and to prevent disease in vulnerable individuals. These epigenetic discoveries have the potential to reveal the complex etiologies of neurologic diseases, illuminating preventive and intervention strategies (Figure 9.11).

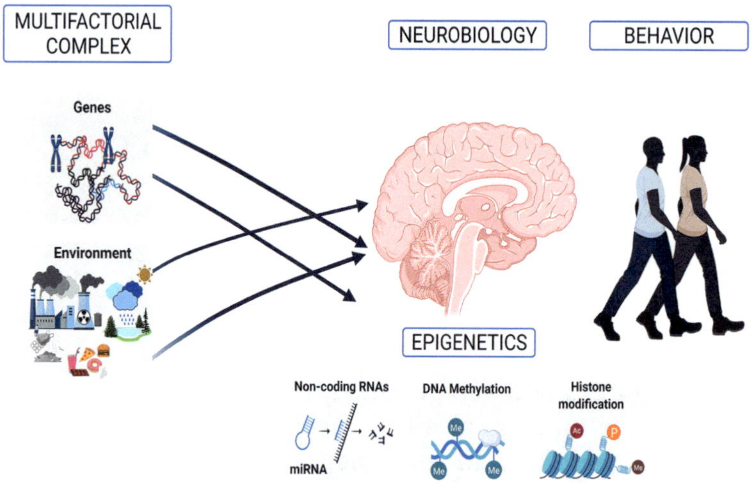

Figure 9.11. Impact of epigenetics on brain development.

Source: https://www.frontiersin.org/files/Articles/917198/fpsyt-13-917198-HTML/image_m/fpsyt-13-917198-g001.jpg.

9.3.2. Epigenetic Factors in Neurodegenerative Diseases

The interaction between epigenetic mechanisms and neurodegenerative disorders is becoming widely known as a key to unraveling the pathogenesis of these disorders. Epigenetic alterations, such as DNA methylation and histone modification, are essential in controlling gene expression without affecting the genetic code per se. These alterations have potent effects on neuronal function and survival. For instance, research has indicated that the methylation status of some genes may be associated with cognitive decline in diseases like Alzheimer's and Parkinson's. Dysregulation of epigenetics triggers pathological processes that can lead to neuronal dysfunction and thereby contribute to the clinical manifestations of neurodegenerative disorders. Consequently, the study of these alterations not only illuminates disease pathogenesis but also offers potential lines of therapeutic attack on the epigenetic context of the brain, a subject of intense investigation interest within the discipline (Im, 2022).

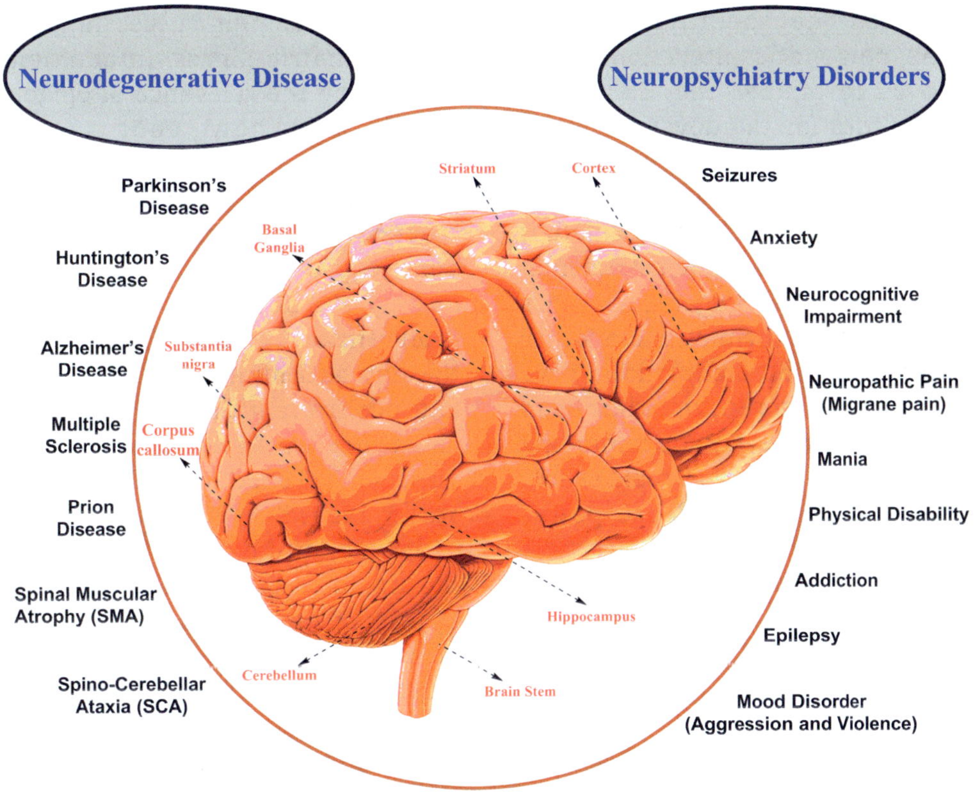

Figure 9.12. Neurodegenerative diseases.

Source: https://www.researchgate.net/publication/345466566/figure/fig1/AS:1023319168012292@1620989710896/Fig-1-Major-human-neurodegenerative-diseases-and-neuropsychiatry-disorders.jpg.

In support of the goal to illuminate the relationship between epigenetics and neurodegeneration, some research has emphasized the role of key epigenetic modulators like MeCP2 and TET1. The results indicate that MeCP2 alterations may impact the expression of genes like ZBTB16, which has a role in cognitive function in the development of Alzheimer's disease. Experimental models demonstrate that loss of the normal epigenetic regulation of gene expression underlies synaptic dysfunction and neuronal loss. In addition, the function of TET1 in repressing the SNCA gene linked to Parkinson's disease suggests a mechanism through which epigenetic regulators may determine the etiology of the disease. This growing body of work highlights the importance of examining epigenetic modifications as potential biomarkers for diagnosis and therapeutic targets in neurodegenerative disorders, as summarized in a number of recent publications (Im, 2022). The therapeutic potential of epigenetic mechanisms in neurodegenerative illnesses is profound. As epigenetic alterations have been shown to be reversible, they hold very promising possibilities for the development of new therapies aimed at normalizing patterns of gene expression. The new findings suggest that the manipulation of some epigenetic regulators can potentially enhance some of the detrimental impacts associated with neurodegeneration. For example, in models of Alzheimer's and other neurodegenerative diseases, modulation of the activity of certain epigenetic enzymes has been promising for reducing pathology and improving cognition. These kinds of approaches could enable new non-invasive treatments with the power to modulate disease at the molecular level, a new paradigm for therapy of neurodegenerative disease. Further research is required to develop these therapeutic approaches further and lead them into the clinic (Figure 9.12).

9.3.3. Implications for Treatment of Mental Health Disorders

The epigenetic significance of treating mental illnesses, particularly depression and anxiety, supports the relevance of accounting for metabolic health in therapy. There is increasing evidence that obesity—a frequently accompanying condition to metabolic dysfunction—encourages the emergence and severity of mood disorders. These correlations are mediated through mechanisms, such as neuroinflammation and hormonal changes that alter neural connections within brain structures engaged in mood regulation. Identifying these interconnections recommends that clinicians treat the psychological aspects of illness, like depression, may not be sufficient unless metabolic status is also treated. Therefore, interventions aiming at lifestyle alterations, e.g., diet and exercise, can be of great benefit to increase outcomes for mental illness as these interventions aim at both psychological and biological mechanisms of mood dysregulation. This interdisciplinary strategy provides a critical view in developing successful treatment plans for psychiatric illness. In addition, counselors are finding the relevance of epigenetic studies, particularly how poor experiences can manipulate gene expression linked to mental well-being outcomes. Laboratory tests demonstrate that poor psychosocial environments can change gene expression linked with schizophrenia, anxiety, and depression. Conversely, therapeutic interventions , such as cognitive behavioral therapy and mindfulness that are therapeutic and positively lifting have also been shown to cause positive epigenetic modifications that improve psychological well-being. From this study, mental health interventions not only target symptom reduction but also address the underlying biological mechanisms altered by psychosocial mechanisms. Counseling therapists can apply this knowledge to facilitate interventions that foster resilience and psychological well-being while considering environmental influences on epigenetic control. Translating epigenetic findings to counseling intervention can lead to more integrated and effective treatment. Finally, the integration of epigenetic theory into counselor training can further specify the skills of future therapists with knowledge that bridges psychological and biological frameworks. Counselor trainers might benefit from incorporating content regarding the epigenetic consequences of environmental stressors, as well as the potential for interventions to have positive epigenetic consequences. Interdisciplinary working by health practitioners could lead to complex care models that incorporate both psychological and physiological aspects of mental health. Preventative measures based upon early life experiences can also play an important role in the minimization of risk for mental disorder. Educating future counselors in the recognition and reversal of the impact of both environmental and individual biological factors can empower them to develop more suitable and effective therapies. Such a paradigm shift in education has the likelihood of reconceptualizing counseling practice to more effectively deliver desired results for the individuals with mental illnesses while understanding the multifaceted interaction between genetics and the environment in their manifestation (Fulton et al., 2021; Jones et al., 2021) (Figure 9.13).

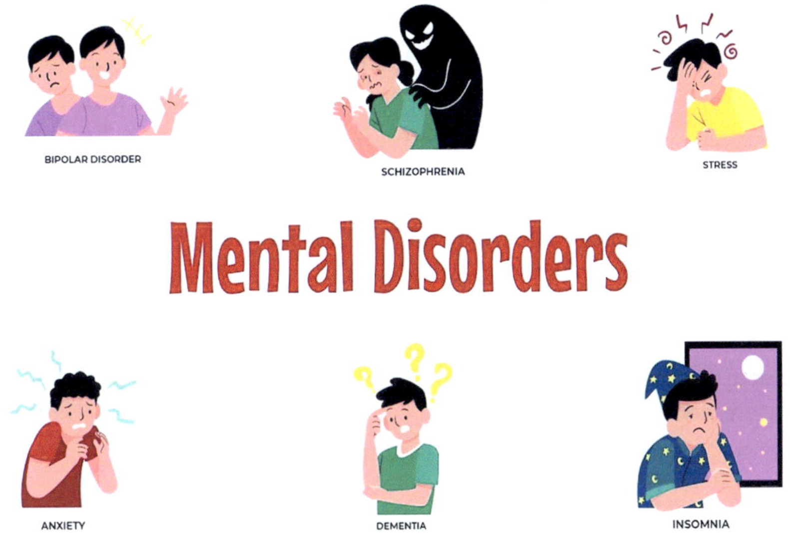

Figure 9.13. Mental health disorders.

Source: https://i.ytimg.com/vi/hRdaasafhYs/maxresdefault.jpg.

9.4. Epigenetics and Cardiovascular Diseases

The intricate relationship between cardiovascular disease and epigenetics is currently one of the areas of interest in the study of environmental factors and how these affect gene expression and subsequent disease pathophysiology. Epigenetic changes, such as DNA methylation and histone modification, play a significant role in regulating cardiovascular function-related genes. Dietary intake, physical activity, and stress, for instance, can activate epigenetic changes that make an individual susceptible to hypertension and atherosclerosis. Particularly, the dysregulation of adipose tissue function is central to this, as visceral fat deposition leads to insulin resistance that is associated with the etiology of cardiovascular disease. Recent evidence suggests that extracellular vesicles (EVs) from adipose tissue facilitate interorgan cross-talk through the transfer of regulatory miRNAs, which can sustain metabolic derangement and influence cardiovascular health (Wang et al., 2025). This new field of investigation emphasizes the requirement for more targeted therapeutic interventions modulating these epigenetic mechanisms to lower cardiovascular risk. Research into epigenetic mechanisms steps into the field of cardiovascular imaging, which itself has advanced considerably to encompass molecular data. Traditional imaging modalities are essentially interested in the structural and functional assessment of the cardiovascular system. However, the evolution of molecular nuclear imaging modalities—single-photon emission computed tomography and positron emission tomography—is now able to image disease mechanisms at a molecular level. These modalities are able to provide information on how cellular function can be affected by epigenetic changes and contribute to cardiovascular disease pathologies (Joshi et al., 2024). The use of epigenetic science in cardiovascular imaging may be able to improve the accuracy of diagnosis and provide valuable insights into the mechanisms of disease. This integrative approach could potentially enable the identification of cardiovascular disease high-risk patients but, more importantly, guide individualized treatment protocols aimed at reversing some epigenetic alterations. With ongoing research deciphering the complexity of epigenetics and its interaction with cardiovascular diseases, the merits of interdisciplinary research become evident. Integration of cardiologists, geneticists, and molecular biologists is important to help us understand how far epigenetic modification can be made to serve a therapeutic benefit. For instance, the discovery of important miRNAs responsible for controlling insulin sensitivity and lipid metabolism can potentially identify new drug targets. Secondly, utilization of technologies , such as CRISPR for targeted epigenetic editing may unveil avenues for novel therapy that may potentially reverse disease mechanisms driven by errant epigenetic alterations. More research down this path not only increases our understanding regarding cardiovascular disease but may also unveil revolutionary prevention and therapeutic approaches that blur the line between genetic predisposition and environmental influence (Figure 9.14).

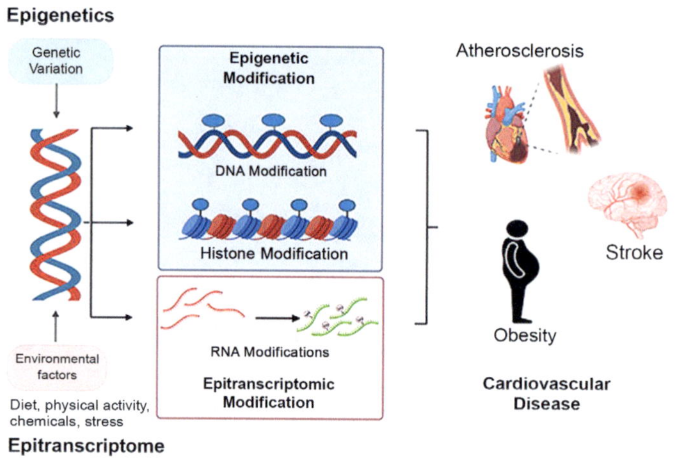

Figure 9.14. Epigenetics and cardiovascular diseases.

Source: https://icahn.mssm.edu/files/ISMMS/Assets/Research/Cardiovascular/ISMMS-Research-Cardiovascular-Slider-750x400.jpg.

9.4.1. Influence of Lifestyle Factors on Epigenetic Changes

This linkage between lifestyle factors and epigenetic changes underscores the importance of understanding how our daily choices affect genetic expression and susceptibility to disease. Factors , such as diet, exercise, and stress management can lead to dramatic shifts in the epigenome, impacting biological processes and health. For example, specific nutrients alter DNA methylation patterns, which are critical for regulating gene expression. By this process, nutritional interventions can play an important role in managing the epigenetic marks responsible for most diseases, including metabolic disease and some cancers. As advances are being made in modern-day science, it is evident that lifestyle changes can alter these epigenetic marks and hence have the potential to prevent disease progression and promote longevity, reflecting a change in paradigm in our approach to disease treatment and prevention (Alzeer, 2025).

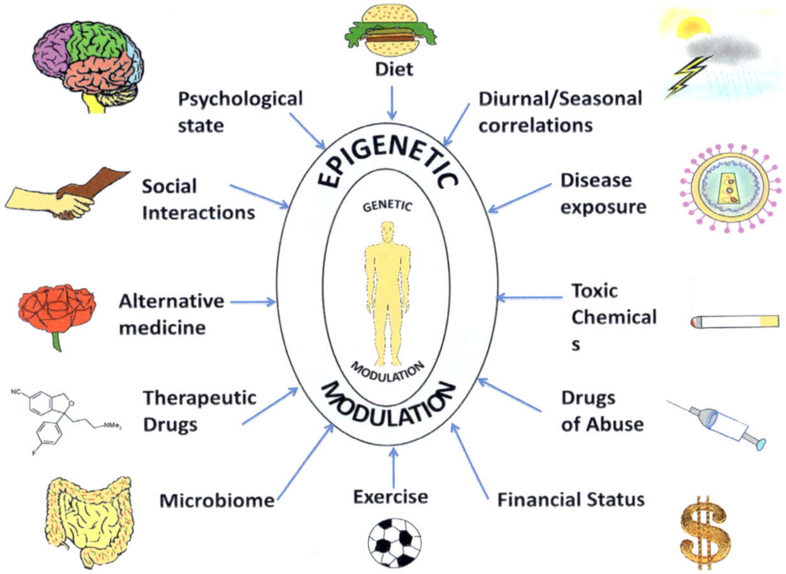

Figure 9.15. Influence of lifestyle factors on epigenetic changes.

Source: https://www.frontiersin.org/files/Articles/105911/fcell-02-00049-HTML/image_m/fcell-02-00049-g001.jpg.

Secondly, the contribution of environmental exposures, such as toxin or pollutant exposure, to epigenetic processes cannot be overemphasized. Exposures to cigarettes and heavy metals have been shown through research to bring about harmful epigenetic alterations leading to disease risk, particularly in vulnerable populations. More deplorable is the fact that these alterations have a transgenerational impact, which not only affects current health but also that of subsequent generations. Pregnant women, for instance, are especially susceptible since the lifestyle could influence fetal growth and eventual health outcomes (Sargent & Reed, 2024). This awareness renders the necessity of promoting public health programs for averting harmful environmental exposure, especially among pregnant women, even more urgent in the maintenance of the next generation's epigenetic health. Lifestylopathy, as a concept, emphasizes the interconnectedness of biological, psychological, and environmental factors in influencing gene expression and health outcomes. Recognizing that lifestyle interventions have the potential to modulate epigenetic processes, we can create an integrative model of healthcare to enhance individual resilience and well-being. This model encourages a harmonious lifestyle that integrates nutrition, physical exercise, stress handling, and awareness of the environment to optimize gene regulation and improve long-term health. With continuous research on the relationship between lifestyle and epigenetics, medical practitioners can create targeted interventions that not only prevent disease but also promote healthier gene expression (Alzeer, 2025). Marketing this integrative model of public policy is likely to lead us towards more sustainable health, ending up with a reduction in the burden of disease within our population (Figure 9.15).

9.4.2. Epigenetic Markers in Heart Disease

Recent research has further highlighted the intrinsic role of epigenetic markers in unraveling heart disease since such alterations have the ability to significantly influence gene expression without altering the DNA sequence. The epigenetic mechanisms of DNA methylation, histone modification, and ncRNA regulation have been shown to play a role in cardiac pathophysiology. These regulatory pathways can control the expression of key genes that mediate inflammation, cardiac hypertrophy, and fibrosis, which are the basic mechanisms in the pathogenesis and development of heart disease. For instance, aberrant DNA methylation patterns are identified in ischemic heart disease and heart failure patients, suggesting that epigenetic changes contribute not only as biomarkers but also as potential targets in intervention. The identification of epigenetic markers specific to the individual may refine risk stratification of patients and enhance the personalized treatment strategy, ultimately contributing to enhanced clinical outcomes in the treatment of heart disease. Furthermore, environmental exposure and lifestyle factors have been reported to influence epigenetic changes, further enhancing the horizon of prevention and therapy for heart disease. Various studies have established that dietary components, exercise, and toxin exposure have been reported to cause DNA methylation and histone modification changes, which impact cardiovascular health. For example, a methyl-donating nutrient-rich diet can modulate the epigenetic state positively, potentially reducing cardiovascular disease risk. Smoking and obesity have been linked to undesirable epigenetic alterations that lead to undesirable cardiovascular events. Explaining the interaction between these lifestyle factors and epigenetic markers contains valuable data to the prevention of cardiovascular disease. It highlights the importance of adopting healthy lifestyle choices as a means of eliminating epigenetic cardiovascular disease risk factors, which could lead to new prevention strategies and treatment. Moreover, new information suggests that epigenetic marks not only hold diagnostic promise but may also have a role to play in the treatment of heart disease. For instance, modification of specific epigenetic targets with pharmacologic agents or modifiable lifestyle has been shown to reverse pathological epigenetic changes of cardiac pathophysiology. Histone deacetylase (HDAC)-targeting or DNA methyltransferase (DNMT)-targeting drugs are under investigation for cardioprotection. In addition, because epigenetic marks are dynamic in nature, it follows that these changes are reversible and thus offer potential therapeutic opportunities to remodel the epigenetic landscape in the direction of improved heart performance. With studies exposing the complex interaction between epigenetics and cardiovascular disease, the prospect of clinical application of epigenetic markers as diagnostic and treatment agents in cardiovascular medicine is an exhilarating and rapidly developing field of study in need of continued research and interdisciplinarity from clinicians and scientists (Stanley et al., 2016; Brabletz et al., 2021) (Figure 9.16).

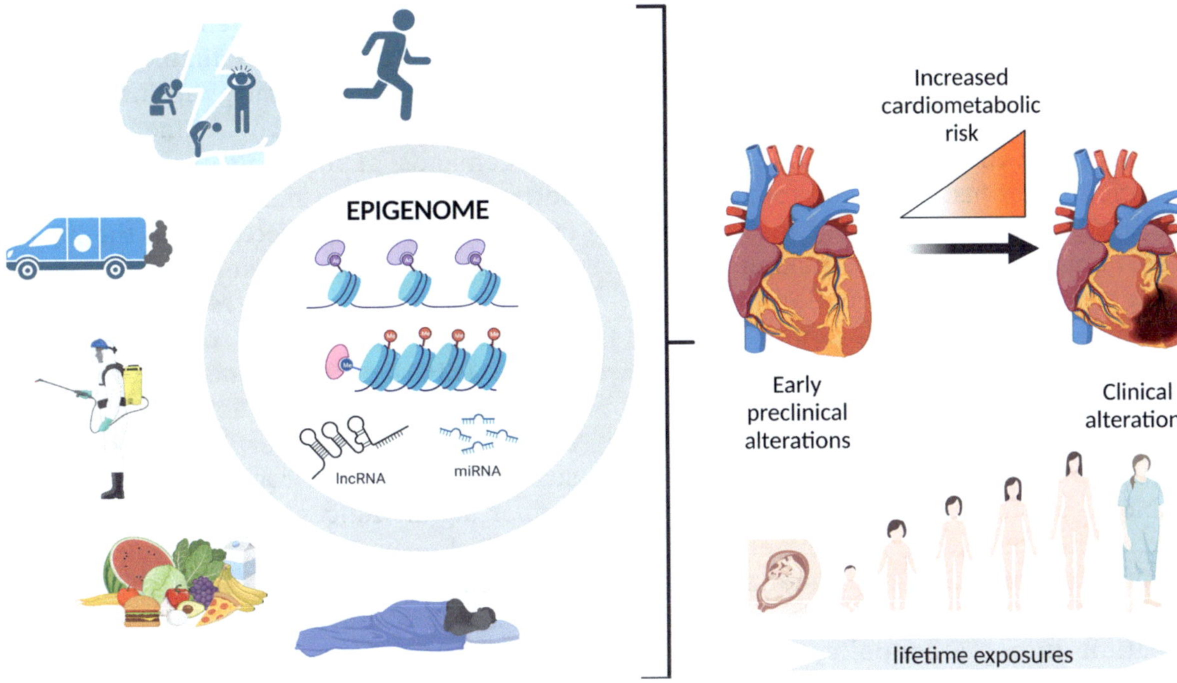

Figure 9.16. Epigenetic markers in heart disease.

Source: https://www.ahajournals.org/cms/10.1161/CIRCRESAHA.123.322135/asset/9953cb2c-9c95-4331-bb13-20c11e1aa1c0/assets/graphic/circresaha.123.322135.fig01.jpg.

9.4.3. Potential for Epigenetic Interventions in Prevention

The potential of epigenetic therapy as a preventive strategy against disease is increasingly better substantiated by scientific evidence, and it represents a shift in the vision of health care. Central to this concept is recognition that gene expression can be affected by environmental cues, lifestyle, and the interaction of systems. This revision of health not only contradicts the determinism of genetics but also allows individuals to modify their lifestyle in a manner that can reverse gene expression to their benefit. As established in research on Lifestylopathy, carefully planned lifestyle interventions have the capability to refine gene regulation, underscoring the interplay of biological and environmental variables in ensuring sustainable health. These strategies support the application of epigenetic mechanisms, such as DNA methylation, to enhance immune resilience and cognitive stability and pave the way for a more personalized approach to preventive healthcare and prevention of disease, individualized to lifestyles and environmental exposures (Alzeer, 2025). Current research also emphasizes the role of epigenetic modifications in obesity, a disease that has far-reaching implications for public health. The epigenome, subject to environmental exposures, directly controls gene expression that includes metabolic processes and therefore offers promising targets for intervention. The work demonstrates lifestyle factors—nutrition, exercise, and the like—to be capable of triggering profound epigenetic changes contributing to obesity prevention. The findings illuminate the importance of learning more about the interaction between epigenetic mechanisms and life choices and opportunities for guided preventive intervention. With the focus on epigenetic determinants, public health interventions can include interventions that encourage more healthy lifestyles and act on the root environmental causes of obesity and thus establish a proactive model of disease prevention and health promotion (Yang, 2024). Moreover, the application of epigenetic intervention is not just restricted to individual health, but perhaps also to more macroscopic socioeconomic disparity. By making use of epigenetic mechanisms, prevention programs can be crafted to help provide equity in health through ensuring adequate support to vulnerable populations in making enough change in lifestyle predictors that may result in poor health outcomes. The approach embraces the need for equitable access to material and social aspects supporting healthy living, thus reversing the environmental determinants promoting health inequities. Moreover, integrating epigenetic information into public policy can enable one to develop programs directed towards education, community assets, and changes in lifestyle. With the globe facing the challenges of managing chronic diseases, tapping into the full potential of epigenetic treatments may not only revolutionize tailored medicine but also usher in an even more sustainable and equitable model of health care (Alzeer, 2025; Yang, 2024).

9.5. Environmental Influences on Epigenetics

The interface between environmental determinants and epigenetic modifications has attracted significant attention towards understanding the etiology of disease. Environmental agents , such as diet, toxins, chemicals, and psychosocial stressors, could lead to epigenetic modifications that influence gene expression without altering the DNA sequence itself. For instance, dietary deficiencies or excesses could alter the DNA methylation pattern, thus influencing pathways critical in diseases , such as coronary artery disease (CAD). It has been implicated by research that certain genes involved in CAD are epigenetically regulated by the environment. This finding emphasizes adopting a preventive strategy against risk factors based on lifestyle and environmental exposure and demands public health policy supporting better diet and environmental conditions to aid in altering disease trajectories in the high-risk populations (Abdelkader et al., 2025). Moreover, emerging evidence underscores the role of epigenetics in the etiology of congenital heart defects (CHD), such as conotruncal congenital heart defects (CTDs). Such defects develop due to an elaborate interplay between genetic susceptibility and environmental insults, further supporting the concept of multifactorial etiology for CHD. Epigenetic alterations can potentially alter gene expression in cardiac development, demonstrating how environmental influences contribute to disease etiology. For example, maternal nutrition and fetal in-utero exposure to environmental toxins have been linked with gene expression modifications that subsequently influence fetal heart development. Systematic reviews to comprehend the epigenetic profile of CTD reveal a significant knowledge gap on how these modifications vary across various populations and settings (Aburawi et al., 2024). Therefore, investigation of these correlations not only enhances scientific knowledge but also informs effective prevention strategies within disparate demographic groups. Integration of the consideration of environmental factors within the epigenetics model is of profound importance in disease prevention as well as in management. Epigenetic markers can also be utilized as predictive indicators, which will serve to inform susceptibility to environmentally related diseases in individuals. For instance, it has been shown that the use of polygenic risk scores together with epigenetic analysis can increase the specificity of CAD risk prediction, allowing for a more sophisticated appraisal of patient risk profiles. Furthermore, novel epigenetics-targeting therapies , such as histone deacetylase inhibitors and microRNA mimics, have the potential to reverse or attenuate disease mechanisms fueled by maladaptive epigenetic regulation. These advances are indicative of a paradigm shift towards personalized medicine, where interventions are tailored not only to genetic risk but also to environmental contexts conditioning epigenetic profiles (Abdelkader et al., 2025) (Figure 9.17).

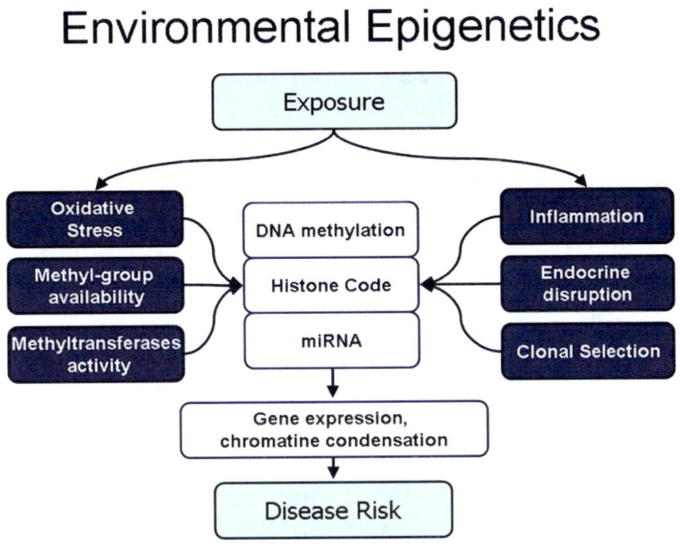

Figure 9.17. Environmental influences on epigenetics.

Source: https://images.squarespace-cdn.com/content/v1/5f717ce9769f9e2f4d6f373c/1603137838594-AXB4YWAES9AX3GNYIGY1/Good+Image+epigenetics+Potential-mechanisms-linking-environmental-exposures-to-epigenetic-effects.jpg.

9.5.1. Effects of Diet on Epigenetic Modifications

The intricate interaction between diet and epigenetic modification provides a compelling viewpoint from which to view the mechanistic basis of the majority of diseases. Diet is progressively regarded as a vital environmental factor that can influence gene expression without altering the fundamental DNA sequence. This is done through a multitude of mechanisms , including DNA methylation, histone modification, and non-coding RNA action. Recent studies have suggested that components of the diet, such as polyunsaturated fatty acids, vitamins, and phytochemicals, may induce some epigenetic changes that will be advantageous to health or cause the onset of disease. This intersection of nutrition and epigenetics forms the starting point for research on dietetic interventions that may emerge as preventive or therapeutic measures against cancer, obesity, or neurodegenerative diseases. Gut microbiotas play an important role in mediating the epigenetic effects of diet, emphasizing how intertwined these systems are. As the intricate community of microbes that inhabit the gastrointestinal tract, gut microbiota is regulated by diet and, in turn, contributes to physiological function in its own way through the production of metabolites. These metabolites can be used as signaling molecules, modulating the activity of epigenetic modifiers, which in turn have an impact on the host's gene expression. For instance, certain bacterial metabolites have been shown to regulate histone acetylation and methylation profiles, showing a direct association between gut integrity, dietary consumption, and epigenetic modification that can establish unique health profiles in individuals. This interaction shows the potential of precision diets to manage gut microbiota structure to achieve specific epigenetic outcomes, paving the way for novel therapeutic mechanisms founded on nutritional science (Reva et al., 2023). Alzheimer's disease (AD) is a dramatic reminder of the interaction between dietary factors and epigenetic modification in determining disease susceptibility and progression. The apolipoprotein E (APOE) gene, particularly its ε4 allele variant, has emerged as a significant risk factor for AD, with epigenetic control of its expression being the area of research focus. Research indicates that diet is a factor that could influence methylation of the crucial CpG sites in the APOE promoter to influence its balance of isoforms and consequently the pathophysiological pathways of AD. By learning how diet affects epigenetic regulation of the APOE gene, researchers can better understand the complex interaction between environmental factors and genetic susceptibility, thereby pinpointing key points of intervention for lifestyle treatment to reduce AD risk (Lozupone et al., 2023).

9.5.2. Role of Toxins and Pollutants

Exposure to environmental toxins and pollutants is increasingly recognized for its widespread implications for human health, particularly if viewed in the light of epigenetics. Toxins , such as heavy metals and organic chemicals have been associated with several diseases, mostly neurodegenerative diseases. Studies have identified that over 127 environmental toxins are most likely associated with such conditions as Alzheimer's Disease, Parkinsons Disease, and amyotrophic lateral sclerosis. These toxins exert their actions through mechanisms , such as DNA methylation, which alters gene expression but not the underlying DNA sequence. This identifies an important juncture at which environmental exposures not only create direct health threats but also cause permanent epigenetic marks that have the potential to make a person predisposed to illness in the long run, hinting at an interactive dynamic between our environmental exposures and gene code that needs serious investigation and public health scrutiny (Newell et al., 2025). In understanding the role that toxins play in disease causation, particular emphasis is placed on the aryl hydrocarbon receptor (AhR). AhR is well characterized as an environmental sensor for a variety of pollutants but is also recognized to mediate the effect of endogenous toxins associated with conditions , such as chronic kidney disease. Upon activation by toxic chemicals, AhR exerts a regulatory impact on numerous areas of biological function, including cellular metabolism and differentiation, leading to tissue injury and organ failure. Significantly, the accumulation of uremic compounds within the body can instigate significant health issues, and hence it is critical to explore the mechanisms through which AhR mediates such reactions. These investigations may yield new clinical strategies aimed at reversing the toxic action of uremic toxins and improving health outcomes, and thereby interlink the tale of chronic disease and environmental exposure (Xie et al., 2024). The results of toxin-induced epigenetic changes are not only at the level of disease outcomes in individuals but also extend to population-level trends in disease. The geographic disparity in exposure to toxins and disease occurrence highlights the necessity of mitigating environmental health disparities. For instance, the occurrence of neurodegenerative disease can often mimic the geographic concentration of heavy industry and pollution that disproportionately affects vulnerable populations. It is through the understanding of such environmental determinants that not only are public health policies informed, but also the necessity for strict regulations that protect vulnerable populations from being exposed to harm. Through prioritizing research over the interfaces between toxins and epigenetics, more effective preventive measures can be instituted, ultimately contributing to healthier environments and fewer aggregate cases of chronic diseases that develop as a result of environmental toxins (Newell et al., 2025) (Figure 9.18).

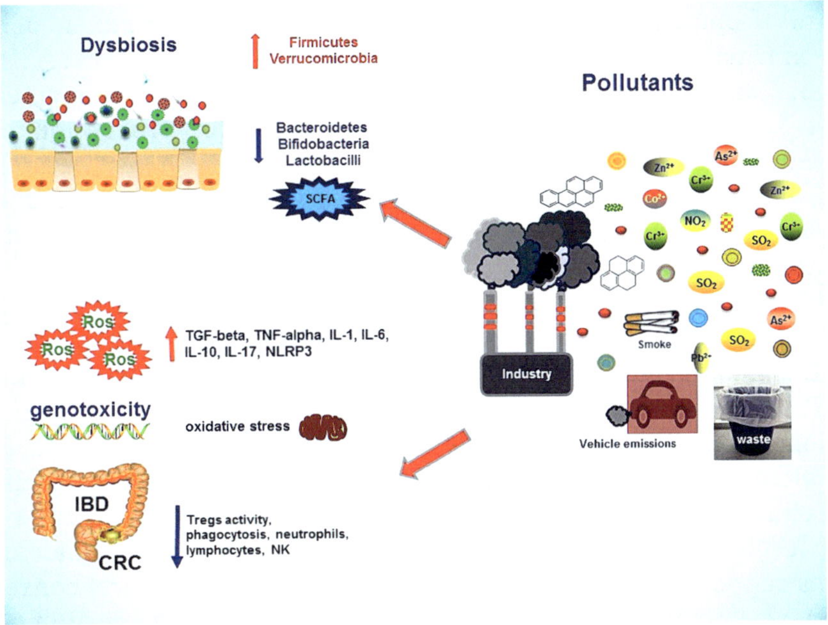

Figure 9.18. Role of toxins and pollutants is becoming increasingly.

Source: https://scienceinfo.com/wp-content/uploads/2023/07/image-148-768x432.png.

9.5.3. Impact of Stress and Lifestyle Choices

The relationship between stress and lifestyle choices is increasingly understood to contribute significantly to health outcomes. Chronic stress, for example, has been proven to trigger a cascade of physiological reactions that can lead to the development of a range of non-communicable diseases (NCDs). Evidence supports that stress impacts the balance of oxidative stress in the body, which consequently can lead to cell damage and inflammation. This biochemical chain reaction has also been implicated in diseases , such as cardiovascular disease, diabetes, and certain cancers. Lifestyle variables like nutrition and exercise can also contribute to or act as a buffer for the effects of stress. Regular physical activity and consuming a healthy well-balanced diet rich in antioxidants might serve as protective factors against the impact of stress on health, ultimately demonstrating that lifestyle choices might make us more resistant and enhance the state of our health with, for instance, lower oxidative stress levels in those who adopted healthier lifestyles, as demonstrated by the outcome of the HLCP-2 program (Husain et al., 2025). Also, the role of epigenetics in linking lifestyle and health effects underscores the value of choosing an informed lifestyle. Epigenetic mechanisms can lead to changes in gene expression without changing the underlying DNA sequence, often affected by the environment in the guise of diet, stress, and poisons. Importantly, the epigenetic changes may be transmitted across generations, which underscores the persistence of lifestyle choices. For instance, maternal stress during pregnancy has been associated with epigenetic modification in the offspring, which can condition them to a variety of diseases in life. This highlights the need for preventative interventions targeting stress reduction and promotion of healthy lifestyle choices at critical stages of development, specifically pregnancy. Attainment and improvement of these factors can reduce the risk of epigenetically affected disease, therefore enhancing the overall health of future generations as proposed in current research (Sargent & Reed, 2024). Lifestyle and stress management effects in epigenetics are not only confined to individual health but also have effects on public health policy and interventions. Community-based interventions that promote healthy living through education regarding nutrition, physical activity, and mental strength are essential in the management of the rising burden of NCDs. Interventions , such as Healthy Lifestyle Community Program-2 (HLCP-2) illustrate the effectiveness of structured interventions in enhancing people's health through reduced levels of oxidative stress. These interventions support a broad approach to health with the four elements of well-being: diet, physical activity, mental well-being, and social connections. By establishing an enabling community environment, individuals are better able to cope with stress and make healthier choices, leading to improved population health. Thus, considering the epigenetic implications of such life changes may provide an important avenue for reducing disease risk at both the individual and the population level (Husain et al., 2025).

9.6. Future Directions in Epigenetic Research

The future of epigenetics holds the promise to transform our knowledge of complex diseases, especially in the manner in which environmental influences interface with genes. As diseases , such as breast cancer are multifactorial in origin, a systems approach must be applied, incorporating a vast number of determinants, from social and behavioral to hormonal ones. According to recent findings, the incorporation of environmental exposures—primarily estrogen-mimetic exposures—suggests that there is a need for more sophisticated risk assessment modalities in the treatment of breast cancer. This combined approach can assist us in identifying modifiable risk factors more easily and, thereby, offer areas for prevention. By systematically expanding our investigations into individual susceptibility, researchers can connect the dots between epigenetic modifications and disease initiation, allowing for the development of tailored interventions that address the individual's own experiences in their own way over time, as summarized in recent work on hormone-sensitive tumors (Stanley et al., 2016). The field of epigenetics is also experiencing exciting advances in agriculture applications, more specifically about the reproductive well-being of dairy cows. Subfertility in dairy cows not only has welfare consequences for the animal but also financial implications for farm profitability and sustainability. New trends in functional genomics point towards the use of genomic selection that can be pivotal in enhancing reproductive performance. Transcriptomic-derived knowledge can enable understanding of the complex physiological mechanisms of fertility traits, particularly through epigenetic changes. This type of research has value in developing effective management strategies that would decrease subfertility issues in dairy cattle herds. Moreover, the discovery of interactions among genetic and epigenetic factors can explain new ways to increase reproductive success in farms; therefore, the integration of these data into sustainable agricultural business can lead to economic and environmental sustainability (Beerda et al., 2008). In the coming years, the convergence of epigenetics with other new and rising fields of science, such as nutrigenomics and RNA interference, provides a promising field for future work. These inter-disciplinary approaches hold the promise for more understanding of how lifestyle and dietary factors influence epigenetic change and ultimately disease susceptibility and progression. For instance, the elucidation of nutritional determinants of gene expression has the potential for the development of individually tailored dietary advice designed to modify disease risk profiles. In addition, integrating approaches that address variable copy numbers within the genome will further advance our understanding of genetic diversity and how it influences health. The more scientists unravel the subtlety of epigenetic regulation, the more dramatic the breakthroughs can be expected that not only will elucidate the pathophysiology of many diseases but also unlock the field to new therapeutic avenues, changing paradigms in healthcare forever (Figure 9.19).

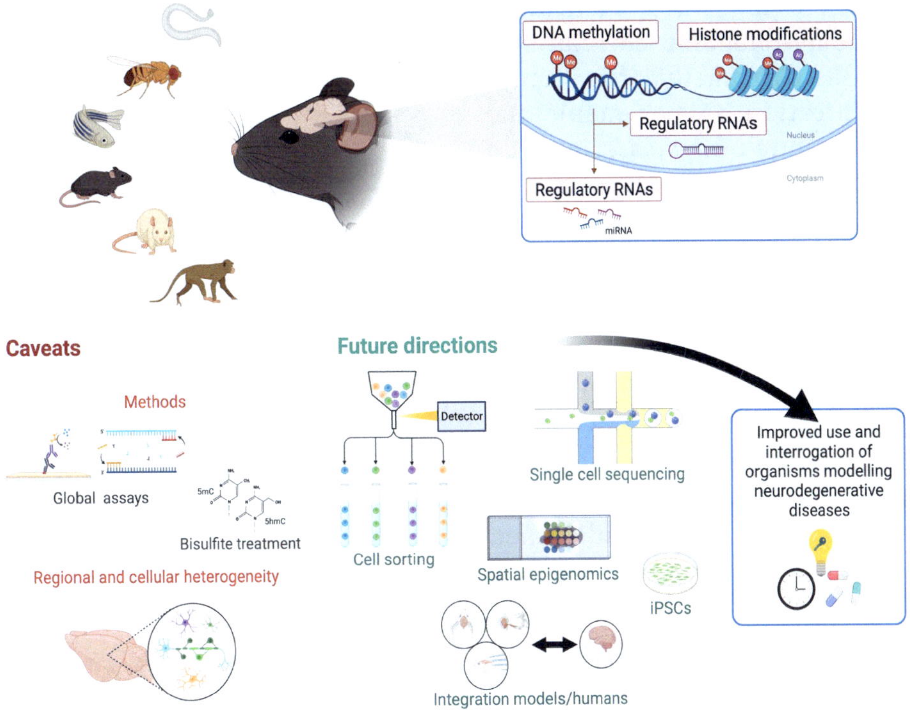

Figure 9.19. Future directions in epigenetic research.

Source: https://www.researchgate.net/publication/365132320/figure/fig1/AS:1143128113187 5362@1680189605732/Vertebrate-and-invertebrate-models-useful-for-epigenetics-research-of-neurodegerative.tif.

9.6.1. Advances in Epigenetic Technologies

The field of epigenetics has witnessed paradigm-shifting advances in the recent past, significantly enhancing our comprehension of molecular mechanisms underlying diseases. Technologies , such as CRISPR-Cas9 and next-generation sequencing have accelerated the manner in which scientists engineer and study epigenetic marks. CRISPR, for instance, enables one to edit epigenetic marks with accuracy, allowing researchers to investigate their functional significance in disease pathology. Such precision has been particularly useful in studies examining the impact of environmental influences—like smoking—on gene expression and disease susceptibility. For instance, research has identified that specific types of DNA methylation associated with smoking patterns can have cardiovascular disease risks, and this knowledge is crucial to understanding lifestyle-related epigenetic alterations (Cao et al., 2025). Not only do these advances illuminate disease pathogenesis, but they also pave the way for future therapeutic approaches. Apart from genome editing, advances in high-throughput epigenomic technologies have facilitated large-scale epigenome-phenome correlations. Techniques , such as DNA methylation arrays and histone modification assays enable the epigenome to be scanned *en masse* over an entire genome at one time. These reagents have been instrumental in uncovering correlations between epigenetic modification and numerous diseases, including cancers, neurodegenerative diseases, and heart disease. New findings indicate that some epigenetic marks are linked with disease susceptibility, illuminating how environmental and genetic stimuli talk to one another at the epigenetic level. Furthermore, with this comprehensive insight into the epigenome, new biomarkers can be identified for early diagnosis and prognosis, ultimately giving rise to personalized medicine programs (Kumar, 2025). With advancing technology, its impact on healthcare and disease management is increasingly obvious. New epigenetic technologies not only redefine research but also impact therapeutic strategies in the clinic. The ability to target epigenetic changes opens new doors for the therapy of disease, particularly those diseases where traditional means have failed. Epigenetic drugs, such as histone deacetylase inhibitors, are already used in cancer treatment, demonstrating the clinical significance of these advancements. In addition, the creation of small molecules with the ability to modulate epigenetic enzyme activity has promising therapeutic potential for the treatment of various diseases where epigenetic dysregulation is of significant importance. With ongoing research revealing the complexities of epigenetic regulation, the incorporation of such cutting-edge technologies into therapeutic strategies will be vital to tackle complex diseases, maximize treatment efficacy, and eventually improve patient outcomes. The ongoing exploration of epigenetics promises to deliver dramatic advances in understanding disease cause and the development of new approaches to therapy (Figure 9.20).

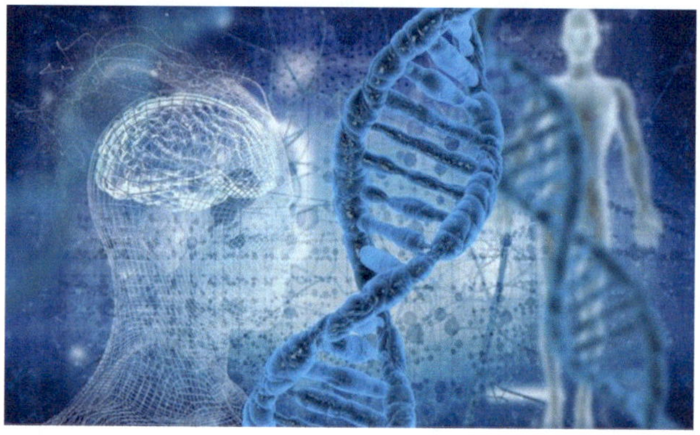

Figure 9.20. Advances in epigenetic technologies.

Source: https://assets.technologynetworks.com/production/dynamic/images/content/389152/exploring-the-new-insights-revealed-by-epigenetics-389152-640x360.jpg.

9.6.2. Ethical Considerations in Epigenetic Studies

The field of epigenetics has unleashed a new era of understanding the complex interplay between genetics and the environment in shaping human health. With the scientific advance, however, also came ethical concerns, particularly in the realm of implications arising from epigenetic mark manipulation. Unlike traditional genetic changes, where the alteration of DNA code is involved, epigenetic changes are reversible and subject to external influences, triggering ongoing debates in responsibility and consent. Ethically, the potential for unintentional outcomes concerns the long-term impacts of such interventions on patients and their offspring. This raises its head further with the potential to apply epigenetic changes as therapeutic applications for disease, which underscores the need to develop distinct guidelines and ethical standards to control the research and its applications in the clinic so that the safety and well-being of patients and even future generations are assured. As scientists employ increasingly sophisticated technologies like CRISPR for epigenetic editing, ethical questions become increasingly complicated. The ability to edit the epigenome offers broad tools for modification of gene expression without modifying underlying DNA, which speaks of revolutionary treatment methods for a variety of diseases. But with that comes ethical questions surrounding human germline editing, in which changes would be passed to future generations. Ethical frameworks need to incorporate equity and fairness considerations to deal with concerns surrounding access to these advanced treatments and the threat of societal health care inequalities. Furthermore, the lack of full regulatory authority in most sectors provides unlimited research protocols, raising questions of accountability and the need for a responsible plan in bringing about such groundbreaking technology. Resolution of these issues is required to safeguard public trust and guarantee the ethical development of epigenetic studies. Ethical aspects of epigenetics extend to societal and cultural domains, considering that epigenetics can potentially influence public perceptions of disease and health. The confluence of epigenetics and chronic and complex disease is troubling in that it raises stigma and discrimination issues, particularly if people are held accountable for their epigenetic status due to environmental factors. There needs to be a careful discussion of agency and blame when thinking about the role of social determinants in influencing epigenetic disease, which can have implications for public health practice and policy. Ethical considerations must take into account the broader social context of epigenetics research, involving stakeholders across sectors to enrich an ongoing open discussion. Regular sessions with ethicists, clinical practitioners, and representatives from the general public are needed to foster a responsible research environment with ethical considerations in mind, without missing out on the potential rewards of epigenetics research in mitigating cancer and metabolic disorders.

9.6.3. Potential for Personalized Medicine

The emergence of personalized medicine represents a paradigm shift in the field of medicine, focusing on the need for individualized therapies to match the unique genetic and epigenetic environment of a person. This approach has profound implications for understanding diseases at the molecular level, particularly diseases with an epigenetic twist. By analyzing gene expression changes due to environmental factors, lifestyle, and epigenetic changes, clinicians can develop personalized interventions that treat not only the symptoms but also the cause of many diseases. For instance, an integration of personalized medicine and genomic data enables the identification of specific biomarkers of treatment response at a personal level, facilitating the efficacy and safety of the available therapeutic choices. Furthermore, the promise of personalization is expressed more starkly in conditions , such as Systemic Lupus Erythematosus (SLE). This condition illustrates well the manner in which personalization can lead to improved outcomes through regard for genetic polymorphisms and epigenetic changes, as well as traditional clinical assessment. Current treatments have limited success for many patients, highlighting the necessity for approaches that appreciate the individual variation in each patient. Through examining the interactions between environmental stimuli and genetic susceptibility, researchers are acquiring informative data on SLE pathogenesis. This information is critical for building tailored biologics that are congruent with specific patient profiles with the ultimate goal of enhancing remission rates and health quality for patients with this complex disease (Wais & Agrawal,

2024). Moreover, personalized medicine is not contained to one discipline; instead, it continues on to include the holistic approach, such as in the case of Ayurveda, wherein it considers a person's unique constitution or Prakriti. This process of integrating ancient knowledge with modern genomic science enhances our insight into disease and health. It offers exciting possibilities for the identification of specific diet and lifestyle modifications that can be uniquely tailored to the individual based on their genetic and epigenetic backgrounds. The convergence of these disciplines has the potential to breed new modalities of therapy that not only honor the complexity of human biology but also provide us with a template for stewardship of long-term health. Hence, the pursuit of personalized medicine, by dint of its advanced recognition of epigenetics, is a step towards enhanced and tailored patient outcomes (Priya & Nair, 2025).

SUMMARY

The nuances of epigenetics significantly enhance our understanding of disease mechanisms and perhaps offer routes to new therapeutic strategies. As the research continues to develop, the interrelatedness between epigenetic modulation and multifaceted diseases, such as cancer, metabolic disease, and neurodegenerative disease, becomes increasingly apparent. For instance, regulation of pathways of cell death, such as ferroptosis pathways, shows how epigenetic factors can explain disease development and therapeutic responses. By illuminating the intricate molecular machinery involved, researchers are paving the way for targeted therapies that could neutralize the adverse effects of such diseases and customize treatment regimens (Tang et al., 2020). Moreover, the relevance of epigenetic research goes beyond personal health; it involves intergenerational effects that can influence disease susceptibility in children. Maternal well-being and how it affects the epigenetics of the offspring are also prominent concerns, particularly in relation to obesity and metabolic syndrome (Moholdt & Hawley, 2020). Therefore, treatment of the disease is not sufficient, and prevention of the risk factors through early intervention is just as crucial. By addressing maternal lifestyle and promoting health before conception, we can potentially halt cycles of disease transmissible through generations in a paradigm shift of public health. In the end, the study of epigenetics in disease represents an exciting frontier with deep implications for population and individual health. It emphasizes the need to integrate genetic, environmental, and lifestyle information in creating comprehensive health strategies (Moholdt & Hawley, 2020). Future research should aim towards the creation of intervention methods targeted at these epigenetic levels with a focus on prevention and early management of disease. Through the development of an interdisciplinary approach, we can expand our understanding of disease etiology and create new treatments that have the potential to transform the landscape of health care in significant ways (Tang et al., 2020). The intricate relationship between disease and epigenetics is brought into perspective by current findings that illustrate the function of some mutations and cascade signals in pathophysiological conditions. Adenomyosis is a good illustration of the condition, characterized by invasion of the myometrium by endometrial tissue, which is extremely challenging to diagnose and manage. The KRAS gene has been identified with mutations in invaded endometrial tissues in adenomyosis, supporting the invagination hypothesis of etiology. This suggests that epigenetic regulation may be centrally active in the growth and survival of these abnormal cells, particularly with respect to ovarian steroids. Moreover, the study highlights the importance of knowing about such molecular interactions to address the unique estrogen-mediated inflammatory pathways typical of adenomyosis and possibly other related gynecologic conditions (Serdar et al., 2021). Besides adenomyosis, the SARS-CoV-2 outbreak has revealed the critical function of epigenetics in viral pathogenesis and host interaction. The identification of durable protein-protein interactions between SARS-CoV-2 and human proteins demonstrates the complexity between the virus mechanism and the host cellular mechanism response. Significantly, the identification of druggable human proteins involved in such interactions opens novel therapeutic windows for intervention. By targeting these host factors, there is potential for researchers to develop strategies that are able to enhance host resistance to infection and thereby advance our understanding of epigenetic regulation of disease susceptibility and disease progression. This is a very good example of how epigenetics can be employed to study and treat infectious diseases since the molecular dynamics of host-pathogen interaction are crucial in the design of effective antiviral therapies (Jones et al., 2021). The crossroads of adenomyosis and COVID-19 findings underscore the polyvalent value of epigenetic studies in disease models. The results not only emphasize how demystifying genetic and epigenetic elements in chronic disease states is a priority, but also summarize the value of the possibility of the development of targeted drugs that consider the root biological mechanisms. With ongoing advances as a scientific discipline, epigenetics' uses hold the potential to revolutionize strategies for disease prevention and management on a wide variety of medical conditions. More studies on genetic mutations and epigenetic alterations will enable the scientific community to develop more holistic treatment models that could cure the symptoms and etiology of diseases (Jones et al., 2021; Serdar et al., 2021).

A LOOK TO THE FUTURE:

EPIGENETIC ALTERATIONS:

Epigenetic alterations have emerged as a central, transformative concept in modern biology, offering a framework for understanding how gene activity can be regulated beyond the static sequence of DNA itself. Unlike genetic mutations that change the underlying code of nucleotides, epigenetic alterations refer to heritable changes in gene expression that do not involve modifications to the DNA sequence but instead influence whether genes are turned "on" or "off" in different contexts. These alterations are mediated through biochemical mechanisms such as DNA methylation, histone modification, chromatin remodelling, and non-coding RNA activity, all of which shape the epigenomic landscape of a cell and guide its functional identity.

At the most fundamental level, epigenetic mechanisms regulate gene expression patterns that determine cell type, developmental timing, and responsiveness to environmental stimuli. DNA methylation—typically involving the addition of methyl groups to cytosine bases—can silence genes by impeding the interaction of transcriptional machinery with DNA, while specific histone modifications can either loosen or tighten chromatin structure, thereby facilitating or repressing access to genetic information. These reversible chemical marks act in concert as part of an "epigenetic code" that dynamically modulates genomic activity without altering the genetic blueprint.

The biological significance of epigenetic alterations extends across the life course. During normal development, epigenetic programs help orchestrate cell differentiation, ensuring that neurons, muscle cells, and immune cells adopt distinct functional identities while sharing the same DNA sequence. Environmental exposures—such as diet, stress, toxins, and lifestyle factors—can leave epigenetic imprints that affect gene expression patterns and influence physiological processes. Because these changes do not alter DNA sequence, they are reversible and, in some cases, can be passed from one cell generation to the next, adding a layer of complexity to inheritance and phenotypic variation.

Epigenetic alterations also play a profound role in disease. Aberrant methylation or histone marks can disrupt normal gene control systems, contributing to pathological states such as cancer, aging-related disorders, diabetes, and neurological dysfunction by mis-regulating tumor suppressor genes or other key pathways. Indeed, in many cancers, widespread epigenomic changes occur early in disease development and are now recognized as both biomarkers and potential therapeutic targets.

As epigenetic research continues to advance through new sequencing technologies and analytical tools, the study of epigenetic alterations offers unprecedented insight into the interplay between genes, environment, and disease. By integrating epigenomic data with clinical and environmental information, scientists and clinicians aim to develop novel diagnostic markers, personalised treatments, and preventative strategies that harness the full complexity of gene regulation for improving human health.

REFERENCES

1. Abdelkader, R. R. M., & Almubarak, E. M. (2025). Genomic and epigenetic influences on coronary artery disease. *International Journal of Chemical and Biochemical Sciences.* https://www.semanticscholar.org/paper/fa585ce261d6467c808f259b54820c5a7969be17 (accessed on 17th July 2025).
2. Aburawi, E., Östlundh, L., Aburawi, H. E., Al Rifai, R. H., Bhagavathula, A., & Bellou, A. (2024). Epigenetics of conotruncal congenital heart disease: Protocol for a systematic review and meta-analysis. *PLOS ONE, 19*(4), e0302642. https://www.semanticscholar.org/paper/dbb4ebe6272483bcdbb7f8ac7cab1112aa407e9f (accessed on 17th July 2025).
3. Alzeer, J. (2025). Personalized health through epigenetics: The lifestylopathy approach. *Medical Research Archives.* https://www.semanticscholar.org/paper/47b1578529d112c15d2382d40385029cd5a00ce9 (accessed on 17th July 2025).
4. Beerda, B., Wyszynska-Koko, J., Te Pas, M. F., de Wit, A. A., & Veerkamp, R. F. (2008). Expression profiles of genes regulating dairy cow fertility: recent findings, ongoing activities and future possibilities. *Animal : an international journal of animal bioscience, 2*(8), 1158–1167. https://doi.org/10.1017/S1751731108002371(accessed on 17th July 2025).
5. Brabletz, S., Schuhwerk, H., Brabletz, T., & Stemmler, M. P. (2021). Dynamic EMT: A multi-tool for tumor progression. *The EMBO Journal, 40.* https://doi.org/10.15252/embj.2021108647 (accessed on 17th July 2025).
6. Budin-Ljøsne, I., Mowinckel, A., Friedman, B. B., Ebmeier, K. P., Drevon, C., Carver, R., Zsoldos, E., et al. (2022). Public perceptions of brain health: An international, online cross-sectional survey. *BMJ Open, 12.* https://www.semanticscholar.org/paper/4fc8604c703c74a0138d6e8cf9663b02cc037b8a (accessed on 17th July 2025).
7. Bulun, S. E., Yıldız, Ş., Adli, M., & Wei, J. J. (2021). Adenomyosis pathogenesis: Insights from next-generation sequencing. *Human Reproduction Update, 27,* 1086–1097. https://doi.org/10.1093/humupd/dmab017 (accessed on 17th July 2025).
8. Cao, S., Zeng, Y., Pang, K., Chen, M., Guo, R., Wu, N., Fang, C., et al. (2025). Unraveling the causal impact of smoking and its DNA methylation signatures on cardiovascular disease: Mendelian randomization and colocalization analysis. *Clinical Epigenetics, 17.* https://www.semanticscholar.org/paper/4f2857919baedb6cd37bdf902cf2347b7a391dff (accessed on 17th July 2025).
9. Caputo, V., Tarantino, G., Santini, S., Fracassi, G., & Balsano, C. (2023). The role of epigenetic control of mitochondrial (dys)function in MASLD onset and progression. *Nutrients, 15.* https://www.semanticscholar.org/paper/b461950f31cc78db1cf0fe3599eeb36b94d5e6ae (accessed on 17th July 2025).
10. De Plano, L. D., Saitta, A., Oddo, S., & Caccamo, A. (2024). Epigenetic changes in Alzheimer's disease: DNA methylation and histone modification. *Cells, 13.* https://www.semanticscholar.org/paper/0aefa89391bc413098ec6046df7e6f962c808c91 (accessed on 17th July 2025).
11. Fulton, S., Décarie-Spain, L., Fioramonti, X., Guiard, B. P., & Nakajima, S. (2021). The menace of obesity to depression and anxiety prevalence. *Trends in Endocrinology and Metabolism, 33,* 18–35. https://doi.org/10.1016/j.tem.2021.10.005 (accessed on 17th July 2025).

12. Gausman, J., & Langer, A. (2020). Sex and gender disparities in the COVID-19 pandemic. *Journal of Women's Health, 29*, 465–466. https://doi.org/10.1089/jwh.2020.8472 (accessed on 17th July 2025).

13. Gordon, D. E., Jang, G. M., Bouhaddou, M., Xu, J., Obernier, K., White, K. M., O'Meara, M. J., et al. (2020). A SARS-CoV-2 protein interaction map reveals targets for drug repurposing. *Nature, 583*, 459–468. https://doi.org/10.1038/s41586-020-2286-9 (accessed on 17th July 2025).

14. Husain, S., Anand, C., Kranz, R. M., Hengst, K., Gellner, R., Bordewick-Dell, U., & Englert, H. (2025). Lifestyle medicine as a pathway to longevity: The impact of the Healthy Lifestyle Community Program (Cohort 2, HLCP-2) on oxidative stress biomarkers in the adult rural German population. *American Journal of Lifestyle Medicine*. https://www.semanticscholar.org/paper/0d6c2c9067f78c1c9b4604d66a286b5249097a1d (accessed on 17th July 2025).

15. Im, H. I. (2022). Epigenetic dysfunction of neurodegenerative diseases, MeCP2 and more. *International Neurourology Journal, 26*, S83–S84. https://www.semanticscholar.org/paper/48c8399368388fcaaa7d8e44aabbddef504fe3b5 (accessed on 17th July 2025).

16. James, S., Ijar, S., Shubhalakshmi, S., & Sithara, K. (2020). Epigenetics in oral pathology. *International Journal of Advanced Research*. https://www.semanticscholar.org/paper/0986ced99807852231d3233dcada56797d4e7031 (accessed on 17th July 2025).

17. Jones, B., Varambally, S., & Arend, R. C. (2018). Histone methyltransferase EZH2: A therapeutic target for ovarian cancer. *Molecular Cancer Therapeutics, 17*, 591–602. https://doi.org/10.1158/1535-7163.mct-17-0437 (accessed on 17th July 2025).

18. Jones, D. E., Park, J. S., Gamby, K., Bigelow, T. M., Mersha, T. B., & Folger, A. T. (2021). Mental health epigenetics: A primer with implications for counselors. *The Professional Counselor, 11*, 102–121. https://doi.org/10.15241/dej.11.1.102 (accessed on 17th July 2025).

19. Joshi, S., Geers, J., Gimelli, A., Hyafil, F., Habib, G., Erba, P., Gheysens, O., et al. (2024). Current and emerging radiotracers in molecular cardiovascular imaging. *Circulation: Cardiovascular Imaging, 17*, e016323. https://www.semanticscholar.org/paper/1fece8a841d54a491ad17d23b0dd0f344abf2e32 (accessed on 17th July 2025).

20. Kang, H. J., Min, B. K., Choi, W. I., Jeon, J. H., Kim, D. W., Park, S., Lee, Y., et al. (2021). Pyruvate dehydrogenase kinase 1 and 2 deficiency reduces high-fat diet-induced hypertrophic obesity and inhibits the differentiation of preadipocytes into mature adipocytes. *Experimental & Molecular Medicine, 53*, 1390–1401. https://www.semanticscholar.org/paper/aa60de52b486697881d4e822f31ba1e4abddc487 (accessed on 17th July 2025).

21. Karabaeva, R., Vochshenkova, T., Mussin, N., Albayev, R., Kaliyev, A., & Tamadon, A. (2024). Epigenetics of hypertension as a risk factor for the development of coronary artery disease in type 2 diabetes mellitus. *Frontiers in Endocrinology, 15*. https://www.semanticscholar.org/paper/c0fe2ba04fc786d4a35e237edebc313f13b5a793 (accessed on 17th July 2025).

22. Katu, A. H. (2024). The role of epigenetics in disease development. *Research Invention Journal of Public Health and Pharmacy*. https://www.semanticscholar.org/paper/8fdbb9da95b34556e48c72af047083e236b8d9d9 (accessed on 17th July 2025).

23. Khavkin, A. I., Loshkova, E., Doroshenko, I. V., Kondratyeva, E., & Erokhina, M. I. (2024). Vitamin D and the epigenome: Basic definitions, mechanisms and clinical effects. *Experimental and Clinical Gastroenterology*. https://www.semanticscholar.org/paper/dba964fbcaf4c85c84bb0be13e4445e7009533e5 (accessed on 17th July 2025).

24. Komarova, A. D., Vorobyeva, N. L., Dzhurtubaeva, D. R., Potapov, A., & Savostyanov, K. (2025). Intrafamilial phenotypic variability of the Wilson–Konovalov disease in pediatric patients. *L.O. Badalyan Neurological Journal*. https://www.semanticscholar.org/paper/cca1e88769bb15ada674ec1b3b986f18d147e566 (accessed on 17th July 2025).

25. Kumar, D. (2025). Assessing the impact of renewable energy technologies on urban air quality: A comparative analysis. *Journal of Scientific Advances*. https://www.semanticscholar.org/paper/531296eb92dc6deb3437783ad25e8f86ba937424 (accessed on 17th July 2025).

26. Larsson, L., Giraldo-Osorno, P. M., Garaicoa-Pazmino, C., Giannobile, W., & Asa'ad, F. (2024). DNA and RNA methylation in periodontal and peri-implant diseases. *Journal of Dental Research, 104*, 131–139. https://www.semanticscholar.org/paper/8bd1649061ac5eb09455aada74185110d0c7c667 (accessed on 17th July 2025).

27. Lozupone, M., Dibello, V., Sardone, R., Castellana, F., Zupo, R., Lampignano, L., Bortone, I., et al. (2023). The impact of apolipoprotein E (APOE) epigenetics on aging and sporadic Alzheimer's disease. *Biology, 12*. https://www.semanticscholar.org/paper/25f9e262915df3205768afb6abd25347d3644cb2 (accessed on 17th July 2025).

28. Lu, Y. (2024). CRISPRi: A promising RNA-guided CRISPR-dCas technology for Alzheimer's disease and glioma therapy. *Highlights in Science, Engineering and Technology*. https://www.semanticscholar.org/paper/6f31bbb30a9ebbbe5389b73a08ed644c773a99e8 (accessed on 17th July 2025).

29. Lundin, J. I., Peters, U., Hu, Y., Ammous, F., Avery, C., Benjamin, E. J., Bis, J., et al. (2024). Methylation patterns associated with C-reactive protein in racially and ethnically diverse populations. *Epigenetics, 19*. https://www.semanticscholar.org/paper/cc91dc15c44db9a1a15ec81e8ceef0246664b8f5 (accessed on 17th July 2025).

30. Ménézo, Y., Elder, K., Clément, A., & Clément, P. (2022). Folic acid, folinic acid, 5 methyl tetrahydrofolate supplementations for mutations that affect epigenesis through the folate and one-carbon cycles. *Biomolecules, 12*, 197. https://doi.org/10.3390/biom12020197 (accessed on 17th July 2025).

31. Moholdt, T., & Hawley, J. A. (2020). Maternal lifestyle interventions: Targeting preconception health. *Trends in Endocrinology and Metabolism, 31*, 561–569. https://doi.org/10.1016/j.tem.2020.03.002 (accessed on 17th July 2025).

32. Monteiro dos Santos, S., Romeiro, C. F. R., Rodrigues, C. A., Lima Cerqueira, A. R., & Monteiro, M. C. (2019). Mitochondrial dysfunction and alpha-lipoic acid: Beneficial or harmful in Alzheimer's disease? *Oxidative Medicine and Cellular Longevity, 2019*, 1–14. https://doi.org/10.1155/2019/8409329 (accessed on 17th July 2025).

33. Newell, M., Aravindan, A., Babbrah, A., & Halden, R. U. (2025). Epigenetic biomarkers driven by environmental toxins associated with Alzheimer's disease, Parkinson's disease, and amyotrophic lateral sclerosis in the United States: A systematic review. *Toxics, 13*. https://www.semanticscholar.org/paper/5ca91de75da95368ed0a82e2b485a334213dac0e (accessed on 17th July 2025).

34. Nicheperovich, A., Schuster-Böckler, B., & Ní Leathlobhair, M. (2025). Gestational trophoblastic disease: Understanding the molecular mechanisms of placental tumors. *Disease Models & Mechanisms, 18*. https://www.semanticscholar.org/paper/868739b3f281fc090bc2fad13c153fcdda9fbe99 (accessed on 17th July 2025).

35. E. Stanley, J. Plant, N. Voulvoulis. Environmental chemical exposures and breast cancer[J]. AIMS Environmental Science, 2016, 3(1): 96-114. doi: 10.3934/environsci.2016.1.96(accessed on 17th July 2025).

36. Lakshmi Priya R, Devi S. Nair. Ayurvedic Personalized Healthcare: Integrating Genomics, Epigenomics and Traditional Wisdom. J Ayurveda Integr Med Sci [Internet]. 2025 Feb. 3 [cited 2026 Jan. 31];9(11):192-7. Available from: https://jaims.in/jaims/article/view/3757(accessed on 17th July 2025).

37. Quagliano, A., Gopalakrishnapillai, A., Kolb, E., & Barwe, S. (2020). CD81 knockout promotes chemosensitivity and disrupts *in vivo* homing and engraftment in acute lymphoblastic leukemia. *Blood Advances, 4*(18), 4393–4405. https://www.semanticscholar.org/paper/e47c779ee39f13d4bde8d2762890bfddd3ace963 (accessed on 17th July 2025).

38. Rani, R. (2025). Screening of ceramide-dependent exosomal cargoes in terms of their vesicular abundance in colorectal cancer. *International Journal for Research in Applied Science and Engineering Technology*. https://www.semanticscholar.org/paper/eb70eab72e7c5388134d914992debab3c0b241de (accessed on 17th July 2025).

39. Reva, K., Laranjinha, J., & Rocha, B. S. (2023). Epigenetic modifications induced by the gut microbiota may result from what we eat: Should we talk about precision diet in health and disease? *Metabolites, 13*. https://www.semanticscholar.org/paper/d07e7d0127a84a76a118321d4c96fe016060e61d (accessed on 17th July 2025).

40. Saliev, T., & Singh, P. B. (2025). Age reprogramming: Innovations and ethical considerations for prolonged longevity (Review). *Biomedical Reports, 22*. https://www.semanticscholar.org/paper/2de8551a25d1bff63341699ffdcdbbf1cba6a749 (accessed on 17th July 2025).

41. Sargent, M., & Reed, A. (2024). The impact of lifestyle factors during pregnancy on the epigenome and subsequent risk of disease. *Journal of Student Research*. https://www.semanticscholar.org/paper/94f03a82341b81f90d84c96d8ee29dd83ff87b33 (accessed on 17th July 2025).

42. Skvortsova, K., Stirzaker, C., & Taberlay, P. C. (2019). The DNA methylation landscape in cancer. *Essays in Biochemistry, 63*, 797–811. https://doi.org/10.1042/ebc20190037 (accessed on 17th July 2025).

43. Takahashi, H., Kojima, D., & Watanabe, M. (2024). Therapeutic potential of trained immunity for malignant disease. *Immunological Medicine*. https://www.semanticscholar.org/paper/05c6da6d1a17ac4b6ca3837ab507a4a9801e2ed7 (accessed on 17th July 2025).

44. Tang, D., Chen, X., Kang, R., & Kroemer, G. (2020). Ferroptosis: Molecular mechanisms and health implications. *Cell Research, 31*, 107–125. https://doi.org/10.1038/s41422-020-00441-1 (accessed on 17th July 2025).

45. Tavajoh, S., Clark, M., Becerril Campos, A. A., Suur, B. E., Jansson, P. A. E., Soták, M., & Börgeson, E. (2025). 1741-P: Resolving inflammation in cardiometabolic health and disease. *Diabetes*. https://www.semanticscholar.org/paper/39cfac5e0caa11fc107649e731d40782c9d38aa1 (accessed on 17th July 2025).

46. van der Hee, B., & Wells, J. M. (2021). Microbial regulation of host physiology by short-chain fatty acids. *Trends in Microbiology, 29*, 700–712. https://doi.org/10.1016/j.tim.2021.02.001 (accessed on 17th July 2025).

47. Wais, N., & Agrawal, D. K. (2024). Systemic lupus erythematous: Gene polymorphisms, epigenetics, environmental, hormonal and nutritional factors in the consideration of personalized therapy. *Archives of Internal Medicine Research, 7*, 331–340. https://www.semanticscholar.org/paper/428678c501f775ebbda0f98b50dec6df4e84ea3f (accessed on 17th July 2025).

48. Wang, Z., Ma, T., Bai, G., Fang, Q., Ou, B., Chen, M., Xu, P., et al. (2025). Adipose tissue-derived extracellular vesicles loaded with miR-141-3p regulate obesity-induced insulin resistance by targeting glycogen synthesis and gluconeogenesis. *International Journal of Nanomedicine, 20*, 5709–5726. https://www.semanticscholar.org/paper/710eecc822c579c4f27d19d1b85723dd6ec05faa (accessed on 17th July 2025).

49. Whelton, P. K., Carey, R. M., Aronow, W. S., Casey, D. E., Collins, K. J., Himmelfarb, C. D., DePalma, S. M., et al. (2017). 2017 ACC/AHA/AAPA/ABC/ACPM/AGS/APhA/ASH/ASPC/NMA/PCNA guideline for the prevention, detection, evaluation, and management of high blood pressure in adults: A report of the American College of Cardiology/American Heart Association Task Force on Clinical Practice Guidelines. *Hypertension, 71*. https://doi.org/10.1161/hyp.0000000000000065 (accessed on 17th July 2025).

50. Xie, H., Yang, N., Yu, C., & Lu, L. (2024). Uremic toxins mediate kidney diseases: The role of aryl hydrocarbon receptor. *Cellular & Molecular Biology Letters, 29*. https://www.semanticscholar.org/paper/265fca68b9ab5522e8f662df85c17a83b2d3fe36 (accessed on 17th July 2025).

51. Yang, Z. (2024). Research on the relationship between obesity and epigenetics and its application. *Theoretical and Natural Science*. https://www.semanticscholar.org/paper/7d1fd5363c01d0ace55b749299d50c9a5c64f1b4 (accessed on 17th July 2025).

52. Yüksel, F. (2024). Comprehensive exploration of CRISPR and gene editing technologies: Applications, ethical considerations, and future implications in genetic research. *Next Frontier for Life Sciences and AI*. https://www.semanticscholar.org/paper/5964dc1df8adfb85b1e38e0d0291b34afa266e6e (accessed on 17th July 2025).

53. Zhang, E., & He, P. (2024). The function of histone methyltransferase SETDB1 and its roles in liver cancer. *Frontiers in Cell and Developmental Biology, 12*. https://www.semanticscholar.org/paper/775e9dd157e3b9dd836833865f11fe90ae06aaa7 (accessed on 17th July 2025).

54. Zhanqiang, L., Huoqiang, H., & Dianxiang, L. (2023). Epigenetics mechanism and therapeutic potential of approved epi-drugs in pulmonary hypertension disease. *Current Topics in Medicinal Chemistry*. https://www.semanticscholar.org/paper/f236206d8307ecf990a4fe218407a632168b3c3f (accessed on 17th July 2025).

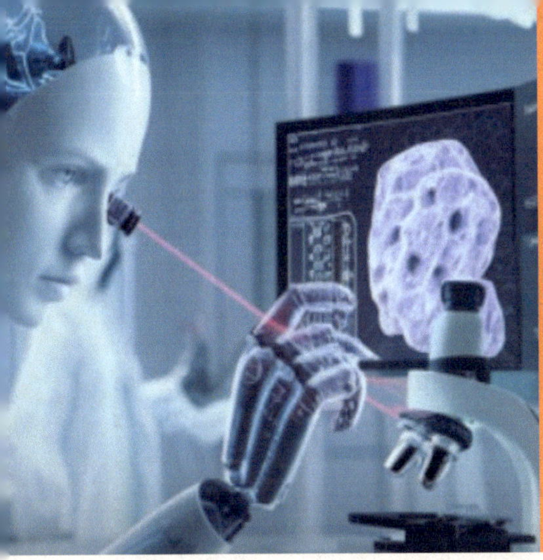

Chapter 10
BIOINFORMATICS IN MOLECULAR PATHOLOGY

Contents

Introduction

The field of bioinformatics is the force that propels molecular pathology as a bridging interface between computer technology and biological understanding. With large biological databases having to be managed increasingly, bioinformatics has emerged as an essential tool in disease diagnosis, prognosis, and treatment. Such convergence not only enriches our knowledge of various genetic and molecular mechanisms of disease but also points towards the importance of data integration in pathology. Access to bioinformatics tools is transforming traditional diagnostic strategies, allowing clinicians and researchers to visualize complex sets of data that can drive precision medicine initiatives. Against this background, the integration of bioinformatics into pathology brings about a new era of innovation, wherein powerful algorithms and methods of analysis result in improved patient outcomes and tailored therapeutic strategies, revising the standards of care in the specialty. Additionally, the evolution of technologies , such as next-generation sequencing (NGS) has revolutionized the paradigm of diagnosis in molecular pathology. With clinical labs expanding the number of targeted NGS panels for the identification of genetic variants associated with various inherited disorders, the requirement for rigorous assay design and validation has emerged. Validation of the tests ensures their effectiveness and reliability, generating trust in their use in clinical decision-making. Implications from such validations enforce the key function of bioinformatics in the analysis of NGS data, where algorithms detect relevant variants among extensive genomic data. Through establishing stringent performance criteria before implementation, clinical laboratories can capture the full power of NGS technology, thereby resulting in more accurate diagnoses and customized treatment strategies that are critical in modern medicine. Finally, the role of crowdsourcing within bioinformatics is another innovative element within the broader landscape of molecular pathology. Engaging a broad population, even those with minimal formal education, has been found to expedite data curation and analysis. Democratization of research input not only increases participation but also accelerates human pathology discovery. Crowdsourcing has various uses, from data annotation to crowdsourced research, which can yield interesting information regarding disease mechanisms. While such dynamics have been addressed in previous studies, their views have a tendency to omit a comprehensive review of previously published works. The systematic review of crowdsourcing applications has the potential to unveil its advantages and drawbacks, guiding future research activities and solidifying bioinformatics position as a driving force behind molecular pathology (Figure 10.1).

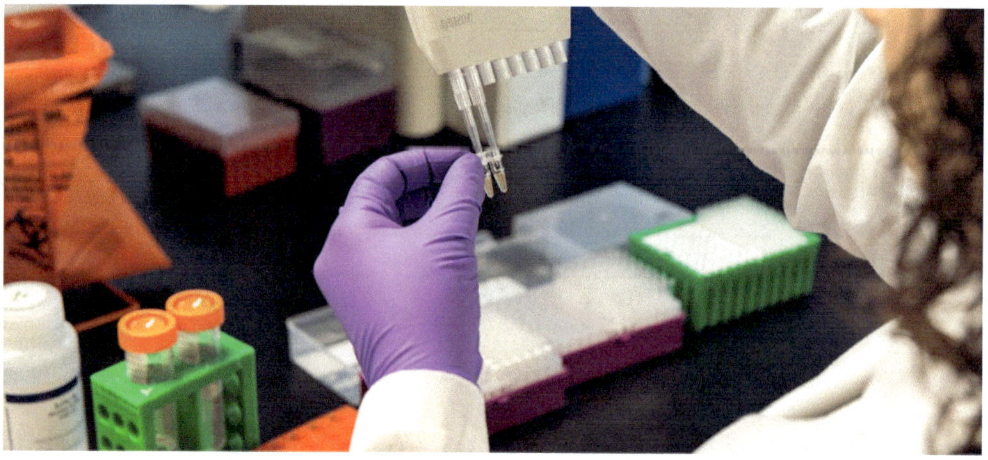

Figure 10.1. Bioinformatics in molecular pathology.

Source: https://pathology.jhu.edu/build/assets/department/_image1200/molecular-pathology-research.jpg.

Definition of Bioinformatics

In molecular pathology, bioinformatics comes to play a significant cross-disciplinary field incorporating biology, computer science, and mathematics to facilitate the analysis and interpretation of high-level biological data. Bioinformatics can be defined as the development of algorithms, computational tools, and databases required for understanding variability and biological processes at the molecular level. This is particularly relevant in fields like genomics and transcriptomics, where lots of data need to be handled and analyzed quickly. Through the use of bioinformatics, scientists are able to extract useful conclusions from large datasets, thus allowing for increased accuracy in molecular pathology diagnostics. For instance, the use of deep learning techniques in bioinformatics has transformed computational pathology and enabled accurate high-resolution mapping of tissues and cells, which is vital to identifying cancer regions and directing the treatment decision-making process (Amgad et al., 2021). Bioinformatics also plays an important role in the personalization of medicine through genetic screening, which has gained increased clinical relevance. The field is an umbrella for a wide range of genetic sequencing techniques, including targeted gene sequencing and whole exome sequencing (ES). The methods facilitate comprehensive assessment in the identification of genetic variants that lead to various diseases, thereby making it possible to have accurate diagnoses and tailored treatment plans. The use of exome sequencing highlights the position of bioinformatics due to its need for sophisticated data interpretation methods to detect pathogenic variants amidst many genetic sequences. Accurate interpretation matters as it affects clinical outcome and family members' risk evaluation (Kiryluk et al., 2019). With the development of bioinformatics, it has become pivotal to crack the codes of human genetic complexities and improve molecular pathology results. Moreover, the utilities of bioinformatics are more than mere data analysis; they symbolize a progressive synergy between human expertise and machine learning methods. With the advent of collaborative platforms integrating artificial intelligence, bioinformatics enables the efficient generation of high-quality annotation datasets required for computational pathology. This integration not only accelerates annotation processing, such as identifying cell nuclei in cancer histology, but also enhances diagnostic outcomes' reliability. Further, crowd-sourcing methods founded on the common and expert intelligence ideally depict an innovative approach that bioinformatics can undertake. Through teamwork in data tagging and implementation of algorithmic suggestions, the domain continues to evolve to handle increasing data loads, ultimately leading to increased diagnostic accuracy and treatment results in molecular pathology (Amgad et al., 2021).

Overview of Molecular Pathology

Molecular pathology is the point at which molecular biology and pathology meet, and it involves the molecular cause of disease. Molecular pathology is a developing field, revolutionizing how diseases are interpreted since it enables researchers and clinicians to examine the genetic, epigenetic, and proteomic changes that occur in the progression of disease. By applying techniques like next-generation sequencing, transcriptomics, and proteomics, molecular pathology is involved in the detection of biomarkers that guide diagnosis, prognosis, and therapeutic approaches. This information is crucial for developing strategies for personalized medicine, where treatment is tailored based on a patient's individual molecular disease profile. Moreover, the integration of molecular pathology with bioinformatics allows for the analysis and interpretation of integrated data, enhancing our ability to form valid conclusions from complex biological data sets and ultimately closing the discovery-to-clinical utility gap. Molecular pathology is making strides, but much remains to be done in harmonizing methodologies and nomenclatures in research and in practice. Diverse definitions and classifications, especially in research domains like microbiome science, have been the cause of inconsistencies holding back progress. An international experts' workshop in microbiome science demonstrated the necessity for a shared framework, highlighting how important clarity in term definition and normal practice are (Berg et al., 2020). Similarly, in molecular pathology, there is a need for consensus on biomarkers, their validation, and how they can be utilized across different diseases. Such harmonization would not only facilitate easy communication among researchers and clinicians but also enhance confidence in the results obtained from molecular studies. Such harmonization would be critical in the establishment of molecular pathology as an authentic diagnostic and therapeutic tool. Besides, spatiotemporal molecular imaging is emerging as a pressing innovation in molecular pathology, extending disease mechanism knowledge at an evolutionary level. Through imaging techniques being combined with molecular information, researchers can visualize and analyze the exact localization and timing of molecular events in tissues. This new approach enables the observation of cell-cell contact and changes in the environment in real time and significantly improves the comprehension of disease development and therapeutic outcome (Wang & Fan, 2021). The spatiotemporal focus not only improves the context of molecular events but also calls attention to the complex nature of pathophysiological processes as they take place. The convergence of molecular pathology with bioinformatics and advanced imaging modalities is thus an area of crossing the divide of laboratory findings to tangible clinical application and ultimately to more effective treatment.

Importance of Integrating Bioinformatics in Molecular Pathology

The integration of bioinformatics in molecular pathology is a new way of understanding complex diseases at a molecular level. With the application of whole computational strategies, researchers can analyze a huge amount of genomic, transcriptomic, and proteomic data derived from various biological samples. This new method of analysis not only makes data interpretation easier but also provides greater insight into disease mechanisms. For instance, the gene analysis of atopic eczema (AE) has revealed key inflammatory pathways for the pathology of the disease. Discovering such key genes as IL10 and TGFB1 illustrates how bioinformatics can help determine molecular targets that will give rise to new therapies and improve patient outcomes through personalized medicine (Sindhu et al., 2025). Furthermore, bioinformatics plays a major role in peri-implantitis (PI) diagnosis and treatment. Through the intersection of ferroptosis-associated genes and differentially expressed genes, researchers can explore important biomarkers that can greatly enhance disease development knowledge. With the use of advanced machine learning approaches, bioinformatics can recognize key indicators like FLT3 and TLR4, determining their function in the immune response and inflammation of PI. The capacity to conduct gene set enrichment analysis serves to further characterize the underlying mechanisms, illustrating how immune cell profiles define the diseased and healthy samples. By accurate mapping of these pathways, bioinformatics significantly facilitates the development of targeted therapies, thus facilitating a better method of disease treatment (Huang et al., 2025). Incorporation of bioinformatics into molecular pathology not only increases our insight into disease processes but also leads to innovation in the development of drugs. Being capable of deciphering large data sets effectively and efficiently allows the detection of patterns and correlations previously undetectable. As illustrated by AE and PI case studies, bioinformatics bridges the experimental research-clinical practice gap. Such convergence fosters a three-dimensional understanding of diseases via the harmonization of molecular data and clinical results. Hence, embracing bioinformatics as the fundamental component of molecular pathology is vital for diagnosis and therapeutic progress, hence enhancing the practice of medicine and patient care in the forthcoming years. Such cross-disciplinary techniques allow scientists to utilize the power of information in an attempt to tackle frequent medical problems more effectively.

10.1. Historical Context

The background history of bioinformatics in molecular pathology dates back to the deep advances in genomic technology and computational biology. The human genome was completely sequenced in the early 2000s, setting the pace for the integration of bioinformatics in various fields of biology and medicine. This magnum opus not only presented a complete atlas of human genetic material but also indicated the need for sophisticated data analysis tools to translate complex biological information. As researchers understood the function of dissecting large amounts of genomic data, bioinformatics has evolved from a background tool to becoming central in interpreting molecular pathology. The interaction between computer science and molecular biology has enabled it to develop algorithms and software that streamline data management, hence providing increased insight into the disease process and possible areas of therapeutic intervention. In the early days of molecular pathology, standard diagnostic approaches utilized histopathology and cytogenetics heavily. As the limitations of these technologies became more obvious, particularly in the case of proper diagnosis of heterogeneous diseases, the need for advanced technologically innovative approaches arose. With the implementation of bioinformatics, molecular pathologists have begun incorporating multi-omics information—i.e., genomics, transcriptomics, and proteomics—into their analyses. The advent of next-generation sequencing technologies played a crucial role in this revolution, providing an unparalleled understanding of pathogen behavior and host-pathogen interactions. Nearly all pathogens contain DNA or RNA genomes and thus sequencing is a very promising way of pathogen identification (Gu et al., 2018). The rapid pace at which bioinformatics software has evolved has consequently played an instrumental role in the simplification of diagnosis methods to more precise and personalized disease treatment.

Moreover, the integration of bioinformatics into molecular pathology has accelerated the shift towards standardization and data sharing among the global research community. Previous collaborations, both through global workshops and consortia, have facilitated the exchange of knowledge and best practices development in microbiome science (Berg et al., 2020). With the developments in frameworks over time, there is a focus on the use of a shared approach to bioinformatics applications. Not only does this enhance the credibility and reproducibility of the research results but also helps in overcoming constraints of the time. For instance, higher standards of microbiome will be instrumental in tackling pressing global healthcare problems, particularly those driven by anthropogenic changes. The development of bioinformatics from its humble beginnings is a mirror to the journey towards cooperation, innovation, and progressive refinement of methods that eventually enhance our understanding of molecular pathology (Figure 10.2).

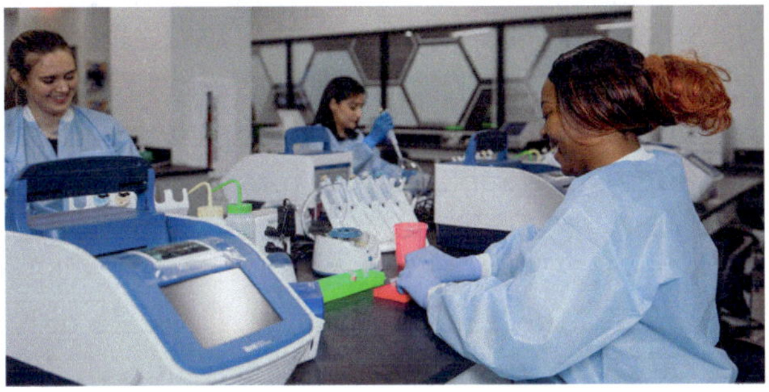

Figure 10.2. Molecular pathology.

Source: https://www.ttuhsc.edu/health-professions/images/master-of-science-molecular-pathology/MP_98.jpg.

10.1.1. Evolution of Bioinformatics

Bioinformatics has significantly transformed the discipline of molecular pathology through the availability of refined tools for data analysis and interpretation. Bioinformatics first concentrated on the handling of biological data in the form of databases, such as nucleotide and protein sequences. Upon the development of high-throughput sequencing technologies, bioinformatics evolved to a new phase by producing vast quantities of datasets requiring advanced analytical techniques. As these databases grew in volume and sophistication, there came the need for sophisticated software solutions that enabled genomic, proteomic, and clinical information to be integrated. This was a breakthrough, as researchers began tapping computer power to draw meaningful conclusions from data and dictate diagnostic methods and treatment plans in molecular pathology ahead of time.

The convergence of computational innovation and biological expertise opened up an unparalleled revolution in personalized medicine, which made it possible to have tailored therapeutic interventions based on the unique molecular profile of a patient. Furthermore, the advancement of artificial intelligence (AI) in bioinformatics is a landmark achievement in the history of science. AI algorithms are capable of enhancing the accuracy and precision of cancer diagnosis and therapy, particularly in precision oncology that seeks to customize treatment protocols to the personal characteristics of patients. Incorporating AI applications streamlines the analysis of large, intricate data sets to identify certain molecular and cellular traits of various malignancies. This shift is located in applications like digital pathology and immune checkpoint inhibitors, which achieve maximum therapeutic effects through targeted precision against cancer-specific attributes. However, the addition of AI is not without challenges; challenges regarding algorithmic bias and the reliability of conclusions generated by AI point to a need for ongoing evaluation and refinement of these technologies. Resolution of such issues will enable the application of AI more rigorously in molecular pathology, creating potential for future breakthroughs. In addition, collaborative platforms have become a vital aspect of bioinformatics development, making it possible to achieve more efficiency in data generation and annotation. For instance, recent studies chronicle the successful use of crowdsourcing techniques in annotating cell nuclei on histological images, enabling large-scale computational pathology applications. The NuCLS dataset is an example of how incorporating medical students and expert pathologists can provide dramatic gains in label quality without imposing clinician drudgery. This groundbreaking approach not only provides higher-quality training data available for machine learning purposes but also demonstrates the efficacy of harnessing collaborative expertise in bioinformatics. These advances signify the potential of machine learning for revolutionizing the field so that more sophisticated models can be developed that efficiently depict tissue architectures and cellular structures in pathology for facilitating further diagnostic and therapeutic endeavors in molecular pathology (Figure 10.3).

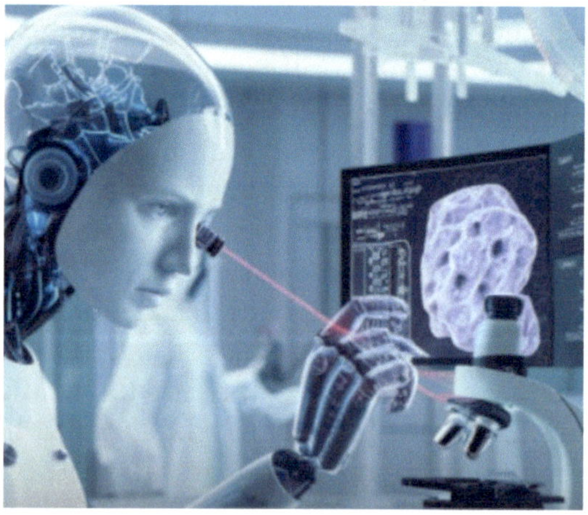

Figure 10.3. Evolution of bioinformatics.

Source: https://pathobot.in/website/wp-content/uploads/2024/08/the-role-of-ai-in-pathology.jpg.

10.1.2. Development of Molecular Pathology

Molecular pathology is an innovative branch of clinical diagnostics that amalgamates the principles of molecular biology with traditional pathology to provide a better understanding of disease mechanisms. It is a method of assessing biological samples at the molecular level, allowing us to attain in-depth knowledge regarding the etiology and course of a disease. As technology in bioinformatics tools and methods continues to advance, they increasingly become essential for the interpretation of vast sets of data generated by workflows , including next-generation sequencing (NGS) and various omics approaches. This has been particularly important in unraveling complex diseases , such as cancer, whose treatment and prognosis are determined to a great extent by molecular heterogeneity. Notably, the development of bioinformatics protocols is a top priority in ensuring valid interpretation of data, as emphasized in the NGS workflows that identify quality assurance at all stages of analysis, paving the way for improved diagnostics and personalized medicine strategies (Arroyo et al., 2021).

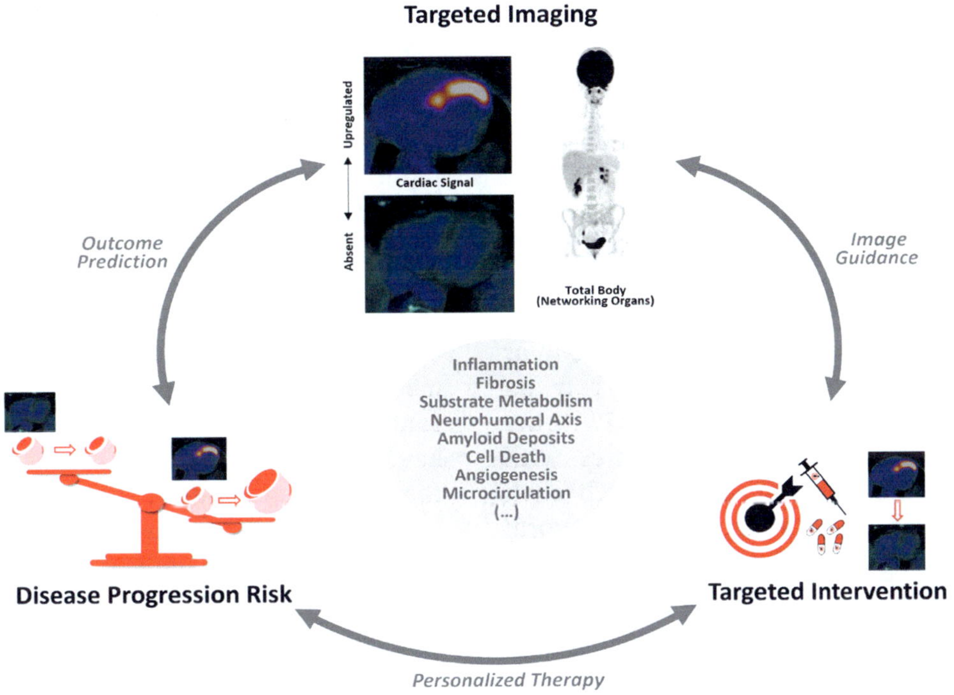

Figure 10.4. Development of molecular pathology.

Source: https://www.researchgate.net/publication/360409366/figure/fig2/AS:1184420639846400@1659399294388/Novel-molecular-imaging-techniques-Schematic-display-of-molecular-imaging-guided.png.

The establishment of spatiotemporal molecular pathology also represents a watershed in the way we understand interactions between molecular processes and clinical outcomes. By bridging space and time into molecular profiling, researchers are better able to understand disease in terms of how it takes place in the human organism. This multi-component approach demands the merging of numerous distinct methodologies—e.g., imaging techniques, molecular diagnostics, and modeling strategies—to know how cell-cell interactions promote disease progression. The potential is vast, from the dissection of tumor microenvironment to the real-time monitoring of treatment responses. The difficulty is in making the transition between intangible molecular information and concrete clinical imagery since a precise modeling of spatiotemporal parameters may significantly contribute to therapeutic approaches and patient care (Wang & Fan, 2021). With the advancement of the field of molecular pathology, the cooperation between technical progress and clinical application continues to take center stage. The development of imaging and computing technologies allows for the creation of high-resolution, multidimensional datasets to visualize molecular events within their original tissue architecture. The marriage of bioinformatics and molecular pathology allows not only for exquisite delineation of disease phenomena but also the untangling of the subtleties involved in intra- and intercellular variations. Future development will rely on the development of robust databases with the capability to blend clinical phenomics with molecular profiles uninterrupted. With such integration, the full potential of spatiotemporal analyses in molecular pathology can be realized, ushering in a new era of diagnosis and tailor-made therapeutic regimens based on an integrated vision of disease biology and patient-specific variations (Arroyo et al., 2021; Wang & Fan, 2021) (Figure 10.4).

10.1.3. Milestones in the Integration of Bioinformatics and Molecular Pathology

The integration of bioinformatics with molecular pathology has recorded giant steps that have reinterpreted our understanding and reaction to disease diagnosis and treatment. The most dominant aspect of this integration, arguably, is the development of genomic data analysis tools that simplify the decoding of complicated genetic variations that are associated with diseases. With the aid of computational algorithms and machine learning techniques, researchers have been able to identify biomarkers that are necessary for the diagnosis and treatment of various cancers and genetic disorders. For instance, the analysis of next-generation sequencing data has facilitated personalized medicine, and drugs have been formulated based on the genetic makeup of a tumor patient, leading to improved therapeutic responses. It has not only streamlined the diagnostic procedures but also provided a clearer insight into molecular disease mechanisms, which is essential to developing novel therapeutic strategies. Furthermore, bioinformatics has played an important role in streamlining the work process of molecular pathology, particularly through the introduction of automated systems and databases to manage high-throughput data. The ability to store and process vast quantities of biological data has led to the identification of patterns and correlations otherwise not revealed through traditional methodology. Comparative expression data from cancer and non-cancerous tissues, for instance, have facilitated the identification of potential therapeutic compounds and an understanding of tumor growth and behavior. The synergy between bioinformatics and molecular pathology speeds up the tempo and accuracy of diagnosis, as can be seen with the application of bioinformatics algorithms in the detection of rare diseases through correlating genomic information with big databases. Such technological innovations are thus a pillar to enhance patient care and hasten research work in the medical science field. Against the background of novel therapeutic interventions, bioinformatics integration has enabled exploration of novel gene therapy vectors, such as adeno-associated viruses (AAV). The vector system has shown potential by its ability to transfer genes that are of low pathogenicity, which is vital in developing safe therapeutic options. The bioinformatics-based design of recombinant AAV (rAAV) for increased specificity shows the ways in which bioinformatics not only aids the design of effective delivery systems but also the evasion of potential safety concerns related to gene therapy. As in recent reviews, the exploration of AAV requires a high-level understanding of immune responses and resulting side effects accounted for by bioinformatics tools at trial phases of rAAV-based treatments (Wang et al., 2024). Also, research on γδ T cell-based immunotherapy continues to bring attention to the contribution of bioinformatics to the identification and normalization of immune responses in the immune system, presenting yet another opportunity for the integration of bioinformatics with molecular pathology (Hu et al., 2023) (Figure 10.5).

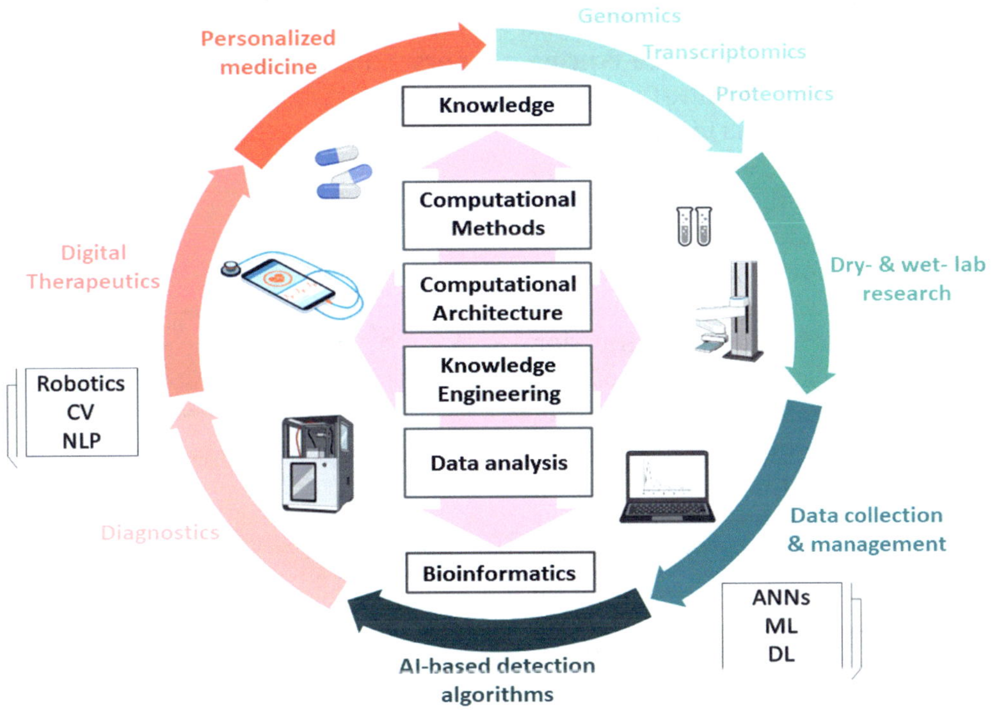

Figure 10.5. Milestones in the integration of bioinformatics and molecular pathology.

Source: https://pub.mdpi-res.com/biomedinformatics/biomedinformatics-02-00049/article_deploy/html/images/biomedinformatics-02-00049-g002.png?1671604398.

10.2. Key Technologies in Bioinformatics

The addition of advanced technologies in bioinformatics is a pivotal aspect towards the enhancement of molecular pathology, transforming diagnostic practices drastically. Quantitative Trait Loci (QTL) mapping and Genome-Wide Association Studies (GWASs) are a few of the techniques through which genomic markers for various diseases can be discovered, which ultimately leads to enhanced classification of molecular subtypes. These methods enable researchers to link some genetic variations to phenotypic traits, thereby enabling the early detection and diagnosis of diseases. In addition, the discovery of genomic selection (GS) simplified and accelerated breeding of organisms with desirable characteristics, hence enhancing crop resistance and productivity, which is crucial in mitigating food security concerns. Systematic application of these bioinformatics resources offers a robust foundation for unraveling complex molecular interactions, thereby driving progress in precision medicine and personalized therapeutic strategies, particularly in precision diagnostics as evident in bioinformatics applications in molecular pathology. Use of genome-editing technologies, particularly CRISPR-Cas9, has transformed bioinformatics. This technology not only allows precise alterations at specific loci in the genome but also allows for the interrogation of gene functions and regulatory networks. The impact on molecular pathology is immense since targeted alteration can lead to enhanced insights into disease mechanisms and the identification of effective treatments. By applying such editing techniques along with bioinformatics analysis, scientists can predict and interrogate outcomes of genetic changes and therefore transform laboratory results into clinical practice. For instance, the accurate manipulation of tumor-related genes can enable efficient research on tumorigenesis and the development of novel therapies. Thus, the integration of CRISPR technology with bioinformatics platforms is a reflection of the extent of innovation leading the field of molecular pathology towards more precise diagnosis and treatment personalization in clinical settings. The future of molecular pathology bioinformatics is unprecedented, particularly with the advent of next-generation diagnostic pathology (NGDP) paradigms. NGDP integrates traditional histopathology with molecular detection and next-generation bioinformatics analysis, making the diagnostic input of pathologists more valuable. The new method is designed such that diagnostic reports contain in-depth multi-omics details, which are extremely valuable in the understanding of complex disease mechanisms and enhanced predictive value for disease outcome and treatment responsiveness. As noted, the role of artificial intelligence in the analysis of large datasets also propels this advancement further, making intelligent diagnoses and remote consultations efficiently performed. The anticipated milestones in this field highlight the significance of continuing study and inter-disciplinary coordination, aiming to establish new golden standards of clinical medicine while addressing the current challenges within the health system, particularly in terms of personalized patient treatment as highlighted by future technologies (Bian et al., 2022) (Figure 10.6).

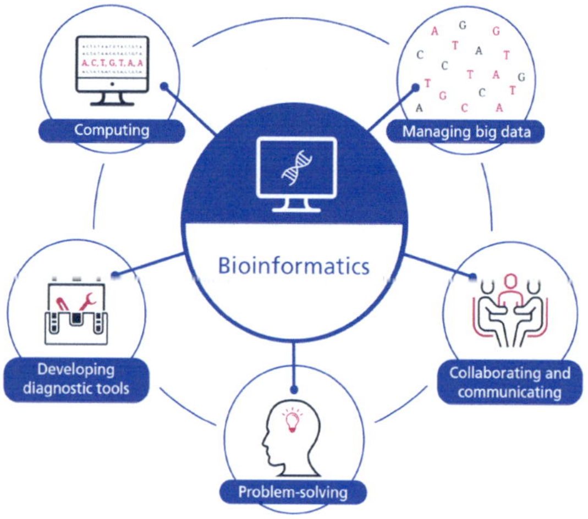

Figure 10.6. Key technologies in bioinformatics.

Source: https://www.genomicseducation.hee.nhs.uk/wp-content/uploads/2021/04/Bioinformatics-graphic-01-983x640.png.

10.2.1. Genomic Sequencing Technologies

The advent of genomic sequencing technologies has revolutionized molecular pathology significantly by offering the ability to conduct extensive analysis of genetic material in numerous biological specimens. The technologies, primarily the next-generation sequencing (NGS), offer for the rapid and cost-effective sequencing of extremely large gene panels that potentially contain hundreds of genes. The capacity to analyze vast amounts of genetic information significantly enhances the diagnostic process and leads to the timely and correct identification of the pathogen. Employing sequencing for diagnostic purposes, physicians can diagnose complex genetic changes that cause disease and thereby make it feasible for customized treatment protocols to be formulated according to the genetic profile of individual patients. Incorporation of genomic sequencing in routine clinical work thus marks a significant milestone for molecular pathology, consistent with the evolutionary transformation towards precision medicine. Furthermore, genomic sequencing plays a crucial role in the detection and management of infectious diseases. Genomic surveillance, a simple use of sequencing technology, provides critical information on the genetic nature of pathogens, facilitating the investigation of plant-pathogen interactions as well as the tracking of disease outbreaks.

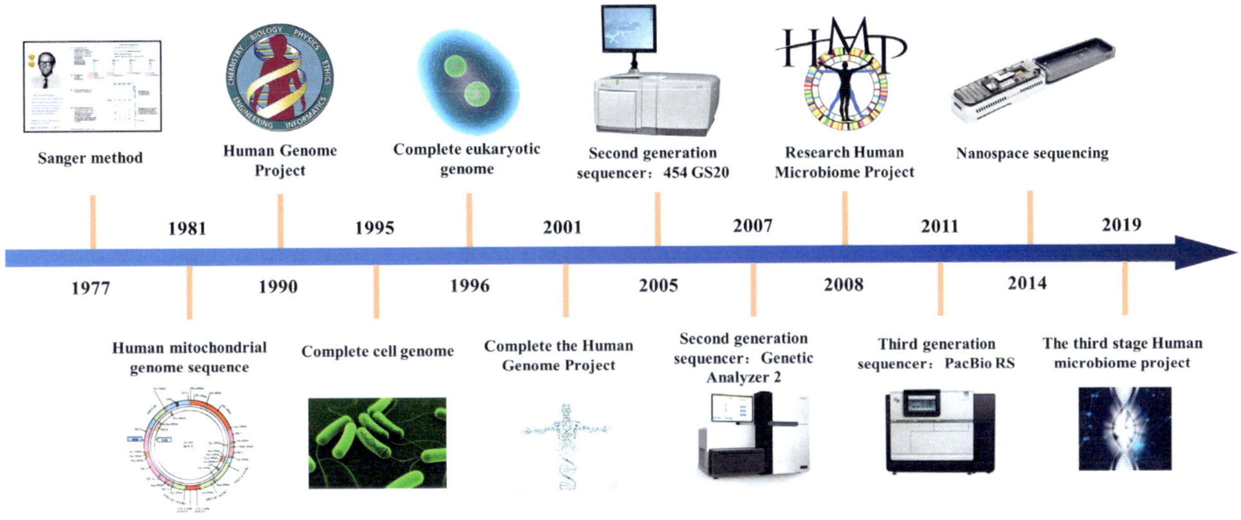

Figure 10.7. Genomic sequencing technologies.

Source: https://substackcdn.com/image/fetch/f_auto,q_auto:good,fl_progressive:steep/https://bucketeer-e05bbc84-baa3-437e-9518-adb32be77984.s3.amazonaws.com/public/images/3f3c3d4a-7a25-44bf-b92a-fdeb185f4b60_880x364.png.

For instance, the use of metagenomics as genomic surveillance provides early detection of impending threats and characterization of pathogen populations. These observations are crucial in developing effective management strategies during times when food security is increasingly under attack from plant diseases, causing substantial crop yield losses, estimated at between 20% and 40% globally. By the potential of genomic data, bioinformatics technology promotes point-of-care disease management, thus promoting agricultural resilience and health. But despite numerous advantages in genomic sequencing technologies, challenges remain, particularly in the interpretation of sequencing data. The complexity involved can make variant interpretations different between labs due to the sheer volumes of data provided by NGS require robust analytical frameworks. Such problems are resolved by applying criteria established by organizations , such as the American College of Medical Genetics and Genomics (ACMG) to standardize variant classification so that comparability is enhanced and errors reduced. Software like GenOtoScope makes certain aspects of this classification easier, particularly for conditions like hereditary hearing loss, where direct examination of variants can be time and labor-intensive. This enhancement of data interpretation processes is a testament to the intersection of bioinformatics and molecular pathology, showcasing the way technology can provide relief for the workload of genomic data analysis tasks while allowing for a more streamlined diagnostic setting (Figure 10.7).

10.2.2. Data Analysis Tools and Software

The success of bioinformatics in molecular pathology is also greatly increased with the utilization of various data analysis software and tools that can handle large volumes of biological data. These resources facilitate the processing, visualization, and interpretation of the complex information that ultimately leads to the recognition of the significant genetic variations as well as interactions. For instance, bioinformatics software , such as STRING and ShinyGO offer sophisticated network analysis capabilities that allow researchers to detect the relationship between genes and their corresponding biological processes. In the case of neuroprotective therapy for neurodegenerative disorders like multiple sclerosis, as mentioned by Kapadia et al. (2023), the selection of proper bioinformatics tools becomes a critical factor in detecting and targeting specific molecular pathways implicated in disease pathogenesis.

Also, public databases , such as Gene Expression Omnibus (GEO) are helpful when it comes to accessing publicly released genomic information, which, when analyzed, offers knowledge regarding diseases. The application of meta-analysis programs , such as the bi-level meta-analysis (BLMA), is particularly pertinent in enhancing differential gene expression between studies (Horan et al., 2023). Through the integration of a combination of high-throughput sequencing data and aggressive statistical models, researchers are able to increase the power of their tests as well as gain a better understanding of molecular mechanisms. The interaction between cutting-edge computational techniques and bioinformatics tools is thus pivotal in moving the field of molecular pathology ahead. Further, the continuous development of bioinformatics tools has facilitated the addition of user-friendly interfaces and reproducible analysis pipelines, allowing researchers to join the community more easily. The R language, in the case of open tools like through packages , such as DESeq2, demonstrates how open tools can be transformed to be used for gene expression data analysis so that analyses can be tailored to fit the specific research goals. This flexibility will be essential in ongoing research in identifying gene targets for complicated diseases, as seen in the case of oocyte quality studies under endometriosis (Horan et al., 2023). As technology progresses, the refinement of these tools in data analysis will be essential for developing new treatment modalities and improving patient outcomes in molecular pathology (Figure 10.8).

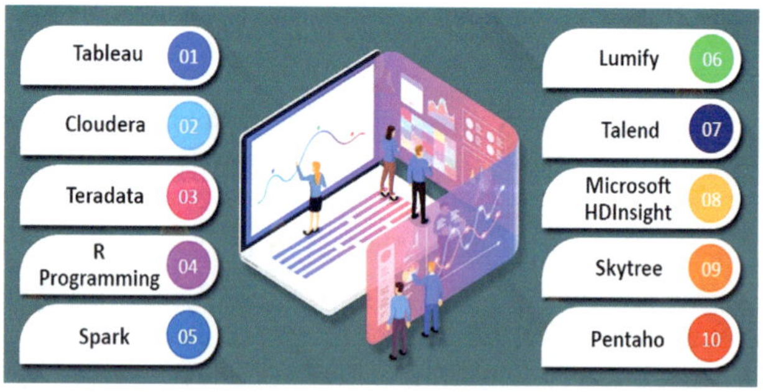

Figure 10.8. Data analysis tools and software.

Source: https://www.acte.in/wp-content/uploads/2022/01/Top-Tools-of-Big-Data-Analytics-with-its-Features-ACTE.jpg.

10.2.3. Databases and Repositories for Molecular Data

In the rapidly expanding area of bioinformatics, molecular information repositories and databases are at the heart of the integration and analysis of large-scale biological data sets. Online repositories , such as The Gene Expression Omnibus (GEO) and The Cancer Genome Atlas (TCGA) are portals to rich genomic and transcriptomic data available for researchers to utilize in an effort to comprehend disease mechanisms and therapeutic strategies. The ability to construct, annotate, and analyze vast collections of molecular data enhances the understanding of complex disease, including various forms of cancer and metabolic syndromes. Scientists increasingly rely on such repositories in uncovering patterns and relationships in multilayered data sets to help identify novel biomarkers and drive personalized medicine approaches. Molecular data repositories not only make it easier to access crucial information but also promote collaboration and reproducibility between scientists. By making the datasets interoperable across scientific communities, databases open up the potential for integrative analysis and meta-analysis. For instance, integrating multiple RNA sequencing datasets can make it feasible to have a stronger understanding of differential gene expression between conditions. The network-based integrative analysis (NBIA) approach shows this possibility, highlighting how researchers can integrate data from various experiments to generate insightful results. This is especially useful in the context of multifactorial disease etiology, such as endometriosis, where oocyte quality is impaired through intricate biological processes and cell-to-cell interactions, as in the case of oocyte, granulosa, and cumulus cells (Horan et al., 2023). Recent advances in computational biology underscore the value of these databases in finding new biomarkers for prognosis and diagnosis in molecular pathology. As an example, research into Ribonucleoprotein (RNP) complexes as PSC biomarkers shows how public repositories can be utilized to determine dysregulated transcripts related to disease development. By taking data from databases like TCGA and NCBI GEO, researchers have detected non-canonical RBPs, which show differential expression in PSC as well as Cholangiocarcinoma (CCA) (Ala & Fagoonee, 2024). The finding points toward the potential application of bioinformatics tools for creating non-invasive screening tools for disease early detection and tracking. With biomedical research in its ongoing development, the need for available and extensive databases will grow more and more critical to driving innovation in molecular pathology.

10.3. Applications in Disease Diagnosis

Use of bioinformatics in molecular pathology has greatly influenced the diagnosis of multifaceted conditions to allow for a more accurate understanding of pathophysiological mechanisms. For example, for multifactorial illnesses , such as primary hypertension (PHTN) and IgA vasculitis (IgAV), bioinformatics tools are used to analyze differentially expressed genes (DEGs) that account for varied biological processes for each disease. The functional enrichment analysis and the identification of DEGs enable clinicians to determine exact genetic markers responsible for the state of disease and therefore enhance the accuracy of diagnosis and direct therapeutic approaches. As the intersection of DEGs in PHTN and IgAV suggests, there are implied common molecular pathways, pointing out that bioinformatics not just enables the identification of diseases but also what they share, opening the door for improved management strategies (Wei et al., 2025). Moreover, bioinformatics application goes beyond genetic data, such as integrative approaches that promote disease diagnosis through the identification of immune cell profiles. The application of platforms , such as CIBERSORT allows scientists to analyze immune cell infiltration within affected tissue, enabling informative details about the immune landscape that is correlated with diseases , such as PHTN and IgAV. Traditionally, histopathological examinations were limited to morphological examination, but with the integration of bioinformatics, these examinations are formulated into comprehensive examinations that inform clinical interventions. Through enabling the identification of immune cell compositions that correlate with various pathologies, bioinformatics not only enhances diagnostics but also assists in the formulation of targeted intervention and personalized medicine approaches in the treatment of chronic diseases (Garg et al., 2025). On a larger scale of disease diagnosis, bioinformatics has revolutionized the application of personalized medicine, tailoring treatment strategies based on individual patient profiles. This is particularly relevant in cardiovascular disease management, where genetic and molecular underpinnings can dictate therapeutic approaches. The combination of genomics and proteomics through bioinformatics enhances the stratification of risk for cardiovascular disease and guides clinical decision-making. Therefore, diagnostic techniques have turned towards more personalized paradigms based on the concept of considering variations in disease pathology among individuals. The challenges that persist, however, are overcoming the gaps in applying bioinformatics results in clinical contexts, which requires the development of evidence-based guidelines and effective biomarker detection methods to guarantee the successful use of such novel diagnostic tools in daily practice (Wei et al., 2025) (Figure 10.9).

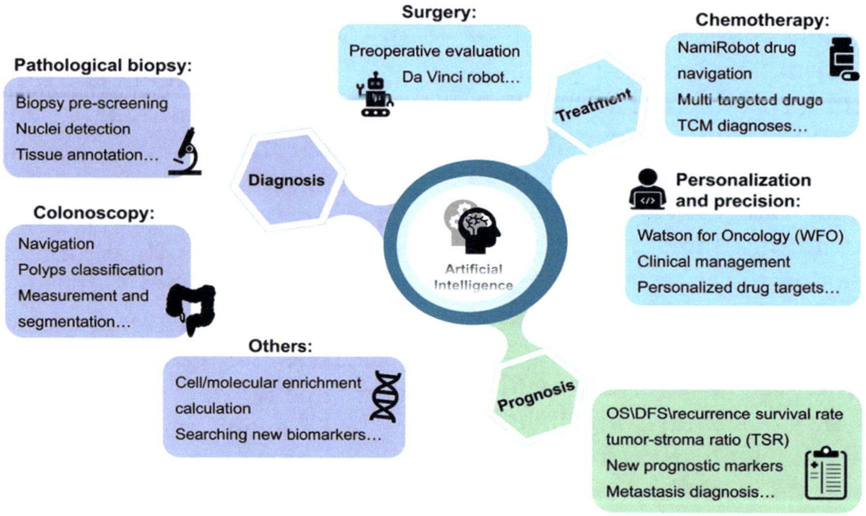

Figure 10.9. Applications of bioinformatics in disease diagnosis within molecular pathology.

Source: https://www.researchgate.net/profile/Chunlin-Ou/publication/348248058/figure/fig1/AS:983762179469313@1611558589109/The-application-of-AI-in-CRC-diagnosis-and-treatment.png.

10.3.1. Identification of Genetic Mutations

Genetic mutation detection is perhaps the most critical field of bioinformatics and molecular pathology, with a wide range of implications in disease diagnosis and therapeutic choice. Advances in sequencing technology, including next-generation sequencing by nanopores, revolutionized the identification and characterization of genetic variation rapidly and accurately. For instance, in one of their recent articles based on orthohantavirus Hantanense (HTNV), high-fidelity genomic sequence information was generated to identify the origins of infection through careful monitoring in rodents. Not only did the method illuminate the genomic diversity of HTNV, but it also provided a foundation for future epidemiological studies, demonstrating the importance of correct genetic identification in public health (Park et al., 2025). Furthermore, the use of bioinformatics also enhances the resolution of genetic variation studies by the integration of biological information into computational analysis. A good example is provided in research on Kleefstra Syndrome type 2 (KLEFS-2), wherein *KMT2C* gene mutations were extensively tested via multidimensional computation techniques. This involved combining genomic analysis with advanced bioinformatics methods to study the structural and dynamic features of genetic differences. By this collaborative method, researchers were able to classify variants into distinct groups, and it was revealed that slight genetic changes are capable of generating colossal impairments in the activity of the *KMT2C* enzyme (Jorge et al., 2023). Hence, the convergence of bioinformatics and molecular pathology explains the complexity of genetic mutations and their effect on human wellness. The implications of being able to identify genetic mutations successfully extend beyond mere scientific curiosity to affect treatment practices and outcomes. As discovered in both HTNV and KLEFS-2 studies, the ability to track mutations back to their functional impact may influence treatment and public health intervention. For instance, accurate typing of viral isolates can guide epidemiological intervention in epidemic situations, whereas complete characterization of variants in genetic disorders can guide individualized medicine interventions. The enhancement in bioinformatics tools further refines the identification of mutations, and soon our capacity to manage genetic diseases as well as infectious pathogens is enhanced. With the might of computational biology, it is increasingly likely that health outcomes can be improved by targeted interventions, making the field of bioinformatics a key area of study in molecular pathology (Figure 10.10).

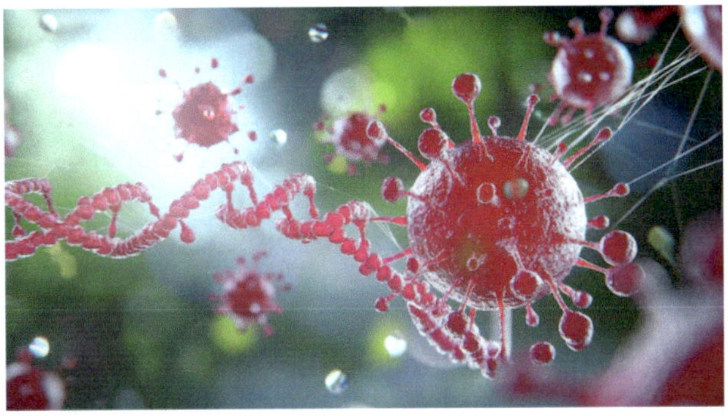

Figure 10.10. Identification of genetic mutations.

Source: https://img.freepik.com/premium-photo/revealing-intricate-anatomy-genetic-mutation-through-molecular-visualization_1326207-10493.jpg.

10.3.2. Biomarker Discovery for Cancer

With the onset of bioinformatics, the landscape of cancer biomarker discovery has been radically altered. Advanced computational tools enable one to interrogate large-scale genomic and proteomic data and identify molecular signatures that correlate with various cancers. High-throughput sequencing and mass spectrometry-driven data can be processed using bioinformatics tools to identify patterns that may indicate tumor presence, progression, or treatment response. For instance, liquid biopsy's cfDNA analysis has also emerged as a noninvasive method of detecting potential biomarkers. cfDNA fragments with unique methylation patterns and fragmentation are significant to explore the biology of tumors, to discern cancer cells from normal cells, hence enhancing diagnostic sensitivity and guidance of targeted therapy (Lo et al., 2021). With their efforts to discover new cancer biomarkers, the integration of various omics sciences—genomics, proteomics, and metabolomics—has been revolutionary. The integration of approaches allows researchers to investigate intricate biological processes and uncover biomarkers that remain masked when isolated molecular systems are examined. Moreover, the recent advances in data mining techniques provide the scope to combine humongous biological datasets to facilitate the discovery of previously unexplored pathways and molecules that may be implicated in cancer. Not only do these advances enhance the understanding of the pathogenesis of cancer, but they also allow the detection of particular biomarkers to inform therapies and predict patient outcomes (Kaushic, 2018). These combined approaches demonstrate how bioinformatics is shaping molecular pathology and facilitating the advancement of cancer biomarker discovery. In addition, clinical application of discovered biomarkers is immense, with the potential to revolutionize cancer diagnostics and therapeutics. For instance, analysis of liquid biopsies for the detection of specific cfDNA methylation signatures not only provides insight into tumor behavior but also has immediate implications for early detection and surveillance of cancer. With the evolving field of bioinformatics, personalized medicine is increasingly possible with biomarkers setting the tone for personalization based on individual patient profiles. The joining of cutting-edge analytics and validated biomarkers into clinical practice will enhance patient management by allowing for anticipatory treatment and simplifying therapeutic strategies (Lo et al., 2021). Therefore, the collaborative effort of molecular pathology and bioinformatics brings in a new era of precision oncology with emphasis on the vital role played by biomarkers to improve the care and outcomes of patients (Figure 10.11).

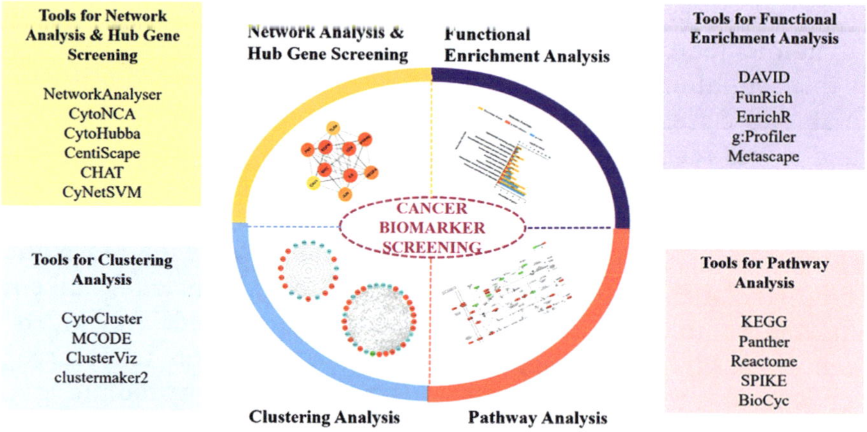

Figure 10.11. Biomarker discovery for cancer.

Source: https://www.researchgate.net/publication/364024684/figure/fig4/AS:11431281094041731@1667358349690/Graphical-illustrations-of-the-tools-for-cancer-biomarker-discovery-using-network.png.

10.3.3. Personalized Medicine Approaches

Personalized medicine is an essential paradigm change in medicine, particularly in molecular pathology. By emphasizing the individuality of the patient's characteristics, personalized medicine endeavors to optimize treatment modalities based on genetic, environmental, and lifestyle determinants. This individualized approach has gained traction in cardiology, where awareness of the personal genomic and proteomic status in cardiovascular disease (CVD) facilitates more effective and directed therapy. Personalized treatment regimens aim to join diagnosis and treatment together perfectly, enhancing patient outcomes with the application of molecular diagnostics and biomarkers. As personalized strategies become a reality, there are opportunities and threats in the wings; the promise of enhanced diagnosis and therapy is immense, but addressing heterogeneity in patients must remain in the hands of sophisticated bioinformatics techniques that can handle huge amounts of data on the fly (Garg et al., 2025).

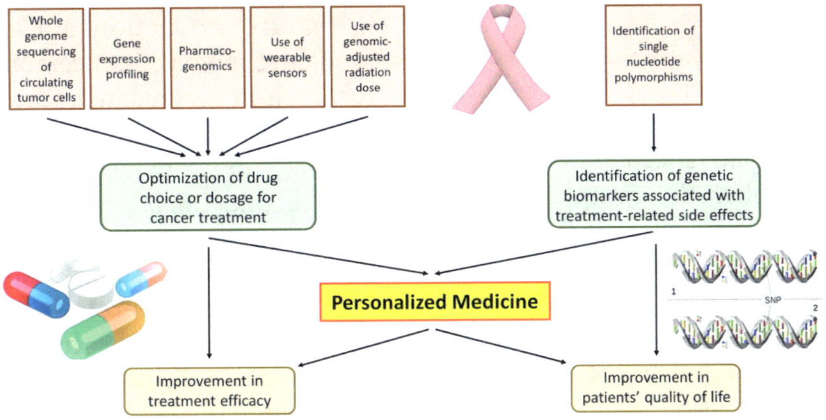

Figure 10.12. Personalized medicine approaches.

Source: https://pub.mdpi-res.com/ijms/ijms-18-02423/article_deploy/html/images/ijms-18-02423-ag.png?1569665173.

In addition, the application of bioinformatics in personalized medicine is the foundation for application in other fields of medicine aside from cardiology to encompass liver disease and others. For instance, one area of focus today is how long noncoding RNAs (lncRNAs) are involved in liver pathology. By applying developments in sequencing platforms and bioinformatics pipelines, scientists can identify and map new lncRNAs that might be crucial biomarkers or therapeutic targets. This is particularly relevant in conditions , such as hepatocellular carcinoma and metabolic-associated liver diseases, in which the lncRNAs play important roles in fibrosis and inflammation. The ability to assess these molecular traits through an individualized setting not only enhances pathophysiological understanding but also opens up windows for RNA-based treatments, which can change therapeutic paradigms through targeted interventions (Anwar et al., 2024). The future of targeted medicine depends to a large extent on new methods and extensive datasets, and therefore, the continued partnership of bioinformatics with patient care is crucial. To assist health systems in their transition to this personalized modus vivendi, it is increasingly imperative to establish robust frameworks that support the ethical use of genetic data while facilitating convergence among multidisciplinary groups. The future of targeted medicine relies on the integration of bioinformatics effectively, which enhances the precision of disease classification and responsiveness to treatment. Overcoming obstacles to implementation in practice, such as data protection and standardization, will be critical in pursuing these measures. Lastly, personalized medicine is a new age leap in healthcare that leverages the power of bioinformatics to create strategies tailored to fit the individual patient needs, maximizing therapeutic effects and maximizing health gains in disease groups (Anwar et al., 2024; Garg et al., 2025) (Figure 10.12).

10.4. Role in Research and Development

The integration of bioinformatics and molecular pathology powerfully increases the research and development potential within cancer biology. Through using advanced genomic data, researchers can decipher the complexity that exists within tumorigenesis, thereby facilitating personalized medicine approaches. Recent innovations, including high-profile efforts , such as The Cancer Genome Atlas, have functioned as a central tool for mapping genomic alterations in numerous types of cancer.

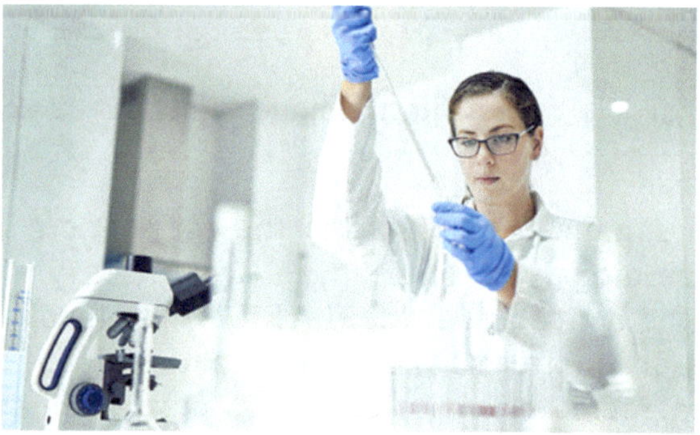

Figure 10.13. Role in research and development.

Source: https://www.onthejob.education/images/4th_level/Pathologist/Pathologist_atwork.jpg.

This has led to the identification of molecular subtypes that not just enhance diagnostic accuracy but also enhance therapeutic strategies. As elucidated by Uhl Mén et al. (2017), the development of an interactive data resource enables researchers to find how certain gene expressions influence patient outcomes, thereby enhancing the knowledge of cancer's molecular mechanisms. Furthermore, the power of bioinformatics in analysis is in its ability to handle multimodal data, which is increasingly significant in health informatics. Machine learning and deep learning have revolutionized the way scientists handle enormous datasets to guarantee that findings based on such data not only hold but are also feasible. Deep learning techniques have been of immense potential in feature extraction automation as well as predictive model enhancement, thereby changing research in molecular pathology. As explained by Rav Dì et al. (2016), the application of deep learning in translational bioinformatics and medical imaging is providing new opportunities in the understanding of disease onset and treatment response, thereby showcasing the bioinformatics key role in increasing research development. Lastly, bioinformatics plays a critical role in the translational phase of research by bridging the laboratory findings with clinical applications. By integrating genomic data with clinical outcomes, researchers can construct models that can predict treatment response and patient survival. Such translational studies are particularly pertinent in personalized therapy, where treatment is tailored based on individual genetic makeup. By providing the techniques and tools needed in extended data analysis, bioinformatics enables the whole research platform in molecular pathology. Not only does this help improve diagnostic processes, but it also stimulates the discovery of new drug targets, thereby highlighting the importance of bioinformatics in advancing research and development within the field (Figure 10.13).

10.4.1. Drug Discovery and Development

The multifaceted process of drug discovery and development has been transformed with the arrival of bioinformatics, particularly with regards to molecular pathology. The integration of large amounts of high-throughput genomic and proteomic data enables researchers to identify new therapeutic targets as well as biomarkers of disease progression. For instance, initiatives , such as The Cancer Genome Atlas have listed genomic alterations in various forms of tumors, supplying data on the molecular mechanisms underlying cancer. Through an understanding of such genetic alterations, bioinformatics aids in the identification of molecular subtypes, thereby enhancing diagnostic precision and treatment methods. Notably, Uhlen et al. approaches offer open-access materials that facilitate investigation of whether certain expressions of genes correlate with survival statuses, thereby providing a method of making treatments patient-specific based on individual genetic composition (Uhl Mén et al., 2017).

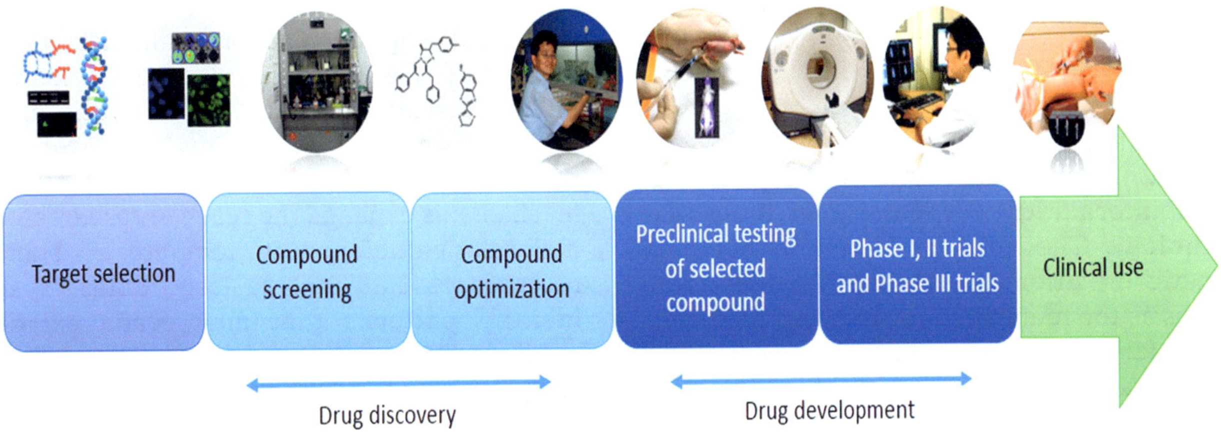

Figure 10.14. Drug discovery and development.

Source: https://pub.mdpi-res.com/ijms/ijms-18-01639/article_deploy/html/images/ijms-18-01639-g001.png?1569465833.

Moreover, the rapid pace of data analysis has encouraged the application of sophisticated computational models in drug discovery. As the field shifts toward multimodal data, machine learning techniques—like deep learning—are increasingly becoming go-to tools for analyzing large datasets generated from drug screening and patient information. These advanced algorithms have been shown in various contexts to predict drug interactions or simulate the effectiveness of new compounds based on historical data and biological considerations. By enabling feature extraction through machine learning from complex sets of data, deep learning assists researchers in discovering patterns that could be employed to enhance the optimization process for patients and drug leads, as well as enhance understanding of disease processes. This shift towards an analytics-oriented process not only accelerates the drug development process but also enhances chances of clinical success by identifying potential candidates sooner during development (Rav Dì et al., 2016). As bioinformatics continues to transform the drug discovery and development process, its impact on molecular pathology is profound and far-reaching. With the capacity to analyze and understand vast biological datasets, bioinformatics programs are well-positioned to redefine personalized medicine. By customizing therapy to the unique genetic blueprint of a disease, clinicians can maximize the effectiveness of treatment and minimize side effects. In addition, the forward-looking identification of patients that are most likely to respond to given medications based on their molecular profile is a signature of a significant advance in precision medicine. Finally, integration between bioinformatics and molecular pathology not only facilitates the identification of potential new drug candidates but also creates a better understanding of disease mechanisms, paving the way for new therapies with applicability to the particular patient's individual biological setting (Figure 10.14).

10.4.2. Understanding Disease Mechanisms

The appreciation of the intricacy of disease mechanisms is extremely crucial in bioinformatics, particularly in molecular pathology. The complex dynamic between genetic mutation and clinical manifestation serves as the foundation for targeted medicine. For instance, pathogenic mutations in genes like *KMT2C* have been shown to cause conditions like Kleefstra Syndrome, whose manifestations cover a range of neurodevelopmental impairments. The application of sophisticated bioinformatics methods assists researchers in dissecting these mutations at the molecular level. Methods like molecular modeling and simulations assist in understanding how particular variations affect protein functions, thus providing clues into the underlying pathological processes. This data not only encourages the identification of disease-causing variants but also directs potential therapeutic strategies according to individualized genetic patterns, advancing the mission towards precision medicine in molecular pathology (Jorge et al., 2022). Unveiling disease mechanisms also involves an inquiry into pharmacogenomics, analyzing how genetic variations influence drug responses among individuals. Bioinformatics plays a pivotal role in this area, as the potential exists to combine genomic data and drug response profiles. An example is the investigation of herbal medication, such as FDY003, in breast cancer treatment, where the complex interaction between different biochemical components and the target of therapy is displayed. Through the implementation of network pharmacology approaches, researchers can identify how these drugs interact with various molecular mechanisms, including cell growth and cell death. Through the identification of such system processes, bioinformatics enhances our capability to design drugs that target specific diseases with decreased side effects but increased therapeutic efficacy. This holistic concept of drug action not only validates existing models of treatment but also paves the way for the discovery of novel therapeutic drugs in cancer therapy (Lee et al., 2021). Further, the integration of bioinformatics in disease mechanisms expands the reach of research into molecular pathology. With computer assistance, researchers can analyze large datasets and identify patterns that may evade existing methods. This capability facilitates the detailed analysis of genetic variation, interactions among them, and the resulting phenotypic impact. As an example, the scoring systems developed to classify variants associated with Kleefstra Syndrome allow systematic comprehension of their structural and dynamic impacts on protein function. These advancements in bioinformatics not only enhance our knowledge about disease at a molecular level but also enhance the clinical diagnostic precision. Consequently, this facilitates earlier detection and intervention, thus ultimately improving patient outcomes by translating molecular insight into tangible clinical utility, which evidences the powerful impact of bioinformatics on modern medicine (Jorge et al., 2022).

10.4.3. Clinical Trial Design and Optimization

Clinical trials planning and optimization are very critical in the evolution of bioinformatics within the field of molecular pathology. Properly planned clinical trials can determine the efficacy and safety of therapeutic interventions, allowing the exploration of new treatments grounded in molecular knowledge. The last few years have seen dramatic advances in bioinformatics resources, which have made the clinical trial design process significantly better by enabling researchers to decipher intricate biological information and identify patient subgroups that will respond differently to therapies.

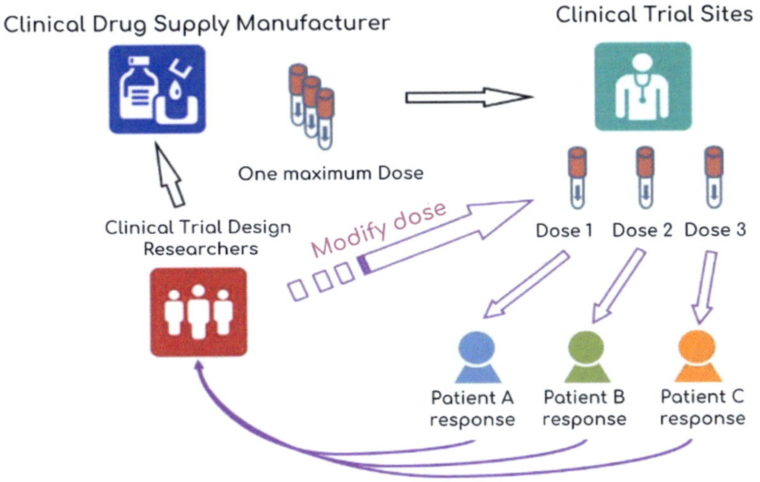

Figure 10.15. Clinical trial design.

Source: https://www.jliedu.com/blog/wp-content/uploads/2018/11/Adaptive-Clinical-Trials.png.

The stratification achieved by it makes trials more precise, which can result in more effective trials. Moreover, the integration of bioinformatics enables adaptive trial designs so that procedures can be modified in light of interim results, with an eye to optimizing use of resources and enhancing participant outcomes as additional information becomes available. Lastly, regulatory bodies increasingly focus on transparency and reproducibility in clinical trials, a principle with important implications for designing and optimizing trials. The ARRIVE guidelines stressed that transparent reporting should be made in research with animals, and it can be extended to use on human subjects. Complete and detailed descriptions of methods from researchers allow others to replicate the experiments, hence enhancing the validity of results in molecular pathology. In the context of optimizing clinical trials, adherence to these standards helps determine effective approaches and strategies that can eliminate bias and variability. With the development of the discipline, integration of these standards in the process of designing trials will be crucial in building confidence in biomedical research results and translating such outcomes to clinically applicable uses. Also, optimization of clinical trial design relies very much on computational modeling in combination with experimental validation. Bioinformatics is also used to analyze patients' data but predictive modeling that can mimic various scenarios of trials so that researchers can experiment with potential outcomes before actual realization. This computational approach enables the identification of key biomarkers capable of influencing patient response to therapy, thus helping in the selection of the appropriate therapy for specific groups of patients. With further research, this integration between bioinformatics and clinical trial design will play a key role in addressing the challenges associated with the development of new therapies. Continuing to refine trial methods by incorporating serial data analysis iteration will be an asset in molecular pathology, with the enhanced potential for more effective and targeted treatments in the clinic, as has been seen in such ventures as examined by and Percie et al. (2020) and Wang et al. (2022) (Figure 10.15).

10.5. Challenges and Limitations

The incorporation of bioinformatics into molecular pathology brings with it a wide range of challenges and limitations that can have a significant impact on the accuracy and effectiveness of diagnostic and therapeutic applications. The first of these challenges involves the intricacy of biological information, traditionally defined by high dimensionality and heterogeneity. High-throughput technologies generate vast amounts of information, from genomic, proteomic, and metabolomic information, which require sophisticated analysis tools to explain. This complexity may result in problems in the integration and standardization of information, so that useful conclusions are hard to come by for researchers as well as clinicians. The need for sophisticated computational expertise also presents a hurdle for pathologists and laboratory technologists, deterring its widespread application in the clinical field. This is the reason, therefore, that it is extremely essential to address these issues in making bioinformatics even more beneficial in molecular pathology.

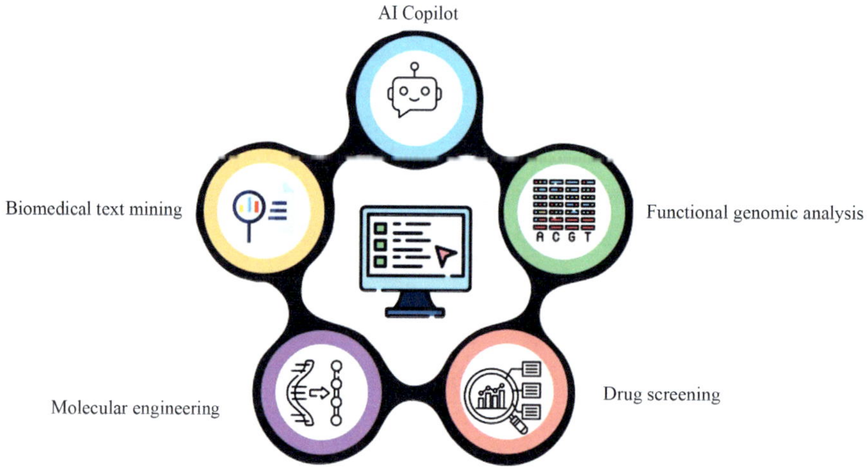

Figure 10.16. Challenges and limitations of bioinformatics.

Source: https://cbirt.net/wp-content/uploads/2024/03/LLMs-in-bioinformatics.webp.

The precision of bioinformatics analysis largely relies on database and reference library completeness and quality. Incomplete and poorly curated data can lead to defective interpretations and misclassifications within clinical settings. A case in point would be the identification of disease-associated molecular signatures, such as Alzheimer's, which requires access to robust databases that can perform diverse biological variations. Lacking a comprehensive set of reference data, the chances of drawing inappropriate conclusions increase, hence undermining diagnostic specificity as well as treatment efficacy. Bioinformatics methods also typically rely on machine learning models, which need large training sets to facilitate successful model development. The absence of high-quality annotated datasets hastens worries of bias as well as overfitting, resulting in less-than-ideal predictive model performance on actual-world datasets. Thus, improving the quality of existing bioinformatics tools is a priority for molecular pathology reliability growth. The second significant limitation is the translational aspect of bioinformatics findings from the study to the clinical setting. While computational methods have shown promise in the discovery of potential biomarkers for the diagnosis of early disease, e.g., those of Alzheimer's, transferring these findings into clinically meaningful tools faces a number of hurdles. Regulatory pathways and approval processes for new diagnostic technologies can be time-consuming and bureaucratic and cause delays that disrupt prompt patient care. There is also typically a gap between the research world and clinical practice, and, as a result, a lack of agreement about which bioinformatics approaches are most suitable for incorporation into standard diagnostics. Creating effective training programs that bridge this gap is essential to making healthcare practitioners learn the appropriate skills for the appropriate application of bioinformatics tools. With ongoing research, overcoming these translational challenges will be key to realizing the maximum potential of bioinformatics in molecular pathology (Figure 10.16).

10.5.1. Data Management and Storage Issues

The rapidly advancing field of bioinformatics in molecular pathology has mandated the need for efficient data storage and management technologies, particularly because scientists are increasingly relying on sophisticated genomic data for diagnosis as well as therapy. With data generated by processes , such as next-generation sequencing (NGS) rising exponentially, institutions must navigate the complexities of storing gigabytes of raw and processed data. For instance, the Swiss HIV Cohort Study Viral NGS Database (SHCND) is a systematic response to this challenge that has identified a central database to hold NGS data due to data storage and computational analysis challenges. This database is an effective tool not only for therapeutic investigation but also for enhancing understanding of viral dynamics, thus signifying the central role that systematic management of data plays in the pursuit of successful scientific investigation in molecular pathology (Zeeb et al., 2025). In addition to this, challenging genomic data processing is further compounded by ensuring reproducibility and the application of advanced bioinformatics tools. With advancing bioinformatics methods, researchers are now faced with escalating complexity in the analysis of big data sets generated from various omics technologies. For instance, genomic monitoring of plant pathogens using extensive analysis of data in the healthcare of emerging plant diseases is hindered by data management complexities. Standardization is required in procedures and the establishment of open data-sharing platforms. Collaborative networks have begun to emerge as one of the solutions, trying to meet the obstacles faced in genomic data analysis and the capacity to make the enormous amounts of generated data substantially useful for driving molecular pathology innovation (Islam, 2024). Lastly, discussions on the ethicalities involved in data management remain crucial in the bioinformatics scenario. With the acquisition of sensitive genomic data from populations of mixed race, researchers have to cope with protecting data privacy as well as honoring ethical standards. This challenge calls for the integration of high-security features in bioinformatics software to be able to keep participants anonymous without compromising data integrity. Forecasts , such as open data sharing and international collaboration present promising directions toward balancing access and ethics, leading to a more collaborative scientific environment. With guidelines emphasizing responsible data use, not only will the overall quality of research be enhanced, but participants' confidence will also be fortified, ultimately facilitating vital advancement in molecular pathology research (Islam, 2024; Zeeb et al., 2025) (Figure 10.17).

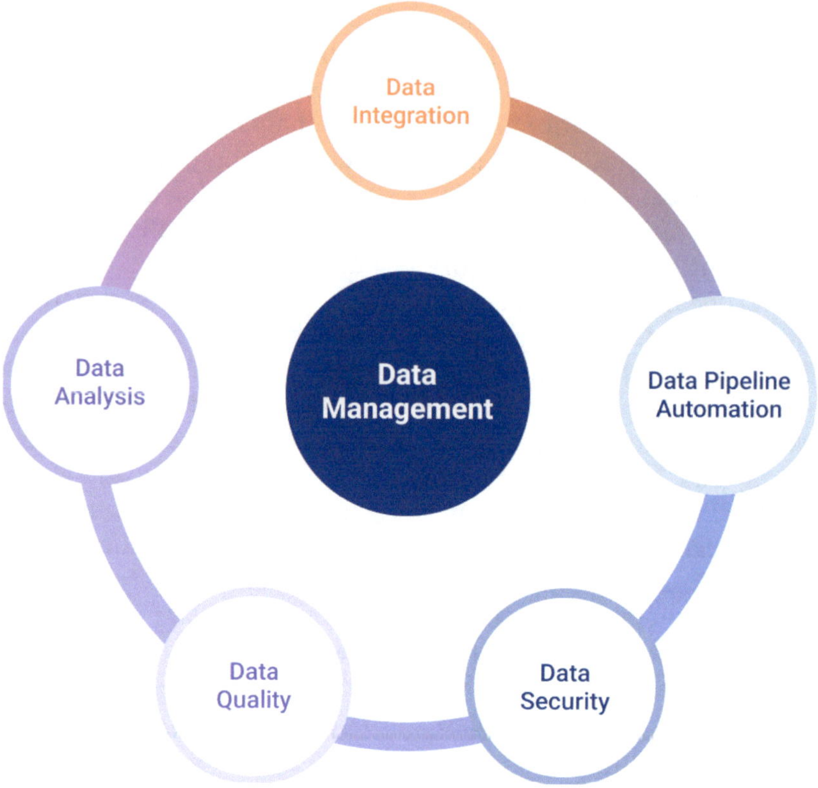

Figure 10.17. Data management.

Source: https://nexla.com/n3x_ctx/uploads/2023/02/article-data-management-best-practices_Img0.png.

10.5.2. Interpretation of Complex Data

Analysis of advanced data, particularly bioinformatic analysis, is a critical component of molecular pathology and highly relevant to practice. The advent of next-generation sequencing (NGS) has transformed the world of genetic testing to enable the simultaneous analysis of hundreds of genes. With thousands of sequence variants generated, however, come huge challenges in their interpretation. As stated, the labor-intensive and error-prone nature of this task has resulted in organizations like the American College of Medical Genetics and Genomics and the Association for Molecular Pathology (ACMG/AMP) establishing standards and guidelines to enhance consistency among laboratories. These frameworks, however, are meant to simplify the variant classification such that pathologists can identify which changes are clinically significant and those that are benign, and consequently enhance diagnostic accuracy in patients and guide treatment (Damianos et al., 2021). In addition, improvements in computational tools play a critical role in mediating the complexities involved in data interpretation. A prime example is the GenOtoScope tool, which automates pathogenicity classification of genetic variants found with congenital hearing loss. The tool is an example of how bioinformatics helps reduce clinicians' cognitive effort in a manner that allows batch processing of large numbers more efficiently. By incorporating ACMG/AMP criteria even when individual patient information is not available, GenOtoScope enhances speed and accuracy in variant classification. Its established supremacy of precision and accuracy over competing tools also signifies the importance of using machine learning and automation for interpreting complex genetic data, a breakthrough in moving beyond the bounds of traditional analysis in molecular pathology (Damianos et al., 2021). In tissue analysis, deep learning techniques have emerged as breakthrough drivers for interpreting complex sets obtained from histological images. A novel collaboration paradigm between pathologists and medical students has emerged as a strong contender for achieving high-quality cell nucleus labels for breast cancer tissues. Creation of the NuCLS dataset that holds over 220,000 annotations demonstrates that the marriage of crowdsourcing and algorithmic assistance can effectively label complex cell structures with high accuracy. This approach not only facilitates high-quality segmentation data but also enhances the precision of annotations made by non-specialists, hence democratizing data annotation in computational pathology. Through the proof-of-concept shown through the value of combining human oversight with machine smarts, the study identifies a major step forward in the way we can better analyze intricate data in molecular pathology, setting the course for improved diagnostic tools and therapy interventions.

10.5.3. Ethical Considerations in Bioinformatics

The intersection of bioinformatics and molecular pathology brings with it significant ethical implications deserving of extensive inquiry. With advancing bioinformatics leading to the analysis of intricate biological data, issues surrounding the handling of data become increasingly critical. The most important ethical concerns are mainly those of consent, specifically in utilizing patient data to perform research beyond the original purpose. The genetic data must also be anonymized to ensure patient confidentiality. Researchers must tread carefully between applying valuable data towards scientific progress and not infringing on citizens' right to privacy. Further, the transparency of algorithms used in bioinformatics is essential to avoid potential biases in analysis or outcomes that may negatively affect patient care and equity in healthcare access, thus the need for efficient ethical standards to guide research practices in molecular pathology (Okpo et al., 2024). Further, growing reliance on the use of bioinformatics tools in molecular pathology raises ethical issues about data ownership and intellectual property. At a time when knowledge is one of the most precious commodities, the rights to information generated by bioinformatics is a matter of concern. Is it that of individual donors, research institutions, or private companies that produce the software? This conflict becomes further entangled with collaborative research, wherein pooled data can have a significant effect but concurrently create concerns over the appropriation of intellectual resources as well as work. In addition, the consequences of genetic engineering, when coupled with bioinformatics, justify a detailed moral review of the potential unforeseen effects of such advancements on biodiversity and public health. Coupling innovation with ethical reasoning is imperative for the moral advancement of bioinformatics in molecular pathology (Chen, 2024). Last but not least, holographic integration of artificial intelligence into bioinformatics opens new ethical issues that need to be recognized. AI software can considerably enhance the velocity of data processing and interpretation; however, reliance on these machines raises concerns over responsibility and dehumanization in treating patients. Algorithmic judgments, particularly in predicting disease outcomes, can inadvertently include or reflect already existing biases or assumptions within the training data. For this reason, it is vital that such algorithms are developed and audited rigorously to uphold ethical standards for bioinformatics protocols. Moreover, the ethical concerns involved in access and utilization of such technology come into play, raising the question of equity, as healthcare inequality may increase if sophisticated bioinformatics tools are not made available to everyone. Hence, it is essential to set up ethical policies and guidelines to guide through these quickly changing arenas in molecular pathology (Okpo et al., 2024).

10.6. Future Directions

With continued growth in molecular pathology, future innovation is more and more driven by the intersection of bioinformatics and artificial intelligence (AI). Specifically, multimodal Gen-AI models applied in anatomic pathology represent a paradigm-shifting potential for diagnostic accuracy and precision. These models are designed to analyze histopathology images in combination with other types of data, including genomic and clinical data, thereby enhancing the predictive power of diagnostic technology. Literature suggests that such multimodal approaches can achieve moderate to high accuracy on a variety of tasks, such as image classification and segmentation. But reliance on data from certain specialized academies places a premium on robust validation on a range of real-world datasets. A federated learning approach, encouraging multicenter consortia, can contribute to the generation of consensus models attempting to offer reliability and generalizability for clinical application, an enormous advance for the field (Ullah et al., 2025). Of no lesser value is the exploration of new cellular pathways that can re-engineer therapeutic strategies in molecular pathology. Current research has established the significance of programmed cell death, or more specifically, a novel pathway called disulfidptosis. It is a situation where cancer cells are loaded with cystine as a reaction to some stress conditions and detach and die. Because greater attention is currently given to disulfidptosis in oncology and other diseases, there is still a need to understand more of its regulatory pathways and molecular targets. By utilizing bioinformatics tools for the investigation of these complex cellular responses, researchers can come across potential therapeutic targets by utilizing bioinformatics to correlate omics data with experimental outcomes. Understanding disulfidptosis not only can provide an insight into cancer biology but could also provide an insight into innovative strategies towards intervention of neurodegenerative and metabolic disorders, thus expanding the vista of molecular pathology (Chen, 2024).

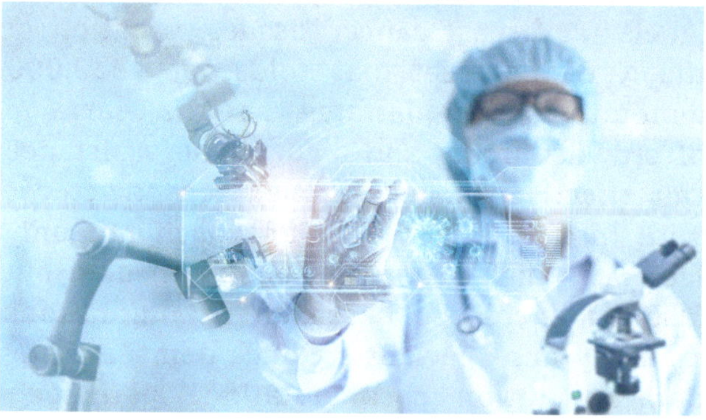

Figure 10.18. Future directions.

Source: https://mma.prnewswire.com/media/1478999/Digital_Pathology_Artificial_Intelligence.jpg?p=facebook.

In the coming years, the meeting of bioinformatics with molecular pathology will also mean that educational frameworks need to be framed to equip the next generation of pathologists with the appropriate competencies. As bioinformatics continues to be felt in diagnostic practices and research methods, training courses will have to adapt to include computational skills and data interpretation as core components of pathology training. This expansion will facilitate clinicians to effectively employ new technologies, facilitating greater data-driven patient care. Moreover, enhanced inter-disciplinary cooperation among bioinformaticians, molecular biologists, and pathologists will also be important in closing gaps between research findings and clinical practice. By fulfilling such educational requirements, the field can ensure that future health professionals are prepared to handle the challenges of bioinformatics in molecular pathology, thereby improving patient outcomes and practice (Chen et al., 2024; Ullah et al., 2025) (Figure 10.18).

10.6.1. Advances in Artificial Intelligence and Machine Learning

The rapid development of machine learning (ML) and artificial intelligence (AI) technologies has dramatically influenced the field of bioinformatics, which is now better able to tackle intricate biological information. In molecular pathology, these developments are essential to unraveling the intricacies of cellular function and disease mechanisms. Bioinformatics software, now supplemented with sophisticated algorithms, allows for massive data sets accumulated from genomic and proteomic studies to be analyzed. This integration allows researchers to uncover molecular patterns and interactions, which were otherwise hidden. For instance, the application of machine learning to proteomic data has helped identify critical biomarkers associated with various diseases, including cancer. Therefore, AI-driven bioinformatics platforms can transform treatment strategies, above all by guiding personalized medicine programs that individualize treatments according to patients' unique molecular signatures, thus enhancing patient outcomes and survival rates (Kimu, 2025). Furthermore, the application of AI and ML in disease forecasting and disease development based on biomarkers is a significant area of concern in molecular pathology. The challenge of determining the risk of oral epithelial dysplasia (OED) and the development to oral squamous cell carcinoma (OSCC) is a testament to the necessity for this kind of innovation. Traditional risk evaluation in OED patients has been unreliable, leading to delayed diagnosis and less-than-optimal treatment results. In diagnostic histopathology, however, machine learning algorithms have begun to hold out the promise of predicting biomarkers. With immunohistochemistry data along with genomic sequencing, researchers are utilizing AI models yielding more accurate prognosis prediction of OED and potential malignancy development. Alongside offering considerable insight into the stratification of patients, these technologies also assist in enhancing therapy strategy optimization according to anticipated outcomes (Chi et al., 2024). Further, the union of deep learning (DL) and bioinformatics is transforming the field of molecular pathology.

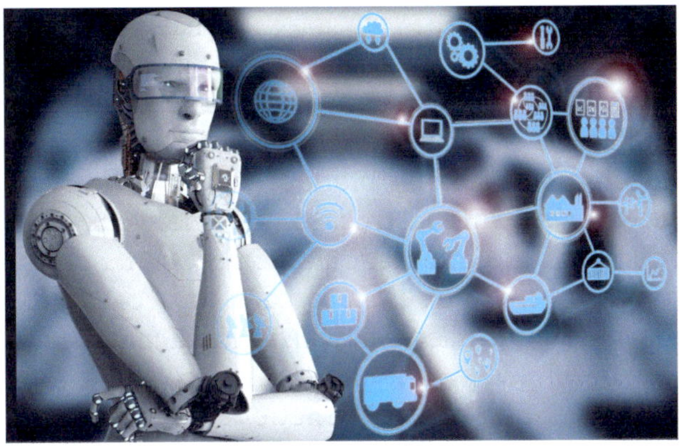

Figure 10.19. Advances in artificial intelligence and machine learning.

Source: https://www.cio.com/wp-content/uploads/2021/12/artificial_intelligence_machine_learning_network_thinkstock_671750598-100724432-orig.jpeg?quality=50&strip=all.

10.6.2. Integration of Multi-Omics Data

Integration of multi-omics data is an innovative approach in the field of bioinformatics and molecular pathology. Through the integration of various levels of biological information—genomics, transcriptomics, proteomics, metabolomics, and more—researchers can potentially derive an integrated perspective of disease processes. This integrated outlook allows researchers to comprehend complex biological systems and interactions among various molecular components. Through this, one is subsequently able to correlate molecular alterations with specific pathological states, enabling more precise phenotyping of disease. Successful convergence of this information not only further clarifies our comprehension of the pathogenesis of disease but also towards the identification of new biomarkers, which can prove invaluable in diagnosing and monitoring disease and in personalized medicine and targeted therapeutic interventions. Moreover, network medicine use provides a framework for multi-omics data integration. The approach encases diseases as disruptions of broader biological networks, hence enabling identification of key drivers that can fuel disease development. Using bioinformatics resources, researchers can construct complex networks that represent the interaction among various omics data types, which is necessary to account for diseases' multifactorial causality, such as atrial fibrillation. Network-based research illustrates the cross-talk among genetic, epigenetic, and environmental determinants in the cell culture and their ultimate effect on disease processes. As illustrated in the case of atrial fibrillation research, unraveling the cross-talk imparts a hint to therapeutic manipulations, including repurposing medication and crafting novel combination treatment protocols, and thus improving patient outcomes (Martins et al., 2023). The challenge of integrating multi-omics data cannot be overstated. Despite technological progress, the size and intricacy of the generated datasets pose formidable computational and analytical issues. Powerful bioinformatics tools to process, analyze, and visualize multi-scale data effectively are a necessity. Current efforts have sought to apply big data analytics for probing intricate biological systems, particularly for processes like autophagy that are implicated in various diseases. Development of multi-omics platforms allows a precise description of the autophagy system, optimizing our knowledge of its role in disease and health. As emphasized in recent studies using network biology approaches, interaction between various omics data types can lead to insights on crucial pathways involved in cellular homeostasis and pathology, thereby enhancing knowledge about molecular mechanisms of human diseases (Jacomin et al., 2018).

10.6.3. Potential for Real-Time Data Analysis in Clinical Settings

Real-time data analysis in clinical situations greatly enhances the functionality of bioinformatics in molecular pathology. It makes clinicians able to make more informed diagnosis and treatment plan decisions since it gives them real-time access to patient information. Real-time analytics enable the processing of genomic and molecular information, which is crucial since it is formidable in comparison to what it generates using high-throughput approaches. For example, applying algorithms , such as the Mapper, where patient data is mapped as a similarity graph, can be utilized to facilitate subgroup discovery in cancer patients. Not only does this type of analysis identify clinically or molecularly differentiated profiles, but it may potentially identify new prognostic markers. However, parameter selection challenges in the Mapper algorithm currently discourage everyday use, indicating the need for improved methodologies during real-time data processing and translation in the clinical environment (Loughrey et al., 2025). In addition, the advent of open-source bioinformatics tools is revolutionizing the potential for real-time data analysis in resource-limited contexts. With such technologies, medical practitioners are able to apply advanced computational methods at low cost, dramatically enhancing clinical functions. The technologies enable real-time computation of genomic data with access to real-time knowledge in real time to inform treatment options. For instance, the monitoring of viral mutations in real time, as was used in the Nextstrain project during the COVID-19 pandemic, illustrates how real-time analysis can be used to inform public health responses. By integrating bioinformatics effectively into clinical models, healthcare systems can respond rapidly to shifting patient conditions and epidemiological trends and position tailored treatments to the needs of each patient with breathtaking accuracy (Mbisva, 2025). Lastly, the applications of real-time data analysis are not merely limited to near-clinical applications; they hold long-term potential for personalized medicine breakthroughs. The integration of bioinformatics and molecular pathology encourages novel mechanisms by which duplicated data retrieval is done, potentially leading to new biomarkers and therapeutic targets. This, in turn, enables the integration of real-time analytics into clinical practice not only to enhance patient outcomes but also drive research progress. Through repeated cycles of data collection, analysis, and use, researchers can improve diagnostic tests and treatment protocols and ultimately transform medicine. Indisputably, the ongoing development and optimization of bioinformatics software, particularly for platforms that facilitate real-time analysis, will play an indispensable part in the advancement of personalized medicine initiatives (Loughrey et al., 2025; Mbisva, 2025).

SUMMARY

The combination of bioinformatics with molecular pathology is a paradigm change in the diagnosis and treatment of diseases, particularly cancer and liver disease. With the use of advanced computational techniques, researchers are able to examine large datasets derived from genomic and transcriptomic profiling, revealing intricate patterns of gene expression and molecular interactions. Bioinformatics supports the enhanced understanding of disease mechanisms, such as the role of long noncoding RNAs (lncRNAs) in liver disease, which reflects the potential of these molecules for biomarker and therapy applications. The ongoing study of lncRNAs as documented also reflects their regulatory function in processes , such as inflammation and tumorigenesis, supporting the necessity for further research in this direction (Terzi, 2024). Thus, not only does bioinformatics enhance our grasp of molecular pathology, but it also introduces the possibility of treatment approaches tailored to individual disease settings. As we conclude this investigation of bioinformatics in molecular pathology, it is worth highlighting the growing importance of spatial transcriptomics and its impact on research in cancer. This innovative platform allows for spatial mapping of gene expression in tumor tissue to significantly advance an understanding of the tumor microenvironment (TME) and of the complex interactions between immune cells and tumor cells. Through the use of advanced bioinformatics tools, researchers can examine these interactions and identify significant biological patterns that help tumorigenesis as well as immune evasion. Development of new algorithms to analyze spatial transcriptomic data, as exemplified by recent studies, is a significant advancement in our ability to map intra-tumor heterogeneity and immune signaling dynamics (Deshpande et al., 2022). Not only does this precise information aid in deciphering the pathogenesis of disease, but it also informs future treatment strategies, underlining the invaluable contribution of bioinformatics to modern pathology. Against the backdrop of the developments outlined, it is evident that the future of molecular pathology is tied to the progress of bioinformatics. The commitment to raising the analytic potential of bioinformatics will certainly lead to an enhanced appreciation of disease at the molecular level. With continued evolution, multidisciplinary interaction between pathologists, bioinformaticians, and clinicians will be paramount in facilitating science into practice. The potential of bioinformatics to drive innovation in treatment and diagnostics—especially through the discovery of new biomarkers and targets for therapy—is high. Ongoing investment in research in bioinformatics will not just assist in demystifying intricate disease mechanisms but also contribute to our overall ability to deliver effective and personalized patient care, cementing its place as a cornerstone of the molecular pathology of the future.

In molecular pathology, bioinformatics is a valuable tool for the analysis of complex biological information to improve the understanding of disease processes on the molecular level. Integrating heterogeneous data types , such as genomic, transcriptomic, and proteomic data, bioinformatics makes it possible for us to detect genetic mutations and their relationships with various pathologies. This multi-faceted approach not only streamlines the identification of disease but also allows for the identification of putative targets for therapy. As research moves toward personalized medicine, bioinformatics takes center stage in the process of adapting treatment based on an individual's molecular profile, in keeping with changing healthcare paradigms. In the big picture, integration of bioinformatics into molecular pathology is essential to the understanding of disease progression and improving patient outcomes. Besides, advances in methodology and tools over the recent past have contributed significantly to the efficiency of bioinformatics in molecular pathology. For instance, the way network pharmacology illustrates how bioinformatics may elucidate therapeutic mechanisms of action of traditional medicines for complex compounds like FDY003, an herbal medicine, is a case in point. Here, the compound was revealed to interact with multiple breast cancer-related targets by systematic data mining and computational methods. These data help scientists discover concealed channels that are activated in cancer biology and hence unlock how compounds can convert their anticancer activity. The implications are vast, as such data can guide future use in the clinic and motivate new therapy approaches. This convergence of traditional modes of medicine and bioinformatics shows how new strategies still enhance our understanding of molecular pathology. Lastly, bioinformatics is instrumental in ongoing discoveries of new biological compounds and their applications. For instance, the recent discovery of α-dioxygenases (α-DOXs) from cyanobacteria is the best demonstration of the application of bioinformatics for unveiling new enzymatic activities and their potential use. The identification of enzymatic activities linked to fatty acid oxidation not only extends knowledge of biochemical pathways in various organisms but also has industry applications, for example, in the synthesis of fragrance and flavor chemicals. The endeavor is evidence of the potential of bioinformatics to bridge the divide between basic science and applied science. With interdisciplinary collaboration, bioinformatics makes significant contributions to the frontiers of molecular pathology, enabling greater exploration of biological processes and assistance with the manufacture of targeted therapeutic treatments.

A LOOK TO THE FUTURE:

AMERICAN COLLEGE OF MEDICAL GENETICS AND GENOMICS (ACMG):

The American College of Medical Genetics and Genomics (ACMG) is a leading professional organization dedicated to advancing the science and practice of medical genetics and genomics. Established in 1991, ACMG was created to provide national representation for providers of genetic services and the patients they serve, and to promote the development and implementation of methods for diagnosing, treating, and preventing genetic disease. It brings together a diverse membership of biochemical, clinical, cytogenetic, medical and molecular geneticists, genetic counselors, and other health care professionals unified by a commitment to translate genetic and genomic knowledge into improved health outcomes.

From its inception, ACMG has played a pivotal role in shaping the landscape of medical genetics. Early efforts included the development of clinical standards and laboratory guidelines, as well as the foundation of the professional journal Genetics in Medicine, which has since become a respected platform for disseminating cutting-edge research, practice standards, and policy analyses. Over the years, ACMG's influence has grown through its collaboration with other medical specialty societies and federal health agencies, contributing to initiatives such as newborn screening programs and proficiency testing frameworks that have wide-ranging impacts on public health.

A central aspect of ACMG's mission is education—both for genetics professionals and for the broader medical community. Through continuing medical education, conferences, workshops, and expert resources, the College supports the development of a skilled workforce capable of integrating genetics and genomics into routine clinical care. This focus on education was recently reaffirmed in ACMG's 2025-2029 strategic plan, which emphasizes leadership in genetics education, advocacy for policy initiatives that advance the field, and the expansion of the genetics workforce.

In addition to educational efforts, ACMG is widely recognized for its evidence-based practice guidelines and policy statements. These include technical standards for clinical genetics laboratories, recommendations for genetic testing practices, and ethical frameworks for areas such as pediatric genetic screening. By developing consensus-based guidance, ACMG helps ensure that genetic and genomic testing is performed with rigor, accuracy, and clinical relevance.

As genetics and genomics become increasingly central to diverse fields of medicine—ranging from oncology to rare disease diagnostics and personalized therapeutics—ACMG continues to serve as a critical authority. Its work reinforces the responsible and equitable integration of genetic knowledge into healthcare, ultimately aiming to improve individual and public health outcomes through scientific excellence and clinical innovation.

REFERENCES

1. E. A., Okpo, Agboke, A. A., Udobi, C. E., John, G. E., and Andy, I. E. 2024. "The Synergy of Molecular Docking and Bioinformatics: An in Depth Review in Drug Discovery". Biotechnology Journal International 28 (4):119-36. https://doi.org/10.9734/bji/2024/v28i4732.
2. (accessed on 17th July 2025).
3. Ala, U., & Fagoonee, S. (2024). RNA-binding protein transcripts as potential biomarkers for detecting primary sclerosing cholangitis and for predicting its progression to cholangiocarcinoma. Frontiers in Molecular Biosciences, 11. https://www.semanticscholar.org/paper/4f9e738910d62818a7c9a7a14383e8987ea0770d (accessed on 17th July 2025).
4. Amgad, M., Atteya, L. A., Hussein, H., Mohammed, K., Hafiz, E., Elsebaie, M. A. T., Alhusseiny, A., et al. (2021). NuCLS: A scalable crowdsourcing approach and dataset for nucleus classification and segmentation in breast cancer. GigaScience, 11. https://www.semanticscholar.org/paper/da47e34533dbf914335393562e4e1d0e7a0316fd (accessed on 17th July 2025).
5. Anwar, A. A., Jalan-Sakrikar, N., & Huebert, R. (2024). LncRNAs, RNA therapeutics, and emerging technologies in liver pathobiology. Seminars in Liver Disease. https://www.semanticscholar.org/paper/01d4c37348d3276715a3473e8b6e4c447f9e968b (accessed on 17th July 2025).
6. Arroyo Mühr, L. S., Guerendiain, D., Cuschieri, K., & Sundström, K. (2021). Human papillomavirus detection by whole-genome next-generation sequencing: Importance of validation and quality assurance procedures. Viruses, 13, 1323. https://doi.org/10.3390/v13071323 (accessed on 17th July 2025).
7. Berg, G., Rybakova, D., Fischer, D., Cernava, T., Champomier Vergès, M. C., Charles, T. C., Chen, X., et al. (2020). Microbiome definition re-visited: Old concepts and new challenges. Microbiome, 8. https://doi.org/10.1186/s40168-020-00875-0 (accessed on 17th July 2025).
8. Bian, X., Zhang, P. P., Ping, Y., & Yao, X. (2022). [Next-generation diagnostic pathology]. Zhonghua Bing Li Xue Za Zhi = Chinese Journal of Pathology, 51(1), 3–6. https://www.semanticscholar.org/paper/50ade59405e90edda062f9a93bbed703d7b3c6df (accessed on 17th July 2025).
9. Chen, J., Ma, B., Yang, Y., Wang, B., Hao, J., & Zhou, X. (2024). Disulfidptosis decoded: A journey through cell death mysteries, regulatory networks, disease paradigms and future directions. Biomarker Research, 12. https://www.semanticscholar.org/paper/0af95aefb65992d6d1553c20dec0edc780062ace (accessed on 17th July 2025).
10. Chen, S. (2024). Advances in molecular breeding of forage crops: Technologies, applications and prospects. Agriculture. https://www.semanticscholar.org/paper/bf24ef30042f8a784a52fc89fa626b2a73aa3bc9 (accessed on 17th July 2025).
11. Atul Deshpande, Melanie Loth, Dimitrios Sidiropoulos, QingFeng Zhu, Genevieve Stein-O'Brien, NIkhil Rao, Cedric Uytingco, Stephen Williams, Cesar Santa-Maria, Daniele M. Gilkes, Lei Zhang, Elizabeth Jaffee, Robert Anders, Ludmila Danilova, Luciane T. Kagohara, Elana J. Fertig; Abstract 2130: Uncovering the spatial landscape of tumor-immune interactions using latent spaces from spatial transcriptomics. Cancer Res 15 June 2022; 82 (12_Supplement): 2130. https://doi.org/10.1158/1538-7445.AM2022-2130(accessed on 17th July 2025).
12. Garg, I., Kumar, H., Verma, M., Chauhan, I., & Panwar, V. (2025). Treating cardiovascular disorders with personalized medicine. Cardiovascular & Hematological Disorders Drug

Targets. https://www.semanticscholar.org/paper/657d9ae387bd19447ce360baf2bd9086f61db3e3 (accessed on 17th July 2025).

13. Gu, W., Miller, S., & Chiu, C. Y. (2018). Clinical metagenomic next-generation sequencing for pathogen detection. Annual Review of Pathology: Mechanisms of Disease, 14, 319–338. https://doi.org/10.1146/annurev-pathmechdis-012418-012751 (accessed on 17th July 2025).

14. Horan, M., Glover, L., Hokamp, K., & Wingfield, M. (2023). P-372 RNA sequencing studies evaluating oocyte quality in women with endometriosis: A meta-analysis. Human Reproduction. https://www.semanticscholar.org/paper/e73735d3589014c643d63f10e934d7af4541ae15 (accessed on 17th July 2025).

15. Hu, Y., Hu, Q., Li, Y., Lu, L., Xiang, Z., Yin, Z., Kabelitz, D., et al. (2023). γδ T cells: Origin and fate, subsets, diseases and immunotherapy. Signal Transduction and Targeted Therapy, 8. https://doi.org/10.1038/s41392-023-01653-8 (accessed on 17th July 2025).

16. Huang, J., Zou, Y., Deng, H., Zha, J., Pathak, J. L., Chen, Y., Ge, Q., et al. (2025). Integration of bioinformatics and machine learning strategies identifies ferroptosis and immune infiltration signatures in peri-implantitis. International Journal of Molecular Sciences, 26. https://www.semanticscholar.org/paper/776706e7cd45dd411fd64b45eb3d5785daca6e5f (accessed on 17th July 2025).

17. Islam, T. (2024). Genomic surveillance for tackling emerging plant diseases, with special reference to wheat blast. CABI Reviews. https://www.semanticscholar.org/paper/a2ea44978ee4da63b8de7d20dd287372966fd17f (accessed on 17th July 2025).

18. Jacomin, A. C., Gul, L., Sudhakar, P., Korcsmáros, T., & Nezis, I. (2018). What we learned from big data for autophagy research. Frontiers in Cell and Developmental Biology, 6. https://www.semanticscholar.org/paper/d11a2fb2be74a6e76dbdc0df2c2e2d71ef462ab1 (accessed on 17th July 2025).

19. Jorge, S., Chi, Y. I., Lizarraga Mazaba, J., Haque, N., Wagenknecht, J. B., Smith, B. C., Volkman, B., et al. (2023). Deep computational phenotyping of genomic variants impacting the SET domain of KMT2C reveal molecular mechanisms for their dysfunction. Frontiers in Genetics, 14. https://www.semanticscholar.org/paper/59b0ac8679bfb58cf0444acb70df7acd42ac00b7 (accessed on 17th July 2025).

20. Jorge, S., Chi, Y., Assunção, T., Mathison, A., Volkman, B., Smith, B., Lomberk, G., et al. (2022). Integrative modeling, molecular mechanics, and molecular dynamics evaluation of genomics variants in KMT2C (MLL3), a gene involved in Kleefstra syndrome type 2. The FASEB Journal, 36. https://www.semanticscholar.org/paper/6c08e7c74034c13864f690b3aa43af26a1e2ccb4 (accessed on 17th July 2025).

21. Kapadia, H., Vora, D., Manjegowda, D. S., Nair, A., Sharma, S., & Dinesh, S. (2023). Integrating network pharmacology and molecular docking for the identification of key genes and therapeutic targets of Nigella sativa in multiple sclerosis treatment. Biomedicine. https://www.semanticscholar.org/paper/2f167e354f34094c161afd5a7f472c6db75b809b (accessed on 17th July 2025).

22. Kaushic, C. (2018). Special issue on "omics data in reproductive immunology". American Journal of Reproductive Immunology, 80. https://www.semanticscholar.org/paper/23eec4a5a9f7130bbdc5a015499a39815fb51a10 (accessed on 17th July 2025).

23. Kim, H. K., Cho, I. H., Hwang, E. A., Han, B. H., & Kim, B. H. (2024). Advancing river health assessments: Integrating microscopy and molecular techniques through diatom indices. Water. https://www.semanticscholar.org/paper/a69b342c87a8b95a8cf3b94da978dd4fca72a85e (accessed on 17th July 2025).

24. Kim, I. J., Brack, Y., Bayer, T., & Bornscheuer, U. (2021). Two novel cyanobacterial α-dioxygenases for the biosynthesis of fatty aldehydes. Applied Microbiology and Biotechnology, 106, 197–210. https://www.semanticscholar.org/paper/e190681d10cf284ae14e6e84e1c96d88a64ffe66 (accessed on 17th July 2025).

25. Kimu, A. K. (2025). A comprehensive review of harnessing bioinformatics in biochemistry: A new era of data-driven discoveries and applications. Control Systems and Optimization Letters. https://www.semanticscholar.org/paper/c4ebe2bcbe0e67efdc1351772286b9a913448981 (accessed on 17th July 2025).

26. Kiryluk, K., Goldstein, D., Rowe, J., Gharavi, A., Wapner, R., & Chung, W. (2019). Precision medicine in internal medicine. Annals of Internal Medicine, 170, 635–642. https://www.semanticscholar.org/paper/c7199e8a5226f8d9d55777da0e15e91797bb459a (accessed on 17th July 2025).

27. Lee, H. S., Lee, I. H., Kang, K., Park, S. I., Moon, S. J., Lee, C. H., & Lee, D. Y. (2021). A network pharmacology study on the molecular mechanisms of FDY003 for breast cancer treatment. Evidence-Based Complementary and Alternative Medicine: eCAM, 2021. https://www.semanticscholar.org/paper/4fae0f182885da3412b1b39900a57d86260af896 (accessed on 17th July 2025).

28. Lee, S., Jang, K. I., Lee, H., Jo, Y. S., Kwon, D., Park, G., Bae, S., et al. (2024). Multi-proteomic analyses of 5xFAD mice reveal new molecular signatures of early-stage Alzheimer's disease. Aging Cell, 23. https://www.semanticscholar.org/paper/ae613c563ea8a6e98bd6016882ceb458fda50ff0 (accessed on 17th July 2025).

29. Lo, Y., Han, D. S., Jiang, P., & Chiu, R. (2021). Epigenetics, fragmentomics, and topology of cell-free DNA in liquid biopsies. Science, 372. https://www.semanticscholar.org/paper/b90e4bc77836e6d0b46360862bce78487a6f04fc (accessed on 17th July 2025).

30. Loughrey, C. F., Maguire, S., Dłotko, P., Bai, L., Orr, N., & Jurek-Loughrey, A. (2025). A novel method for subgroup discovery in precision medicine based on topological data analysis. BMC Medical Informatics and Decision Making, 25. https://www.semanticscholar.org/paper/63ba50fde47547ec8400d52378856e422704b82e (accessed on 17th July 2025).

31. Martins, I. L. F., Almeida, F. V. S., Souza, K. P., Brito, F., Rodrigues, G., & Scaramello, C. B. V. (2023). Reviewing atrial fibrillation pathophysiology from a network medicine perspective: The relevance of structural remodeling, inflammation, and the immune system. Life, 13. https://www.semanticscholar.org/paper/95fda524eef7212c2330bd2118d390b46d70d8f2 (accessed on 17th July 2025).

32. Mbisva, S. (2025). The role of open-source bioinformatics tools in resource-limited African settings. Innovative Medicines & Omics. https://www.semanticscholar.org/paper/01f31f3a94171425e1d947e22aa2e2fd5d67d26b (accessed on 17th July 2025).

33. Melidis, D. P., Landgraf, C., Schmidt, G., Schöner-Heinisch, A., von Hardenberg, S., Lesinski-Schiedat, A., Nejdl, W., et al. (2021). GenOtoScope: Towards automating ACMG classification of variants associated with congenital hearing loss. PLoS Computational Biology, 18. https://

www.semanticscholar.org/paper/622f7821be59a5d0aada88d2fd8f614dda38a9f2 (accessed on 17th July 2025).

34. Park, K., Kim, J., Noh, J., Kim, S. G., Cho, H. K., Kim, K., Seo, Y. R., et al. (2025). Epidemiological surveillance and phylogenetic diversity of Orthohantavirus hantanense using high-fidelity nanopore sequencing, Republic of Korea. PLOS Neglected Tropical Diseases, 19. https://www.semanticscholar.org/paper/ef36bebd1844a8b311235a2e4057766038033fa2 (accessed on 17th July 2025).

35. Percie du Sert, N., Ahluwalia, A., Alam, S., Avey, M. T., Baker, M., Browne, W. J., Clark, A., et al. (2020). Reporting animal research: Explanation and elaboration for the ARRIVE guidelines 2.0. PLOS Biology, 18, e3000411. https://doi.org/10.1371/journal.pbio.3000411 (accessed on 17th July 2025).

36. Ravì, D., Wong, C., Deligianni, F., Berthelot, M., Andreu-Pérez, J., Lo, B., & Yang, G. Z. (2016). Deep learning for health informatics. IEEE Journal of Biomedical and Health Informatics, 21, 4–21. https://doi.org/10.1109/jbhi.2016.2636665 (accessed on 17th July 2025).

37. Sindhu, B. S., Adiga, U., Kumar, K. P., Sindhuja, N., Ravikanth, E. V., & Sneha, K. H. (2025). Genetic and molecular characterization of atopic eczema: A comprehensive bioinformatics analysis of gene interactions and pathways. Biomedical and Biotechnology Research Journal. https://www.semanticscholar.org/paper/3bb1a4c23620f6f1d080c0cda0fc853b67a3bf68 (accessed on 17th July 2025).

38. Terzi, T. A. (2024). Using artificial intelligence for personalized cancer treatment. Next Frontier for Life Sciences and AI. https://www.semanticscholar.org/paper/8eea521d91d3fa06bddacbf4e2117fb0edb766b2 (accessed on 17th July 2025).

39. Uhlén, M., Zhang, C., Lee, S., Sjöstedt, E., Fagerberg, L., Bidkhori, G., Benfeitas, R., et al. (2017). A pathology atlas of the human cancer transcriptome. Science, 357. https://doi.org/10.1126/science.aan2507 (accessed on 17th July 2025).

40. Ullah, E., Baig, M., Waqas, A., Rasool, G., Singh, R. S., Shandilya, A., GholamHossieni, H., et al. (2025). Multimodal generative AI for anatomic pathology—A review of current applications to envisage the future direction. Advances in Anatomic Pathology. https://www.semanticscholar.org/paper/d43d118488994132a7b2c8d4e6571ba0a8b94157 (accessed on 17th July 2025).

41. Viet, C. T., Zhang, M., Dharmaraj, N., Li, G. Y., Pearson, A. T., Mañón, V., Grandhi, A., et al. (2024). Artificial intelligence applications in oral cancer and oral dysplasia. Tissue Engineering. Part A. https://www.semanticscholar.org/paper/6360511bc56457781d90f5bd9528887450d259e3 (accessed on 17th July 2025).

42. Wang, J. H., Gessler, D. J., Zhan, W., Gallagher, T. L., & Gao, G. (2024). Adeno-associated virus as a delivery vector for gene therapy of human diseases. Signal Transduction and Targeted Therapy, 9. https://doi.org/10.1038/s41392-024-01780-w (accessed on 17th July 2025).

43. Wang, L., Wang, N., Zhang, W., Cheng, X., Yan, Z., Shao, G., Wang, X., et al. (2022). Therapeutic peptides: Current applications and future directions. Signal Transduction and Targeted Therapy, 7. https://doi.org/10.1038/s41392-022-00904-4 (accessed on 17th July 2025).

44. Wang, X., & Fan, J. (2021). Spatiotemporal molecular imaging is a critical part of spatiotemporal molecular medicine. Clinical and Translational Medicine, 11. https://doi.org/10.1002/ctm2.347 (accessed on 17th July 2025).

45. Wei, Q., Feng, J., Mu, Y., Shen, Q., Xu, H., Sun, L., & Liu, H. M. (2025). Exploring the shared molecular mechanisms of primary hypertension and IgA vasculitis through a case report and combining bioinformatics analysis. Frontiers in Immunology, 16. https://www.semanticscholar.org/paper/c1c0bfe5b8a6941ef8db7cc618d885b4fdb3fd06 (accessed on 17th July 2025).

46. Zeeb, M., Frischknecht, P., Balakrishna, S., Jörimann, L., Tschumi, J., Zsichla, L., Chaudron, S. E., et al. (2025). Addressing data management and analysis challenges in viral genomics: The Swiss HIV cohort study viral next generation sequencing database. PLOS Digital Health, 4. https://www.semanticscholar.org/paper/f1ae2695568c7b9933f404942071b7dfee9c31bf (accessed on 17th July 2025).

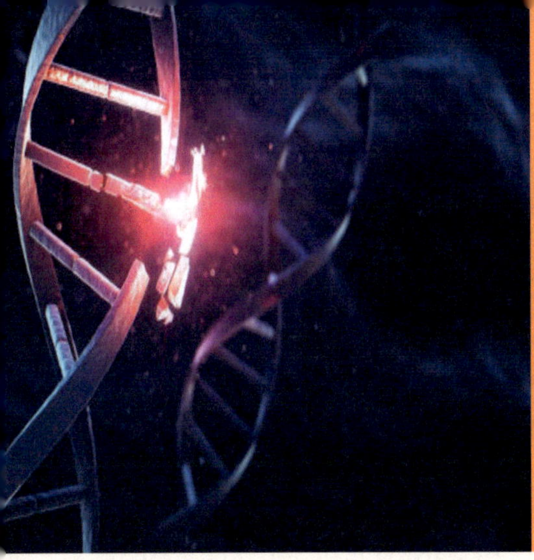

Chapter 11

CRISPR AND GENOME EDITING TECHNOLOGIES

Contents

Introduction

The evolution of novel genome editing technologies has transformed a number of fields of science, including agriculture, medicine, and biotechnology. Among these technologies, CRISPR/Cas9 stands out for its high specificity and flexibility, whereby scientists have the ability to drive specific changes into an organism's genome with ease. This cutting-edge tool operates by inducing double-stranded DNA breaks that enable the addition, excision, or modification of specific genetic sequences. With a growing global need for food production in combination with ecological concerns , such as climate change, CRISPR has excellent future potential to enhance the resistance and yield of crops. This introduction of CRISPR and genome editing technologies is the precursor to the discussion of their applications, implications, and roles to come for many of the big issues , such as food security and control of genetic disease. The impact of CRISPR goes beyond farming, with enormous potential in the field of human health. Being able to edit genes that cause different genetic disorders, CRISPR has the capability of transforming therapeutic approaches in medicine. The technology allows for the generation of animal models specific to disease, which help improve our understanding of disease-causing mechanisms and play a part in drug discovery procedures. As research goes on, cases of successful use of CRISPR in clinical trials point to its promise as a therapeutic drug for the treatment of genetic disorders. However, despite its promise, the application of CRISPR technologies is problematic on the grounds of how it will influence human genetic alteration and species diversity. An appropriate understanding of both the benefits and drawbacks provided by CRISPR is therefore paramount to the well-informed development of this powerful technology. Moving forward, the optimization of CRISPR and the emergence of next-generation genome editing technologies hold promising opportunities for researchers and industry players. Advances like prime editing and advanced delivery systems could further the efficiency, accuracy, and breadth of genome editing, overcoming some of the limitations of current CRISPR approaches. Further, global cooperation between scientists, ethicists, and policymakers will be needed to establish responsible guidelines for the application of CRISPR in medicine and agriculture. As we proceed further into this new era of genetic technology, continued monitoring of the wider societal implications of CRISPR will be required to exploit its full potential without risking its misuse. This combined comprehension of CRISPR and genome editing technologies will allow us to chart the complexities of modern genetics sensibly and proficiently (Figure 11.1).

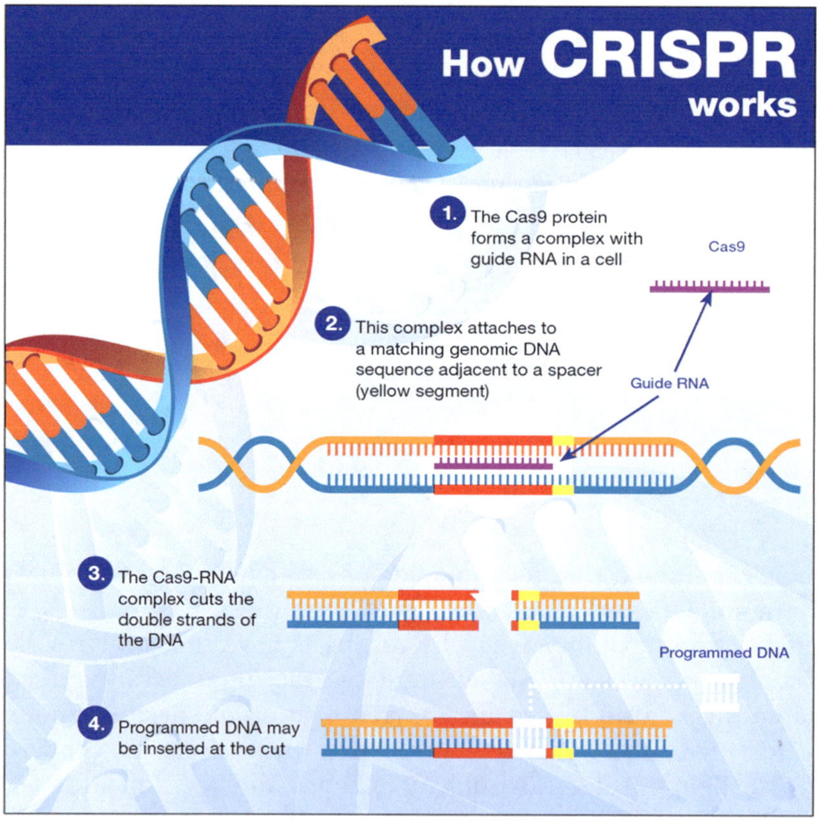

Figure 11.1. CRISPR and genome editing technologies.

Source: https://www.cambridge.org/core/services/aop-file-manager/file/582df76221b559de0536a2c2/CRISPR-1.jpg.

Definition of CRISPR and Genome Editing

The development of CRISPR technology has transformed genome editing, and it has never been more accurate and efficient to modify genetic material. Essentially, CRISPR, or Clustered Regularly Interspaced Short Palindromic Repeats, is a defensive mechanism that is a part of bacteria's adaptive immune system. It allows for the identification and removal of viral genetic material, and that opened the door to the development of genome editing technology. By tapping into this natural mechanism, researchers have developed the CRISPR/Cas9 system, in which the Cas9 enzyme and a specially designed guide RNA are used to find and slice particular DNA sequences. Not only does this targeted approach enable the insertion, deletion, or substitution of genes, but it also eliminates unwanted off-target effects that had beleaguered previous genome editing techniques. As such, CRISPR technology has grown to become a cornerstone in genetic study and therapeutic application, enabling researchers to explore and tinker with the complexity of the genome , such as never before (Zhang et al., 2024). Apart from application in human diseases, CRISPR technology is also making strides in agriculture, where genome editing is employed to enhance crop resilience and productivity. The demand for food globally is likely to increase exponentially, and sustainable farming methods will be needed to meet this demand. Scientists have started designing crops with specific characteristics through the CRISPR/Cas9 technology, including increased abiotic stress tolerance and improved yields. Not only can this method enhance food security with rising populations, but it can also counteract the negative impacts of climate change on agriculture. The efficiency of CRISPR in plant breeding, in contrast to traditional means, speaks volumes about its capacity to generate the preferred crop varieties in a few minutes rather than days and is currently a pivotal aspect of modern agricultural science. Through the capacity to demystify gene editing, CRISPR/Cas9 is ushering in a new era in food production (Ahmad, 2023). With advancing science, the implications of CRISPR and genome editing technologies extend from intellectual interest to encompass ethical, social, and regulatory concerns. The potential for editing genes with accuracy raises critical questions about long-term consequences on biodiversity, health, and ecosystems. The potential for germline editing—alterations that are transmissible to future generations—raises heated debate among scientists, ethicists, and the public about potential misuse and unintended consequences. Therefore, continuous dialogue is important to develop ethical standards and regulatory guidelines that facilitate the responsible use and application of CRISPR technology. Moreover, making these breakthroughs accessible in an equitable manner, particularly for medical and agricultural purposes, continues to be a glaring concern while societies wrestle with managing the balance between innovation and safe deployment. Resolving these complex issues is imperative to tap into the full potential of CRISPR and genome editing technologies responsibly and sustainably.

Historical Context of Genome Editing Technologies

Genome editing technologies are an important avenue of scientific inquiry, beginning with the identification of the first methods of genetic engineering in the 1970s. Early methods, such as recombinant DNA technology, allowed for the alteration of genetic material but were limited by requirements regarding efficiency and specificity. The arrival of zinc-finger nucleases (ZFNs) and transcription activator-like effector nucleases (TALENs) in the early 2000s was a turning point towards more targeted editing tools. But the complexity and high cost of these technologies prevented them from widespread use. The historical transition from rudimentary genetic engineering to more sophisticated approaches mirrors the growing imperative for accurate genome editing tools to address complex scientific and societal challenges, which, in turn, enabled the emergence of CRISPR/Cas systems as the front-runner of genomic technology. CRISPR/Cas systems originated from the adaptive immunity of prokaryotes, initially described in 1987. Its discovery stimulated a record-breaking wave of research, turning CRISPR from a bacterial immunity mechanism into an unmatched genome editing tool. The discovery of CRISPR-Cas9—characterized by its capability to introduce double-strand breaks in DNA in a specific position—has transformed the area of genetic research. As opposed to its predecessors, CRISPR/Cas9 provides unparalleled convenience and affordability, significantly lowering barriers to entry for researchers of all disciplines. This historical context not only identifies the technological advancements that resulted in the development of CRISPRs but also highlights their tremendous potential for use in agriculture and medicine, including the prevention of diseases and the improvement of crops to tolerate climatic change, as discussed further in the literature (Lin & Yang, 2024; Amombo et al., 2025). The implications of CRISPR technology are far greater than the one-function editing capability; they include critical concerns regarding world food security and medicine. As highlighted by recent studies, CRISPR/Cas genome editing can make climate-resilient crops that are critical for filling nutrition gaps in regions of the world heavily affected by climatic stressors , such as drought and salinity. With the help of precise gene editing technology, scientists anticipate that they will improve crop nutritional content in conditions of dryness, addressing malnutrition and hunger with excellent results. Supporting policy frameworks and capacity development efforts for the activation of CRISPR/Cas technology will help achieve the maximum benefit from this scientific breakthrough. Having it will ensure that biosafety regulations are up to date with these advancements, which will facilitate a more efficient and safer application of genome editing tools, which will also benefit vulnerable populations and promote sustainable agriculture (Amombo et al., 2025).

Importance of CRISPR in Modern Science

The importance of CRISPR in modern science cannot be overstated, with the gene-editing tool having transformed genetic research and therapeutic development. First discovered as a natural defense mechanism among microbes, CRISPR now stands as a potent tool for fine-scale genome editing among various organisms. Scientists employ CRISPR in creating precise DNA sequence alterations, enabling exploration not hitherto possible. This methodology enables scientists to more accurately model human disease and unlocks the potential for novel therapeutic modalities. Furthermore, CRISPR technology has also been optimized in its specificity and efficiency, making it an important tool in basic and applied sciences. Aside from research purposes, CRISPR has great potential in agricultural biotechnology. By its editing capability, scientists can design crops that are immune to pests, diseases, and environmental stresses, increasing food security. Such technologies are critically essential with the rising growth of global populations and increased climate change impacts on agriculture. Furthermore, the reality that traits can be designed specifically minimizes the impacts of unintended consequences, a significant advance from traditional genetic modification technologies. By doing so, CRISPR not only advances scientific expertise but also addresses actual problems of productivity and sustainability in agriculture, highlighting its social repercussions at large. The intersection of CRISPR technology with public health further highlights its innovative position in modern science. With antibiotic resistance emerging as an urgent global health threat, novel solutions will be required to combat multidrug-resistant (MDR) pathogens. As cited by Uddin et al. (2021), synthetic biology, as well as molecular work, makes important contributions to the discovery of novel antimicrobial compounds. CRISPR possesses the ability to introduce precision therapies to fight specific pathogens, which can revolutionize treatment protocols. Furthermore, CRISPR's capability to edit microbial genomes allows for the engineering of probiotics that facilitate rebalancing of microbiota to counteract disease-related dysbiosis (Hou et al., 2022). In so doing, the value of CRISPR goes beyond laboratory settings, delivering solutions that attest to the overwhelming necessity for novel solutions in medical and public health programs (Figure 11.2).

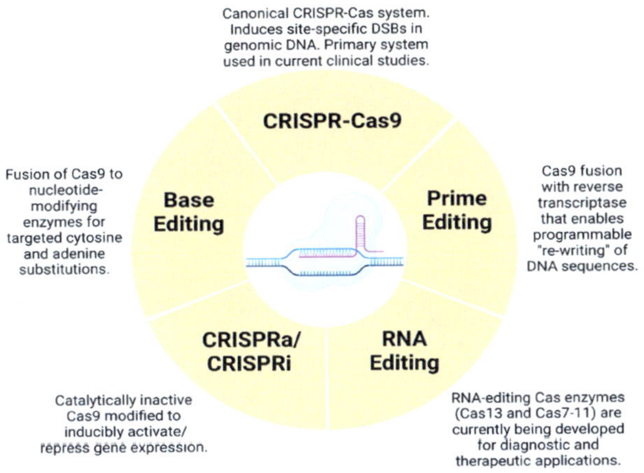

Figure 11.2. Importance of CRISPR in modern science.

Source: https://www.mdpi.com/cells/cells-12-01103/article_deploy/html/images/cells-12-01103-g001.png.

11.1. Mechanism of CRISPR

The CRISPR system, underpinning its design largely based on bacterial adaptive immunity, facilitates genome editing on target by leveraging the natural processes of RNA-programmed endonucleases. It begins with target DNA sequence selection, whereby a guide RNA (gRNA) complementary to the target is anchored to the DNA for the Cas9 nuclease to cause a double-strand break. The significance of this process is not only due to its accuracy but also because it possesses the ability to initiate some genetic changes through subsequent repair processes, e.g., non-homologous end joining or homology-directed repair. This two-pronged approach enables scientists to knock out, insert, or modify genes in the genome, thereby expanding the possible applications of CRISPR to numerous different fields, from agriculture to medicine, to make crops more resistant and design gene therapies for genetic disorders. Application of CRISPR technology is revolutionizing farming practice since it facilitates the modification of genes that are associated with agronomic characteristics. For instance, scientists apply CRISPR to enhance crop disease resistance, abiotic stress tolerance, and improve the quality of yields. Compared to traditional breeding involving random selection of characteristics, CRISPR offers a more direct and efficient route by allowing accurate modifications at certain genomic locations. Using this specific approach, it becomes less ambiguous than traditional breeding. Additionally, the elimination of foreign DNA from genome-edited organisms solves regulation problems to allow easier approval of new crop varieties. These advantages are highly applicable against the backdrop of the need to mitigate climate change and food security concerns in modern agriculture (Nerkar et al., 2022). Alongside agricultural enhancement, the application of CRISPRs also reaches industrial biotechnology, such as its application in the use of fungal strains for the production of enzymes. By specifically editing specific genes in fungi, scientists can design maximum production of enzymes , such as proteases, which are of fundamental importance across several industries, such as food processing and waste treatment. The CRISPR/Cas9 system has been effectively used in filamentous fungi, which indicates its usability outside plants (Naeem et al., 2022). Additionally, this new engineered use of CRISPR has the potential to produce more effective industrial processes with increased sustainability by leveraging improved enzyme effectiveness and specificity. The latest research on CRISPR's mechanism highlights its revolutionary potential within multiple domains, fostering developments that can surmount environmental and economic challenges in the bioindustries of the contemporary era (Figure 11.3).

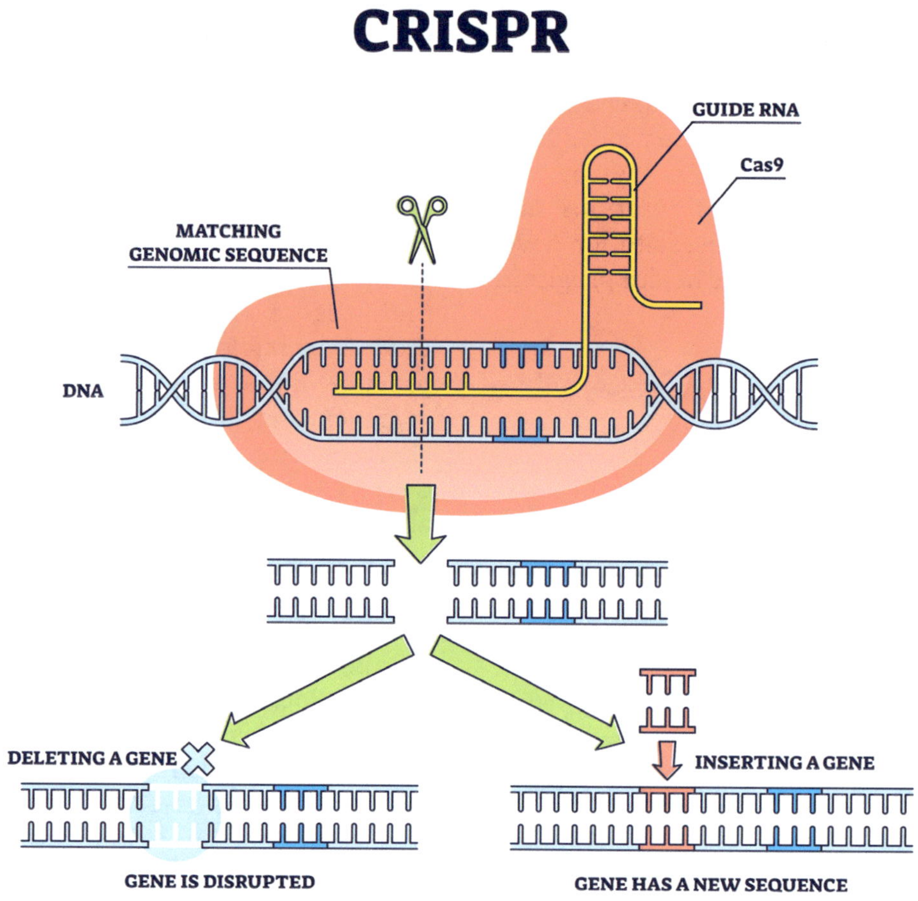

Figure 11.3. Mechanism of CRISPR.

Source: https://mutans.biologia.unipd.it/wp-content/uploads/2023/06/crispr-720x720-1.jpg.

11.1.1. Components of the CRISPR System

The CRISPR system, another game-changer within genome editing technologies, consists of various critical components cooperating to achieve point genetic modifications. Central to the system is the CRISPR-associated protein 9 (Cas9), which is a molecular scissor that induces double-strand breaks in DNA at targeted sites. This ability to cut DNA is accompanied by the guidance of a single guide RNA (sgRNA), which is carefully designed to bind complementarily to the target DNA sequence. The Cas9-sgRNA complex is essential to the specificity and efficacy of the system in recognizing and altering targeted genes. Other crucial factors involve CRISPR arrays that include RNA sequences from past infections by viruses, which allow organisms to recognize and defend against such infections in subsequent infections, thus playing a role in the adaptive nature of the system. In practical application, the CRISPR system's exceptional performance permeates various organisms, symbolizing its broad applicability in various fields of biology. For instance, its use has been demonstrated by genome editing in fruit crops like apples, where stable transformation relies on introducing both Cas9 and sgRNA into the plant genome. However, in such instances, the factors of self-incompatibility and extended generation times add complexity to the processes such that new approaches are needed to effectively deliver strategies. Current studies illustrate the potential of geminivirus-derived replicons (GVRs) in facilitating transient expression of CRISPR elements without foreign DNA integration. This study highlights the continuous innovation of the CRISPR system, allowing more efficient genome editing while circumventing loopholes of traditional transgene insertion techniques, as illustrated by Negishi et al. (2024). Despite the innovation of CRISPR technologies, studies continue to overcome the obstacles that have arisen, particularly off-target effects and overall delivery systems. The development of better Cas9 nucleases and novel delivery platforms, such as functional biomaterials and synthetic carriers, represents a paradigm shift toward higher precision and fidelity in genetic modification. Apart from this, the understanding of the potential of CRISPR technologies in medicine, focusing on the treatment of genetic diseases, brought the technology to the forefront. While full of potential, ethical considerations and regulatory challenges are significant barriers to its adoption universally. Thus, a systematic review of delivery systems available is crucial to the realization of the full potential of CRISPR/Cas9 technology and translating bench-top research into clinical success, as covered by Kaupbayeva et al. (2024).

11.1.2. How CRISPR Targets Specific DNA Sequences?

It is at the core of CRISPR technology that the accuracy with which it can target DNA sequences lies. The system depends largely on two key components: guide RNA (gRNA) and Cas protein, of which the most well-known is Cas9. The gRNA is engineered to be complementary to the target DNA sequence such that it can bind specifically where one wishes to edit. Once it is complexed, the Cas9 endonuclease acts to induce a double-strand break (DSB) on the target sequence site, paving the way for other gene editing processes , such as gene knockout or repair. The specificity of the system is enhanced further by the presence of protospacer adjacent motifs (PAMs) flanking target sequences that are required for Cas9 activity and recognition. Thus, the interaction of gRNA, Cas9, and PAM yields precise genome editing, making CRISPR an effective method in molecular biology and medicine (Feng, 2024). Editing specific DNA sequences via CRISPR-Cas9 involves not only specificity but also versatility of application. Cas9's ability to cause DSBs enables multiple downstream alterations, including insertion of larger deletions or insertions facilitated by homologous recombination mechanisms. In addition, advances in CRISPR technologies have also led to a range of adaptations , such as CRISPR interference (CRISPRi) and CRISPR activation (CRISPRa), which utilize engineered Cas proteins that are non-cutting. Instead, they inhibit or activate genes but retain the same level of targeting specificity. Such diversity opens new doors to gene regulation study and therapeutic strategies, particularly in fields like cancer research and genetic disorders. Breakthroughs beyond CRISPR-Cas9, such as base editing and prime editing, are developments within the genome modification field indicating the widescale uses of CRISPR-based systems (Feng, 2024). While effective, CRISPR technology in certain environments, such as plant genome editing, has challenges that require alternate approaches. For instance, CRISPR traditional systems are hindered when the chloroplast genome is targeted since gRNAs fail to deliver efficiently to chloroplasts. As highlighted in recent research, the traditional approaches involving homologous recombination are often employed for long-term changes in the chloroplast genome. Progress is being made towards overcoming the challenges using artificial enzymes that incorporate targeting transit peptides that enable the targeted editing of chloroplast DNA. These breakthroughs not only demonstrate the dynamic character of CRISPR technologies but also emphasize the necessity for establishing certain strategies for various contexts of genes, ultimately facilitating the goal of efficient and precise genome editing in various organisms (Figure 11.4).

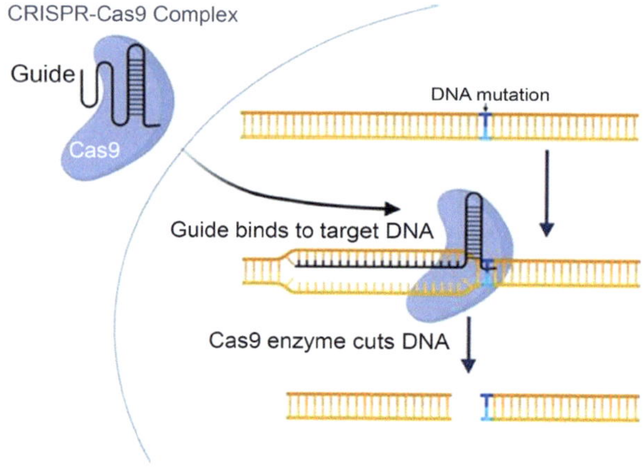

Figure 11.4. How does CRISPR target specific DNA sequences?

Source: https://external-content.duckduckgo.com/iu/?u=https%3A%2F%2Ftse1.mm.bing.net%2Fth%2Fid%2FOIP.2jYlM6czMXNC64IpEzkdwQHaFM%3Fpid%3DApi&f=1&ipt=a6604ba5c90054a0db4eca17d15b7b5a4716eecbf755817692ebd660fe9e3cb8.

11.1.3. The Role of Cas Proteins in Genome Editing

The Cas proteins constitute the basis of the functionality and diversity of CRISPR systems in editing genomes. The proteins, which are classified into different types and subtypes, possess distinct mechanisms for the targeting and cleaving of specific DNA sequences. Preeminent among these is Cas9, which is a commonly used protein guided by a synthetic RNA molecule to create double-strand breaks in the target DNA, allowing the cellular machinery to repair it and thus facilitating gene disruption or insertion. The ability of Cas9 to identify and bind specifically to the desired DNA sequences makes it useful across a broad spectrum of disciplines , such as therapeutic application and agricultural biotechnology. With continued research, other Cas protein developments , such as Cas12 and Cas13, continue to unscramble the toolkit for genome editing, enabling many applications and increasing the rate of genetic manipulation in a broad spectrum of organisms (Feng, 2024; Mao et al., 2025). Apart from being used as a starting point in gene targeting, Cas proteins have also been improved by innovative strategies in synthetic biology. Recent breakthroughs harness artificial intelligence to optimize the structure of single-guide RNAs (sgRNAs), which are critical for the specificity and efficacy of the Cas proteins. AI-aided approaches facilitate the fast scanning of massive data, allowing for the identification of sgRNA sequences with optimal editing efficiency without off-targets. The integration of computational methods with the traditional molecular approaches represents a revolutionary leap in the enhancement of CRISPR-Cas systems. With the progression of genome editing technologies, Cas protein-sgRNA interactions will also be more intricate and contribute to safe and effective utilization of CRISPR technology in biomedical research and treatment (Feng, 2024; Mao et al., 2025). In addition, the future of genome editing through CRISPR technology is reliant on additional study and Cas protein manipulation. Not only are scientists investigating new uses , such as base editing and prime editing, but they are also aiming at enhancing the abilities of existing Cas systems to have more accuracy and versatility. That Cas proteins can be designed for special purposes—, such as improved targeting accuracy or novel functionalities beyond gene editing per se—opens up new doors for exploration and application. These advances underscore the manner in which creativity in the regulation of Cas proteins can address difficult biological issues and lead to groundbreaking developments in gene therapy, plant engineering, and others, ultimately shaping the destiny of genetic technologies (Feng, 2024; Mao et al., 2025).

11.2. Applications in Medicine

With the invention of CRISPR technology came revolutionary advancements in the field of medicine through its innovative genome-editing capabilities. Initially, a bacterial immune system was conceived. CRISPR/Cas9 has since come to be linked with precise genetic modification, where scientists could target specific genes responsible for fatal diseases. This platform's versatility and affordability position it ahead of therapeutic applications, ranging from genetic disorders to cancer treatment. Therapeutic applications of CRISPR are increasingly being explored in preclinical models and in the clinic with the potential to fix mutations causing inherited disease, such as cystic fibrosis and muscular dystrophy. The simplicity with which CRISPR systems can be tailored makes it a promising prospect for personalized medicine, where drugs are designed based on individual genetic profiles, ultimately providing improved patient outcomes in an era anticipating more efficacious medical interventions (Zang et al., 2025). In cancer therapy, the application of CRISPR extends beyond simple targeting of genetic mutations to optimizing available therapies. By the precise editing of immune cells, researchers are employing the technique to develop novel forms of immunotherapies for detecting and destroying cancer cells. CRISPR can utilize T-cells to destroy cancer cells by providing them with receptors capable of recognizing and killing tumor cells more efficiently. Further, research in the integration of CRISPR with other types of genomic editing, such as base editing and prime editing, shows a method for making the editing more targeted and less subject to off-target activity. These advancements are critical to not only increasing efficiency in cancer treatment but also ensuring patient safety for those who undergo such genomic treatment, leading eventually to even more targeted approaches to cancer treatment (Chaudhari & Ranjan, 2024). CRISPR applications in the field of medicine also involve groundbreaking advances in infectious disease treatment, especially through the potential for engineering resistance in human cells. The technology allows scientists to meddle with the genes of viruses and render them harmless or less virulent. For instance, HIV studies have been promising in utilizing CRISPR for eliminating proviral DNA in infected cell genomes, providing a new avenue to destroy the virus's hidden reservoir. Apart from HIV, CRISPR's engineerability can be applied to engineer antiviral therapy against other viral diseases, which is a paradigm shift in the approach towards infectious diseases. Such achievements reveal that CRISPR cannot only cure lifelong diseases but also can respond dynamically to newly-emerging viral pathogens, thus revolutionizing the paradigm for global health interventions (Zang et al., 2025) (Figure 11.5).

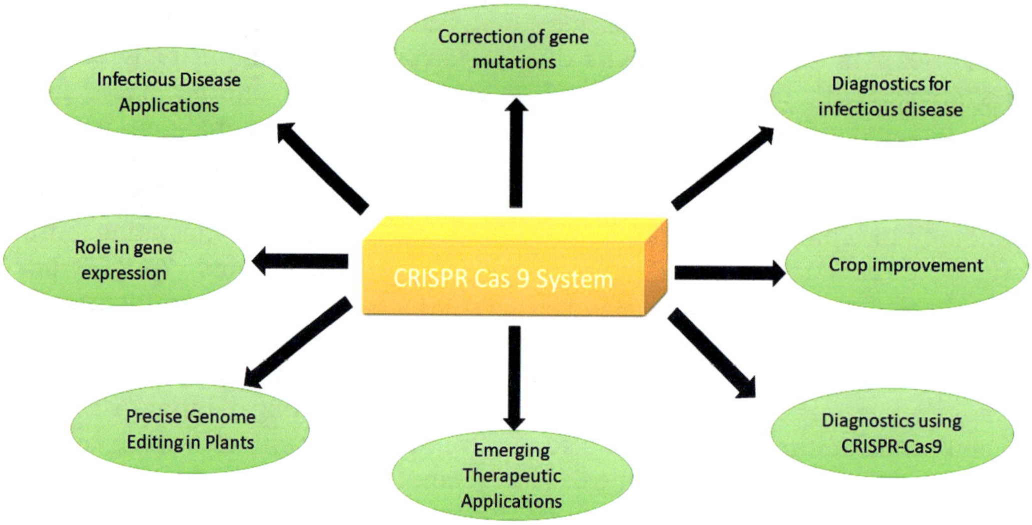

Figure 11.5. Applications in medicine.

Source: https://encyclopedia.pub/media/item_content/202308/64c9a1ddda744antibiotics-12-01075-g002.png.

11.2.1. Gene Therapy for Genetic Disorders

Gene therapy has emerged as a revolutionary way to treat genetic disorders with the aid of advanced technologies , such as CRISPR and other genome editing tools. The most important thing in gene therapy is that it can introduce, remove, or change genetic material into or from a patient's cells, addressing the root cause of various conditions, from monogenic illnesses to more complex ones. By shrewd targeting of defective genes, gene therapy holds the key to individually tailored treatment programs that have the potential to significantly improve patient outcomes. The potential of the new approach has been underscored by ongoing research and clinical trials documenting its capacity not only to cure symptoms but also to provide long-term cures for inherited diseases. This therapeutic promise positions gene therapy at the cutting edge of modern medicine, underscoring the importance of understanding ethical implications and clinical uses as the science evolves (Sen et al., 2025). In addition, the integration of advanced genomic technologies has opened new possibilities for gene therapy, particularly with the development of CRISPR/Cas9 and other related editing tools. These genome editing tools enable precise alterations at desired locations in the genome, making targeted gene correction for genetic mutations possible. The use of CRISPR has revolutionized gene therapy by offering a degree of precision and efficacy in gene modification never before achieved, allowing researchers and clinicians to develop more effective therapies for numerous genetic disorders. These innovations underscore the role of genomic medicine, where genomic data are combined with clinical practice in tailoring interventions based on individual genetic profiles. As genomic technology continues to advance, the future of medicine promises to have drastic implications, promising to streamline and enhance therapeutic interventions across a myriad of medical specialties (Khan et al., 2025). Despite the enormous potential gene therapy holds in genetic disease treatment, some challenges must be addressed. Challenges to gene therapy delivery systems, expense, and ethics surrounding genetic modifications slow down the process. The issue of equal access to these new therapies is essential, but can be prejudiced by the cost of developing and transporting gene therapies. In addition, the moral aspects of gene modification, especially of germline cells, raise issues about long-term consequences on human evolution and potential side effects. In view of such complexities, the entry of gene therapy into daily clinical work must be judiciously assessed and balanced by ongoing debate among scientists, clinicians, ethicists, and policymakers. Overcoming these issues is the key to realizing the maximum potential of gene therapy for genetic disorders and ensuring ethical use for the treatment of patients (Sen et al., 2025) (Figure 11.6).

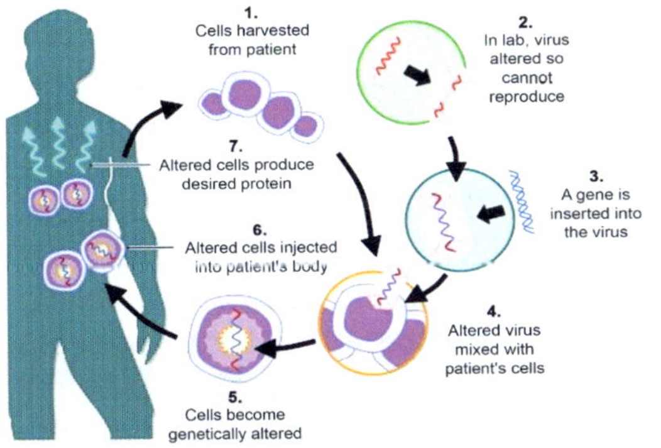

Figure 11.6. Gene therapy for genetic disorders.

Source: https://scienceofhealthy.com/wp-content/uploads/2019/04/the-process-of-gene-therapy-1.jpg.

11.2.2. Potential for Cancer Treatment

The strength of CRISPR and genome editing tools in cancer treatment lies in their ability to specifically target and modify genes that are responsible for tumor activity. New gene-editing techniques have made it much easier to target cancer-causing oncogenes with accuracy, as well as to revitalize tumor suppressor genes. The strongest potential progress is the knockout of genes responsible for drug resistance and malignancy. For example, CRISPR-Cas9 can specifically knock out individual pathways that are utilized by tumors for survival and growth. Consequently, tumors can become sensitized to current treatments. This action not only proves the potency of targeted therapy but also signifies how the ability to edit genomes can be exploited to tackle the intricacies and heterogeneities in cancer biology. Moreover, CRISPR is also expected to find applications in the optimization of the efficiency of immunotherapy methods, including CAR-T cell therapy. While CAR-T cells have been spectacularly successful in the treatment of certain hematologic malignancies, constraints like cytokine release syndrome (CRS) have limited their more extensive application. Gene-editing techniques enable the T cells to be designed so that they knock out the interleukin-6 receptor, thereby blunting inflammatory reactions that have been associated with CRS but retaining highly effective anti-tumor efficacy. Not only does this new technique avert significant safety concerns, but it also aims to improve CAR-T therapy's treatment, thereby presenting a probable breakthrough in the fight against various forms of cancer. These advances reflect the ability of CRISPR technologies to lead to safer and more effective treatments, ultimately changing the course of cancer therapy. Furthermore, CRISPR-Cas9 is also being investigated for its possible application in targeting specific cancer genes, as in the case of head and neck squamous cell carcinoma (HNSCC). Current studies have employed lipid nanoparticle (LNP) delivery platforms for the facilitated targeted delivery of CRISPR reagents specifically designed for the knockdown of oncogenic genes like SOX2. The outcomes have shown significant reductions in the viability of tumor cells, with promising preclinical data demonstrating the repression of tumor growth and enhanced survival in mouse models. These findings point to the power and effectiveness of CRISPR as a therapeutic strategy for highly recurrent solid tumors. In brief, as researchers continue to refine these technologies, the potential of CRISPR to revolutionize cancer therapy is vast, which sets hopes for new therapeutic interventions in previously resistant malignancies.

11.2.3. Use in Infectious Disease Research

The use of CRISPR and genome editing technology has significantly contributed to the study of infectious diseases, allowing researchers to analyze intricate host–pathogen interactions with unprecedented accuracy. The CRISPR/Cas9 system, in fact, has played a critical role in the generation of disease models that accurately reflect human infection responses, which are invaluable for gaining deeper insights into the mechanisms of pathogens. Through the ability to generate targeted gene knockout, researchers can probe the functions of particular genes in both pathogens and host immune systems. For instance, studies using CRISPR tools have clarified the genetic determinants for susceptibility or resistance to numerous infectious pathogens, giving us clues regarding potential therapeutic targets. This strategy not only enhances our knowledge of infectious diseases but also provides an entry point into the development of new interventions that can potentially reduce their contribution significantly to public health. Besides facilitating basic research, CRISPR technologies have also been promising in the development of therapeutic drugs against infectious diseases. The ability to edit the genomes of both pathogens and host cells has opened new avenues for combating viral infections, such as HIV and hepatitis. By employing CRISPR/Cas9 systems in interfering with the genome of viruses or overexpressing antiviral functions of the host cell, researchers are advancing new therapeutic strategies. For instance, CRISPR has been employed to target and eliminate sequences from the genomes of viruses and ultimately block their replication and transfer.

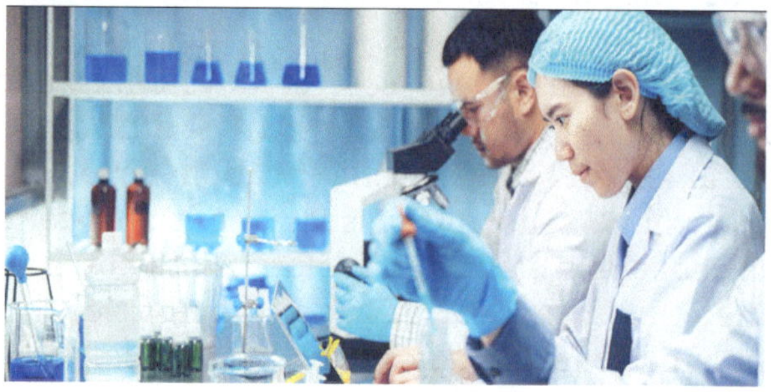

Figure 11.7. Use in infectious disease research.

Source: https://docxellent.com/wp-content/uploads/2024/03/Fostering-Insights-Data-Empowerment-in-Infectious-Disease-Research-.jpg.

Moreover, ongoing research is determining the capacity of CRISPR to engineer immune cells more effectively against refractory viral infections, representing a multidimensional approach to such disease treatment by targeted genomic modification. With regard to the encouraging potential of CRISPR for infectious disease study, however, problems do arise. Off-target activity risk, in combination with the need for successful delivery, offers a special challenge to extensive use of CRISPR-based therapies. Despite the newer advancements , such as base editing and prime editing, improving the specificity of genome editing agents, safe application of such agents in the practice of medicine is a priority. Moreover, ethical considerations of gene editing within humans also need careful consideration and regulation. Owing to the progressing field, overcoming these issues will be critical to realizing the full potential of CRISPR technologies in the combat against infectious diseases and improving global health outcomes. The continuous evolution of CRISPR and its integration with other molecular strategies will surely take this research forward, promising new solutions for previously insurmountable challenges in infectious disease management (Figure 11.7).

11.3. Agricultural Innovations

The past of farming practices has experienced a complete turnaround, one of the driving factors being advancements , such as CRISPR and other genome editing tools. Through allowing scientists to introduce targeted modifications in the crop's DNA, CRISPR technology enhances various agronomic traits—most notably, pest resistance, drought tolerance, and nutritional content. Since its emergence around 2012, CRISPR has consistently demonstrated the potential for promoting agricultural economic productivity in ways of increased yields and reduced reliance on chemical pesticides and fertilizers. Such strategic advancement not only resolves the food security concerns but also adheres to the principles of sustainable agriculture practices in that it reduces environmental pressures stemming from the conventional farming practices as well as promotes ecological balance, thereby bringing about sustainable development for the agricultural sector (Zhu et al., 2025). In addition, the application of advanced genomic sequencing technologies has also upgraded the ability of CRISPR by making it possible to implement genotype and phenotype data in crop improvement. Advances in genome-wide markers and phenotyping methods significantly enhance the process of gene discovery, as well as quantitative trait identification and selection, needed in crop improvement. Notably, techniques , such as DNA sequencing and marker-assisted selection have enhanced the effectiveness and cost-effectiveness of the breeding process, hence democratizing access to biotechnological advancements in most agricultural systems. Resistance of crops to climate change is an emergent global concern, and the advancement of CRISPR into breeding programs has facilitated the generation of climate-resilient varieties, which have demonstrated their importance in innovations for agriculture to guarantee food production in the face of environmental uncertainty (Rehman et al., 2024). The combined impact of genome editing tools is not limited to agriculture but extends to related fields, including biomechanics and other fields of scientific inquiry. Accuracy offered by CRISPR can be utilized to develop genetically engineered organisms (GMOs) with maximized mechanical frameworks, which have significant applications in enhanced performance under various situations, including farm machinery and bioengineering. Moreover, the resulting synergy between biomechanics and agricultural biotechnology underscores the beauty of interdisciplinarity in leading innovations that are central to remediating contemporary complicated challenges. Through continued study of the economic worth and potential impacts of CRISPR, researchers highlight the technology's strategic value not just in agriculture, but in many other areas as well, thus validating the significance of continued advances in gene editing technologies in fostering bio-innovation and driving economic development (Zhu et al., 2025).

11.3.1. Development of Disease-Resistant Crops

With the rising population of the world, the requirement for sustainable agriculture is becoming more essential by the day. Traditional plant breeding methods, while central to crop improvement, have the tendency to create varieties worse than their wild counterparts, particularly against biotic stresses , such as pests and disease. The recent innovation of genome editing tools in the form of CRISPR has enabled researchers to design crops that are resistant to disease with more vigor and fitness. By precisely targeting the genes associated with plant immunity, scientists can design crops that are more resistant to environmental stress and biological assault. This new approach not only promises to stabilize food production but also is likely to reduce the application of chemical pesticides, which are toxic to the environment and human well-being.

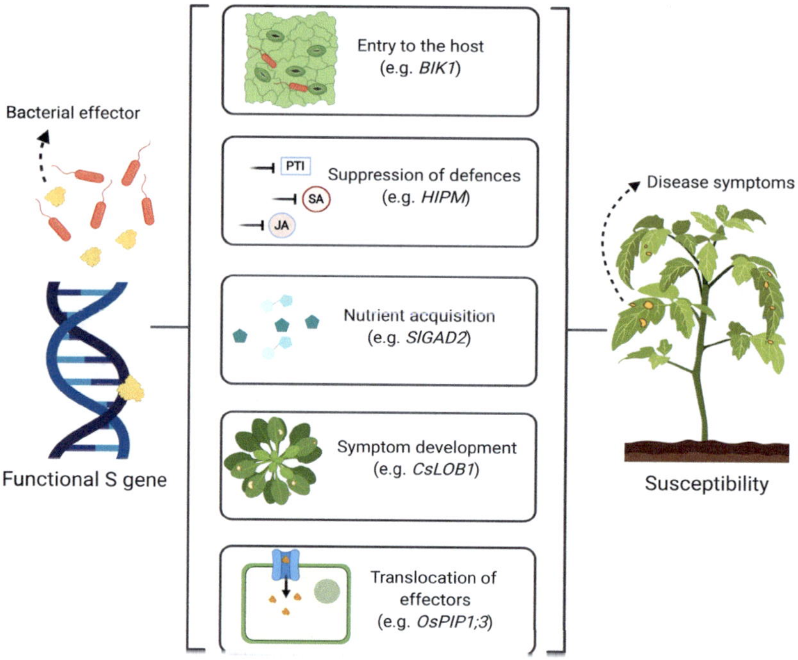

Figure 11.8. Development of disease-resistant crops.

Source: https://www.cell.com/cms/attachment/06c93e39-828d-40d5-8c01-083e8379102a/gr1_lrg.jpg.

Thus, the strategic use of CRISPR and other genome editing tools is a groundbreaking advancement in agricultural biotechnology and food security. CRISPR-Cas technologies, being highly efficient and accurate, have revolutionized plant genetics. The system employs the Cas9 enzyme to induce very accurate double-strand breaks in the DNA, thereby activating the plant's own repair machinery. These developments allow researchers to enhance the resistance of crops to all types of pathogens, including bacteria, fungi, and viruses. By enhancing both ETI and PTI, genome editing can potentially augment the defense systems of crops to a large extent. Most notably, the integration of CRISPR into breeding programs has yielded stunning outcomes for the leading agricultural crops, thus emerging as a core tool in the development of disease-resistant crop varieties. With scientists venturing deeper into the vast potential of CRISPR technology, the potential of bioengineered crops with improved resistance is on the horizon with the advent of shifting agricultural challenges and climate change (Jahan et al., 2025). Furthermore, the quest for disease-resistant crops must also consider the genetic diversity in wild relatives of the domesticated species. Such identification and incorporation of these genetic resources are essential in building robust agricultural systems that can counter challenges from new plant pathogens in the future. Genome editing has made it possible to classify disease-resistant mutants based on their genetic changes, as in studies using *Arabidopsis thaliana* and other crops. Targeted gene modifications allow researchers to discover critical genes linked to plant immunity, paving the way for novel therapies in molecular breeding. With increasing frequency and severity of plant disease due to climate change, employing CRISPR technology offers a responsive means for ensuring food security in the context of an ever-changing environment. Continuing development and application of these genome-editing systems hold a fantastic future for sustainable agricultural development and resistance (Park et al., 2024) (Figure 11.8).

11.3.2. Enhancements in Crop Yield and Quality

Ongoing quest for sustainable agriculture has driven the adoption of CRISPR and gene editing technologies, significantly increasing crop yield and quality. Traditional breeding methods, as effective as they are, have the tendency to involve lengthy processes that can hamper rapid response to environmental demands and consumer preferences. For instance, climate change poses an unprecedented threat to farm output, requiring an immediate response to ensure food security. Gene editing technologies offer precise and efficient solutions by enabling targeted modifications in plant genomes. With the advances of technology , such as CRISPR/Cas9, researchers can now design climate-resilient crops with better attributes, such as drought resistance and disease resistance, needed to thrive in growing hostile environments (Mann et al., 2024). Thus, adopting genome editing technologies can have a significant impact on global agricultural systems. In particular, CRISPR technology has been marked with huge potential for improving specific crops, such as potatoes, which are key to food and nutritional security globally. With the emphasis being on further research, potatoes are subjected to several issues, such as biotic and abiotic stress components, affecting tuber yield and post-harvest quality negatively. Conventional breeding is not usually successful in coping with these complexities since the crops have distinct genetic features and complexities. Nonetheless, CRISPR technology can allow scientists to develop potato varieties better equipped to withstand these stresses as well as enhance their physical and biochemical attributes, including nutritional value as well as storage attributes. Streamlining genome editing techniques in potatoes can allow scientists to pioneer cultivars that meet the needs of consumers as well as promote sustainable agriculture methods (Chincinska et al., 2022). Further, the broader implications of heightening crop yield and quality through genome editing are more than just short-term agricultural benefits. These technologies have ramifications for a more stable and abundant food supply required for an expanding world population. As the World must increase the productivity of agriculture between 25% and 70% to meet future needs, CRISPR and other technologies offer a promising way to meet these goals (Mann et al., 2024). By developing crops that can maintain yield and quality despite changing climatic patterns, genome editing can potentially limit food insecurity and widen economic access to most communities. As this field evolves, continued innovation in CRISPR applications will be crucial in shaping a sustainable agricultural future that prioritizes both efficiency and environmental stewardship.

11.3.3. Ethical Considerations in Genetically Modified Organisms (GMOs)

The moral challenges related to genetically modified organisms (GMOs) are of a two-dimensional nature, encompassing such things as safety, environmental impact, and social concern. One of the challenges is the potential for unintended consequences upon introducing GMOs into the ecosystem. A case in point is where GMO crops have been produced to be herbicide-resistant, and such GMO crops are cultivated, leading to the occurrence of superweeds, which are herbicide-resistant, thereby calling for increased use of more poisonous chemicals. This situation evokes issues concerning whether agricultural production and biodiversity conservation can be sustained in the long term. As realized in relevant research, weighing between driving agricultural productivity by technologies , such as CRISPR and ecological integrity has been a formidable ethical dilemma that requires careful assessment of possible risks posed by genetic modification (Choriyeva, 2024). Further, ethical debates in the case of GMOs also extend to equity and access concerns, most notably concerning food security in poor nations. The possibilities in nutritional content enhancement, disease resistance, and environmental adaptability with genome editing tools , such as CRISPR have triggered discussions regarding their accessibility for the poor. Such technologies have enormous potential in world hunger reduction; however, issues regarding who benefits from these technologies arise. There is a fear of monopolization by the large biotech companies, which could exacerbate inequalities as it limits access to resources for small farmers. It is thus important to develop inclusive policies that make genome editing technologies accessible equally accessible to everyone. As argued in recent literature, such inequities must be redressed in terms of broader ethical principles of biotechnology so that biotechnology inventions in agriculture do not circumscribe marginalized groups (Waghmode et al., 2024). Public perception of GMOs also complicates the ethical situation, as public opinion has the ability to affect regulatory action and the acceptance of these technologies. Misinformation and ignorance about genetic alteration are largely at fault for public skepticism. Public participation in open debate concerning the safety and benefits of GMOs is needed to build people's trust. This includes identifying and addressing the concerns of various stakeholders, including consumers, farmers, and environmentalists. Involving these stakeholders in the debate on the implications of CRISPR and genome editing technologies is crucial to ensure well-informed decision-making. Lastly, an ethical strategy that foregrounds public engagement and fully informed consent could heighten acceptance such that the development and use of GMOs would be within the values and interests of communities (Choriyeva, 2024).

11.4. Ethical Implications

The advent of CRISPR and genome editing technologies has ushered in a new era of scientific promise, namely in the genetic alteration of living organisms for many applications. But with these game-changing technologies comes a profound ethical truth that must be confronted by society. The ability to engineer or eliminate vast categories of species raises questions regarding biodiversity, ecosystem resilience, and the long-term implications that such practices can have. For instance, genetic engineering of vectors, i.e., mosquitoes, could significantly decrease the occurrence of such diseases as malaria. Nevertheless, if not regulated, this kind of manipulation can produce unforeseen consequences, such as the deterioration of an ecosystem relying on the organism of interest. The discussion of such ethical issues is a necessity that needs to be addressed by an interdisciplinary combination, such as scientists, ethicists, and policymakers, to unravel the complexity of ecological disruption with tools explained in the literature, but also emphasizes the need for broad regulatory frameworks (Kumari et al., 2024). Besides ecological issues, the ethical implications of CRISPR technology also encompass its human applications, especially in medical environments. The potential of germline editing offers tantalizing possibilities as much as ethical challenges. For instance, the potential for eradicating disease at the genetic level before birth is to be very much welcomed, but opens the floodgates to smooth slopes of an ethical nature, such as designer babies, where traits are selected by procuring tastes of parents beyond medical necessity. This commodification of human life has the potential to worsen social inequalities by favoring individuals who have access to genetic editing technologies while excluding those who lack the financial capacity to access these technologies.

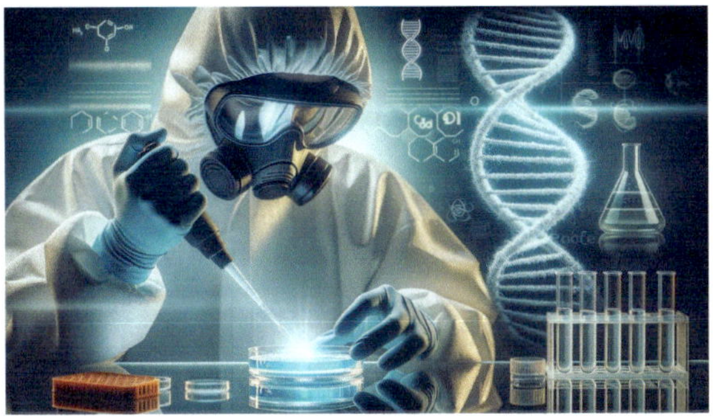

Figure 11.9. Ethical implications of the advent of CRISPR and genome editing technologies.

Source: https://businessner.com/wp-content/uploads/2023/10/crispr-solution-into-a-petri-dish.jpg.

To counter these ethical issues, the educational curriculum must include genome editing discussions. Engaging students in discussion of the ethical implications of these technologies fosters a generation not only scientifically literate but also ethically active, to ensure proper stewardship of biotechnology (Carlos et al., 2023). Moreover, public opinion and acceptability are significant drivers in the ethical debate surrounding CRISPR and genome editing technologies. With advances, social acceptance hinges on forthright information about risk and benefit. Involving the public by means of education and outreach can de-mystify the science and provide arenas for public input on regulatory action. Scientists and organizations must collaborate in putting a system together that will articulate an informed decision-making process with ethics as well as concerns about scientific discovery. It is crucial that research institutions create programs to acquaint students and the public with these technologies while simultaneously discussing their implications and establishing guidelines that take into account societal values. These will not only enhance understanding but also form a framework of ethical practice that guides the continuous development of genome editing technology (Carlos et al., 2023) (Figure 11.9).

11.4.1. Concerns About Designer Babies

The discovery of CRISPR and genome editing technologies has ushered in a fiery controversy surrounding the morality of producing designer babies. Its supporters are convinced that it can be used to eradicate inherited illnesses and enhance desirable traits to bring about a better quality of life. Critics, however, raise a cautionary note about the potential consequences of these manipulations in the form of unintended genetic alterations and the creation of social inequalities. As gene editing becomes more accessible, there is the very real possibility that it will accrue only to wealthy families, further entrenching socio-economic health and opportunity disparities. The long-term effect of gene editing on human diversity can be of essential philosophical concern, inviting consideration of the nature of what it is to interfere with human genetics. Thus, as with the promise of CRISPR being incredible, there needs to be consideration of the implications of applying such technology to human embryos and what ethics would govern its use (Wheatley, 2025). In addition to social injustices, the technical problems with genome editing also need to be overcome, such as those related to safety and efficacy. Data from studies indicate that editing in the initial stages of development has the potential to introduce unpredictable consequences, for instance, loss of heterozygosity (LOH) from a lack of DNA repair. For instance, attempts at targeted editing can create complex genomic rearrangements that may be outside of detection thresholds of standard testing protocols, further adding to the safety profile of CRISPR. Studies show that the majority of LOH that has been noted in CRISPR-treated embryos result from faulty DNA repair mechanisms, rather than the intended interhomolog-homologous recombination processes. The fact highlights the necessity of careful preclinical testing and regulation before CRISPR technologies are applied in reproductive medicine and the importance of coming up with a full set of regulations to address progress and safeguard it (Kubikova et al., 2024). Finally, the argument regarding designer babies transcends the technical and ethical boundaries to encompass societal values as well as individual rights. In our move towards the beginning of a new era of biotechnology, questions of consent and individual autonomy come into play. The possibility of changing human genetic makeup is a concern not just for the implications on those who are being edited but also on the coming generations that would inherit these changes—often without even their own knowledge. The concept of informed consent is complicated when in regard to potential future upgrades to human intelligence, physical capabilities, or physical appearance. Therefore, the designer babies debate needs sophisticated arguments between scientists, ethicists, policymakers, and society so that the advancements in CRISPR and genome editing technologies do not precede our regulatory and ethical frameworks (Wheatley, 2025).

11.4.2. The Debate Over Genetic Privacy

As CRISPR and genome editing technologies continue to develop, they pose deep implications for genetic privacy. While the power to engineer genes means the potential to cure genetic disease, it also raises concerns of ethics regarding what use is put to this information and how it will be safeguarded. With genetic data increasing in availability, citizens are vulnerable to abuse of privacy, particularly in environments where the data is used as leverage by governments, employers, or insurers. The potential that individuals' genetic codes are subject to scrutiny and potential acquisition creates consent and autonomy issues that defeat existing regimes designed to protect personal information in the genomics era. During the debate, the need for clearly stated policies and regulations comes up to ensure strong protection for genetic information, given the fast rate of genomic data integration into health care systems and research study initiatives (Tham et al., 2017). Secondly, the growing genome editing capability drives the debate over what defines proper use of genetic technology. As individuals become more fascinated with the prospect of assuming designer genes—where aspects , such as intelligence or physical strength could be optimized—the issue of genetic privacy matters above everything. Genetic information encompasses not only one's own medical history but also inherited susceptibilities that could affect families generally. The consequences of such information extend to individuals; it holds the prospect of genetic marker discrimination that predicts vulnerability to particular diseases or traits. Thus, warning of genetic privacy loss might result in increased social inequality, fostering a double-edged future that has access to genetic modification and accompanying benefits divided along socioeconomic lines. This highlights the imperative for inclusive discussion that balances genetic technology developments against societal values and ethical issues (Tham et al., 2017). Secondly, while genomic technologies promise hitherto unprecedented opportunities for progress in science, the ethical implications of genetic privacy must be addressed holistically. Not just do manipulations enabled by CRISPR erode traditional ideas of privacy, but they also pose a challenge to rethinking informed consent in genetics research. Individuals are often unaware of the effects of donating their genomic data; thus, the need for transparent and straightforward consent procedures is even more significant. It is particularly pertinent with the possibility of transferring data between different platforms, where information derived from one individual may unknowingly put others in their family line at risk. Active discussion of these matters will encourage a more ethical application of genetic technology that protects privacy and autonomy, which will result in ethical innovation that upholds the rights and dignities of all those who are involved (Gomes & Soares, 2017) (Figure 11.10).

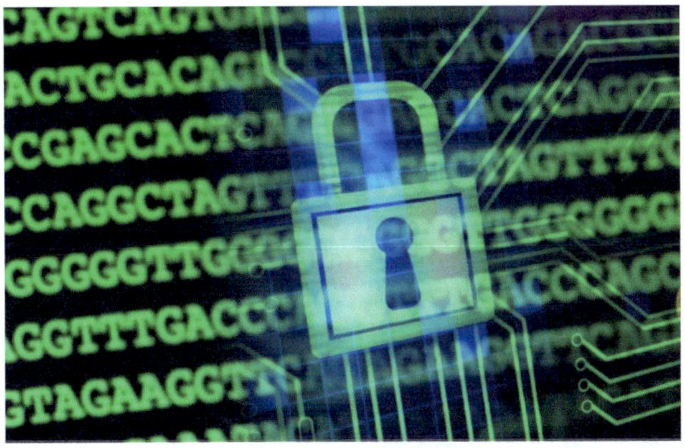

Figure 11.10. The debate over genetic privacy.

Source: https://schoolworkhelper.net/wp-content/uploads/2018/01/Genetic-Privacy.jpg.

11.4.3. Regulatory Challenges and Public Perception

The rapid advancement of CRISPR and genome editing technologies has generated considerable interest in their applications across different fields, e.g., agriculture and aquaculture. Nevertheless, there are regulatory issues that significantly retard the widespread adoption of these technologies. For instance, regulation in the United States is fragmented, with the USDA, FDA, and EPA each regulating different parts of genetically modified organisms (GMOs). This lack of a harmonized regulatory framework creates confusion for scientists and industries aiming to develop CRISPR-engineered organisms. The difficulty in deciphering these complex regulatory requirements not only impedes scientific development but raises the stakes for public approval because there remains general apprehension surrounding GMOs (Zhu et al., 2024). Therefore, an open regulatory system that inspires trust in both consumers and developers alike is an urgent requirement in a bid to realize the full potential of CRISPR technologies. Public opinion plays a vital role in shaping the debate on CRISPR and its use. Despite the promise of improved food security and enhanced environmental sustainability, the majority of individuals have apprehensions concerning safety, ethics, and unintended ecological effects. Evidence shows that public resistance is a result of historical experiences with GMOs, where miscommunication and misinformation have caused significant erosion of consumer confidence (Sampath et al., 2023). Fixing these, therefore, requires a sweeping approach that includes open disclosure about the safety and benefits of CRISPR technologies and overt engagement of all stakeholders in the decision-making process. Public participation in the form of education and outreach will result in greater understanding and acceptance, and thus overcome the scientific advances-public concern gap. Finally, public perception control is essential to ensure the successful use of CRISPR technologies in agriculture as well as in other fields. Moreover, the interplay between public perception and regulatory mechanisms is highly complex. In order for CRISPR technology to gain greater popularity, it is crucial that the regulatory bodies not only streamline their procedures but also become more responsive to the interests of the public. This implies involving the public widely in public discourse regarding the implications of genome editing technology, thereby creating an inclusive dialogue. By publicly addressing ethical concerns and potential risks together with the presentation of the technological benefits, regulatory agencies can strengthen trust in genome editing by the public (Zhu et al., 2024). In addition, through the provision of responsive regulatory systems to new developments in science, such as differences between traditional GMOs and gene-edited organisms, both innovation and public attitudes will be benefited. Finally, an engaged, open style of regulation that balances scientific expertise with social values will be instrumental in ensuring the successful integration of CRISPR and genome editing technologies in our societies.

11.5. Comparison with Other Genome Editing Technologies

The introduction of CRISPR technology has catalyzed phenomenal advances in genome editing, particularly in contrast to earlier methods , such as zinc-finger nucleases (ZFNs) and transcription activator-like effector nucleases (TALENs). Whereas ZFNs must be designed with a particular protein per target sequence, CRISPR/Cas9 utilizes a guide RNA to target Cas9 to the desired site on the chromosome, rendering it quicker to edit. Its versatility ensures it is easier to engineer and use in various organisms, hence speeding up research and applications across sectors from agriculture to therapeutics. Secondly, CRISPR's multiplex ability—edit several genes at once—stands out as a distinguishing characteristic that extends its application in complex genetic engineering processes (Li et al., 2020). Taken cumulatively, the above factors explain the enhanced preference for CRISPR as the technology of choice in genome editing in both research and clinical contexts. In biotechnology involving agriculture, CRISPR presents a revolutionary process compared to traditional breeding and earlier genome editing techniques like ZFNs and TALENs. The accuracy and specificity of CRISPR edits enable crops to be engineered with desired traits more efficiently than previously. For instance, while ZFNs and TALENs involve labor-intensive gene targeting, CRISPR is able to facilitate the rapid generation of genetically modified lines that can enhance yield, disease resistance, and nutritional content (Chen et al., 2019). This rapid advancement means a more efficient agriculture system since CRISPR can minimize the lengthy time required for crop improvement programs. Consequently, this leads to enhanced food security and less reliance on chemical inputs, and hence projects the capability of CRISPR to address world problems in agriculture. Despite the readily apparent superiorities of CRISPR over its predecessors, ZFNs and TALENs, the latter possess merits that might make it the best for some applications in genome editing. For example, both traditional techniques have well-documented and well-characterized gene editing modes with the known and well-established systems, and there has been much studied regarding their mechanisms and impact. This typically entails fewer regulatory issues than with CRISPR, which continues to struggle with controversies surrounding its ethics and potential unwanted effects (Li et al., 2020). In addition, in instances where off-target effects of CRISPR editing may pose a major risk, scientists would prefer utilizing TALENs or ZFNs to maintain greater control over genomic changes. Accordingly, even though CRISPR is a revolutionary tool, the finicky aspects related to genome editing tool selection demand an extensive knowledge of every technique's particular characteristics and uses.

11.5.1. Overview of TALENs and ZFNs

The landscape of genome editing tools is dynamic, with systems like Transcription Activator-Like Effector Nucleases (TALENs) and Zinc Finger Nucleases (ZFNs), which have gained popularity because they are both precise and accurate in targeting a DNA sequence. TALENs employ designed DNA-binding modules derived from plant transcription factors, hence enabling them to specifically bind to a sequence of DNA with great affinity. The technique allows researchers to trigger double-strand breaks in loci of their preference, which are either fixed through non-homologous end joining or homology-directed repair processes. Hence, TALENs represent a versatile platform for gene editing applications across various organisms. Their ability to introduce specific genetic modifications has profound applications in therapeutic treatment and agricultural biotechnology and has the connotation of redirecting the way specific traits are introduced into crops or genetic illnesses addressed in medicine, with the increasing global challenges in biotechnology innovation (Waghmode et al., 2024).

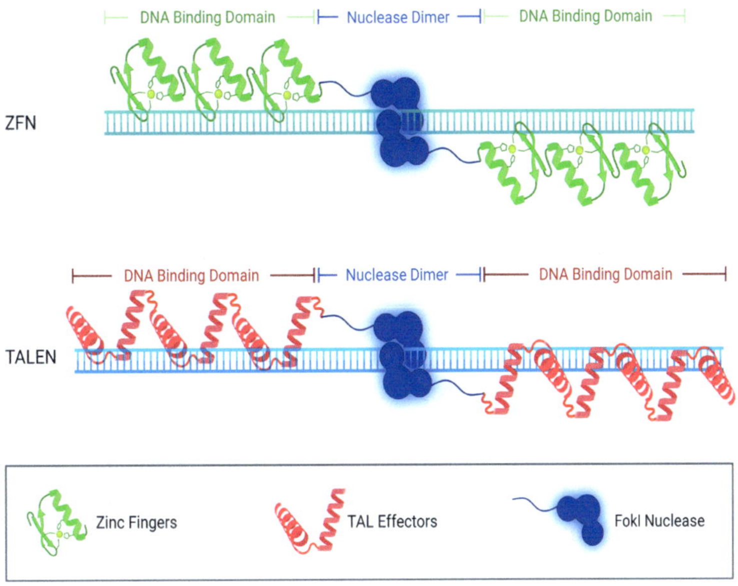

Figure 11.11. Overview of TALENs and ZFNs.

Source: https://images.aatbio.com/universal/catalog/GenomeEditing/ZFN%20and%20TALEN%20Nucleases%20for%20Gene%20Editing.png.

On the other hand, ZFNs employ a unique mechanism based on zinc finger proteins that are amenable to engineering to bind specific DNA sequences. By combining modules of multiple zinc fingers, researchers can construct ZFNs that target specific genomic locations. Double-strand breaks are also triggered in the ZFN technology, which triggers repair machinery capable of integrating desired genetic modifications. Similar to TALENs, the ability to create site-specific gene disruptions or modifications has vast implications for basic and applied research. Therapeutically, ZFNs have been investigated for their ability to correct genetic pathology underlying diseases. While ZFNs are more specific and effective, they are difficult to design and develop, necessitating stringent validation before application. Despite all these hurdles, ZFNs remain a trusted workhorse in the toolkit of genome editing technologies, paving the way for new gene therapies and genetic crop improvement (Patel, 2024). TALENs and ZFNs are merely two of the examples of the breakthroughs beyond the standard genetic engineering methods, paving the way for the prospect of precision genome editing. Notably, the technologies have seen extensive research and development and support various applications in agriculture and medicine. While CRISPR/Cas9 technology has gained popularity due to its ease of use and low cost, TALENs and ZFNs are still very promising.

They have different mechanisms that bring about exceptional advantages where off-target effects should be circumvented or when precise modifications are of significant importance. As the technology of genome editing advances, knowing the position of these tools in the larger picture of biotechnology will be essential to their utilization in addressing global issues like food security, healthcare, and environmental sustainability (Waghmode et al., 2024) (Figure 11.11).

11.5.2. Advantages of CRISPR Over Traditional Methods

The discovery of CRISPR technology is a significant advance in genome editing compared to traditional approaches like homologous recombination. Traditional approaches often take enormous amounts of time and resources to yield desired genetic changes because they entail multiple vector constructions and lengthy developmental periods. On the other hand, CRISPR/Cas9 makes the process easier by utilizing one guide RNA (gRNA) to direct the Cas9 endonuclease to a desired locus in the genome. This ease not only reduces the entire genetic editing timeline but also makes genome modification techniques more accessible across research fields. The accuracy of CRISPR can also be quite useful in biotechnology in agriculture, where rapid response to evolving threats is crucial to keep productivity high and supply food across the world, as reported by Gallala (2025). Another excellent advantage of CRISPR technology is that it is very accurate and precise in generating desired genetic sequences. The traditional techniques tend to provide off-target effects, whereby unwanted changes can be made in the genome, making interpretation difficult and, in some cases, causing harmful mutations. CRISPR's design is such that it provides more accurate edits, essentially limiting the possibility of such off-target effects. This precision is further supported by recent studies demonstrating the high efficiency of CRISPR editing in various organisms, such as 100% editing efficiency in target genes like cyclosporin-resistant-1 (csr-1) in experiments with *Neurospora crassa* (Süttner et al., 2024). The ability to perform accurate changes enables scientists to use CRISPR with confidence for gene function studies, genetically modified organisms (GMOs), and therapeutic developments without the rampant dangers of standard methods. Furthermore, CRISPR technology is a convenient way of genetic modification where several genes can be edited simultaneously—a task quite challenging for standard methods. By the utilization of multiplexing capability, researchers can design more than one gRNA in one vector for more than one locus for one experiment. This renders the process efficient and thereby allows the process from research to execution to be quicker, as illustrated in the advancement in agriculture towards making livestock and plants more resistant to diseases, as explained by Gallala (2025). Moreover, the range of CRISPRs use is also encompassed within the medical domain, where its ability to edit several genes simultaneously is of immense worth in treating complex diseases with numerous genetic factors. The entire strategy of CRISPR techniques presents a groundbreaking path for genome editing, and hence, they are improved choices for research and therapy purposes.

11.5.3. Limitations and Challenges of CRISPR Technology

The application of CRISPR technology, while groundbreaking, is linked to a chain of limitations that pose important challenges to its safety and effectiveness. Among the most critical limitations is the risk of off-target effects, in which the CRISPR/Cas9 complex inadvertently edits genomic locations other than the targeted ones, leading to undesirable mutations. The unforeseen changes have severe implications, including the interference with vital genes or the triggering of toxic phenotypes. Recent advancements in CRISPR design, including the use of high-fidelity Cas9 variants, are designed to surmount such challenges; however, complete specificity remains a primary challenge. Furthermore, unraveling long-term effects of such modifications remains a challenge, and one must use diligence and prudence to avoid harming patients when CRISPR-based treatment is executed in the clinical setting (Zhang et al., 2024). A second pressing issue in the use of CRISPR technology is delivery techniques. Delivery of the CRISPR components, i.e., the guide RNA and Cas9 enzyme, into target cells is needed for genome editing to become effective. Various approaches, such as viral vectors, liposomes, and electroporation, have been explored; each is however, weighed down by its own disadvantages, such as immune responses or toxicity risk for viral delivery systems. Also, not all tissues are as easily accessible to these modes of delivery, which can restrict the potential of CRISPR in specific therapeutic areas.

Although scientists are finding ways to more specifically deliver CRISPR, extending beyond these restrictions will be vital to continue advancing CRISPR applications in disease prevention and treatment (Zhou et al., 2024). Finally, ethical concerns surrounding CRISPR technology cannot be dismissed, along with the further refinement of the technology. The potential for germline editing raises profound ethical questions regarding consent and the implications of genetically altering human beings. Such interventions could have long-term effects that might reach future generations, thus complicating the question of genetic modification. The stakeholders need to determine how to control the application of CRISPR technologies to avoid compromising a standard of ethics while allowing scientific advancement. As society tries to figure out these issues, the worth of public involvement and an open discourse will be key to shaping the course of CRISPR technology and clinical uses in the future (Zhang et al., 2024; Zhou et al., 2024).

11.6. Future Prospects

The future applications of CRISPR and genome editing technologies are vast and expansive in medicine, agriculture, and biotechnology. With improvements in the technologies come their ability to revolutionize treatment regimens for genetic diseases and cancer. For instance, advancements in gene therapy, particularly using CRISPR, enable exact genetic material editing to create tailored treatments based on specific patient needs. The ability to correct genetic errors at the level of DNA not only optimizes the outcomes of treatments but also reduces unwanted side effects that are part of traditional treatments. The global scientific community is working hard to further these technologies, anticipating a better future where diseases long thought to be incurable could be manageable and therefore maximize quality of life for millions (Sen et al., 2025). Besides, CRISPR technologies have optimistic potential in agriculture for food security and sustainability. Genome editing can be used to enhance crops' resistance to environmental stresses, pests, and diseases, ultimately leading to increased yield and reduced use of chemical inputs. These technologies are crucial amidst the growing global population that needs sustainable food. With the accuracy of CRISPRs, the possibility of incorporating beneficial traits into crops without the laborious exercise of traditional breeding methods becomes clear. Not only does this capacity assist in the fight against food shortages, but it also allows the development of crops with enhanced nutritional content, which would contribute positively to public health (Zang et al., 2025). While these advancements continue to grow, the intersection of biotechnology and environmental stewardship is an area of study that must become a top priority for the future. While the potential of CRISPR and genome editing technologies promises much, there is a need to maintain ethics regarding their utilization at the forefront of debate. The potential for human genome editing raises troubling questions regarding consent, equity, and the potential for unintended consequences. As researchers tread the edge of genome editing, it is important to formulate comprehensive frameworks to direct their responsible use. This includes establishing the long-term consequences of genetic modifications, particularly in human germlines, which have long-term consequences for generations to come. The continuous debate on the ethical significance of these technologies will be instrumental in shaping policies offering equitable access to their advantages without opening the door to hazards of genetic manipulation (Sen et al., 2025). Hence, as we set the trajectory for the future, maintaining equilibrium between innovation and ethics will be critical to realizing the full potential of CRISPR and genome editing technologies (Figure 11.12).

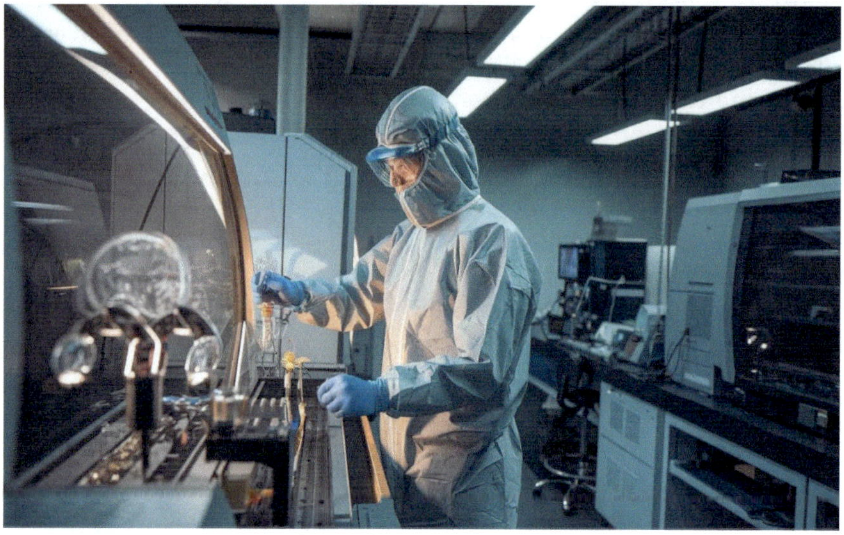

Figure 11.12. Future prospects of CRISPR.

Source: https://goodsciencing.com/wp-content/uploads/2025/01/Future-Prospects-of-CRISPR-Tech.jpg.

11.6.1. Advances in CRISPR Technology

The discovery of CRISPR technology has been a watershed moment in the field of molecular biology and genetics. Initially discovered to naturally exist in bacteria as a mechanism of defense, CRISPR has now been redesigned in a remarkably innovative manner for the purpose of genome editing, allowing for precise modification across a wide range of organisms. The cornerstone of the revolution was CRISPR/Cas9, which allowed scientists to cut to precise locations of DNA with remarkable accuracy. As research continues to develop, subsequent incarnations of the technology have emerged, including CRISPR/Cas13, which targets RNA instead of DNA. This broadens the potential for genetic manipulation and opens up exciting possibilities for therapeutic applications, especially in the fight against RNA viruses. These advances imply that CRISPR is not just a tool for basic research anymore but is increasingly becoming a cornerstone for sophisticated therapies and agricultural enhancement (Chaudhari & Ranjan, 2024). Recent advances in the technology of CRISPR have been centered around improving gene-editing methods' specificity and limiting undesirable effects. One of the biggest challenges to CRISPR/Cas9 use has been off-targeting, where regions of the genome not anticipated to be targeted are modified. Researchers have made great strides to develop engineered Cas9 nucleases that enhance specificity and reduce the possibility of off-target mutations. Tools , such as high-fidelity versions of Cas9 and paired nickases have already shown promise in solving these problems. Besides, the ongoing research on other CRISPR systems, such as CRISPR/Cas12, provides even more potential for genomic manipulation.

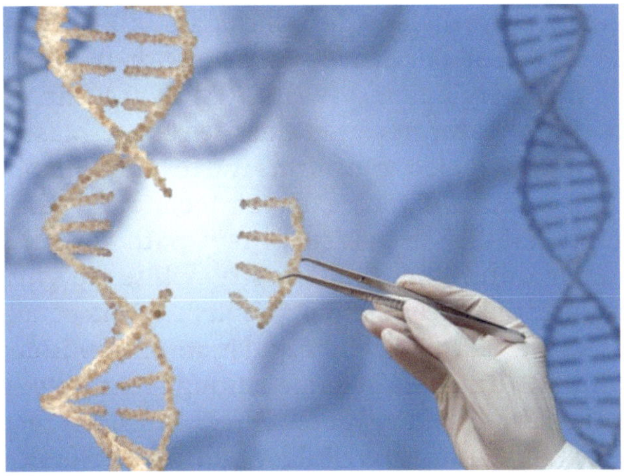

Figure 11.13. Advances in CRISPR technology.

Source: https://synthetic.com/wp-content/uploads/2020/09/DNA_snipped-585x444-1.jpg.

Through their capacity to deliver high accuracy in gene editing, such developments not only enrich scientific understanding but also bring about opportunities for safer clinical use and more reliable agricultural products (Kaupbayeva et al., 2024). The uses of breakthroughs in CRISPR technology extend well beyond the laboratory to potentially revolutionize medicine and agriculture. In medicine, CRISPR promises to upend the treatment of genetic disease, with clinical trials already underway for such diseases as muscular dystrophy and sickle cell anemia. Similarly, in crop biotechnology, CRISPR is being applied to breed plants as pest- or climate-stress-resistant, ultimately fostering food security. However, with these technologies being employed more and more, ethical considerations regarding their utilization also come into play, necessitating holistic debates on potential consequences and regulation. Innovation has to be accompanied by responsibility; thus, the advances in CRISPR technology not only reflect scientific progress but also compel society to engage in critical debate regarding its use and impact (Chaudhari & Ranjan, 2024) (Figure 11.13).

11.6.2. Potential for Personalized Medicine

The CRISPR and genome editing tool discovery is a pivotal point in the evolution of personalized medicine, in which therapy can now be tailored based on an individual patient's unique genetic makeup. Personalized medicine applies genomic information to optimize medical therapy based on a specific individual patient's unique genetic make-up for better efficacy and fewer side effects. With the use of CRISPR, researchers can target and edit genes for various diseases with precision, such that it is now possible to design treatments in consideration of individuals' genetic backgrounds. Integration of technologies , such as DNA sequencing has facilitated increased identification of specific genetic mutations influencing treatment, thereby transforming how conditions , such as cancer and rare genetic disorders are managed in clinical practice. This shift to individualized therapies is an unprecedented time to enhance patient engagement and adherence, which highlights the potential of personalized medicine in contemporary healthcare. With continued developments in genome editing techniques, including breakthroughs with CRISPR/Cas9, there are great advances in personalized medicine. With this technology, one can make targeted alterations in the genome, thus allowing for the development of specific treatments tailored to distinct genetic profiles. Genetic diseases, previously thought to be incurable, may now be treated with direct gene editing. The application of CRISPRs in the treatment of genetic conditions , such as sickle cell disease and muscular dystrophy, is a prime example of the revolutionary power of personalized medicine.

By correcting mutations at the DNA level, CRISPR has the possibility of not only alleviating symptoms but also correcting the fundamental genetic underpinnings of disease, with long-term, if not permanent, therapeutic effects. With this new future, the integration of genomic data into clinical practice becomes fundamental, so that therapy can be designed on the basis of an evidence-based knowledge of a person's genetic make-up. Despite the promising technologies offered by CRISPR and genome editing, there remain obstacles to the large-scale implementation of personalized medicine. The interpretability of genomic information is a monumental hurdle for clinicians and scientists. Moreover, data privacy issues, ethical concerns, and fair access to genetic therapy and testing are also issues in the healthcare field. As established in existing studies, widespread use of genomic medicine in routine clinical practice will entail overcoming the challenges in the form of cost and the requirement of greater genomic literacy on the part of medical doctors. The success of personalized medicine hinges on concerted efforts to establish guidelines and policies to facilitate the ethical application of CRISPR technology. By solving these problems, the full potential of CRISPR in personalized medicine can be fulfilled, and eventually, the future of patient care can be revolutionized and a better understanding of the complex interaction between genetics and the outcome of health (Grüttner & Kempken, 2024).

11.6.3. Global Implications for Biodiversity and Conservation

The plastic pollution epidemic is an urgent environmental threat to global biodiversity and conservation. With plastic manufacture projected to double, to 1800 million tons by 2050, the litter it generates is a critical threat to ecosystems and all the species inhabiting them. Marine and terrestrial life both contend with the detrimental impacts of man-made products, which may lead to destroyed habitats, species loss, and diminished food chains. Emerging technologies like PlastiCRISPR are therefore emerging as potential solutions to address waste management problems biologically. By breaking down polyethylene terephthalate (PET), one of the most pervasive plastics, with the help of microorganisms, PlastiCRISPR presents a two-way path: not only does it reduce plastic waste, but it also transforms waste into valuable bioproducts. This nexus of technology and sustainability provides a new path forward for maintaining biodiversity while solving an acute environmental problem (Palit et al., 2025). Apart from the regulation of pollution, CRISPR and other genome editing technologies hold revolutionary potential to rescue forest ecosystems that are vital for world biodiversity conservation. Forest ecosystems are uniquely hit by climate change, compelling plant and animal life to adapt or become extinct. Traditional conservation measures lose out in the face of rapid environmental changes, particularly given that tree breeding and selection processes are sluggish and circumscribed. With multiplex genome editing, researchers can enhance the longevity of woody plants by targeting multiple traits at once, thereby improving stress tolerance and disease resistance. With such techniques, it becomes feasible to rapidly accelerate the adaptation of forest tree species, ensuring that forest ecosystems continue to provide significant ecological services , such as carbon sequestration and habitat provision. These developments in forest ecology call for integrating CRISPR technologies into overall conservation policies, bringing new hope to biodiversity conservation in an uncertain age of climate change (Sen et al., 2025). Finally, the potential of genome editing technologies extends beyond any one species or ecosystem, impacting overall conservation policies and strategies worldwide. As synthetic biology develops, the ethics of engineering organisms become increasingly complicated. Preserving technological advancement while preserving ecological wholesomeness necessitates redefining conservation goals and practices, driving collaboration among scientists, policy-makers, and stakeholders. Effective use of CRISPR technologies can play a role not only in species recovery and ecosystem restoration but also in enhancing our capacity to manage invasive species and protect endangered populations. In our attempts to understand the intricacies of biodiversity conservation against the global push of rapid technological transformations, we must link such efforts with sustainable ways that uphold the intricate web of life on Earth. The holistic approach is crucial to conserve biodiversity in ways that will establish a strong, productive world for future generations (Sen et al., 2025) (Figure 11.14).

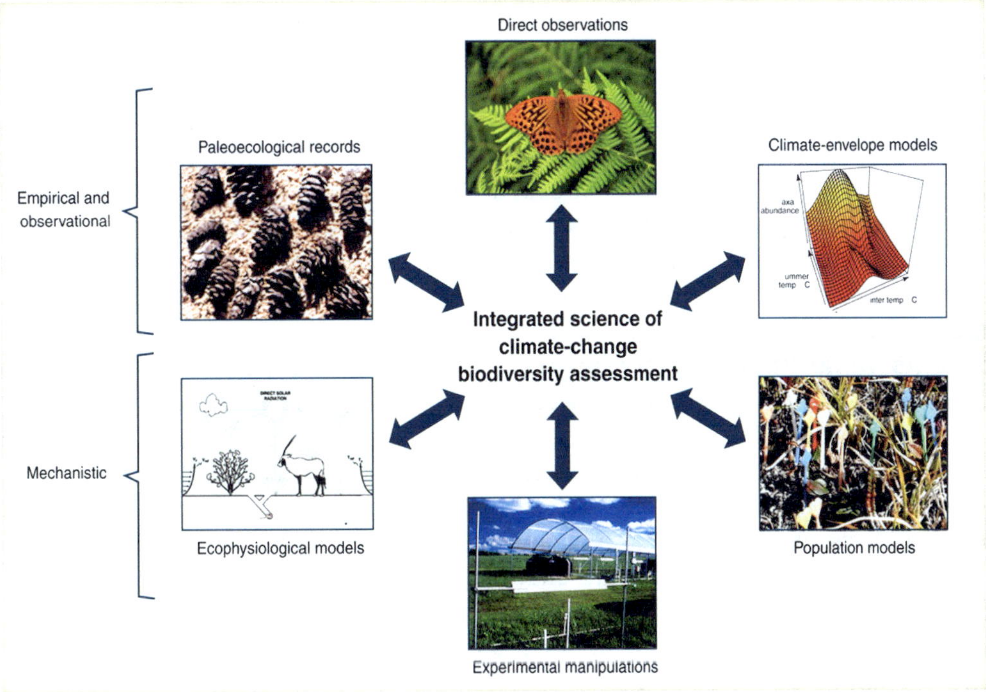

Figure 11.14. Global implications for biodiversity and conservation.

Source: https://www.science.org/cms/10.1126/science.1200303/asset/91ab023d-13ca-447f-9839-3c88489925ae/assets/graphic/332_53_f1.jpeg.

SUMMARY

The rapid evolution of CRISPR and genome editing technologies is a revolutionary period in genetic research and its applications in agriculture, medicine, and environmental management. With capabilities of making precise and efficient changes to the genomic architectures of various organisms, the technologies hold great promise for transforming agriculture, healthcare, and environmental conservation. As the world population struggles with even greater food security challenges and the impacts of climate change, the adoption of CRISPR-led technologies is overdue. Specifically, the potential of genome editing to develop crops with increased resistance to abiotic stresses can be crucial in ensuring sustainable farming practices and ensuring food supplies for many generations to come. It is clear that the stakes of CRISPR technology extend far beyond mere scientific curiosity; they hold the potential to answer some of humanity's most urgent problems, as outlined in existing research work (Ahmad, 2023). Though potential gains are unimaginable, it should be tackled with caution and extensive reviews for potential risks. One of the serious concerns regarding genome editing is the potential for off-target effects, which can lead to unpredictable genetic changes that can make edited organisms useless due to invalidation of safety and efficacy. Next-generation methodologies, such as the DANGER analysis, are being developed to evaluate the dangers of CRISPR applications by attempting to find and quantify the impact of off-target mutations. This bioinformatics approach enhances the safety of genome editing by providing a structured system for predicting phenotypic outcomes due to unexpected edits. To counter these developments, responsible and ethical deployment of genome editing technologies is needed to maximize benefits while limiting potential risks (Nakamae et al., 2023). In short, the future of genome editing tools and CRISPR is poised to have a central role in virtually every aspect of life, from plant farming to medicine. With scientists still discovering the potential of CRISPR systems, innovation must be balanced with ethical consciousness and rigorous checks on safety. The continued conversation around such technologies needs to involve stakeholders from all disciplines, such as scientists, policymakers, and the public, to encourage informed decision-making and enhance public awareness. Ultimately, by surmounting the challenges and duties of genome editing, societies can utilize CRISPR technologies to engineer progress to keep pace with scientific development and social good, leaving behind a blueprint for fresh solutions to approaching international challenges (Ahmad, 2023; Nakamae et al., 2023).

CRISPR and genome editing technology have transformed the science of genetic engineering and molecular biology to its essence. The centerpiece of these technologies is the CRISPR-Cas system, a natural process utilized by bacteria to defend against viruses. The technology operates via RNA-guided nucleases that cut specific sites in DNA selectively, thereby making possible the precise modification of the genome. Clearly, the identification of various Cas proteins, such as Cas9 and the recently reported Cas12l, has pushed the tools into hand to scientists, making programmed gene editing possible as well as advances in genetic research. Cas12l's ability to recognize a C-rich protospacer adjacent motif (PAM) is a significant achievement in eliminating the limitations faced by traditional CRISPR systems that tend to utilize T-rich PAMs, thus opening the frontiers of genomic loci that can be efficiently targeted (Urbaitis et al., 2022). The programmability of CRISPR systems extends beyond gene editing to gene regulation, epigenetic modification, and therapeutic approaches. Recent studies have shown the capability of engineered systems to kill antibiotic-resistant bacteria, showcasing CRISPR's potential for developing new antimicrobial strategies. The application of CRISPR-Cas9 delivered through engineered probiotics, for example, was quite effective in targeting specific resistant bacterial strains found within the gut microbiota. This approach highlights not only the therapeutic potential of CRISPR technologies for battling bacterial infections but also underscores the necessity of developing efficient delivery systems to achieve effective use in intricate biological situations (Neil et al., 2021). Ethical concerns regarding CRISPR and gene editing technologies remain pivotal in informing research and use. As these powerful resources become increasingly accessible, the danger of off-target side effects and unforeseen consequences raises significant issues about safety and regulation to the table. Regulators and scientists must establish comprehensive guidelines to address the implications of genome editing for human well-being, agriculture, and ecology. This is especially so with the rapid pace of advances achieved in CRISPR technology, with ongoing exploration into next-generation CRISPR systems and their associated applications. Discussion of ethical frameworks will be indispensable to ensure the future trajectory of genome editing to reach the responsible use while harnessing the full potential of benefits these technologies have to offer (Urbaitis et al., 2022).

A LOOK TO THE FUTURE:

GENE-EDITING TECHNIQUES:

Gene-editing techniques represent some of the most transformative innovations in molecular biology and medicine, enabling precise, targeted modifications of DNA or RNA within living cells. These techniques allow scientists not merely to observe genetic information but to actively alter it by inserting, deleting, or substituting sequences at defined locations in the genome, thereby advancing research, diagnostics, and therapeutic strategies across diverse biological fields. Gene editing has evolved from early protein-based methods to highly efficient RNA-guided systems, fundamentally changing how genetic manipulation is applied in basic science, agriculture, and clinical medicine.

One of the earliest programmable gene-editing methods is based on zinc finger nucleases (ZFNs)—engineered proteins that combine DNA-binding domains with a nuclease to create specific double-strand breaks at targeted genomic sites. ZFNs laid the groundwork for targeted editing by exploiting custom-designed zinc finger arrays to recognize specific sequences and trigger cellular repair mechanisms that introduce desired changes. While effective, ZFNs are technically challenging to design, requiring unique protein engineering for each target sequence.

Building on this foundation, transcription activator-like effector nucleases (TALENs) were developed, offering greater ease of customization. TALENs consist of programmable DNA-binding repeats fused to a nuclease domain, enabling them to induce site-specific double-strand breaks via a modular arrangement of DNA-recognition motifs. TALENs are more straightforward to assemble than ZFNs and have been widely used to edit genomes in various organisms for both research and applied purposes.

The advent of CRISPR-Cas systems marked a major leap in gene editing technology. Originating from bacterial adaptive immunity, CRISPR (Clustered Regularly Interspaced Short Palindromic Repeats) combined with Cas nuclease proteins uses a short guide RNA (gRNA) to direct the nuclease to virtually any desired DNA sequence, where it creates a precise cut. This RNA-guided approach dramatically simplified target design, increased efficiency, and reduced costs relative to previous methods, making CRISPR-Cas9 the most widely adopted gene-editing tool in both basic research and clinical development.

More recent advancements expand on CRISPR's versatility. Prime editing, for example, introduces desired changes without creating double-strand breaks, acting like a "search-and-replace" system for DNA with potentially fewer undesired edits. Additionally, emerging RNA-editing methods such as LEAPER harness endogenous cellular enzymes to precisely edit messenger RNA rather than the genome itself, offering alternative paths for therapeutic modulation.

Taken together, gene-editing techniques illustrate a remarkable progression from labor-intensive protein engineering to programmable, versatile systems that are rewriting the boundaries of biology. Their continued refinement promises deeper understanding of genetic mechanisms and unprecedented opportunities for treating genetic diseases, enhancing crop resilience, and addressing some of the most pressing challenges in medicine and biotechnology.

REFERENCES

1. Abdulsalam, M., Hamza, F. U., Saddeeq, F. A., Ibrahim, H. H., Isa-Dutse, H. A., & Falaki, A. M. (2024). Unveiling the molecular symphony: Exploring mechanisms, diversity and applications of restriction enzymes in biology. *International Journal of Applied and Scientific Research.* https://www.semanticscholar.org/paper/d3ccb1c61eae9bf46efda77a07bccd779735b4c7 (accessed on 17th July 2025).

2. Ahmad, M. (2023). Plant breeding advancements with "CRISPR-Cas" genome editing technologies will assist future food security. *Frontiers in Plant Science, 14.* https://www.semanticscholar.org/paper/30efad3c8ef0d27e39b89f434e3deba025babfb8 (accessed on 17th July 2025).

3. Amombo, E., Mumm, R.H., Nilahyane, A., Hirich, A., Hijri, M. and Ntui, V.O. (2025), Enhancing Crop Nutrition in Arid and Semiarid Regions of Africa Through Genome Editing Using CRISPR/Cas. Food Energy Secur, 14: e70068. https://doi.org/10.1002/fes3.70068(accessed on 17th July 2025).

4. Chaudhari P, Ranjan M. Advances in CRISPR-based technologies for genome editing in microorganisms [Internet]. IP Int J Med Microbiol Trop Dis. 2024 [cited 2026 Feb 02];10(1):11-16. Available from: https://doi.org/10.18231/j.ijmmtd.2024.003(accessed on 17th July 2025).

5. Chen, K., Wang, Y., Zhang, R., Zhang, H., & Gao, C. (2019). CRISPR/Cas genome editing and precision plant breeding in agriculture. *Annual Review of Plant Biology, 70*, 667–697. https://doi.org/10.1146/annurev-arplant-050718-100049 (accessed on 17th July 2025).

6. Chencinska, I., Miklaszewska, M., & Sołtys-Kalina, D. (2022). Recent advances and challenges in potato improvement using CRISPR/Cas genome editing. *Planta, 257.* https://doi.org/10.1007/s00425-022-04054-3 (accessed on 17th July 2025).

7. Choriyeva, Z. (2024). Genetically modified ecosystems: Innovative approaches in agriculture and their environmental impact. *BIO Web of Conferences.* https://www.semanticscholar.org/paper/9f6ee53e8bdf2ba0280833a790244ab86e9fe06d (accessed on 17th July 2025).

8. Feng, J. (2024). Instrumentation and application of the CRISPR-Cas system. *Theoretical and Natural Science.* https://www.semanticscholar.org/paper/3aa933735195ce49a672269e1ca3cdd845ba9f7b (accessed on 17th July 2025).

9. Gallala, M. (2025). Application of CRISPR/Cas gene editing for infectious disease control in poultry. *Open Life Sciences, 20.* https://www.semanticscholar.org/paper/80c86a53e28e5beb84911137118926984001 2ade (accessed on 17th July 2025).

10. Gomes, A. Q., & Soares, H. (2017). Metodologias emergentes de larga escala na era pós-genómica: Benefícios e questões éticas. https://core.ac.uk/download/94085599.pdf (accessed on 17th July 2025).

11. Grüttner, S., & Kempken, F. (2024). A user-friendly CRISPR/Cas9 system for mutagenesis of *Neurospora crassa. Scientific Reports, 14.* https://www.semanticscholar.org/paper/14948a155c00dd4c7faa10957395df5b36ed3576 (accessed on 17th July 2025).

12. Hou, K., Wu, Z. X., Chen, X. Y., Wang, J. Q., Zhang, D., Xiao, C., Zhu, D., et al. (2022). Microbiota in health and diseases. *Signal Transduction and Targeted Therapy, 7.* https://doi.org/10.1038/s41392-022-00974-4 (accessed on 17th July 2025).

13. Irfan, M., Majeed, H., Iftikhar, T., & Ravi, P. K. (2024). A review on molecular scissoring with CRISPR/Cas9 genome editing technology. *Toxicology Research, 13*(4), tfae105. https://www.semanticscholar.org/paper/7ed7fdb88727bf00643d3b4bda9aa4dbf20f4ec3 (accessed on 17th July 2025).

14. Jahan, I., Angon, P. B., Mou, S. J., Zannat, M., Antu, U. B., Alam, M. M., Sweety, A. A., et al. (2025). The potential of CRISPR-Cas genome editing technologies to mitigate biotic stress in plants. *CABI Agriculture and Bioscience*. https://www.semanticscholar.org/paper/f065428f9fe56120ca8424d20eb5db8015559425 (accessed on 17th July 2025).

15. Kaupbayeva, B., Tsoy, A., Safarova (Yantsen), Y., Nurmagambetova, A., Murata, H., Matyjaszewski, K., & Askarova, Sh. N. (2024). Unlocking genome editing: Advances and obstacles in CRISPR/Cas delivery technologies. *Journal of Functional Biomaterials, 15*. https://www.semanticscholar.org/paper/92f48b7ca74d07164220798fdaf5162c1c81d881 (accessed on 17th July 2025).

16. Khan, A., Barapatre, A. R., Babar, N., Doshi, J., Ghaly, M., Patel, K., Nawaz, S., et al. (2025). Genomic medicine and personalized treatment: A narrative review. *Annals of Medicine and Surgery, 87*, 1406–1414. https://www.semanticscholar.org/paper/a48c7f88008ee3f6f5e730cd7155fc1a412d588b (accessed on 17th July 2025).

17. Kubikova, N., Savash, M., Esbert, M., Titus, S., Fagan, J., Scott, R., & Wells, D. (2024). O-095 Assessment of genome editing outcomes in human preimplantation embryos subjected to CRISPR-Cas9–most loss of heterozygosity (LOH) events is caused by DNA repair deficiency. *Human Reproduction*. https://www.semanticscholar.org/paper/2a8f86e4362109a7878a6cbdf799e3a71713b2b0 (accessed on 17th July 2025).

18. Kumari, P., Verma, T., Yadav, M., Pawar, P., Mounika, J., & Singh, B. (2024). Advancements in genome editing for insect control–A comprehensive review. *Environment and Ecology*. https://www.semanticscholar.org/paper/771cfb418d82fa01aa66059a0da2651d9446ba35 (accessed on 17th July 2025).

19. Li, H., Yang, Y., Hong, W., Huang, M., Wu, M., & Zhao, X. (2020). Applications of genome editing technology in the targeted therapy of human diseases: Mechanisms, advances and prospects. *Signal Transduction and Targeted Therapy, 5*. https://doi.org/10.1038/s41392-019-0089-y (accessed on 17th July 2025).

20. Lin, J., & Yang, J. (2024). CRISPR-Cas systems: A revolution in genome editing and its diverse applications. *Journal of Biomed Research*. https://www.semanticscholar.org/paper/ca1561c375c8975b8fea2092545c8a745c059dfc (accessed on 17th July 2025).

21. Mahtab Uddin, T., Chakraborty, A., Khusro, A., Zidan, B. R. M., Mitra, S., Emran, T. B., Dhama, K., et al. (2021). Antibiotic resistance in microbes: History, mechanisms, therapeutic strategies and future prospects. *Journal of Infection and Public Health, 14*, 1750–1766. https://doi.org/10.1016/j.jiph.2021.10.020 (accessed on 17th July 2025).

22. Mann, A., Ranga, P., Choudhary, P., Yadav, S., Kaul, N., Dahiya, A., Prakash, N. R., et al. (2024). Genome editing technologies for enhancing plant resilience to biotic and abiotic stresses–Brief review. *Journal of Soil Salinity and Water Quality, 16*, 180–193. https://doi.org/10.56093/jsswq.v16i2.156291 (accessed on 17th July 2025).

23. Mao, Y., Chu, G., Liang, Q., Liu, Y., Yang, Y., Liao, X., & Wang, M. (2025). [Artificial intelligence-assisted design, mining, and modification of CRISPR-Cas systems]. *Sheng wu gong cheng xue bao = Chinese Journal of Biotechnology, 41*(3), 949–967. https://www.semanticscholar.org/paper/0f9058538c70b37da60101b07d9287792c339949 (accessed on 17th July 2025).

24. Masarwy, R., Breier, D., Stotsky-Oterin, L., Ad-El, N., Qassem, S., Naidu, G., Aitha, A., et al. (2024). Targeted CRISPR/Cas9 lipid nanoparticles elicits therapeutic genome editing in head and neck cancer. *Advanced Science, 12*. https://www.semanticscholar.org/paper/14a5d3133816dc1dccb78ca9a0b0a5dc9028a33a (accessed on 17th July 2025).

25. Naeem, M., Manzoor, S., Abid, M. U. H., Tareen, M. B. K., Asad, M., Mushtaq, S., Ehsan, N., et al. (2022). Fungal proteases as emerging biocatalysts to meet the current challenges and recent developments in biomedical therapies: An updated review. *Journal of Fungi, 8*, 109–109. https://doi.org/10.3390/jof8020109 (accessed on 17th July 2025).

26. Nakamae, K., & Bono, H. (2023). DANGER analysis: Risk-averse on/off-target assessment for CRISPR editing without a reference genome. *Bioinformatics Advances, 3*. https://www.semanticscholar.org/paper/ab63ccac6d12021260f130d9e04a2eb68acb0647 (accessed on 17th July 2025).

27. Nakazato, I., & Arimura, S. (2024). Genome editing in angiosperm chloroplasts: Targeted DNA double-strand break and base editing. *The Plant Journal: For Cell and Molecular Biology*. https://www.semanticscholar.org/paper/f29ff3580ac8d50ca97d660831e2c46fc1dc7cbe (accessed on 17th July 2025).

28. Namata, M. J., Xu, J., Habyarimana, E., Palakolanu, S. R., Wang, L., & Li, J. (2025). Genome editing in maize and sorghum: A comprehensive review of CRISPR/Cas9 and emerging technologies. *The Plant Genome, 18*. https://www.semanticscholar.org/paper/03e3c97c1ecb853a14f95a557e1a557e1ee59aba (accessed on 17th July 2025).

29. Negishi, K., Endo, M., Endo, T., & Nishitani, C. (2024). Genome editing in cells of apple cultivar 'Fuji' using geminivirus-derived replicons for transient expression of CRISPR/Cas9 components. *Plant Biotechnology, 41*, 425–436. https://www.semanticscholar.org/paper/cace6686c830a12635f3fa5f951b6d0b676f786c (accessed on 17th July 2025).

30. Neil, K., Allard, N., Roy, P., Grenier, F., Menéndez, A., Burrus, V., & Rodrigue, S. (2021). High-efficiency delivery of CRISPR-Cas9 by engineered probiotics enables precise microbiome editing. *Molecular Systems Biology, 17*. https://doi.org/10.15252/msb.202110335 (accessed on 17th July 2025).

31. Nerkar, G., Devarumath, S., Purankar, M. V., Kumar, A., Valarmathi, R., Devarumath, R. M., & Appunu, C. (2022). Advances in crop breeding through precision genome editing. *Frontiers in Genetics, 13*. https://doi.org/10.3389/fgene.2022.880195 (accessed on 17th July 2025).

32. Palit, P., Minkara, M., Abida, M., Marwa, S., Sen, C., Roy, A., Pasha, M. R., et al. (2025). PlastiCRISPR: Genome editing-based plastic waste management with implications in polyethylene terephthalate (PET) degradation. *Biomolecules, 15*. https://www.semanticscholar.org/paper/5f4bac5c51f2c3969d4289195a1318a17cb57801 (accessed on 17th July 2025).

33. Park, H. J., Kim, M., Lee, D., Kim, H., & Jung, H. W. (2024). CRISPR-Cas9 and beyond: Identifying target genes for developing disease-resistant plants. *Plant Biology*. https://www.semanticscholar.org/paper/7ad36106d07649770c337a88ade6e2ca4859a01b (accessed on 17th July 2025).

34. Patel, D. (2024). Genome editing technologies in the treatment of diabetes. *Journal of Student Research*. https://www.semanticscholar.org/paper/0560b3f2993d2439fb7443b5b4f0c2419e2109a1 (accessed on 17th July 2025).

35. Rehman, A., Abbas, A., Arshad, A., Raza, G. M., Umar, M., & Bukhari, M. S. (2024). Advancements in genomic technologies and their impact on crop improvement and breeding methods. *Bulletin of Biological and Allied Sciences Research*. https://www.semanticscholar.org/paper/75e1cf271c7132a0711ffae4fd9c1204bf809fa8 (accessed on 17th July 2025).

36. Sampath, V., Rangarajan, N., Sharanappa, C. H., Deori, M., Veeraragavan, M., Ghodake, B. D., & Kaushal, K. (2023). Advancing crop improvement through CRISPR technology in precision agriculture trends - A review. *International Journal of Environment and Climate Change, 13*, 4683–4694. https://doi.org/10.9734/ijecc/2023/v13i113647 (accessed on 17th July 2025).

37. Sen, A., Singh, V., Dwivedi, S., Agrawal, R., Bansal, A., Shekhar, S., & Kushwaha, S. S. (2025). Gene therapy and gene editing: Current trends and future prospects of molecular medicine. *Current Gene Therapy*. https://www.semanticscholar.org/paper/25fcf14d7421a285bda69ccae261660da8cc8fcc (accessed on 17th July 2025).

38. Sen, M. K., Mondal, S., Bharati, R., Severová, L., & Šrédl, K. (2025). Multiplex genome editing for climate-resilient woody plants. *Frontiers in Forests and Global Change*. https://www.semanticscholar.org/paper/850987b158cc0156b6b1c0500315bf13d1691577 (accessed on 17th July 2025).

39. Tham, J. (2017). Resisting the temptation of perfection. https://core.ac.uk/download/141204588.pdf (accessed on 17th July 2025).

40. Urbaitis, T., Gasiūnas, G., Young, J. K., Hou, Z., Paulraj, S., Godliauskaitė, E., Juskeviciene, M. M., et al. (2022). A new family of *CRISPR*-type V nucleases with C-rich *PAM* recognition. *EMBO Reports, 23*. https://doi.org/10.15252/embr.202255481 (accessed on 17th July 2025).

41. Vasquez, C. A., Evanoff, M., Ranzau, B. L., Gu, S., Deters, E., & Komor, A. C. (2023). Curing "GFP-it is" in bacteria with base editors: Development of a genome editing science program implemented with high school biology students. *The CRISPR Journal*. https://www.semanticscholar.org/paper/bc84b6eec241fd02a34b9059df0c7f81fa67d2bd (accessed on 17th July 2025).

42. Waghmode, P., Pitha, C. C., & Banka, V. (2024). The role of genome editing technologies in sustainable agriculture. *Journal of Advances in Biology & Biotechnology*. https://www.semanticscholar.org/paper/c3a7b93ab064f31876c675e54d217d2e499b7b09 (accessed on 17th July 2025).

43. Wang, Z. (2025). The feasibility of using CRISPR-Cas9 to knock out IL-6 receptor in CAR-T cells to mitigate cytokine release syndrome in cancer therapy. *Theoretical and Natural Science*. https://www.semanticscholar.org/paper/c2f7401161a6069ba8245d4505d68dfc98e30045 (accessed on 17th July 2025).

44. Wheatley, M. C. (2025). Gene editing: CRISPR and beyond. *Premier Journal of Biomedical Science*. https://www.semanticscholar.org/paper/3d3edac3be6de29dcddbb09184c91781afbc8e3c (accessed on 17th July 2025).

45. Zang, S. S., Zhang, R., Zhang, J. R., Zhang, X., & Li, J. (2025). Progress, applications and prospects of CRISPR-based genome editing technology in gene therapy for cancer and sickle cell disease. *Human Gene Therapy*. https://www.semanticscholar.org/paper/2d5091bbb50a58b99c0d0d29fe316c867de14c3f (accessed on 17th July 2025).

46. Zhang, M. L., Li, H. B., & Jin, Y. (2024). Application and perspective of CRISPR/Cas9 genome editing technology in human diseases modeling and gene therapy. *Frontiers in Genetics, 15*. https://www.semanticscholar.org/paper/d146b388595f6bde483179f00c214caebbf01a0b (accessed on 17th July 2025).

47. Zhou, L., & Simonian, A. L. (2024). CRISPR/Cas technology: The unique synthetic biology genome-editing tool shifting the paradigm in viral diagnostics, defense, and therapeutics. *Annual Review of Biomedical Engineering*. https://www.semanticscholar.org/paper/81c848b55e5a024831c98659110a55e887255df2 (accessed on 17th July 2025).

48. Zhu, H., Wu, X., Zheng, R., & Zhu, Y. (2025). The impact of gene editing technology on agricultural economic efficiency: An empirical analysis based on international CRISPR patent data. *Molecular & Cellular Biomechanics*. https://www.semanticscholar.org/paper/739b5f07675bff1daa8039913b2867365a3e8d1d (accessed on 17th July 2025).

49. Zhu, M., Sumana, S. L., Muhammad, A. M., Falayi, O. C., Shui, Y., Zhang, C., Zhu, J., et al. (2024). CRISPR/Cas9 technology for enhancing desirable traits of fish species in aquaculture. *International Journal of Molecular Sciences, 25*, 9299–9299. https://doi.org/10.3390/ijms25179299 (accessed on 17th July 2025).

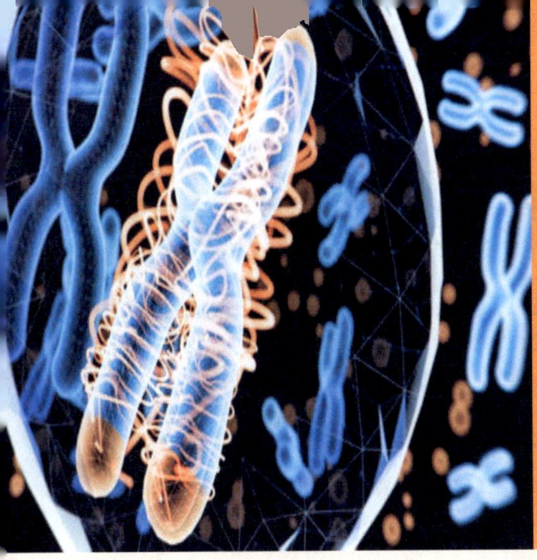

Chapter 12

MOLECULAR CYTOGENETICS

Contents

Introduction

The area of molecular cytogenetics has improved considerably, especially in the last decade, due to the development of methods in genome studies. This area combines traditional cytogenetic methods and molecular biology to allow researchers to analyze the genetic material of cells at a level of precision. Molecular cytogenetics focuses on chromosomal structure, function, and behavior in cellular genetics, illuminating genetic abnormalities and their implications in disease. As is clear from recent reviews, the use of molecular cytogenetics in the clinic has provided new possibilities for more specific diagnostic and prognostic assessment, particularly in oncology and genetic disease. With advanced software and future technologies, the field moves towards an improvement in the genetic basis of disease and health, foreseeing its pivotal role in present genomic medicine (Weier et al., 2012). Among the significant applications of molecular cytogenetics is the ability to decompose complex genetic disorders through techniques , such as fluorescence in situ hybridization (FISH) and comparative genomic hybridization (CGH). Such technologies enable precise visualization of chromosomal anomalies, such as aneuploidies and structural rearrangements, which are most often linked with cancer and other genetic diseases. Recent research has emphasized that the way such technologies have accelerated risk evaluation and early diagnosis and, in turn, transformed patient management (Crocker, 2003). For instance, the description of some chromosomal alterations can direct therapeutic decisions in CML and other types of cancer, illustrating the concrete clinical utility of molecular cytogenetics. The association of these methods not only permits better recognition of genetic abnormalities but also offers support for individualized medicine plans tailored to a patient's genomic signature. Besides, the application of bioinformatics in molecular cytogenetics has sped up the progress of the discipline by enabling large genomic data sets to be analyzed.

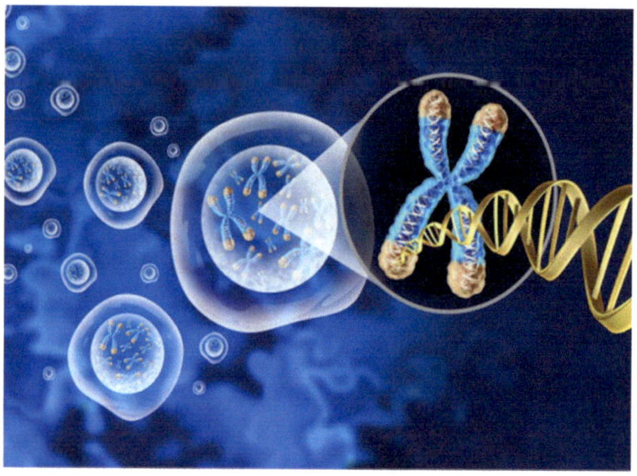

Figure 12.1. Molecular cytogenetics.

Source: https://visualvistaventures.weebly.com/uploads/1/4/9/2/149215425/molecular-cytogenetics_orig.jpg.

This allows scientists to develop predictive models as well as identify biomarkers associated with disease, thereby enhancing the diagnostic yield and therapeutic impact. Bioinformatics has been demonstrated by current studies to unleash the potential of its capability to explain genetic instability and radiosensitivity, which can be utilized in prognosis and treatment choice (Weier et al., 2012). By leveraging the use of computational tools and genomic data, scientists are now able to tease out the intricate relationships between disease phenotypes and genetic variations. With further research, the future will inevitably shed new light on what is happening at the molecular level of genetic disease, reinforcing the importance of molecular cytogenetics in clinical and translational research. The future also promises even more innovation that will increase our capability in genetic analysis as well as patient treatment (Figure 12.1).

Definition and Scope of Molecular Cytogenetics

The field of molecular cytogenetics combines the two sciences of molecular biology and cytogenetics by utilizing hi-tech techniques to study chromosomes at a molecular level in terms of their structure and functions. This science utilizes FISH and CGH methods primarily to identify chromosomal abnormalities that lead to various genetic disorders and cancers. Chromosomal structure definition by these techniques empowers researchers with deep insight into the detection of submicroscopic changes , such as deletions, duplications, and translocations, which are essential in clinical genetics. These levels of accuracy in the identification of chromosomal abnormalities enhance risk stratification in conditions like acute myeloid leukemia (AML), where identification of the cytogenetic profile influences treatment strategies and predicts patient outcomes, illustrating the central role of molecular cytogenetics in modern medical diagnosis (Brodersen et al., 2020). Expanding beyond its clinical application, the scope of molecular cytogenetics extends to research frontiers that aim to elucidate the mechanisms of genomic instability and oncogenesis. Researchers employ molecular cytogenetic techniques to examine the function of specific chromosomal alterations in the process of tumorigenesis. Through the convergence of molecular profiles and cytogenetic data, researchers can uncover the relationships between chromosomal abnormalities and clinical phenotypes, thus improving our understanding of cancer formation. For instance, the identification of specific translocations associated with certain cancers enables the creation of directed therapies to correct or exploit these genetic weaknesses. Besides that, this discipline also trains public health policy and genetic counseling, issuing information on hereditary syndromes and cancer risk that they bring, and subsequently, expanding the scope of molecular cytogenetics from the laboratory to the practice of preventive medicine and personalized health care.

Furthermore, the definition and the scope of molecular cytogenetics encompass an evolving array of techniques and applications that cope with the complexity of human genetics. With advancing technology, the integration of traditional cytogenetic methods with high-throughput sequencing narrows down the resolution at which geneticists are able to analyze chromosome configurations. These advancements facilitate the ease of identification of the structural variants that are linked with various pathologies, paving the way for the chances of more therapeutic interventions. Along with these technological advancements, increased studies emphasize the influence of environmental determinants on the genetic abnormalities, and hence towards the complexity of the genetic diseases. This integrative knowledge of the human genome stimulates interdisciplinary cooperation among geneticists, oncologists, and bioinformaticians, thereby enhancing the combined capacity to unravel complex genetic diseases and further solidify the relevance of molecular cytogenetics in contemporary biological and medical research.

Historical Development and Key Milestones

The history of molecular cytogenetics can be dated as early as the mid-20th century, when there was revolutionary advancement in genetic research. The advent of this science to a great extent was influenced by the development of chromosome banding techniques in the 1970s, which allowed scientists to investigate chromosomal defects to an unprecedented level of accuracy. The introduction of G-banding, where chromosomes are identified based on their unique light and dark staining patterns, was central to the identification of chromosomal rearrangements in various genetic disorders and cancers. This fundamental technology set the stage for subsequent discoveries, as it opened up further investigations into the dynamics between chromosomal architecture and disease phenotypes. Consequently, the specificity that these approaches brought about transformed the understanding of genetic material and inaugurated a new era of genetic diagnostics and investigation into oncology and developmental biology. With the advancing science, the advent of fluorescence *in situ* hybridization (FISH) during the 1980s was a significant milestone that enhanced molecular cytogenetic analysis. FISH employs fluorescently labeled DNA probes to precisely localize specified DNA sequences onto chromosomes. Not only did this technology amplify the detection of chromosomal abnormality but it also promoted research in gene amplification and translocations, particularly cancer studies. The ability to visualize the spatial organization of genes in the nuclear architecture provided better insight into the association of genetic alterations with clinical manifestations. For instance, the achievements in the integration of FISH with cell line models, mainly in oncology, unveiled the need to maintain accurate cellular contexts for further insight into oncogenic processes. The proven usefulness of FISH has resulted in its extensive application in diagnostic use, which has allowed more comprehensive genetic evaluation in clinical settings (Mirabelli et al., 2019). In the last few years, molecular cytogenetics has developed further with technological progress in genomic technologies. One of the most significant developments is the use of next-generation sequencing (NGS) in the field of cytogenetics, which enabled high-throughput analysis of genetic material with outstanding sensitivity and resolution. This advancement not only enhanced the detection of novel genetic changes but also optimized the assessment of complex genomic rearrangements previously difficult to explain. The combination of NGS with traditional cytogenetic methods , such as FISH, has further enhanced diagnostic utility, especially in rare and childhood hematologic malignancies whose treatment response is extremely heterogeneous (Gore et al., 2018). With advancing technologies, the integration of newer technologies is the key to unlocking the intricate cellular mechanisms in causing various diseases and highlights the role of molecular cytogenetics in personalized medicine.

Importance in Modern Genetics and Medicine

The advancements in molecular cytogenetics have completely transformed the discipline of modern genetics and medicine, enabling rich insight into chromosomal structure and function. Molecular cytogenetics is an advanced division of genetics integrating molecular biology techniques to study chromosomal anomalies, which are responsible for most genetic disorders. For instance, the potential to identify specific chromosomal aberrations with techniques , such as fluorescence *in situ* hybridization (FISH) has been proven essential for diagnosis and therapy. The emerging technologies in this field have made it possible for clinicians to establish precise genetic diagnoses, enabling molecular-level insight into genetic diseases and paving the way to targeted therapies. Molecular cytogenetics has, therefore, moved from being a specialized research field to an integral component of clinical practice, with no doubt indicating its central place in modern genetics and medicine. Further, the use of molecular cytogenetics in clinical care has enormously improved prenatal screening capacity. Methods , such as amniocentesis and chorionic villus sampling have allowed for preterm diagnosis of chromosomal defects in fetal development, providing prospective parents with helpful information regarding genetic risk. Seminars and past controversies among geneticists have highlighted the emotional considerations of genetic diagnosis, necessitating family communication and counseling when making such tough decisions (Jones & Tansey, 2014). Such access to these prenatal diagnostics not only informed family planning decisions but also generated broader debates over ethics in genetic tests. Finally, the impact of molecular cytogenetics in prenatal medicine marks its pivotal role in shaping the evolution of present-day medical practice and enhancing patient outcomes. In addition, the growth of molecular cytogenetics has motivated the increase in multidisciplinary working teams that include genetics, medicine, and patient advocacy. As noted in the professionals' community, professional associations have evolved to provide greater knowledge exchange and offset the complexities of genetic diseases, for instance, the establishment of clinical genetics as a recognized specialty (Harper et al., 2010). The multidisciplinary nature facilitates integration of genetic data into practice to facilitate comprehensive understanding of genetic disease by clinicians. The provision of genetic counseling services also broadens the field of molecular cytogenetics further since they provide necessary support to patients and families who struggle with genetic information. Through such a partnership, therefore, not only is medical intervention improved in terms of accuracy, but patient care continues to be paramount in the fast-evolving world of genetics and medicine (Figure 12.2).

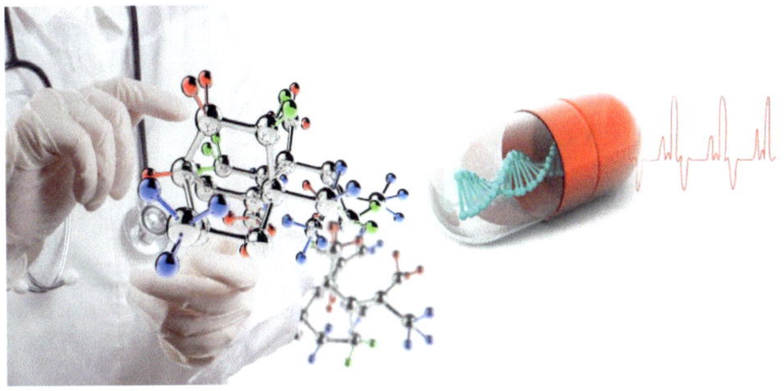

Figure 12.2. Importance in modern genetics and medicine.

Source: https://health.uconn.edu/genetics/wp-content/uploads/sites/124/2015/11/genx.jpg.

12.1. Techniques in Molecular Cytogenetics

The field of molecular cytogenetics employs a variety of sophisticated techniques to investigate chromosomal content and function at a molecular level to gain insight into genetic disorders and cell behavior. One of the simplest techniques is fluorescence *in situ* hybridization (FISH), in which fluorescent probes that hybridize to specific regions of a chromosome are employed for genetic abnormality visualization. This technique is particularly valuable in the identification of chromosomal rearrangements and aneuploidies, both common in cancer and genetic diseases.

In addition, enhanced multi-color FISH has made it possible to identify several genetic loci simultaneously in a single specimen, significantly enhancing diagnostic specificity and clarifying complex genetic interactions. By complementing these techniques with conventional chromosome analysis, researchers can develop a clearer picture of chromosomal dynamics and how they function in disease and health. The second key technique in molecular cytogenetics is array comparative genomic hybridization (aCGH), which allows for high-resolution investigation of genomic imbalance in the whole genome. The technique has revolutionized the identification of microdeletions and duplications, which may be beyond the ability of routine karyotyping. aCGH involves reference versus test comparison of a sample genomic DNA to a reference sample to detect copy number variations (CNVs) with unmatched precision. With advancing technology in aCGH, researchers have developed custom platforms that increase detection sensitivity and resolution, making it a valuable asset for clinical diagnostics and research. In addition, higher throughput of aCGH allows large-scale research, in which researchers are able to map specific genomic alterations to disease development and phenotypic consequences and hence uncover the genetic architecture of complex diseases.

Lastly, NGS gives unrivaled information regarding the genomic topography and is a novel technique in molecular cytogenetics. By allowing the simultaneous sequencing of millions of DNA fragments, NGS gives a comprehensive examination of chromosomal alterations. This approach not only enhances the detection of single-nucleotide changes (SNVs) and small insertions/deletions (indels) but also facilitates the understanding of larger structural alterations like chromosomal rearrangements and translocations. The integration of bioinformatics analysis with NGS data enables researchers to effectively handle vast amounts of genomic data, leading to useful insights for personalized medicine and targeted therapies. As NGS technology continues to advance, its application in molecular cytogenetics continues to expand, holding out to offer new dimensions to genetics and oncology research and treatment, in line with the advancement in related methodologies , such as those covered by Aguiar & Camps (2025) and Basu et al. (2025) (Figure 12.3).

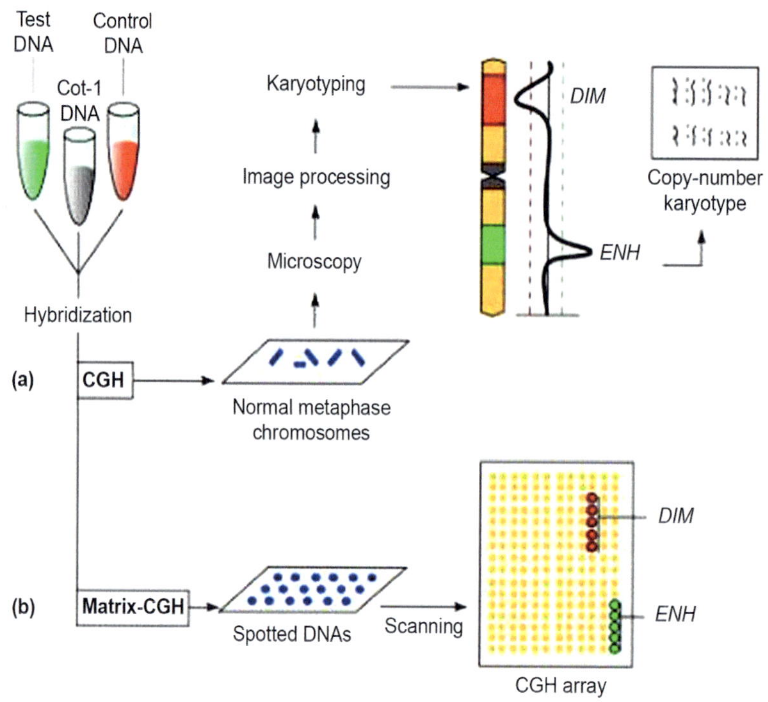

Figure 12.3. Molecular cytogenetics and its use of sophisticated techniques.

Source: https://www.cell.com/cms/10.1016/S1471-4914(02)02335-3/asset/0cf3c3b7-5534-42ae-8f29-059d0eedce61/main.assets/gr2.jpg.

12.1.1. Fluorescence In Situ Hybridization (FISH)

Fluorescence *in situ* hybridization (FISH) is a core method of molecular cytogenetics, providing data on the structure and function of chromosomes that traditional karyotyping cannot offer. FISH makes it possible to visualize particular DNA sequences within the chromosomes using fluorescently labeled DNA probes, allowing detection of chromosomal aberrations with high specificity. This is particularly critical in clinical settings where precise diagnosis needs to be attained, as some cytogenetic abnormalities cannot be resolved by conventional methods. The technique's specificity to target particular areas significantly expands the genetic understanding of a variety of ailments, and it is a critical instrument for applied and basic research. To this effect, FISH not only clarifies genetic architecture but also facilitates the establishment of targeted therapeutic interventions, thereby bridging the gap between practice and molecular biology. The overall applications of FISH range across several biological sciences, with high-impact implications being in domestic animal research as well as cancer diagnosis. In this context, molecular cytogenetics, specifically with FISH, in animal genetics can play a physical mapping of DNA sequences onto chromosomes that is critical for breeding and conservation strategies. FISH-based diagnostics have confirmed the existence of chromosome defects known to be detrimental to fertility, hence affecting animal husbandry significantly. In cancer, FISH-based diagnostics have transformed the practice of diagnosis, particularly in the detection of chromosomal abnormalities found in leukemias and solid tumors. By facilitating the correction of complex karyotypic aberrations, FISH-based techniques , such as comparative genomic hybridization (CGH), have aided the detection of genomic imbalances, thus personalizing patient-specific treatment protocols that optimize the use of personalized medicine (Wan & Ma, 2012). Despite all the impeccable advancements brought forward by FISH, difficulties remain inherent to its application. FISH interpretation can be complex, requiring close awareness of both biological background and technicalities of methodology. Beyond that, while FISH circumvents many of the disadvantages of conventional cytogenetic methods, it does possess an opposite side. Probe specificity is critical because cross-hybridization can yield false results. In addition, reliance on expert microscopy may hinder extensive application, particularly in settings with limited resources. However, the progressive developments in FISH technology, such as multicolor karyotyping and cross-species comparative genomics, are creating opportunities for more complex genomic research and diagnostic applications (Iannuzzi et al., 2023). This advances the pivotal role that FISH plays in the evolution of molecular cytogenetics as a science and its capacity to illuminate intricate genetic events (Figure 12.4).

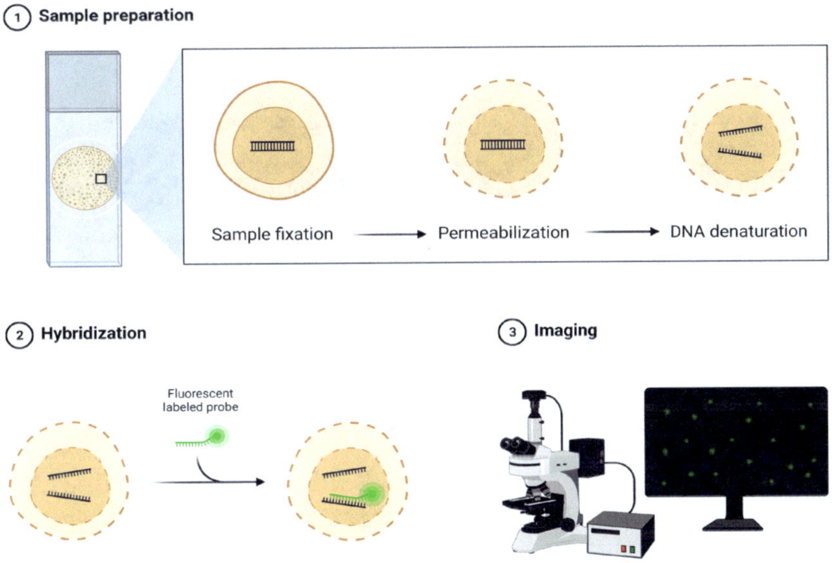

Figure 12.4. Fluorescence *in situ* hybridization (FISH).

Source: https://images.aatbio.com/universal/catalog/FISH/Fluorescence_In_Situ_Hybridization_(FISH).png.

12.1.2. Comparative Genomic Hybridization (CGH)

Comparative genomic hybridization (CGH) is an important method in molecular cytogenetics for a general analysis of chromosomal alterations across the genome. Based on this methodology, an efficient means of identifying genomic gain or loss can be achieved through a comparison of test sample DNA, typically from tumor cells, against a reference sample. Unlike traditional karyotyping, CGH is used to examine all of the chromosomes at once and, therefore, to identify many genetic aberrations that can be the cause of disease pathology. As studies , such as the ones presented in recent reviews clearly illustrate, CGH has been instrumental in illuminating the complexity of supernumerary marker chromosomes (sSMCs) and their etiology, and results are important for genetic counseling and prenatal diagnosis (Jang et al., 2016). This broadens our definition of chromosomal instability in most diseases, and CGH therefore assumes a central role in both research and clinical practice.

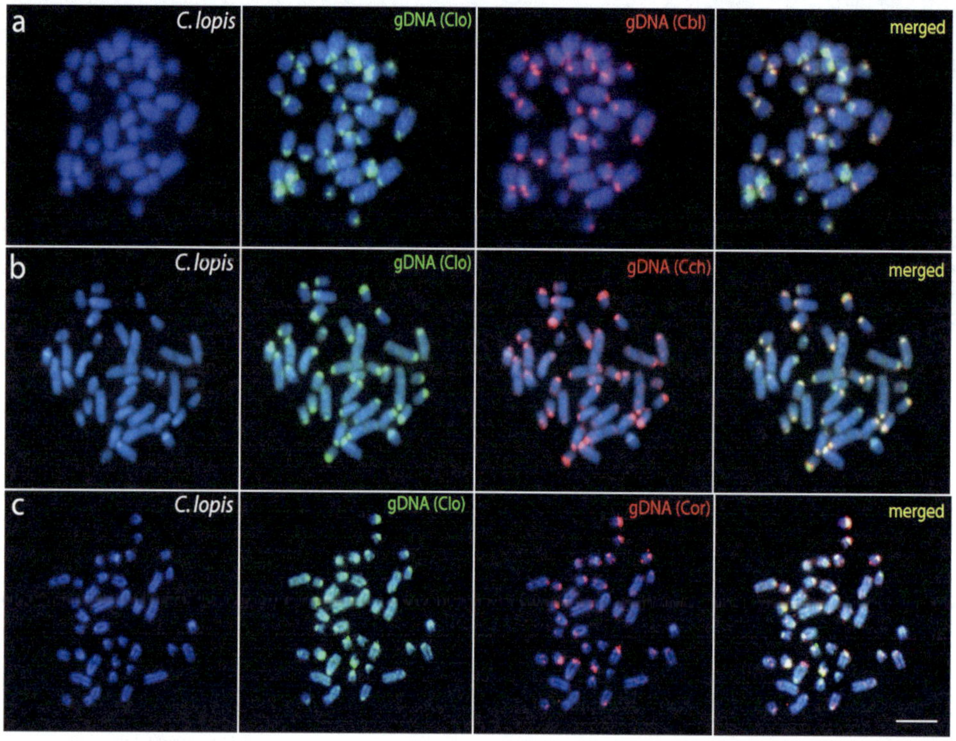

Figure 12.5. Comparative genomic hybridization (CGH).

Source: https://www.researchgate.net/publication/330852576/figure/fig2/AS:723843249344513@1549589087940/Comparative-genomic-hybridization-CGH-using-the-gDNA-of-C-blanci-a-C-chitala-b.jpg.

Advances in the CGH methodology have enabled the addition of molecular approaches to cytogenetic analysis, enhancing resolution and specificity of genetic studies. The technology of array CGH allows for the more accurate analysis of genomic intervals, so that weak chromosomal imbalances that are not available by conventional methods can be identified. This has far-reaching implications of particular significance in the field of oncology, where frequent chromosomal changes commonly serve as markers of disease advancement and prognosis. The capability of deciphering high-throughput data generated by CGH experiments provides improved insight into cancer biology through the identification of genes and tumorigenesis pathways. An increasing body of cancer genetic data requires robust analytical tools to untangle complex CGH datasets, an issue confronted by novel software solutions (Liu et al., 2007). In molecular cytogenetics, in addition to offering more insight into genetic abnormalities, CGH is also involved in the direction of therapeutic interventions. Identification of some genomic abnormalities may lead to the development of specific targeted drugs to treat cancer patients. The application of CGH is not just for the diagnosis of cancer but also for prenatal diagnosis in ascertaining the occurrence of genetic disorders in a fetus and therefore allowing early therapies. Recent research emphasizes the merit of CGH in the identification of sSMCs as predicting a probable parental origin and clinical significance to hereditary disease (Jang et al., 2016). With advancing science, the utility of CGH as a research and clinical tool will expand further and open up promising avenues for investigating intricate genetic landscapes in neoplastic and non-neoplastic disease (Figure 12.5).

12.1.3. Next-Generation Sequencing (NGS)

With the emergence of next-generation sequencing (NGS) technology, molecular cytogenetics has witnessed revolutionary changes and enhanced dramatically the investigation of chromosomal aberrations and inherited diseases. Traditional cytogenetic techniques , such as karyotyping and fluorescence *in situ* hybridization (FISH) have conventionally provided information about chromosomal number and structure but are still deficient in identifying fine genomic changes. With NGS, it is now possible to obtain a more definitive image, allowing for single-nucleotide polymorphisms and copy number variations across the genome to be detected. At a more sensitive level, this allows detection of cryptic changes that are central to the understanding of mechanisms behind genetic disorders. By filling the gap between traditional cytogenetics and molecular genomics, NGS plays a significant role in our knowledge of the genetic origin of diseases, allowing progress in diagnosis and individualized medicine in the field of molecular cytogenetics (Shinde et al., 2025). In addition, applications of NGS in molecular cytogenetics go beyond simple detection of chromosomal abnormalities; they allow for detailed examination of genomic structure that is critical to successful therapeutic approaches. For instance, the integration of NGS with other cytogenetic techniques has improved crop management against biotic stresses through the identification of the genetic basis of stress resistance. Integration of molecular genetics and cytogenetics allows one to determine specific molecular markers that can enhance breeding programs to generate tolerant crop varieties. By applying such integrated strategies, scientists can better understand the adaptive processes of plants under environmental stress and devise interventions that are able to amplify agricultural yields.

Synthesizing NGS with cytogenetics ultimately fosters a space that favors innovation, opening doors to sustainable approaches in agricultural science (Olivucci et al., 2024). In the clinical environment, NGS has emerged as a crucial tool in the field of genetic diagnosis, and its capacity to analyze challenging genomic areas previously problematic to study is unmatched. While conventional methods like Southern blotting and PCR have been sufficient for some cases, they are not very sensitive and efficient, particularly with repetitive or GC-rich sequences. NGS surmounts these limitations by enabling high-throughput, long-range sequencing that more accurately captures allelic and structural variation information. With the direction in which the field is moving towards third-generation sequencing platforms, NGS's capacity to impact diagnostic yield continues to gain speed. By facilitating the detection of structural variations and repeat expansions, NGS will propel the diagnostic procedures for hitherto undiagnosed genetic conditions, thereby presenting hope for improved patient outcomes and the expansion of the realm of genetic medicine within the perspective of molecular cytogenetics (Olivucci et al., 2024) (Figure 12.6).

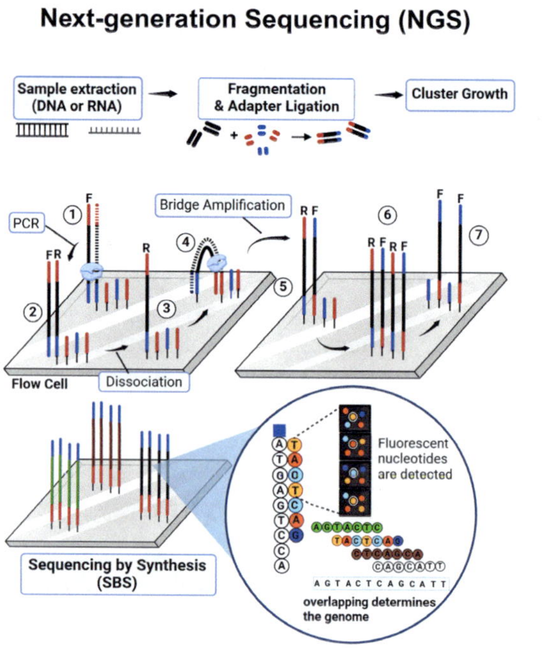

Figure 12.6. Next-generation sequencing (NGS).

Source: https://cdn.prod.website-files.com/621e95f9ac30687a56e4297e/6616e431969cb09a484ad825_V2_1710736280155_6bea9c2c-7e31-4b5c-8d1b-ef5863d5d6af_HIGH_RES.png.

12.2. Chromosomal Abnormalities

Chromosomal abnormalities are significant issues in molecular cytogenetics, influencing the understanding of genetic diseases, as well as their diagnostic and therapeutic approaches. Abnormalities arise due to structural changes in chromosomes or by numerical fluctuations, such as aneuploidies, where there is a defective number of chromosomes. The consequences of these abnormalities are enormous, with the ability to lead to various clinical manifestations, including developmental retardation, infertility, and conditions like Down syndrome. Clarification of the mechanisms by which these chromosomal changes occur is essential to the institution of proper diagnostic reagents and therapeutic intervention, and hence a call for meticulous molecular analysis in their identification. Advances in molecular cytogenetic techniques in the recent past have made the detection and identification of chromosomal abnormalities significantly easier. For example, fluorescence *in situ* hybridization (FISH) and high-throughput whole-genome sequencing (WGS) have become essential techniques in detecting complex chromosomal rearrangements that may be missed by conventional karyotyping. He et al. (2022) highlight the advantages of these multi-technique approaches in unravelling the genetic etiology underlying recurrent spontaneous abortions, proposing that combining several different methods gives all-around insight into chromosome structure.

The multi-faceted methodology allows researchers to gain an improved understanding of complex chromosomal aberrations, useful not only for diagnostics but also for application in genetic counseling practice among participating families. Impacts of chromosomal aberrations extend not only to direct healthcare effects but to prenatal diagnostics as a whole. Cordocentesis, established as the definitive method for fetal karyotyping, is of great value for assessing chromosomal aberrations in pregnancy risk. Sun et al. (2020) address the effectiveness of this test in the detection of abnormal karyotypes and cite the variable aneuploidy detection rates in different diagnostic contexts. Moreover, the study reveals that although NIPT may be suitable under particular circumstances, it cannot be the first screening tool for cases with ultrasound soft markers. This multilayered understanding of prenatal diagnostics supports the conventional karyotyping methods even further, especially for keeping accurate diagnoses in addition to guiding clinical decision-making in complex cases of chromosomal aberrations.

12.2.1. Types of Chromosomal Abnormalities

Chromosomal aberrations are further categorized into two broad categories: numerical and structural, both of which significantly impact the phenotype of an organism as well as overall health. Numerical aberrations involve changes in the overall number of chromosomes, typically as a result of nondisjunction during cell division. This leads to aneuploidy, either excess or deficiency of chromosomes. For instance, Down syndrome occurs due to trisomy of chromosome 21, demonstrating the critical consequences of numeric aberrations. Structural abnormalities, on the other hand, result from alterations in individual chromosomes, e.g., deletions, duplications, inversions, and translocations.

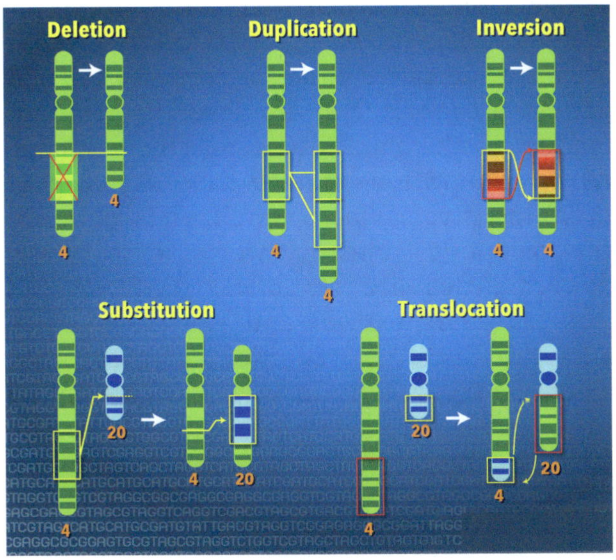

Figure 12.7. Types of chromosomal abnormalities.

Source: https://www.genome.gov/sites/default/files/inline-images/chromosome_abnormalities_factsheet_0.jpg.

These structural changes can interfere with gene function and create a myriad of genetic diseases and contribute to the complexity of diseases , such as cancer. Thus, the determination of the distinction between these forms is important in diagnosis and therapy in the case of molecular cytogenetics. An example of a chromosomal structural abnormality is the translocation, whereby there is a transfer of genetic material between chromosomes that are non-homologous. The t(7;12)(q36;p13) translocation is an example whereby there is engagement of the *ETV6* gene on chromosome 12, and it is a critical abnormality in childhood acute myeloid leukemia (AML), as it can be detected in 20–30 percent of cases. The challenge in the identification of such translocations is often that classical chromosome banding fails to identify them; thus, fluorescence *in situ* hybridization (FISH) is employed for correct identification. This new technique enhances the precision of the diagnosis of translocations, such as cryptic rearrangements, and is significant in proper treatment planning. As supported in t(7;12) research, the negative clinical consequences of such anomalies reaffirm the importance of early diagnosis for the successful treatment of leukemia (Naiel et al., 2013). In molecular cytogenetics, understanding complex chromosomal changes plays a central role in enhancing patient management and prognosis assessment, particularly in hematological neoplasms. This characteristic is illustrated in an example of a patient with acute myeloid leukemia (AML), where identification of a ring chromosome 1 was a prognostic marker for an adverse outcome. Additional chromosomal investigations revealed other numerical abnormalities that helped in the diagnosis and accounted for disease evolution. This tacit awareness of karyotypic evolution emphasizes the manner in which cytogenetic abnormalities may be involved in shaping treatment, such as the utilization of donor peripheral blood stem cells following relapse. This example underscores the significant role of cytogenetic examination within the detection of malignant clones, showing its value in monitoring disease progression and response to therapy as illustrated by this patient's development of MDS to AML (Bennett et al., 2006) (Figure 12.7).

12.2.2. Mechanisms Leading to Chromosomal Abnormalities

The mechanisms leading to chromosomal abnormalities are intricate and consist of complex molecular processes which negatively affect normal cell functioning. One of the primary causes of such abnormalities lies in DNA replication and repair errors. These errors lead to deletions, duplications, and translocations of genetic material, resulting in chromosomal instability. These may be further provoked by some environmental factors , such as radiation and chemical exposure. These outside agents may induce DNA lesions that, if improperly repaired, result in chromosomal rearrangements. The identification of these mechanisms is most significant in unraveling how chromosomal abnormalities arise and how they impact cellular and organismal health. Another significant force behind chromosomal abnormalities exists in the realm of chromosomal segregation during cell division. Errors , such as nondisjunction, where chromosomes are not divided properly during meiosis or mitosis, can lead to aneuploidy—abnormal chromosomal content of a cell. In cancer cells, this event may become frequent, in which case chromosomal instability may be fueling tumorigenesis. Last but not least, the contribution of epigenetic factors cannot be overstated; epigenetic changes , such as DNA methylation and histone modification, can alter gene expression patterns that impact chromosomal stability. The interaction of these mechanisms points to the complexity of chromosomal behavior and the possibility that many disorders can result from such abnormalities. The clinical implications of chromosomal abnormalities are immense, typically owing to genetic disorders as well as cancers. For instance, the Philadelphia chromosome, involving the translocation between chromosomes 9 and 22, is a prototypic example in chronic myelogenous leukemia (CML). The resultant BCR-ABL fusion gene encodes for a constitutively active tyrosine kinase with an unbraked penchant for growth. This describes an immediate correlation of molecular mechanisms of chromosomal aberrations and pathological effects, in the spirit of acknowledging the value of ongoing cytogenetic studies. With the evolution of the International System for Human Cytogenomic Nomenclature (ISCN), an understanding of these mechanisms will remain central to making diagnoses and accurately monitoring the prognosis of chromosomal abnormalities in clinical settings (Benchikh et al., 2022; Minzhenkova et al., 2023).

12.2.3. Clinical Implications of Chromosomal Abnormalities

Clinical correlations of chromosomal abnormalities are of most value in molecular cytogenetics, particularly in cancer prognosis and treatment choice. Abnormal karyotypes are often indicative of disease progression and patient prognosis, and are generally essential markers of the complexity of some malignancies. As an illustration, studies have shown that in Waldenström Macroglobulinemia patients, the frequency and nature of cytogenetic abnormalities are statistical predictors of less favorable overall and progression-free survival. Such a prediction suggests that extensive cytogenetic analyses have the ability to inform clinical decision-making strategies, particularly in individualizing individual treatment modalities that are tailored to the patient's unique genetic makeup of the disease (Danesin et al., 2024). Thus, the identification of chromosomal aberrations forms an integral component of diagnosis and preparation of a therapeutic plan in oncology. In pediatric acute lymphoblastic leukemia (P-ALL), chromosomal abnormalities are highlighted in the formation of fusion oncogenes, which form the central role not only in disease causation but also in prognostic grouping. The oncogenes , such as BCR-ABL and ETV6-RUNX1, are the best indicators of the same, whose presence or absence decides clinical management and impacts survival rates. Research has found considerable ethnic differences in the prevalence of these oncogenes, which suggests that some cancer management schemes should be devised with these variations in mind (Al-Mukhaylid et al., 2024). For instance, BCR-ABL children have poorer prognoses and shorter life expectancies, necessitating aggressive treatment regimens and meticulous follow-up. Such detection of these chromosomal anomalies is also imperative in not only identifying the disease presentation but also in developing the optimal regimens for treatment. Furthermore, the impact of chromosomal abnormalities is not only in malignancy diagnosis but is also applied to inform larger epidemiological information and healthcare policy. Identification of unique chromosomal alterations can further determine disease prevalence patterns in various populations, thereby allowing focused screening and prevention. For example, the identification of the typical chromosomal aberrations frequent among ethnically heterogeneous groups can guide public health strategies to improve availability and outcomes of treatment in disadvantaged groups (Al-Mukhaylid et al., 2024). In the same vein, the ongoing evolution of targeted therapies against particular genetic constellations is a reminder of the necessity for molecular cytogenetic studies to become integral in routine clinical practice. Hence, the clinical significance of chromosomal aberrations is vast, driving continued research and cooperative efforts towards maximizing patient treatment and survival in the arena of personalized medicine.

12.3. Applications in Cancer Research

The application of molecular cytogenetics to cancer studies has revolutionized our knowledge about the biology of tumors. The availability of novel sequencing technologies has helped us decipher the genetic complexities of malignant tumors with very high morbidity and mortality. These methods, particularly spatial transcriptomics, allow researchers to quantify gene expression in the spatial context of tissues, reporting on cellular composition and interactions occurring in the tumor microenvironment. By revealing the more nuanced picture that traditional approaches could not offer, spatial transcriptomics is the first to detect the complex layers responsible for cancer initiation and therapeutic response, thereby offering novel opportunities for targeted intervention approaches in oncology (Jin et al., 2024). In addition, fluorescence *in situ* hybridization (FISH) is the trademark of molecular cytogenetics evolution for the diagnosis of cancer. FISH makes possible the visualization of chromosomal alterations that typically evade the detection of standard karyotyping. With FISH, fluorescent labels on DNA probes can be utilized to identify particular genomic differences that may indicate disease susceptibility or treatment. Development of multicolor karyotyping and comparative genomic hybridization (CGH) has advanced clinical application in facilitating complete analysis of chromosomal abnormalities. Moreover, these procedures facilitate the early monitoring and detection of hematological malignancies, emphasizing the critical importance of precise genetic testing in patient success and personalized medicine (Wan & Ma, 2012). As research continues, the limitations and boundaries of existing molecular cytogenetics techniques call for continual honing and improvement. While advances , such as array CGH and cross-species analysis have improved the application of genetic identification in cancer, issues with resolution and data complexity remain. Yet the science stands at the threshold of imminent technological leaps that will further increase our capacity for diagnosis and therapeutic specificity. With the surmounting of such obstacles, molecular cytogenetics can open doors to epoch-making discoveries in deciphering cancer pathways and making more effective treatment protocols, eventually enhancing patient management and survival rates (Wan & Ma, 2012; Jin et al., 2024) (Figure 12.8).

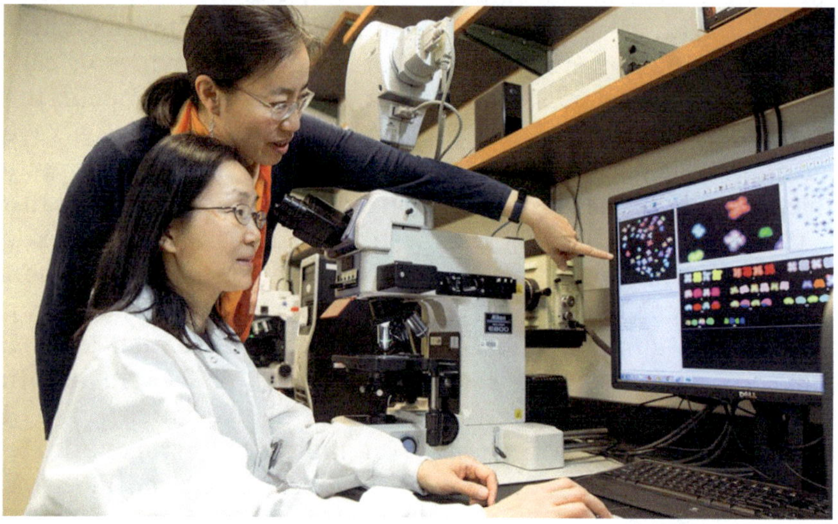

Figure 12.8. Applications in cancer research of molecular cytogenetics.

Source: https://www.cancer.columbia.edu/sites/default/files/styles/cola_media_1280_16_9/public/media/images/2021-04/tlps-4i2acytogenetics-featured-image.jpg?itok=8G7xecAW.

12.3.1. Role of Molecular Cytogenetics in Cancer Diagnosis

Molecular cytogenetics is an important element in cancer diagnosis insofar as it facilitates more precise and finer identification of the genetic abnormalities that underlie various malignancies. Molecular cytogenetics brings together molecular biological techniques with traditional cytogenetic techniques to enable the very detailed analysis of chromosomal structure and function. The integration of these techniques makes the detection of the most frequently implicated chromosomal rearrangements, deletions, and duplications contributing to the pathogenesis of cancer. For instance, the classification of hematopoietic neoplasms according to World Health Organization (WHO) criteria relies heavily on genetic findings, signifying the shift from morphological assessment to an elaborate realization on the basis of genetic etiology (Abduallah et al., 2024). Lastly, the application of molecular cytogenetics for cancer diagnosis enhances clinicians' ability to provide personalized treatment approaches based on the unique genetic characteristics of a patient's tumor. With cancer genetics better understood, machine learning and advanced computational techniques have also taken on a central role in improving diagnostic accuracy. Precision medicine is increasingly supplemented with strong algorithms that evaluate large data sets from sources like the blood transcriptome and imaging. Such advances allow clinicians to identify tumor types and subtypes more effectively, especially in challenging situations where traditional methods may fail. For example, Swarm Learning, a decentralized machine learning, is a perfect example of disparate data that can be merged and synthesized to produce robust classifiers of many diseases, like leukemia. Such technologies not only enhance diagnostic strengths but also are in accordance with privacy legislations, thereby enabling sensitive patient information to be used while maintaining confidentiality (Warnat et al., 2021). Such technological innovations are a revolution in cancer diagnosis, with molecular cytogenetics becoming increasingly integrated with bioinformatics. Second, molecular cytogenetics in cancer diagnosis supports an environment for risk stratification and treatment decisions. With elucidation of discrete genetic changes, the prognosis of patients can be more accurately predicted, and treatment strategies could be individually designed to match the unique biological characteristics of each tumor. For example, identification of certain chromosomal translocations and mutations can guide the use of targeted therapy and the design of new drugs and thus significantly affect patient outcome. The International Consensus Classification of Myeloid Neoplasms and Acute Leukemia illustrates such a paradigm shift since it emphasizes the necessity for genetic incorporation in developing diagnostic criteria. This international cooperative framework by experts emphasizes how robust classification schemes, supported by molecular knowledge, are pivotal to successful hematological malignancy management (Abduallah et al., 2024). Thus, molecular cytogenetics represents the frontier in the diagnosis of cancer and gives an exhaustive understanding of the causative genetic determinants that affect the disease behavior and the treatment response.

12.3.2. Identification of Genetic Markers for Cancer Prognosis

The identification of genetic markers of cancer prognosis is a cornerstone of contemporary molecular cytogenetics, providing valuable information on disease behavior and treatment responsiveness. In acute myeloid leukemia (AML), for instance, some cytogenetic and molecular abnormalities are key determinants of patient stratification and therapy selection. Recent studies illustrate that recurrent somatic mutations, such as those of RUNX1, IDH2, and FLT3, are not only predictive markers for disease onset but also have an important role in separating prognosis. Approximately 22% of patients show mutations in RUNX1, which indicates an inferred poor prognosis but highlights the possibility of targeted treatments owing to the identification of these genetic markers. This genetic classification allows medical professionals to personalize treatment regimens, thereby enhancing the chances of successful therapy in AML patients. The addition of these markers to clinical practice is an advancement towards individualized medicine in cancer (Marrero-León et al., 2023). Moreover, the impact of genetic markers is not only in the diagnosis and immediate management of AML. Prognostic classification systems, like the European LeukemiaNet (ELN) 2022 criteria, incorporate a mix of molecular data and apply it to classify patients into adverse, intermediate, or favorable risk groups. In a recent comprehensive review, 48% of the population of patients were classified as having adverse risk based on genetic and cytogenetic profiles, primarily because of complex cytogenetics and some mutations like TP53. These findings emphasize the importance of characterizing such markers, both due to their ability to inform expected treatment outcomes and due to their influence on the design of surveillance plans following therapy. Therefore, precise characterization of genetic alterations significantly contributes to patient outcome knowledge as well as designing improved, targeted therapeutic strategies (Hang et al., 2023). Furthermore, the role of genetic markers is also evolving with the evolution of new drug therapies and treatment regimens. For example, in AML with core binding factor (CBF) abnormalities, while these have been traditionally associated with a favorable prognosis, those with other adverse risk markers , such as complex cytogenetics or TP53 mutations, complicate treatment. Research has shown that patients with secondary-type mutations or complex abnormalities of the genome are not necessarily worse off in overall survival compared to patients without such abnormalities. This subtle result is contrary to previous assumptions and prompts the prognosis to be reassessed in terms of genetic heterogeneity of AML. Therefore, continuous study of the interaction between various genetic markers and treatment outcomes is required to enhance prognostic models and to ensure that individualized treatments match shifting clinical proof in molecular cytogenetics (Marrero-León et al., 2023) (Figure 12.9).

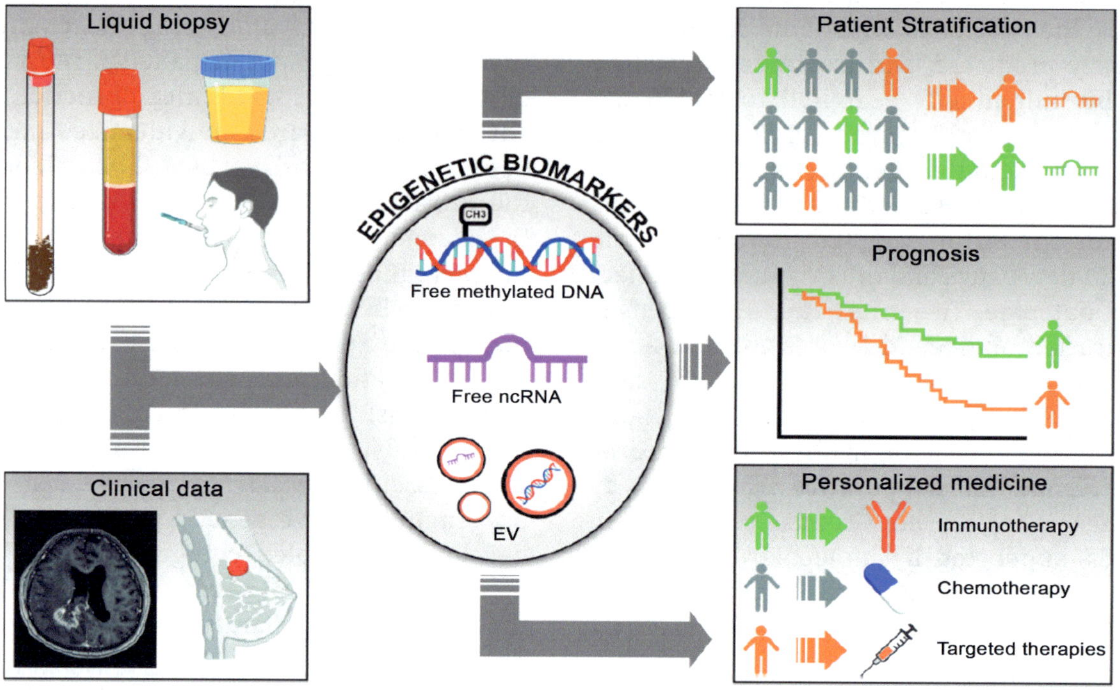

Figure 12.9. Identification of genetic markers for cancer prognosis.

Source: https://pub.mdpi-res.com/cancers/cancers-13-03016/article_deploy/html/images/cancers-13-03016-g001.png?1623915147.

12.3.3. Targeted Therapies Based on Cytogenetic Findings

Development of cancer therapies has been heavily influenced by cytogenetic findings, which provide important information regarding tumor genetics. With the aid of molecular cytogenetics, clinicians can identify specific chromosomal lesions that drive cancer development. Targeted therapy allows for the development of treatments that will attack specifically the intrinsic gene alterations in a patient's tumor. With the advent of technologies , such as next-generation sequencing, oncologists are now able to detect many types of actionable mutations that have potential as a treatment target. Therapies can thus be tailored to the unique molecular profile of a patient's disease, raising the chances of successful treatment and improved patient outcomes. The integration of cytogenetic analysis in the clinic is critical for refining prognostic assessments and tailoring treatment protocols in oncology. Furthermore, models of targeting therapy application are evolving so that clinicians can incorporate molecular cytogenetic results into their routine. Established biomarkers' utilization by precision oncology is evidently identifiable, whereby the biomarkers assist in determining which specific treatments are suitable for individual patients. Advanced databases and precision medicine software have become choice tools for interpreting cytogenetic information and clinical decision-making. Sophisticated options , such as MyCancerGenome and OncoKB are examples of how these platforms have integrated high levels of genomic information and provide actionable data for clinicians. Focused resources like these aid clinicians in making the right choices for treatment plans, thereby enhancing the general standard of care for oncology. The emphasis on integrating cytogenetics into therapeutic choice stems from mounting recognition of the promise of personalized medicine in excel in the management of a wide range of malignancies. In addition, with the expanding division of molecular cytogenetics, the integration of multi-omics approaches is becoming increasingly promoted. This combination of genomics, transcriptomics, proteomics, and metabolomics enables scientists to adopt a holistic perception of tumor biology. By integrating big data analytics and machine learning models, the probability of identifying novel targets and biomarkers significantly improves. Multi-omics investigation not only facilitates the study of complex interplay between molecular alterations but also enhances therapeutic responses through network pharmacology strategies. The combined strategies facilitate simultaneous targeting of multiple disease-controlled networks to create more effective therapeutic responses. As this interdisciplinarity works itself out further, the promise for targeted therapy on the basis of cytogenetic revelations is high, and a new era is opening in the design of useful anticancer drugs that are delicately tuned to the molecular idiosyncrasy of a particular cancer (Figure 12.10).

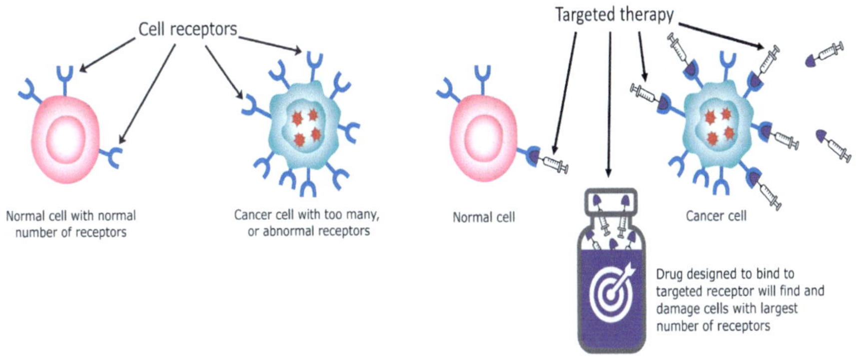

Figure 12.10. Targeted therapies based on cytogenetic findings.

Source: https://www.facingourrisk.org/uploads/targeted-therapy.JPG.

12.4. Genetic Disorders and Molecular Cytogenetics

There is a sophisticated relationship between molecular cytogenetics and genetic disorders through which it becomes possible to form a deeper understanding of disease mechanisms. Molecular cytogenetics is the integration of cytogenetic techniques with molecular biology, which provides data regarding chromosomal mutations resulting in genetic diseases. Molecular cytogenetics has been revolutionized greatly since the 1960s because it now employs high-tech capabilities, with the use of which it detects chromosomal changes more precisely than ever. Genetic illnesses, inherited or acquired, have most commonly resulted from mutations or chromosome structural anomalies, such as deletions, duplications, or translocations. A good example is the case of Chronic Myelocytic

Leukemia (CML), in which mutations in protein tyrosine phosphatases lead to the uncontrolled activation of kinases, ultimately to the disease's pathophysiology (Nader et al., 2016). Thus, molecular cytogenetics is a key methodology in the diagnosis and therapy of genetic disorders, which revolutionizes patient care. Integration of genetic tests into the practice of medicine has significantly enhanced the diagnosis and management of many genetic disorders. Recent advances in molecular cytogenetics have allowed practitioners to employ a variety of methodologies, either cytogenetic or molecular, to detect inherited or acquired genomic alterations. They provide valuable information about the diagnosis, risk prediction, and therapy interventions of most genetic disorders. For instance, a number of studies have shown that the detection of some mutations among patients can be related to treatments, as reported in the research study of PTPRG mutations in patients with CML (Nader et al., 2016). This linkage reflects the potential of genetic testing to inform treatment, particularly in personalized medicine and pharmacogenomics. With the increasing use of genetic testing, the role of genetic testing in the early diagnosis and treatment of genetic diseases is going to increase, leading to better patient outcomes in the long run. Moreover, the evolving science of molecular cytogenetics has the potential to expand our understanding of complex diseases beyond the scope of genetic diseases. With increasingly cheaper and accessible genomic sequencing technology, public health has possibilities for application in broader uses, such as screening for multifactorial etiology diseases, such as cardiovascular disease and most cancers. Genetic testing not only identifies mutations but also assesses the risk of individuals and relatives for the development of certain diseases or for adverse reactions to medications. This capacity is a paradigm shift in healthcare towards prevention, based on genetic knowledge that enables intervention at certain points. Through more research, using the latest knowledge from genetics and epigenetics will be central, as environmental influence impacts gene expression significantly. This integrated process will eventually tell us more about genetic disorders and how to improve disease prevention and control in molecular cytogenetics (Figure 12.11).

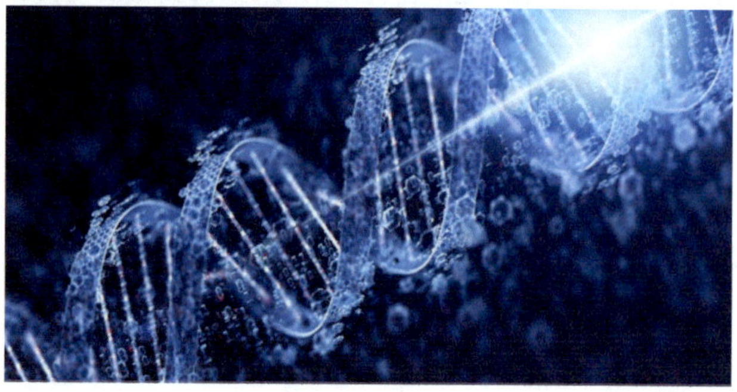

Figure 12.11. Genetic disorders and molecular cytogenetics.

Source: https://knightdxlabs.ohsu.edu/images/default-source/banners/molecular-genetics-banner-mobile.jpeg?sfvrsn=85d1e44f_0.

12.4.1. Common Genetic Disorders Studied Through Cytogenetics

The field of cytogenetics plays an important role in the diagnosis and understanding of common genetic disorders with chromosomal abnormality analysis. One key focus area is aneuploidies, which are conditions resulting from having an abnormal number of chromosomes. A case in point is Down syndrome, which occurs as a result of trisomy 21, showing how cytogenetic technique allows diagnosis by visualizing chromosomal forms. These methods not only serve to establish the clinical suspicion but also permit genetic counseling of the affected families. Further, the study of other diseases with chromosomal abnormalities, such as Turner syndrome and Klinefelter syndrome, demonstrates the variety of phenotypic effects for such genetic variations. Cytogenetics provides information not just regarding the number of the chromosomes but also structural abnormalities that may have a dramatic health impact. Cytogenetic techniques extend from aneuploidies to uniparental disomy (UPD), which is of great significance in imprinting disorders. UPD is a state where an individual inherits two copies of one chromosome from one parent, a state with the potential for gene mutation silencing or activation of recessive gene mutations. UPD has been linked to several genetic syndromes, including Prader-Willi and Angelman syndromes.

Notably, UPD detection can account for complex genetic patterns with particular stress on integrating cytogenetic studies into the framework of molecular genetics. It is evident that frequencies of observed UPD can be non-random and provide unique clinical correlations that are critical in appropriate diagnosis and understanding (Liehr, 2022). In this case, it is important that molecular and cytogenetic strategies be employed to unravel the genetic etiology of these conditions comprehensively. Neurodevelopmental disorders represent another significant category of genetic disorders investigated by cytogenetic strategies. Autism spectrum disorder (ASD), attention-deficit hyperactivity disorder (ADHD), and cerebral palsy are a few disorders that have been exhaustively investigated and best illustrate the intricate interdependence of gene defects and phenotypic manifestations. Earlier studies have implicated a series of vulnerability genes in the pathogenesis of the disorders, citing the possibility of common molecular pathways influencing critical biological processes like brain growth and synapse formation (Cheng, 2024). Prioritization of these genetic factors will lead the way to therapy targeting and improved risk prediction. Therefore, cytogenetics occupies the frontier position of our efforts to unmythologize the complexity of neurodevelopmental disorders, demonstrating its important role in achieving enhanced diagnostic specificity and therapeutic effectiveness for affected individuals.

12.4.2. Prenatal Diagnosis and Screening Techniques

Technological innovation in prenatal screening and diagnostic techniques has become a major pillar within the field of molecular cytogenetics, facilitating early diagnosis of chromosomal abnormalities and congenital defects. Traditional amniocentesis and CVS procedures are now complemented by non-invasive procedures , such as cell-free fetal DNA testing. Such technological innovations have facilitated not only the identification of copy number variations (CNVs) but also the intricate visualization of their phenotypic effects. For instance, there was a report of a family undergoing amniocentesis in which CNV sequencing detected microduplications on chromosomes 15q21.3 and 16p11.2, both previously established to be associated with several developmental disorders and highlighting the importance of such findings for prenatal care (Zhang et al., 2025). The interaction among karyotype analysis, state-of-the-art sequencing technology, and genetic counseling has completely transformed prenatal care, with informed choices being made by prospective parents. Introduction of quantitative cytogenetic techniques has also contributed to the depth of prenatal screening as a field. Non-invasive prenatal testing (NIPT) has been a highly sensitive technique for detecting aneuploidy and other chromosomal abnormalities with a lower need for invasive methods. In one significant case, a study demonstrated the effectiveness of NIPT in a pregnant woman who was a carrier of a balanced translocation. Despite initial concerns following high-risk NIPT results early in pregnancy, subsequent cytogenetic testing to investigate in greater detail revealed complex duplications on chromosomes 18p and 9q, which helped to establish the risk presented (Ardisia et al., 2024). The synergy between cytogenomics and molecular biology techniques has been especially advantageous, demonstrating the excellence of extensive genetic testing in prenatal settings and delivering information beyond the scope of routine techniques. As prenatal diagnosis advances and becomes more precise, the ethical dimensions of such technologies loom larger in the debate. The potential to screen for a multitude of genetic conditions triggers basic questions regarding how genetic information is relevant to parental choice and social expectation.

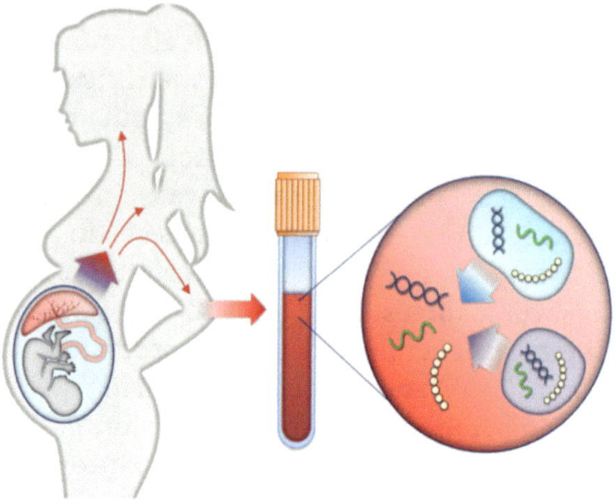

Figure 12.12. Prenatal diagnosis and screening techniques.

Source: https://microbiologynotes.org/wp-content/uploads/2023/05/Prenatal-Diagnosis-An-Overview-e1685268472455.png.

Furthermore, the psychological and emotional impact on families of the threat of congenital anomalies must be considered sensitively. The outcomes of prenatal testing not only direct clinical practice but also decide the path of subsequent reproductive plans for families. Multidisciplinary consultation , including genetic counseling, may help to decrease expected distress associated with indefinite or unfavorable results, providing a more positive environment for pregnant couples facing hard family decisions. Therefore, although the developments in prenatal diagnosis offer unparalleled prospects for early treatment, at the same time they pose also challenges to the social understanding of disease and normalcy, demanding a careful reconciliation between scientific progress and ethical accountability (Figure 12.12).

12.4.3. Ethical Considerations in Genetic Testing

Ethical problems relating to genetic testing are sophisticated and emerge with increasing relevance as molecular cytogenetics progresses. As the ability to identify genetic predispositions to illness grows, practitioners are faced with the significant responsibility of dealing with confidential information. Confidentiality and abuse of genetic information can cause ethical problems for healthcare workers, patients, and families. Notably, instances of genetic discrimination have the potential to result in negative psychological impacts since individuals might feel that the knowledge of their genetic predisposition will lead to stigmatization or exclusion from society. These social impacts necessitate firm policies to protect genetic information, with the principle of non-maleficence being at the center of the debate surrounding genetic testing. Moreover, a lack of education or misunderstandings about genetic testing—particularly among minority groups—must be addressed to mitigate ethical concerns, as outlined in the review of genetic testing for several diseases by Alruwaily (2025). Informed consent is among the most significant ethical aspects of genetic testing, especially with regard to the ability of patients to understand complex genetic details. Genetic test results can have extreme implications not only for the individuals being tested but also for their families, raising the important issue of family and genetic responsibility. In many cases, patients may have difficulty comprehending and fully appreciating the nuances of their genetic information, leading to potential misinterpretations of the implications of the test results. When individuals order genetic tests, they should be properly educated on the risks, advantages, and drawbacks of the tests. Also, access to genetic counseling is the major factor in developing an idea about test outcomes, which allows patients to make their decisions in accordance with both autonomy and family duties (Alharbi et al., 2024). This demand calls attention to a broader demand for educational programs that enhance genetic literacy in the public sphere.

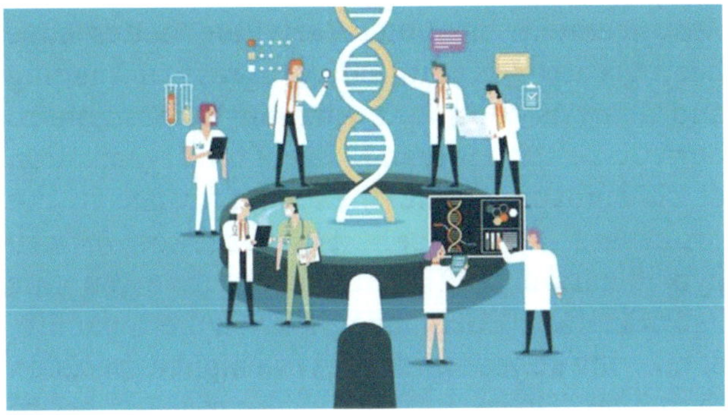

Figure 12.13. Ethical considerations in genetic testing.

Source: https://assets.technologynetworks.com/production/dynamic/images/content/334392/exploring-the-ethics-of-genetic-testing-where-does-duty-begin-and-end-334392-640x360.jpg.

As technological advancements create opportunities for greater genetic testing, ethical concerns extend beyond the technology into the equitable provision of testing capabilities. In the majority of low- and middle-income countries, growth in the availability of genetic testing, as occurring in Malaysia, provokes controversy regarding access and equity in healthcare. The variations in genetic literacy and potential socio-economic barriers may render some groups vulnerable to the appropriate application of genetic services. Hence, cultural competency approaches must be designed that take into consideration certain beliefs and values of certain individuals. Along with this, as providers of health care navigate the ethical landscape of genetic testing, policies are sorely needed to offer access to testing and counseling on a fair basis. This includes projects that require the protection of genetic discrimination with equity in genetic research and hence allow everyone to participate and benefit from developments in molecular cytogenetics (Alruwaily, 2025) (Figure 12.13).

12.5. Advances in Molecular Cytogenetics

In recent years, the emergence of molecular cytogenetics has transformed genetic research and clinical diagnosis. Advances in high-throughput sequencing platforms, such as whole genome sequencing (WGS), have enabled researchers to investigate complex genetic variation to previously unattainable levels of detail. Such detail affords the ability to determine specific genetic loci implicated in numerous diseases, enhancing the understanding of their mechanisms. Thus, they facilitate the application of bespoke therapies based on the unique genetic profile of the patient, highlighting personalized medicine's potential. Being able to integrate population genomics tools along with these sequencing technologies further strengthens selection signals, prior population directions, and structural information. These developments in molecular cytogenetics not only increase our insight into genetic heterogeneity but also provide windows towards more improved diagnostics and treatments in the clinic. In addition, the new field of exposomics enforces the advancements in molecular cytogenetics by examining how the environment influences genetic expression and cell function. This multi-disciplinary approach uses the full repertoire of molecular and environmental data to shed light on gene-environment interactions that manifest as phenotypic variation and susceptibility to disease. Exposomics may help molecular medicine significantly by explaining how these exposures control epigenetic modifications and metabolic pathways. Through the integration of high-throughput omics technologies with rigorous analysis methods, scientists can identify biomarkers important for early diagnosis, detection, and treatment of many ailments. Consequently, the integration of exposomics with molecular cytogenetics provides an integrated understanding of disease and health by bringing into focus the intricate relationship between genetic susceptibility and exposures and thus maximizes personalized healthcare.

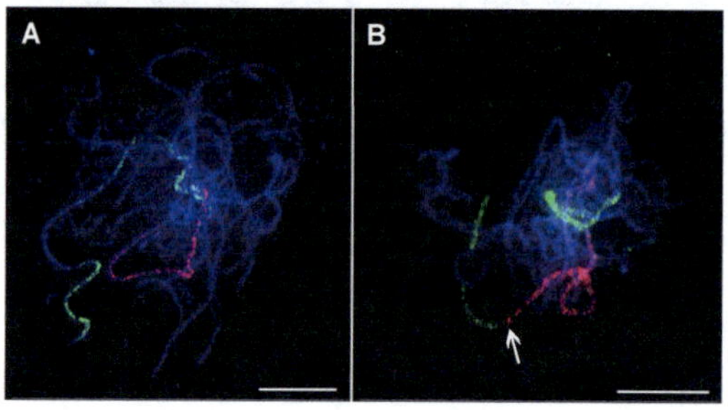

Figure 12.14. Advances in molecular cytogenetics.

Source: https://www.mdpi.com/plants/plants-11-00482/article_deploy/html/images/plants-11-00482-g006.png.

The future of molecular cytogenetics will capitalize on advanced analytical methods, including machine learning models and deep learning models, to further enhance research findings. With improvements in computing power, integrating large-scale data from genomic and environmental sources will enable researchers to develop more complex models that reflect the complex interaction between genetic and non-genetic factors. These technologies have the potential to streamline population genetic epidemiology and population dynamics and help achieve a better understanding of disease mechanisms. Furthermore, these technologies can aid in the prediction of how patients will react to drugs and guide public health planning to diminish the risk of disease associated with certain environmental exposures. By facilitating cross-talk between computer science and molecular cytogenetics, the field can progress with trailblazing research that is highly responsive to pressing public health concerns while paving the way for more effective and targeted therapeutic interventions and, ultimately, reshaping the future of healthcare globally (Figure 12.14).

12.5.1. Innovations in Imaging and Analysis Techniques

Advancements in molecular cytogenetics have been greatly promoted by progress in imaging and analysis techniques, making it possible to derive a better understanding of the organization of chromosomes and their significance in the processes of the cell. Fluorescence *in situ* hybridization (FISH) and comparative genomic hybridization (CGH) have enriched the capability of imaging genetic changes with higher precision than ever. These methods allow researchers to detect and investigate chromosomal diseases on the molecular level, thereby increasing clinical diagnostic accuracy. As these imaging technologies advance, they play a critical role in recognizing unique genetic alterations that are associated with cancers and inherited diseases. Such a fantastic degree of specificity not only assists diagnostics but also precludes therapy, thereby demonstrating the significant impact of imaging technology in molecular cytogenetics. Another critical milestone is the application of high-throughput sequencing technologies, which can enable broad-scale interrogation of genomic variations between populations and disease states. These techniques reduce the time and cost of genetic analysis while increasing the volume of data that can be generated. For instance, NGS can analyze many genes simultaneously, something that is valuable in understanding complex illnesses and heterogeneous tumors. The co-option of NGS with other imaging modalities provides better interpretation of genomic data through the incorporation of spatial context into genomic alteration, facilitating functionally relevant and clinically applicable interpretations. Thus, these technologies not only expand research activities but also enhance personalized medicine strategies within the field of molecular cytogenetics. Furthermore, the inclusion of machine learning algorithms and artificial intelligence in imaging and analysis procedures is revolutionizing the sector by enhancing accuracy and efficiency in interpreting data. Applications developed from artificial intelligence can quickly analyze big data collected from imaging techniques and identify patterns that are imperceptible to human eyes. For instance, image analysis by AI can measure chromosomal aberrations and also predict disease prognosis by genetic profiling and thus inform clinical decisions. AI can streamline the molecular cytogenetics pipeline by automating routine tasks and thereby reducing human error and improving the overall throughput of laboratories. These technologies herald a new revolutionary era of molecular cytogenetics, one where technology not only supplements traditional methods but fundamentally reconfigures the discipline of genetic inquiry and clinical practice.

12.5.2. Integration of Bioinformatics in Cytogenetic Research

The integration of bioinformatics into cytogenetic research is a paradigm shift that augments the analysis and interpretation of complex genomic information. With advancing additional technical enhancements in high-throughput sequencing, bioinformatics tools aid researchers to manage and interpret monstrous datasets generated by methods , such as whole genome sequencing (WGS) and whole transcriptome sequencing (WTS). These tools facilitate tasks , such as variant calling, gene expression profiling, and structural variant detection, which have the potential to elucidate the genetic cause of cancers like leukemia and solid tumors. For instance, the high-throughput genomic analyses used in pediatric leukemia diagnosis showed the promise of applying bioinformatics algorithms to assess copy number variations, ploidy alterations, and gene fusions, which ultimately enables the identification of the most important disease-relevant mutations within days, as shown in recent studies (Voss et al., 2025). The analytical power offered by bioinformatics in cytogenetics not only assists with the classification of genetic alterations but also leads to personalized medicine methods. With high-complexity genomic profiling (CGP) techniques, researchers can systematically map genetic landscapes and define therapeutic targets. For example, in extraskeletal myxoid chondrosarcomas (EMCs), the integration of NGS-based CGP with bioinformatics tools allowed for the complete characterization of genomic alterations, which produced new insight into disease mechanism. The process examined alterations like copy number variants and fusion genes carefully, which are pivotal during tumorigenesis (Schmitthenner et al., 2025). Furthermore, bioinformatics-directed analysis offers an infrastructure for the identification of novel biomarkers that can further refine treatment stratification in treated patients, leading eventually to improved clinical outcomes. With the complexity of genomic data, synergism between bioinformatics and cytogenetics is necessary to progress research protocols. Such integration not only enhances data accuracy and reliability but also enables the creation of efficacious diagnostic and prognostic tools tailored to the patient. As the acute workflows of pediatric leukemia diagnosis have illustrated, bioinformatics facilitates expedited identification of disease-defining genetic mutations, highlighting its value in the clinical setting. Moreover, the ongoing refinement of bioinformatics pipelines holds the capacity to address issues inherent in variant interpretation and clinical decision-making. Hence, the convergence of bioinformatics with cytogenetics is a paradigm in the application of molecular cytogenetics that fosters a culture where precision medicine can prevail based on a greater understanding of genomic subtleties and their facets in disease therapy (Figure 12.15).

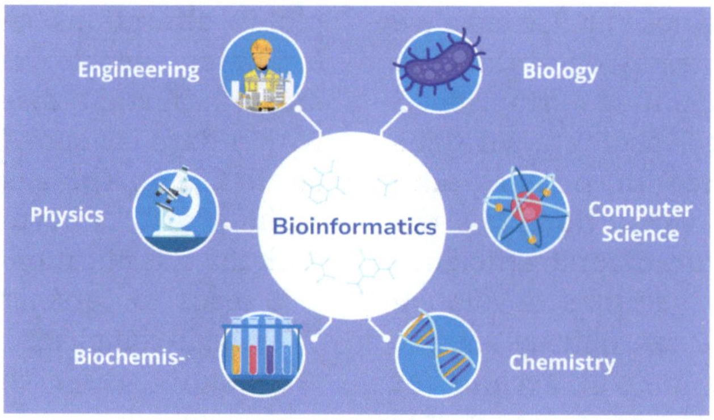

Figure 12.15. Integration of bioinformatics in cytogenetic research.

Source: https://media.geeksforgeeks.org/wp-content/uploads/20240424122635/Bioinformatics.png.

12.5.3. Future Directions and Potential Breakthroughs

As molecular cytogenetics continues to advance, the direction of future trends in the field more and more centers on integrating genomic technologies with traditional cytogenetic methods, which may help to further elucidate chromosomal aberrations. Already, the use of next-generation sequencing (NGS) and high-resolution array comparative genomic hybridization (aCGH) has been promising for making breakthroughs by enabling researchers to detect nanoscale genomic differences that are not always detected with traditional approaches. This resolution improvement allows for the identification of quantitative trait loci (QTLs) in plants , such as the allohexaploid intermediate wheatgrass, in which genetic mapping has revealed critical associations between traits and specific chromosomal locations, as indicated by existing studies. These innovations, as well as accelerating plant domestication, also open up avenues for maximizing traits that lead to more resilient farming varieties, capable of resisting environmental stresses and meeting world food demands (Larson et al., 2019). Another promising field is telomere biology, especially its relevance to health and disease. Recent research highlights the fact that telomere length (TL) can serve as a biomarker for several psychological and physical conditions, particularly for cancer patients. The longitudinal analysis of breast cancer patients at an early stage determined correlations between TL and psychoneurological symptoms and suggested that TL could be impacted by physical stressors, e.g., cancer treatments (Alhareeri, 2016). Subsequent studies can further elucidate the mechanisms through which telomere movement affects disease progression and patient quality of life, potentially leading to interventions that would better mitigate treatment toxicities. In addition, the integration of telomere biology within the broad discipline of molecular cytogenetics can enhance therapeutic strategies based upon individualized genetic profiles, further driving personalized medicine. Furthermore, the future of molecular cytogenetics will likely be more inclined toward the role played by epigenetics in chromosomal dynamics. With researchers increasingly acknowledging that gene expression could be regulated by epigenetic modifications , such as DNA methylation and histone modification, the link with genomic stability and disease susceptibility is apparent. Understanding how such epigenetic elements operate on chromosomal entities has the potential to significantly enhance gene therapy and genetic engineering techniques. For instance, gene editing missions via CRISPR technology can be guided by insights from cytogenetic studies, considering the target site's chromosomal organization and epigenetics. By elucidating these connections, future breakthroughs may enable the design of new strategies that best leverage cellular processes for therapeutic benefit and provide the hope of advances in the treatment of genetic disorders and plant tolerance (Larson et al., 2019) (Figure 12.16).

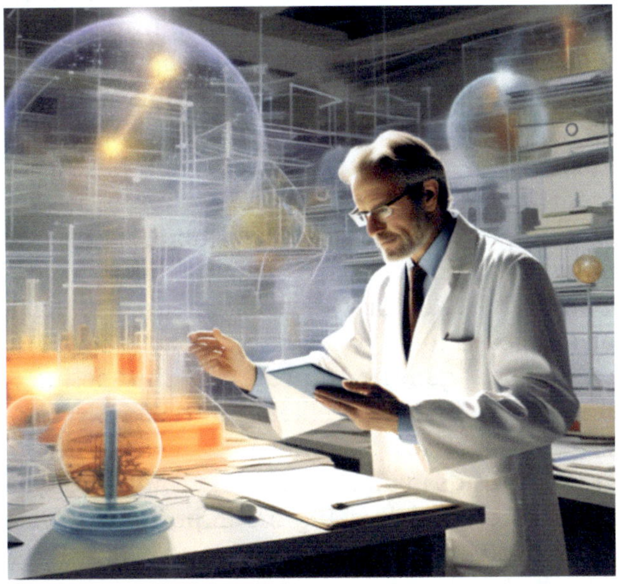

Figure 12.16. Future directions and potential breakthroughs.

Source: https://miro.medium.com/v2/resize:fit:640/1*Nj_TShS1_SbLo-DOlWDy3g.png.

12.6. Case Studies in Molecular Cytogenetics

Molecular cytogenetics is now a key area in deciphering many hematological malignancies, especially in case studies that reveal the intricate interaction of genomic changes and disease course. One such example is chronic myeloid leukemia (CML), in which standard banding cytogenetic analysis is still important. In a single case, a 45-year-old female patient with CML-like symptoms was found to have the Philadelphia chromosome, a marker for the disease, and a rare 5q deletion. The case is significant because it highlights the role of cytogenetic diagnosis not only in the diagnosis of CML but also in identifying rare genetic abnormalities, which play an important part in tailoring treatment strategies. By bringing cytogenetic findings together with clinical presentations, clinicians are able to feel more acutely the course of the disease and adjust treatments, particularly in atypical cases that include those where 5q deletions are concerned (Haidary et al., 2021). Another case that is reminiscent of the value of molecular cytogenetics concerns Li–Fraumeni syndrome (LFS), which occurs with germline mutations of the TP53 tumor-suppressor gene. Patients with LFS also have elevated risks for many malignancies, including hematologic malignancies , such as acute myeloid leukemia (AML) and chronic myeloid leukemia. A review of seven adults with hematologic malignancy that was related to LFS, as done at the Hereditary Hematologic Malignancy Clinic, identified the majority as having therapy-associated illnesses. This underscores the significance of meticulous follow-up of genetically predisposed patients since an early diagnosis and intervention can have significant impacts on the prognosis. All that could be learned from such cases is a better appreciation of how molecular cytogenetic analysis can inform clinical management and family screening and thus respond to the broader concerns of genetic disorders rather than individual patient therapy (Swaminathan et al., 2019). The combined results of several case studies in molecular cytogenetics illuminate the multifaceted mechanisms of hematological malignancies and their implications for therapy. Not only does the integration of cytogenetics and molecular genetics enable a deep understanding of genetic abnormalities, but it also facilitates personalized medicine approaches that maximize patient care. For instance, the identification of the pathogenic Philadelphia chromosome in CML and the complex genetic pattern in cases of LFS demonstrate how accurate cytogenetic analysis can impact patient management of these disorders. With lucid case studies, the utility of molecular cytogenetics is made evident, illustrating how these tests not only contribute to diagnosis and prognosis but also dictate more and more individualized treatment options based on the patient's genetic profile. This experience of personalized medicine is a reaffirmation of the persistence of case studies as a tool for elucidating the dynamics of disease pathology and disease progression in molecular cytogenetics.

12.6.1. Notable Case Studies Illustrating Key Concepts

In molecular cytogenetics, good case examples are extremely useful in providing insights into the practical application of theoretical concepts in real-life situations. A well-known example is the application of the Bobath Concept in hemiplegic patients. This treatment approach emphasizes sensory input, postural alignment, and selective movement control. Emphasizing these concepts, therapists can facilitate neuroplasticity and motor learning, which eventually leads to better functional recovery. One single-case study that employed this method showed significant balance and gait improvements in patients after several sessions of treatment. Findings received indicated a particular correlation between compliance with Bobath principles and observed changes in motor control, illustrating how fundamental concepts in molecular cytogenetics can be used successfully in clinical practice to benefit patient outcomes (Song et al., 2025). Not less interesting is the exploration of virtual reality (VR) as a new tool in molecular cytogenetics education and research. Systematic review of the literature has discovered several barriers and facilitators to the adoption of VR in middle school STEAM education, such as technical limitations, poor teacher training, and policy interventions required. Qualitative synthesis of case studies indicated that with adequate assistance in professional development, as well as collaboration environments, there is considerable potential for VR to enhance educational achievements. In particular, some case studies reported successful implementations that led to increased student participation and understanding of complex genetic ideas. These findings provide evidence not only of the transformative power of VR in molecular cytogenetics but also of the compelling necessity for strategic policy, training programs, and technological resource harmonization to enable effective learning environments (Nemani, 2025). Furthermore, the external validity of these case studies well exceeds their respective contexts, shedding light on underlying principles that can be extended across molecular cytogenetics, as well as related disciplines. The neuroplasticity processes shown with the Bobath Concept emphasize genetic expression and cellular response plasticity. Likewise, research into VR as a tool for learning is a microcosm of greater trends in digital pedagogy and emerging pedagogies, emphasizing the importance given to adaptive methods in scientific learning. By applying these lessons from the case studies to the general context of molecular cytogenetics, researchers and educators alike can better see how fundamental principles, when well operationalized, can lead to enhanced comprehension and functional application. This coalescence of theoretical and applied understanding ultimately lays the groundwork for advancement in the field, validating the potential for future research and innovative methodologies towards enhancing both teaching and clinical care in molecular cytogenetics.

12.6.2. Impact of Findings on Patient Management

The findings of recent research in molecular cytogenetics have tremendous bearings on clinical handling of the patient, particularly in conditions , such as acute myeloid leukemia (AML). In particular, the incorporation of cytogenetic data into clinical prognosis has radically changed treatment strategies. Research identified a rising trend in survival rates of

AML patients due to advances in molecular diagnosis and targeted therapy, indicating a 2% decrease in excess mortality corresponding to each consecutive year of diagnosis. This advanced understanding allows healthcare providers to tailor treatments more precisely, considering factors of individual patients and specific genetic mutations. By applying this information, clinicians can best identify patient-specific treatment plans, maximize efficacious interventions while avoiding excessive exposures to ineffective therapies, in turn improving patient outcomes in a clinically meaningful manner (Abduallah et al., 2024). Moreover, integrating geographic and demographic factors into patient management plans represents an individualized type of healthcare delivery. The data indicate that city patients have better survival prospects compared to their rural counterparts, and this is largely attributed to the greater access to sophisticated medical facilities and care. It is very crucial for medical professionals who aim to have equal standards of treatment among different patient populations to comprehend this disparity. For instance, targeted outreach programs with a view to facilitating greater access to health care in poorer areas could lower death rates in rural communities. In addition, the potential disparities elicited by the research need clinical practices to be adjusted to incorporate these social determinants of health so that all patients receive the advancements in care facilitated by molecular cytogenetics on equal grounds (Abduallah et al., 2024). The applications of molecular cytogenetics extend beyond cancer therapy, as evidenced in the management of surgical site infections (SSIs), particularly in at-risk patients , such as pediatric cardiac surgery patients. The consensus document contains comprehensive guidelines on management of peri-operative antibiotic prophylaxis, rationalizing strategies that reduce SSIs by a wide margin. Increased awareness of genetic predispositions can further educate healthcare professionals regarding the most appropriate prophylactic modalities for their patients. By offering clinicians evidence-based advice and tailoring the application of antibiotics, the attendant risk of these complex procedures can be minimized, with a possible outcome of better postoperative results and lower healthcare costs. The evolving science of molecular cytogenetics demonstrates the imperative to practice individualized medicine to enhance patient care in medicine as a whole (Figure 12.17).

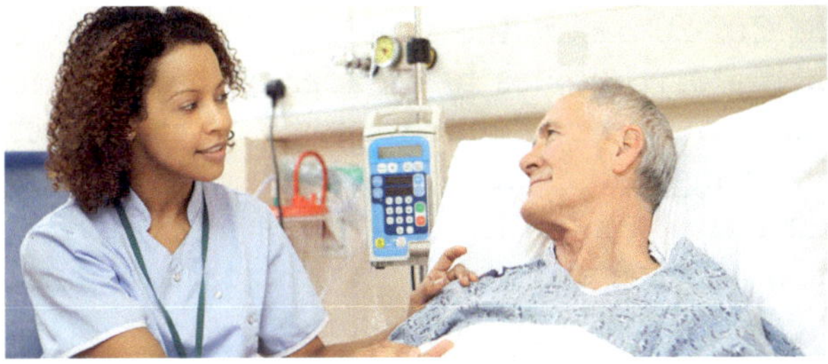

Figure 12.17. Impact of findings on patient management.

Source: https://avanthealthcare.com/file/116/Featured-Image_Patient-Care.png.

12.6.3. Lessons Learned from Case Studies

The sophisticated field of molecular cytogenetics has gained much from a multitude of case studies that have provided insight into successes and problems in its application. For instance, the development of new tools in health and rehabilitation facilities, particularly in settings like South Africa, emphasizes the need for refining methodologies to suit existing conditions. These case studies illustrate that it is not possible to implement one-size-fits-all responses to a population's unique genetic makeup and environmental setting. The findings show that interactions with end-users as well as local stakeholders make it easier to get a grasp on the problems at hand, making sure that developed tools will be relevant and applicable. This collaborative approach is in alignment with the premise that effective service delivery in molecular cytogenetics relies on contextualizing scientific practice, hence making it more reflective of the experienced world of diverse populations (Kathard et al., 2024). Pilot studies as a process in molecular cytogenetics have been highly invaluable in the assessment of new technology and methods. These experiments not only allow researchers to try out new approaches but also to test their efficacy before scaling them further. Piloting enforces the necessity of a systematic, scientific process of tool development again. Through careful analysis of the findings of these initial tests, researchers can recognize potential pitfalls while fine-tuning their methodology based on evidence. This test-crafted cycle of refinement is required to advance the discipline, ultimately resulting in a strict yet adaptable body of knowledge. The knowledge acquired through these pilot tests acts as a blueprint for developing tools that have the ability to empower practitioners in the field, allowing for a healthy feedback loop that continues to strengthen universal scientific progress (Kathard et al., 2024). Lastly, the experience gained via case studies in molecular cytogenetics goes beyond laboratory bubbles to broader issues of concern in society. Outreach to society, for example, in many studies of public response to crisis scenarios , such as the COVID-19 pandemic, depicts an enlarging reach that encompasses health, ethics, and global topics. For example, responses from various communities can create innovative ways of promoting the greater good, demonstrating how cooperative efforts in science and public health are able to provide. When societies look back at their condition and envision a future with no pandemic, what they learn can lead to equitable practice in various scientific fields, including molecular cytogenetics. The general thrust emphasizes the necessity of global cooperation and sharing of resources, which would redesign existing paradigms and promote an inclusive scientific environment.

SUMMARY

In molecular cytogenetics, the blending of chromosomal research and molecular techniques has far advanced our understanding of genetic abnormalities and variation. The results from studies in various species and conditions illustrate the critical role of chromosomal arrangements in establishing taxonomic affiliations as well as in the diagnosis of genetic abnormalities. For instance, *Turcichondrostoma fahirae*, an endemic species, had its karyotype analyzed, which indicated that the diploid chromosome number was 50, in accordance with the maintained karyotype pattern of leuciscid fishes. The research points out the value of molecular cytogenetic markers in enabling future taxonomic comparison and our enhancement of evolutionary relationship insight in different ichthyofaunal settings (Güldane et al., 2025). This serves to emphasize how cytogenetic techniques help to further our knowledge of not only biodiversity, but also the processes of chromosomal evolution. Additionally, advances in molecular technology have a central role to play in our ability to diagnose and understand complex genetic disorders. One particularly poignant example is the study of 46,XX male syndrome and its illustration of the complex interrelationship between chromosomal constitution and phenotypic expression. The translocation of the SRY gene to the X chromosome in patients with a 46,XX karyotype highlights the importance of cytogenetic testing in the clinical arena. It not only helps to establish a definitive diagnosis but also provides pointers towards the mechanisms of gonadal development and associated endocrine imbalance (Rawal et al., 2024). Thus, molecular cytogenetics includes the area between basic research and clinical application, with profound potential for genetic counseling and reproduction management in problem patients. Thus, the future for molecular cytogenetics appears rosy with prospective research likely to unravel the secrets behind genome architecture and function. The continuous advancement in high-resolution techniques, such as chromosomal microarray analysis and fluorescence *in situ* hybridization (FISH), will definitely enhance our ability to detect genetic abnormalities more accurately. These advances will not only facilitate improved understanding of species evolution but also enhance the diagnostic procedures for genetic conditions, resulting in improved patient outcomes. Lastly, the insights of molecular cytogenetic studies must inform conservation, clinical practice, and our wider understanding of genetic diversity, ultimately forming a solid foundation for ongoing research activity in this continually developing field.

The field of molecular cytogenetics has seen profound leaps in understanding the complexity of chromosome form and function, particularly in some organisms. A major area of interest involves comparative cytogenetics of New World monkeys, whose structure of the genome provides clues about evolutionary forces. Scientists have traced the evolutionary history of the ancestral New World monkey karyotype, $2n = 54$ chromosomes, and have documented lineage-specific chromosome rearrangements that have resulted in an enormous range of karyotypes among living species. Karyotypes range from as few as $2n = 16$ in titi monkeys to as many as $2n = 62$ in woolly monkeys. Such heterogeneity testifies to the plasticity of such species within their ecological niches and bears witness to the role of chromosomal evolution in primates as a force of speciation (de Oliveira et al., 2012). Another of molecular cytogenetics' most important uses is research into specific molecular mechanisms behind chromosomal evolution and stability. Recent research points to the importance of chromatin remodeling and genomic imprinting as being crucial for correct gene expression and cellular function. Understanding how these mechanisms function supports a comprehension of development processes and disease, particularly in cancers and genetic diseases. Furthermore, the studies that observe the interaction between chromatin structure and fundamental cellular processes , such as apoptosis, reveal the complex interactions that regulate cellular response to stressors and stimuli. Such studies are not only a fundamental requirement for the understanding of basic biological mechanisms but also for implications in therapeutic intervention and clinical application (Pavan, 2013). The marriage of molecular and cytogenetic data provides the opportunity for further advances in the understanding of mechanisms of genetic diseases and therapy. Studies have shown that alterations in the organization of chromosomes can lead to predispositions for various disorders, such as cancers, where aberrant karyotypes typically result in poor prognostic consequences. One such interaction is the formation of protein kinases, such as CK2, which are responsible for the regulation of anti-apoptotic signals and consequently influence cellular responses to chemotherapy. By investigating in a systematic manner the interaction between epigenetic and genetic elements, researchers will be able to design more effective interventions. These studies not only augment the current volume of knowledge in molecular cytogenetics but also propel the discipline into the development of targeted therapies, thereby enhancing patient care and deciphering the complexity of genetic disorders (Pavan, 2013).

A LOOK TO THE FUTURE

INTEGRATION OF MOLECULAR GENETICS:

The integration of molecular genetics into contemporary biological and medical science marks a transformative evolution in how we understand, investigate, and apply genetic information. Molecular genetics, the study of the biochemical mechanisms that govern gene structure, function, and expression, provides the foundational insights into how genotypes influence phenotypes at the most fundamental level. When integrated with other disciplines—such as genomics, clinical research, systems biology, and bioinformatics—molecular genetics becomes far more than a set of isolated techniques; it becomes a framework for interpreting complex biological systems and translating that understanding into real-world applications.

At its core, integration in molecular genetics seeks to bridge several traditionally distinct areas of inquiry. In research, this involves combining molecular genetic data with high-throughput genomics and proteomics to unravel the intricate networks that underlie cellular function and disease mechanisms. By correlating genetic variation with gene expression profiles and cellular phenotypes, integrated approaches can reveal how molecular pathways interact, adapt, and malfunction in health and disease. This synthesis of methodologies enables more holistic interpretations of genetic information and supports the discovery of new biological insights that single techniques alone might miss.

In clinical medicine, the integration of molecular genetics has spurred unprecedented advances in diagnostics and personalized care. The ability to incorporate DNA- and RNA-based testing into clinical workflows has redefined disease risk assessment, early screening, and therapeutic decision-making. For example, molecular genetic tests that identify specific mutations or variant patterns are now instrumental in diagnosing hereditary conditions, guiding targeted therapies, and predicting drug response. This integration is central to the emerging paradigm of precision medicine, where interventions are tailored to the genetic makeup of individual patients rather than applied universally.

Successful integration also requires thoughtful collaboration across disciplines. Molecular genetics researchers often work closely with clinical scientists, bioinformaticians, epidemiologists, and ethical-legal experts to ensure that genomic data are interpreted correctly and applied safely. This collaborative model enhances both scientific discovery and translational impact, allowing complex genetic information to be incorporated responsibly into patient care and public health strategies. Moreover, integration extends into educational realms, where genetics and genomics are woven into multidisciplinary curricula to train future scientists and clinicians to harness these tools effectively and ethically. As molecular genetics continues to intersect with diverse fields, its integration promises to deepen our understanding of biological complexity, improve clinical outcomes, and broaden the horizons of what genetic science can achieve.

REFERENCES

1. Abduallah, Y., Sriranjan, N., Paulson, K., & Houston, B. L. (2024). Population-based analysis of outcomes in acute myeloid leukemia from a provincial cancer registry and the Canadian Cancer Registry: A population-based retrospective cohort study. *Blood*. https://www.semanticscholar.org/paper/f57190ffbdf935890e11c654d8ce7f45811db1df (accessed on 17th July 2025).
2. Aga Khan University Hospital, Karachi. (2007). *LABRAD: Vol 32, Issue 1–January 2007*. https://core.ac.uk/download/47263432.pdf (accessed on 17th July 2025).
3. Aguiar, C., & Camps, I. (2025). Molecular Docking in Drug Discovery: Techniques, Applications, and Advancements. *Current medicinal chemistry*, *32*(28), 5924–5938. https://doi.org/10.2174/0109298673325827240926081845(accessed on 17th July 2025).
4. Al-Dewik, N. I., Monne, M., Araby, M., Al Sayab, A., Vezzalini, M., Tomasello, L., Modjtahedi, H., et al. (2016). Novel molecular findings in protein tyrosine phosphatase receptor gamma (PTPRG) among chronic myelocytic leukemia (CML) patients studied by next generation sequencing (NGS): A pilot study in patients from the State of Qatar and Italy. *Blood, 128*, 5427–5427. https://www.semanticscholar.org/paper/8eb40d1767148cbc3f9158124a6b3140095bb415 (accessed on 17th July 2025).
5. Alharbi, A. H., Alawi, S., Al-Sadah, A., Abdrabalnabi, F., Altarouti, A., Noha, [3]., Alsharif, M., et al. (2024). Cytogenetics testing: The evolving role of medical lab technicians in genetics labs. *Power System Technology*. https://www.semanticscholar.org/paper/7b48fbcb9d89730407da04439aab4fe7072f6f11 (accessed on 17th July 2025).
6. Alhareeri, A. (2016). Telomere length in women with breast cancer: A longitudinal study of their relationship to chemotherapy and acquired psychoneurological symptoms. https://core.ac.uk/download/51294406.pdf (accessed on 17th July 2025).
7. Al-Mukhaylid, S., Iqbal, Z., Alanazi, N., & Awan, T. (2024). Abstract B039: Investigations on ethnographic disparities in molecular epidemiology of pediatric ALL and its impact on clinical outcome as well as cancer management planning strategies. *Cancer Research*. https://www.semanticscholar.org/paper/1debca641817382328ebb527e7ff000ef74554a3 (accessed on 17th July 2025).
8. Larson, S., DeHaan, L., Poland, J., Zhang, X., Dorn, K., Kantarski, T., Anderson, J., Schmutz, J., Grimwood, J., Jenkins, J., Shu, S., Crain, J., Robbins, M., & Jensen, K. (2019). Genome mapping of quantitative trait loci (QTL) controlling domestication traits of intermediate wheatgrass (Thinopyrum intermedium). *TAG. Theoretical and applied genetics. Theoretische und angewandte Genetik*, *132*(8), 2325–2351. https://doi.org/10.1007/s00122-019-03357-6(accessed on 17th July 2025).
9. Arber, D. A., Hasserjian, R. P., Orazi, A., Mathews, V., Roberts, A. W., Schiffer, C. A., Roug, A. S., et al. (2022). Classification of myeloid neoplasms/acute leukemia: Global perspectives and the international consensus classification approach. *American Journal of Hematology, 97*, 514–518. https://doi.org/10.1002/ajh.26503 (accessed on 17th July 2025).
10. Ardisia, C., De Falco, L., Savarese, G., Ruggiero, R., Suero, T., Petrillo, N., Ianniello, M., et al. (2024). Inherited unbalanced reciprocal translocation with 18p11.32p11.21 tetrasomy and 9q34.3 trisomy in a fetus revealed by cell-free fetal DNA (cffDNA) testing: Cytogenetic and cytogenetic characterization in prenatal diagnosis. *Genes, 15*. https://www.semanticscholar.org/paper/946cf10f1e865d9c2323dae4de60f4882894ab5e (accessed on 17th July 2025).

11. Basu, P., Verma, J., Abhinav, V., Ratnesh, R. K., Singla, Y., & Kumar, V. (2025). Advancements in lithography techniques and emerging molecular strategies for nanostructure fabrication. *International Journal of Molecular Sciences, 26*. https://www.semanticscholar.org/paper/05904a708b7408d39725678d9bea0244539ca3b6 (accessed on 17th July 2025).

12. Benchikh, S., Bousfiha, A., El Hamouchi, A., Soro, S. G. C., Malki, A., & Nassereddine, S. (2022). Chronic myeloid leukemia: Cytogenetics and molecular biology's part in the comprehension and management of the pathology and treatment evolution. *Egyptian Journal of Medical Human Genetics, 23*. https://www.semanticscholar.org/paper/802bfc06a76973365aae59198ddb3b853fe85677 (accessed on 17th July 2025).

13. Bianchini, S., Nicoletti, L., Monaco, S., Rigotti, E., Corbelli, A., Colombari, A., Auriti, C., et al. (2022). Peri-operative prophylaxis in patients of neonatal and pediatric age subjected to cardiac and thoracic surgery: A RAND/UCLA appropriateness method consensus study. *Antibiotics, 11*. https://www.semanticscholar.org/paper/6e49e3a0a9a152f7c1a8d55f79bc6cca4e1890f5 (accessed on 17th July 2025).

14. Brodersen, L., Gerbing, R., Pardo, M., Alonzo, T., Paine, D., Fritschle, W., Hsu, F. C., et al. (2020). Morphologic remission status is limited compared to ΔN flow cytometry: A Children's Oncology Group AAML0531 report. *Blood Advances, 4*(20), 5050–5061. https://www.semanticscholar.org/paper/f5872f330c2ba1e2bca00decc653aef63fdc579f (accessed on 17th July 2025).

15. Cassiman, J. (2011). Molecular diagnostics. *Human Genomics, 5*, 208–209. https://www.semanticscholar.org/paper/1068b79d3d8016493b4a87ef00f22831f4a4ec24 (accessed on 17th July 2025).

16. Cheng, Y. (2024). Genomic relationships and common mechanisms across neurodevelopmental disorders. *Proceedings of the 2024 4th International Conference on Bioinformatics and Intelligent Computing*. https://www.semanticscholar.org/paper/93061115539c156a442f036ada4d44e237850d13 (accessed on 17th July 2025).

17. Crocker, J. (2003). Molecular biology in cellular pathology. https://www.semanticscholar.org/paper/fb919f528a9f7c0478a30c0fc981b539bae8e1fb (accessed on 17th July 2025).

18. Danesin, N., Bonaldi, L., Martines, A., Nalio, S., Bertorelle, R., Compagno, S., Marcato, R., et al. (2024). Impact of the presence and number of chromosomal abnormalities on the clinical outcome in Waldenström Macroglobulinemia: A monocentric experience. *Annals of Hematology, 103*, 2961–2968. https://www.semanticscholar.org/paper/30033a24fd684713882ace8765e0d0d16375fd80 (accessed on 17th July 2025).

19. de Oliveira, E. H. C., Müller, S., & Neusser, M. (2012). Chromosome evolution in New World monkeys (Platyrrhini). https://core.ac.uk/download/16432827.pdf (accessed on 17th July 2025).

20. Gazola, A. A., Lautert-Dutra, W., Archangelo, L. F., Dos Reis, R. B., & Squire, J. A. (2024). Precision oncology platforms: Practical strategies for genomic database utilization in cancer treatment. *Molecular Cytogenetics, 17*. https://www.semanticscholar.org/paper/6ede5dab7db0fc02394243f8c9a629cb8263efd0 (accessed on 17th July 2025).

21. Gerard, J. P., Tan, A. H., Lim, S. Y., Ahmad-Annuar, A., Schee, J., & Gopalan, N. (2025). Genetic testing for Parkinson's disease in an underrepresented population: Knowledge, attitudes, and ethical considerations from a Malaysian perspective. *Journal of Genetic Counseling, 34*. https://www.semanticscholar.org/paper/db0081f2d172b1b221def775822b5fcbdf2e5cde

(accessed on 17th July 2025).

22. Gore, L., Kearns, P., de Martino, M. L., Lee, L., De Souza, C. A., Bertrand, Y., Hijiya, N., et al. (2018). Dasatinib in pediatric patients with chronic myeloid leukemia in chronic phase: Results from a Phase II trial. *Journal of Clinical Oncology, 36*, 1330–1338. https://doi.org/10.1200/jco.2017.75.9597 (accessed on 17th July 2025).

23. Gözen Tavşan, G., Arslan, A., Özçay Ekşi, B., Alpaslan, Z., Arslan, E., & Sember, A. (2025). Karyotype and repetitive DNA analysis in *Turcichondrostoma fahirae* (Cypriniformes, Leuciscidae): A step toward the use of molecular cytogenetics in taxonomy of freshwater fishes in Türkiye. *Cytogenetic and Genome Research, 165*, 39–50. https://www.semanticscholar.org/paper/631fabd7d06f8ec953afb5e6ae14bdbc82d07eec (accessed on 17th July 2025).

24. Haidary, A. M., Ahmed, Z., Abdul-Ghafar, J., Rahmani, S., Noor, S., Erfani, F., Ahmad, M., et al. (2021). Philadelphia chromosome positive chronic myeloid leukemia with 5q deletion at diagnosis. *Molecular Cytogenetics, 14*. https://www.semanticscholar.org/paper/4d9f86ab9f6781b637a4abf7155ba9e8ff5c3dfc (accessed on 17th July 2025).

25. Halim, F. A. (2024). Lessons learned, resilience built, and multipolarism imagined: The Muslim experience of the 2019–2022 pandemic crisis. *Abdurrauf Journal of Islamic Studies (ARJIS)*. https://www.semanticscholar.org/paper/af5459a5d21b869b9552b84e73390a79fee48edf (accessed on 17th July 2025).

26. Hang, Y., Bouligny, I., Murray, G. F., Patel, T., Doyel, M., Boron, J., Tran, V., et al. (2023). Clinical outcomes of core binding factor acute myeloid leukemia in the modern era. *Journal of Clinical Oncology*. https://www.semanticscholar.org/paper/aac8ed570130e49969d29c9bd0cdbc20a5b303f8 (accessed on 17th July 2025).

27. Harper, P. S., Reynolds, L. A., & Tansey, E. M. (2010). Clinical genetics in Britain: Origins and development. https://core.ac.uk/download/30696166.pdf (accessed on 17th July 2025).

28. He, P., Wei, X., Xu, Y., Huang, J., Tang, N., Yan, T., Yang, C., et al. (2022). Analysis of complex chromosomal rearrangements using a combination of current molecular cytogenetic techniques. *Molecular Cytogenetics, 15*. https://www.semanticscholar.org/paper/5797eccf9b8b34743bffc858f99831ddc3c2eaac (accessed on 17th July 2025).

29. Iannuzzi, A., Iannuzzi, L., & Parma, P. (2023). Molecular cytogenetics in domestic bovids: A review. *Animals: An Open Access Journal from MDPI, 13*. https://www.semanticscholar.org/paper/42a46c5ca3f40ac5993d226109c0e51a85345b05 (accessed on 17th July 2025).

30. Jang, W., Chae, H., Kim, J., Son, J., Kim, S., Koo, B., Kim, M., et al. (2016). Identification of small marker chromosomes using microarray comparative genomic hybridization and multicolor fluorescent *in situ* hybridization. *Molecular Cytogenetics, 9*. https://www.semanticscholar.org/paper/318a9d9dab22fe33d435b732445a7e4450493288 (accessed on 17th July 2025).

31. Jin, Y., Zuo, Y., Li, G., Liu, W., Pan, Y., Fan, T., Fu, X., et al. (2024). Advances in spatial transcriptomics and its applications in cancer research. *Molecular Cancer, 23*. https://www.semanticscholar.org/paper/fb8ba6a424922fdea28451ef81ee4284340b35a6 (accessed on 17th July 2025).

32. Jones, E. M., & Tansey, E. M. (2014). Clinical molecular genetics in the UK c.1975–c.2000. https://core.ac.uk/download/30696934.pdf (accessed on 17th July 2025).

33. Kathard, H., Mallick, R. B., Cloete, T. L., Hansen, A., & Thabane, L. (2024). Lessons learned about development and assessment of feasibility of tools for health and rehabilitation services.

Pilot and Feasibility Studies, 10. https://www.semanticscholar.org/paper/9aae6a2288af2886e3b84c93d33bad8cbad6d813 (accessed on 17th July 2025).

34. Liehr, T. (2022). Uniparental disomy is a chromosomic disorder in the first place. *Molecular Cytogenetics, 15*. https://www.semanticscholar.org/paper/2ce54cbe092893865406d711fa52da630c39a90a (accessed on 17th July 2025).
35. Lima-Quintanilha, T. C., Nova, M., & Torres-da-Silva, T. L. (2019). Fake news and its impact on trust in the news: Using the Portuguese case to establish lines of differentiation. *Communication & Society*. https://www.semanticscholar.org/paper/93d433fc45f06bae74d7615a9358fe3593c70df6 (accessed on 17th July 2025).
36. Liu, J., Ranka, S., & Kahveci, T. (2007). A web server for mining comparative genomic hybridization (CGH) data. *953*, 144–161. https://www.semanticscholar.org/paper/bf0a37cfb9849dd0b5c0cea8e5d996ef7129ef48 (accessed on 17th July 2025).
37. Lu, Y., Li, M., Gao, Z., Ma, H., Chong, Y., Hong, J., Wu, J., et al. (2025). Advances in whole genome sequencing: Methods, tools, and applications in population genomics. *International Journal of Molecular Sciences, 26*. https://www.semanticscholar.org/paper/8b9983b5b9de00ec0aaa261a6c62fde6c85d1385 (accessed on 17th July 2025).
38. Marrero-León, W. D., Cintrón-Colón, H., Cruz-Rodriguez, S., Cáceres, W., Rodriguez-Arocho, C. I., & Cruz, A. (2023). Molecular and cytogenetics abnormalities in acute myeloid leukemia at Puerto Rico. *Journal of Clinical Oncology*. https://www.semanticscholar.org/paper/9b785b0ecb9aa72a27f8b918693a5f445ee0e625 (accessed on 17th July 2025).
39. Mirabelli, P., Coppola, L., & Salvatore, M. (2019). Cancer cell lines are useful model systems for medical research. *Cancers, 11*, 1098–1098. https://doi.org/10.3390/cancers11081098 (accessed on 17th July 2025).
40. Mukherjee, A., Abraham, S., Singh, A., Balaji, S., & Mukunthan, K. (2024). From data to cure: A comprehensive exploration of multi-omics data analysis for targeted therapies. *Molecular Biotechnology, 67*, 1269–1289. https://www.semanticscholar.org/paper/04593d2268ccd7c26b5296d8342b468ca84ae7b1 (accessed on 17th July 2025).
41. Naiel, A., Andreasson, A., Beverloo, H., Cho, S., Fleischman, E., Tsaur, G., Hollington, S., et al. (2013). A novel three-color fluorescence *in situ* hybridization approach for the detection of t(7;12)(q36;p13) in acute myeloid leukemia reveals new cryptic three-way translocation t(7;12;16). https://core.ac.uk/download/18488545.pdf (accessed on 17th July 2025).
42. Nemani, S. (2025). Barriers and enablers to adopting virtual reality in lower secondary STEAM curricula. *Journal of Advanced Research in Education*. https://www.semanticscholar.org/paper/75cb48dd50ad20b369b97e2fa43ffca763e83108 (accessed on 17th July 2025).
43. Olivucci, G., Iovino, E., Innella, G., Turchetti, D., Pippucci, T., & Magini, P. (2024). Long read sequencing on its way to the routine diagnostics of genetic diseases. *Frontiers in Genetics, 15*. https://www.semanticscholar.org/paper/a6ba1fe924f5a8b547b145f8e62b542335197675 (accessed on 17th July 2025).
44. Pavan, L. (2013). Overexpression of the protein kinase CK2 increases the survival and resistance to chemotherapy of acute myeloid leukemia cells. https://core.ac.uk/download/18294131.pdf (accessed on 17th July 2025).

45. Rawal, L., Prabhash, S., Kumar, R., Sharma, G., Shariq, M., Jangra, S., Nakra, R., et al. (2024). 46,XX males with *SRY* gene translocation: Cytogenetics and molecular characterization. *Journal of Rare Diseases, 3*, 1–8. https://www.semanticscholar.org/paper/333451047ef7796d5f46513eb7f252658805c818 (accessed on 17th July 2025).

46. Schmitthenner, C. P., Evelt, F., Scholl, L. S., Janke, J., Kuntze, A., Kirmse, S., Falkenberg, K., et al. (2025). Abstract 7173: Comprehensive genomic profiling reveals novel insights into the genomic landscape of extra skeletal myxoid chondrosarcomas. *Cancer Research*. https://www.semanticscholar.org/paper/9c8ed670378170d1a345c678ed4d2ae63e2fa952 (accessed on 17th July 2025).

47. Shinde, S., Mehandi, S., Wakte, S., Wagh, D. T., Eligeti, N., Gheware, A., et al. (2025). Crop-specific biotic stress management: Leveraging cytogenetic insights. *Plant Cell Biotechnology and Molecular Biology*. https://www.semanticscholar.org/paper/295737895ce36329d42ec21e5e73d761ca48aaf7 (accessed on 17th July 2025).

48. Song, J. O., Kwon, Y. D., Jeon, H. J., & Yang, B. I. (2025). Effect of Bobath concept-based rehabilitation on gait and balance in a hemiplegic patient: A case study. *Journal of Clinical Movement Science in Human*. https://www.semanticscholar.org/paper/4a7367b53f4e25c958987125b15cad8abe8a9b2b (accessed on 17th July 2025).

49. Sun, Y., Zhang, P., Zhang, N., Rong, L., Yu, X., Huang, X., & Li, Y. (2020). Cytogenetic analysis of 3387 umbilical cord blood in pregnant women at high risk for chromosomal abnormalities. *Molecular Cytogenetics, 13*. https://www.semanticscholar.org/paper/2098d488481fa081e988d5f215fc2cd98cad17e4 (accessed on 17th July 2025).

50. Swaminathan, M., Bannon, S., Routbort, M., Naqvi, K., Kadia, T., Takahashi, K., Alvarado, Y., et al. (2019). Hematologic malignancies and Li-Fraumeni syndrome. *Cold Spring Harbor Molecular Case Studies, 5*. https://www.semanticscholar.org/paper/dcd8fc3c1d7c207cf72f61fd99b0c15e576e131a (accessed on 17th July 2025).

51. Voss, R., Cardenas, M., Jin, M., Liu, Y. C., Siskar, A. N., Rice, S. V., Edmonson, M. N., et al. (2025). Abstract 7178: Advancing WGS and WTS diagnostic testing for pediatric leukemia: Fast-tracking CNV, ploidy, and fusion oncogene detection in 5 days. *Cancer Research*. https://www.semanticscholar.org/paper/c292de3c8182a5c215f5729d2a73c9bf34716e1d (accessed on 17th July 2025).

52. Wan, M., Simonin, E. M., Johnson, M., Zhang, X., Lin, X., Gao, P., Patel, C. J., et al. (2025). Exposomics: A review of methodologies, applications, and future directions in molecular medicine. *EMBO Molecular Medicine, 17*, 599–608. https://www.semanticscholar.org/paper/f04abe54d3a8340355d359758a2f8b1f0835dd18 (accessed on 17th July 2025).

53. Wan, T. S., & Ma, E. (2012). Molecular cytogenetics: An indispensable tool for cancer diagnosis. *Chang Gung Medical Journal, 35*(2), 96–110. https://www.semanticscholar.org/paper/11f1625f219598fdb4c7f2b018e1475107edd579 (accessed on 17th July 2025).

54. Warnat-Herresthal, S., Schultze, H., Shastry, K. L., Manamohan, S., Mukherjee, S., Garg, V., Sarveswara, R., et al. (2021). Swarm learning for decentralized and confidential clinical machine learning. *Nature, 594*, 265–270. https://doi.org/10.1038/s41586-021-03583-3 (accessed on 17th July 2025).

55. Weier, H., & O'Brien, B. (2012). Genetics and risk assessment. *Current Genomics, 13*, 417. https://www.semanticscholar.org/paper/b89926ac0293b75f8d2cc5d1f67771a3fbfead10 (accessed on 17th July 2025).

56. Wunderlich, B., Poleck-Dehlin, B., Chen, Z., Schmid, C., Cutler, C. S., De Witte, T., Bennett, J. M., et al. (2006). Clonal karyotype evolution involving ring chromosome 1 with myelodysplastic syndrome subtype RAEB-t progressing into acute leukemia. https://core.ac.uk/download/16432948.pdf (accessed on 17th July 2025).
57. Zhang, F., Liao, G., Wen, X., & Zhang, C. (2025). Prenatal diagnosis and molecular cytogenetic analyses of a rare 15q21.3 and 16p11.2 microduplication family. *Molecular Cytogenetics, 18*. https://www.semanticscholar.org/paper/64af92ab0c6b8e21ce724c6ba677e2a6d7810b70 (accessed on 17th July 2025).
58. Minzhenkova M.E., Antonenko V.G., Shilova N.V. International System for Human Cytogenomic Nomenclature (ISCN 2020): Additions and modifications in recording the results of fluorescence *in situ* hybridization and chromosomal microarray analysis in constitutional cytogenetics. *Medical Genetics*. 2023;22(4):11-16. (In Russ.) https://doi.org/10.25557/2073-7998.2023.04.11-16(accessed on 17th July 2025).

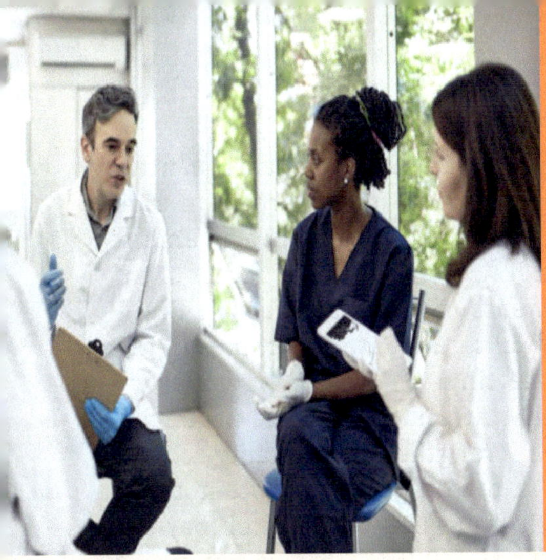

Chapter 13

QUALITY ASSURANCE AND LABORATORY MANAGEMENT

Contents

Introduction

The concept of quality assurance in laboratory management is integral to ensuring accurate and reliable test results, which are essential to patient safety and quality healthcare provision. Modern-day laboratories in the rapidly expanding medical age are under pressure to adapt to innovations in technology and methods while simultaneously imposing stringent quality controls. The challenge lies in the negotiation of the sophisticated regimes of regulation that govern laboratory work, such as the "Guide de Bonne Execution des Analyses" (GBEA) in Morocco, which are the foundation of quality assurance. Despite guidelines, there are discrepancies that could undermine patient safety and laboratory report integrity. Specifically, regulatory protocols of this sort lag behind evolving best practices in quality management and hence require careful reassessment and revision of current protocols to adapt to contemporary healthcare demands (Kharrazi et al., 2025). At the forefront of laboratory quality assurance enhancement is the implementation of systematic internal audits, which serve as a preparatory method for external evaluations and as a tool for ongoing compliance optimization. Regular internal auditing allows laboratories to track operational and quality measurements to guarantee continued conformity to stipulated standards. Through the application of audit procedures to specific clinical settings, e.g., those that happen in ambulatory care clinics, laboratories can gather significant data that inform best practices on operational efficacy as well as efficiency.

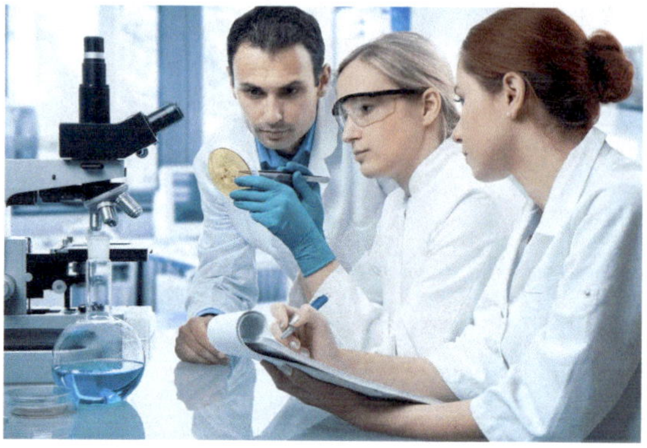

Figure 13.1. Quality assurance and laboratory management.

Source: https://www.learngxp.com/wp-content/uploads/2018/05/q.png.

A recent study has shown that the application of a formal audit process has the potential to bring about spectacular compliance rate increases in certain laboratory activities and has emphasized the importance of continuous inspection to enforce best practice among laboratory staff (Ronny et al., 2024). Such commitment not only maximizes quality assurance outcomes but also secures the laboratory manager's role in establishing accountability and uniformity culture. Last, creating an efficient quality assurance system in laboratory management involves integrative thinking and includes documentation, quality control, and employee education. Continued improvement through a process of iteration enables labs to efficiently manage the nuances of modern healthcare while maintaining patient safety as a central priority. As labs become more prone to risk management and continuous improvement principles, bringing in models of success from other environments, such as the French GBEA and CLIA, can facilitate greater outcomes in the Moroccan lab setting. By aligning regulatory obligations with international best practices, medical labs can strengthen their quality control measures and, in the bargain, promote not just operational efficiency but also better patient care (Kharrazi et al., 2025). Thus, commitment to ongoing improvement and responsiveness remains key in the quest for laboratory management quality assurance (Figure 13.1).

Definition of Quality Assurance

Quality assurance (QA) refers to an orderly process employed to ascertain that the products or services comply with set stipulated requirements and standards. In laboratory management, QA is essential in confirming the reliability and validity of experimental results. QA entails a list of systematic and planned activities, intentionally designed to raise the level of confidence in product development and operating procedures. By the implementation of QA processes, laboratories can minimize risks involved in test errors, which is an element that is very critical in vivarium facilities. Such working environments call for strict management and compliance in reference to animal welfare standards, along with correct utilization of state-of-the-art equipment to facilitate research outputs. As explained, ongoing improvement offered by quality assurance programs is a key element that could improve operating procedures and ensure compliance through systematic monitoring and auditing. Besides direct operational benefits, the integration of quality assurance in laboratories extends to fostering a culture of responsibility and excellence among employees. A standard QA framework allows laboratories to make systematic evaluations and improvements, as seen with activities like Gemba walks and Kaizen events. Such activities encourage participation by everyone on staff, creating a spirit of cooperation and shared responsibility for quality assurance. Subsequent adoption of 5S principles further supports improved organization and efficiency in the lab, facilitating ease of productivity and wastage reduction. Adoption of such practices allows laboratories not only to comply but also to improve utilization of space and operations' workflow, consequently assisting in general research purposes and animal care problems (Devan et al., 2024). The significance of quality assurance also appeals to other disciplines, such as the construction industry, proving its transdisciplinary relevance. Smoothly operating quality control systems, as enforced in construction, serve as mirrors to laboratory procedures, recalling one of the significances of specification and quality compliance in obtaining the best output. The QA ethos is not merely being compliant right from the beginning; it sets a culture for continuous learning so that experience gleaned from past projects or experiments can inform future practices. In the case of labs, it implies an effective QA system that is not only compliant with regulatory standards , such as ISO 9000 and ISO 14000, but also demonstrates dedication to improvement and innovation. By focusing on quality materials and monitoring in laboratory processes, quality assurance is a central pillar that ensures laboratory management's success and reliability (Devan et al., 2024).

Importance of Laboratory Management

Good lab management is the secret to ensuring quality assurance in research laboratories. With prioritized, well-structured workflows, effective communication systems, and adherence to ethical values, laboratory managers can minimize errors and maximize productivity. Structured systems of management enable researchers to maintain accurate records, which encourages reproducibility—a pillar of true scientific research. For instance, implementation of the ARRIVE guidelines places extra emphasis on detailed reporting in animal research so that transparency and accountability are improved (Percie et al., 2020). Laboratories can facilitate better study design through well-defined procedures, allowing subsequent researchers to replicate experiments effectively and build on existing findings even further, making the scientific community richer. Apart from improving reproducibility, effective laboratory management enhances safety culture and adherence to regulatory guidelines. Adherence to laid-down guidelines not only protects researchers but also the research subjects.

For example, updated guidelines for the use of non-domesticated mammalian species in research emphasize the responsibilities of researchers and regulatory bodies in ensuring ethical treatment during research activities (Robert, 2016). Through prioritizing safety protocols, lab management ensures that the risks associated with experimentation are minimized, ultimately creating a more sound and robust research outcome. Further, high commitment to safety encourages researchers to adopt best practices, hence reinforcing the validity of their research and the integrity of the scientific community at large. Finally, the significance of lab management is also evident in the way it optimizes collective effort within the scientific community.

By good management practices, lab leaders can create a culture of teamwork, interdisciplinarity, and sharing of information. This is particularly important in complex research environments where diverse fields of expertise must be mobilized to address complex problems. Effective management ensures an understanding of project goals and plans by the collective, which ultimately means breakthrough solutions and scientific advancements. Thus, integrating quality assurance mechanisms into laboratory management is not just a means to improve the performance of the individual lab but also contributes to the overall scientific community by facilitating setting up high-quality research focusing on the globe's most critical challenges (Figure 13.2).

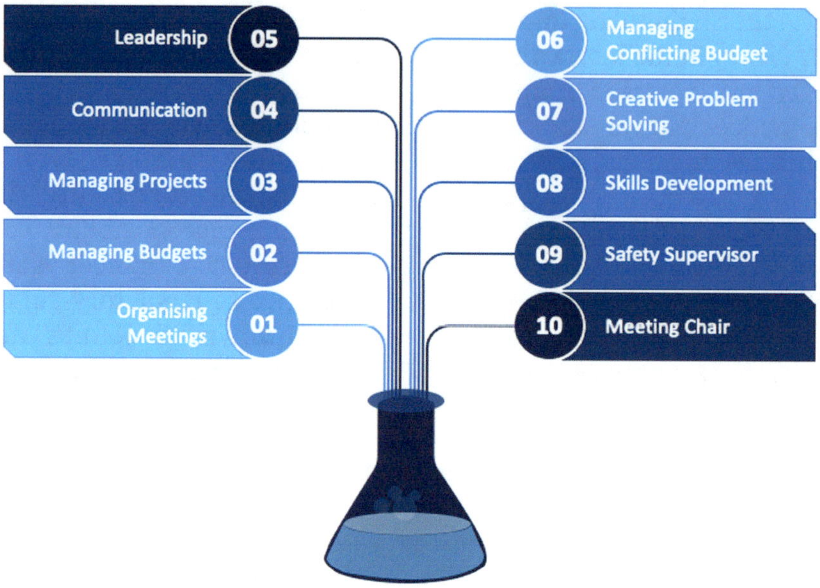

Figure 13.2. Importance of laboratory management.

Source: https://cdn.sketchbubble.com/pub/media/catalog/product/optimized1/9/a/9ae2b2a63ee f840baf7768af5acd3184abf39d05eff6c60baaffd8ddb5ec03f7/lab-management-slide4.png.

13.1. Historical Context of Quality Assurance

The roots of quality assurance (QA) can be traced back to the start of the 20th century, when the industrialization process saw a systematic approach to quality in manufacturing. The introduction of assembly lines and mass production required standardized practices for maintaining product consistency. Visionaries like W. Edwards Deming and Joseph Juran introduced statistical quality control methods, which significantly transformed industry work by highlighting data and measurement in achieving quality outcomes. This innovation was particularly significant in the pharma industry and biotechnology, whose laboratory environment demanded stringent quality requirements to safeguard product integrity as well as public safety. Initial models led to the development of more comprehensive quality assurance programs, and a culture took root in which continuous improvement was essential to maintaining high standards across various industries, including laboratory management. The history of the evolution of quality assurance systems is marked by the development of formalized standards and guidelines designed to enhance laboratory practices. The establishment of the Bethesda Reporting System of Cytological Diagnosis during the 1980s is a perfect example, as it helped to standardize reporting language and implement clearly delineated follow-up practices. The system significantly reduced the vagaries that always crept into medical diagnoses, enabling medical professionals to make well-educated decisions based on objective and credible information. Such standardization not only enhanced the agreement between cytopathologists but also enabled communication between clinical teams, thereby streamlining quality assurance processes. The effectiveness of the Bethesda system promoted further development in quality reporting and consolidated the notion that standardized practices were necessary for laboratories to generate and sustain high-quality outputs within a complex healthcare system (Layfield & Baloch, 2020). As the concept of quality assurance evolved, so did the methods applied to analyze and assure those standards. The application of technology to quality assurance processes became more prevalent, facilitating increased data collection and analysis. Software tools, such as those used to align Course Learning Outcomes (CLOs) with Student Outcomes (SOs), are one indicator of such increasing trends. These tools do the assessments automatically, allowing teachers more abilities for tracking performance and maintaining education programs accredited as needed (Imam & Tasadduq, 2012). This technology is just a part of a larger trend towards data-driven decision-making in laboratory management that promotes transparency and accountability in quality assurance systems. Even as laboratories continue to grapple with an evolving environment of challenges, the past provides some valuable lessons on building quality assurance, underlining the value of systematic and evidence-based practices in working towards laboratory excellence in administration.

13.1.1. Evolution of Quality Assurance Practices

The development of quality assurance procedures in laboratory management is a reaction to the sophistication in accuracy, reliability, and compliance requirements. Evolving from initial roots in basic quality control, there has been a widespread evolution of such processes, particularly with the introduction of systematic approaches , such as Quality Management Systems (QMS). QMS has become inevitable in laboratories by streamlining processes and guaranteeing conformity to local as well as international standards, such as those of ISO. The transition has not only enhanced the productivity of operations but has also played a key role in elevating the standard of patient safety and ensuring that laboratories deliver uniform, quality results. The developmental history of the same practices suggests a continuous pursuit towards improved methodologies that safeguard public health as well as the credibility of laboratory results, contributing significantly to the field of laboratory management (Mishra et al., 2025).

Developments in quality assurance have been greatly influenced by shifts in regulatory environments as well as advancements in technology. As the range of laboratory services and capabilities expanded, quality assurance practices developed to incorporate overall risk control strategies and adherence to Good Manufacturing Practices (GMP). The development of these stringent guidelines has contributed significantly to establishing quality management as a core pillar of laboratory activity. Moreover, the evolution of total quality management (TQM) methodologies has prompted organizations to use a systemic approach to quality that fosters a continuous improvement culture. The need to meet standards set by chief organizations, such as the FDA, has also increased the importance of maintaining high-quality levels in quality assurance processes, imposing responsive adjustments based on evolving industry requirements (Aroon et al., 2024). In today's laboratory settings, the introduction of new technologies has further driven the evolution of quality assurance policies. Automated systems, data analysis, and process improvement tools are increasingly applied to enhance accuracy and timeliness in laboratory operations. This trend is not only streamlining workflow but also enabling real-time monitoring of quality measures, which enables laboratories to respond instantly to deviations and maintain adherence to pre-established standards. Also, technology use allows efficient training and engaging staff in quality assurance processes so that employees are well-equipped to maintain quality standards. Together, these innovations are a revolutionary era in lab management with quality assurance focus being extremely synergistic to the overall goals of operational excellence and patient safety to make the lab's future-proof in combating upcoming challenges (Aroon et al., 2024; Mishra et al., 2025) (Figure 13.3).

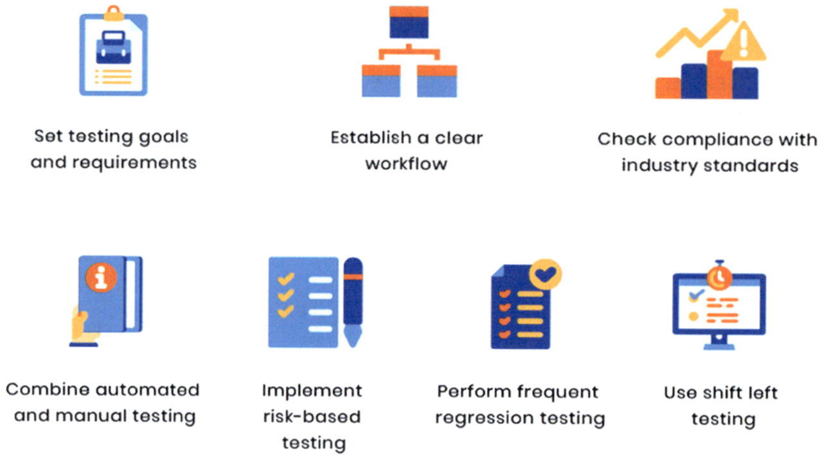

Figure 13.3. Evolution of quality assurance practices.

Source: https://rubygarage-production-production-bucket.s3.amazonaws.com/uploads/article_image/file/3542/3.png.

13.1.2. Key Milestones in Laboratory Management

The history of laboratory management has been marked by a series of milestones that reflect the growing significance of quality assurance in research. One of the significant milestones was the institution of standardized procedures that govern laboratory practice. Standardized procedures ensure laboratories operate at optimal efficiency levels even as they abide by legislation. Evolution towards a more structured approach in project management, like the creation of development plans as well as cost estimations, has been essential in upholding the integrity of lab operations. Organizational management problems concerning planning projects, generating deliverables, and performing audits have also allowed laboratories to have quality assurance standards, as Agresti et al. (1984) state. Therefore, these practices provide the arena through which scientific inquiry can gain a foothold and ultimately impact the larger world. A second pivotal change in laboratory management involves a focus on continuous improvement based upon data-driven decision-making. Effective laboratories are characterized by their ability to track metrics of performance, which can drive operational excellence as well as outcome accuracy. The use of management tools employed to monitor the status of projects and compare performance to standards has become more common.

The systematic approach enables laboratories to act proactively on quality assurance. Notably, the project management guidelines outlined by Koenig et al. (1979) are directives for how one can guarantee proper organization and control of projects, which is essential in optimizing laboratory activity performance. Their compliance reflects the continued resolve of laboratories to uphold high-quality assurance systems.

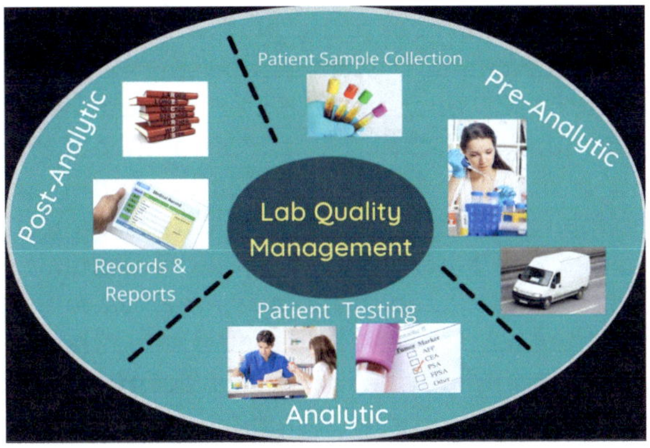

Figure 13.4. Key milestones in laboratory management.

Source: https://img.oercommons.org/oercommons/media/editor/342129/image-20220113003611-2.png.

The impact of information technology in laboratory management is another ground-breaking milestone. The incorporation of sophisticated software systems has revolutionized the gathering, analysis, and reporting of laboratory information. As such, laboratories have experienced increased accuracy and efficiency in their operations. Moreover, combining computer tools allows team members to communicate and collaborate better, a factor that is fundamental in a research environment. Through the utilization of management systems that track project timeliness and costs effectively, laboratories can ride through complex developments in their areas of research. Lastly, the innovations brought about by technology ensure laboratories are responsive and flexible to evolving scientific issues, further solidifying the role of quality assurance in offering stable and reproducible results (Figure 13.4).

13.1.3. Impact of Historical Events on Current Standards

The evolution of quality assurance in laboratory management may be traced through some of the pivotal events in history, which have had an impact on current standards. One such instance is the establishment of regulatory bodies following high-profile medical scandals and mistakes, which highlighted the urgent need for effective quality controls. For instance, the establishment of the Clinical Laboratory Improvement Amendments (CLIA) in 1988 was a reaction to laboratory testing errors. This act necessitated an entire spectrum of quality assurance practices, extending to laboratory testing and quality management. Such milestones in history highlighted the repercussions of lax regulatory control, pointing to the conviction that relentless quality standards have to be guaranteed to safeguard patient well-being and public confidence in healthcare organizations, particularly at a time when advanced technologies and complex methods of testing were the order of the day. Additionally, global health initiatives as well as international crises have played a crucial role in the evolution of quality assurance practices in laboratory management. The HIV/AIDS pandemic during the 1980s and 1990s necessitated the establishment of standardized testing protocols since disparate laboratory procedures led to variability in the treatment regimes and care of patients. This period marked a notable shift towards worldwide standardization of laboratory practice, emphasizing cooperation and shared knowledge amongst professionals. The emphasis on laboratory quality assurance not only improved diagnostic accuracy but also offered a platform for future laboratory management development. These past precursors highlight the demand for laboratories to evolve to adapt to emerging challenges, such that quality assurance is a vital cornerstone in the provision of credible healthcare services among various populations. Moreover, the integration of technological advancements into laboratory management has been influenced by past occurrences and the demand that has hence arisen for proper quality assurance schemes. The recent innovation of patient registries as essential tools for enhancing healthcare delivery has relied on lessons learned from earlier quality assurance initiatives. The registries, as discussed by Devan et al. (2024), are basically created to capture data quantifying patient outcomes, relating traditional means of data collection to contemporary methods. Similarly, the drive for improved health care quality among middle-income and low-income countries has called for greater focus on historical deficiencies in care quality, as encapsulated by Devan et al. (2024). This is the context in which today's standards have evolved, with the addition that genuine quality assurance not just enhances laboratory performance but also helps in addressing more general health system issues, leading to improved patient outcomes and a more efficient allocation of healthcare resources.

13.2. Principles of Quality Assurance

The use of effective quality assurance (QA) practices is central in laboratory management, particularly in health and clinic facilities. Principles of quality assurance include systematic approaches as well as regulatory compliance to guarantee laboratory practices yield credible as well as accurate results. These principles set a formal process to minimize error, uphold standards, and enhance overall service provision. For instance, compliance with protocols guided by clinical laboratory standards , such as those advocated for by CLSI and ISO, can considerably improve the consistency of laboratory findings. The guidelines help laboratories navigate through the complexities of test processes and documentation requirements so that results are not only accurate but timely as well. Aside from this, the application of effective QA frameworks also facilitates ongoing improvement where laboratories are able to maintain pace with emerging technologies and practices and yet maintain high standards of patient care (Srivastava et al., 2020). The presence of quality assurance principles also entails a multidimensional system comprising validation, verification, and monitoring of laboratory operations. Validation ensures methodologies and protocols are scientifically sound and pertinent to their stated use. This is typically achieved by rigorous testing and examination against established standards. Verification, on the other hand, involves the guarantee that the laboratory operations work as desired under real-world conditions. Ongoing oversight and review through internal audits and peer reviews also assist in confirming the commitment to quality, offering means of identifying non-conformities and taking corrective action. By incorporating these aspects, laboratories not only achieve the regulatory requirements but also embrace an ethic of quality improvement that enhances staff accountability and patient safety (Arnold et al., 2019). Encouragement of stakeholder involvement, including laboratory staff, clinicians, and patients, is vital in achieving successful implementation of quality assurance practices. There should be a team-based effort to ensure that all stakeholders understand their roles and responsibilities in ensuring quality standards are maintained. This may entail regular staff training sessions focusing on the importance of adhering to QA protocols and the consequent impact on patient outcomes. Secondly, encouraging open channels of communication among staff allows the flow of feedback and ideas, thus further enhancing procedures and policy. Encouraging a culture of constant quality improvement aids laboratories in remaining responsive to evolving dynamics in healthcare needs. Therefore, by giving QA due priority, laboratories can increase their operational efficiencies and eventually contribute toward better patient care outcomes, mitigating previous constraints in service delivery (Srivastava et al., 2020) (Figure 13.5).

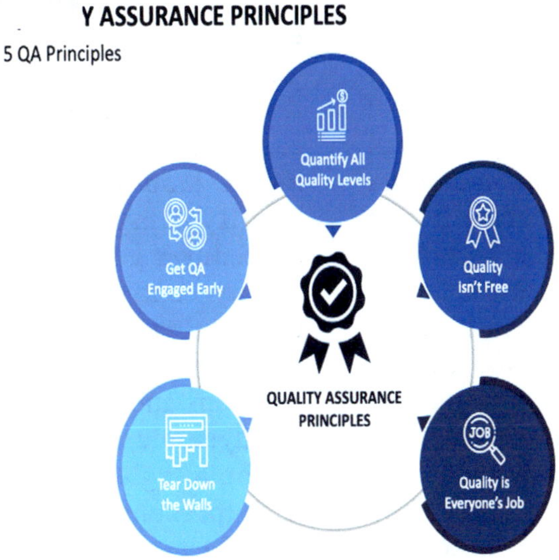

Figure 13.5. Principles of quality assurance.

Source: https://cdn.sketchbubble.com/pub/media/catalog/product/optimized1/a/0/a0960032104d591a712f71c0adfaa1c199fdeed3c4ddc42502befbbf57246c44/quality-assurance-principles-slide1.png.

13.2.1. Accuracy and Precision in Testing

Precision and accuracy in laboratory management are vital to the integrity of test findings. Accuracy refers to how close the results of a test estimate the true value, whereas precision refers to the reproducibility of results under the same conditions. These two variables are critical for proper laboratory testing, particularly in clinical settings where the outcome directly affects patient care. For instance, in a project that analyzed the performance of clinical chemistry laboratories in Ethiopia, none of the participating institutions could maintain accurate test results for a set of parameters on a consistent basis. About 65% of the data presented were outside the tolerable allowable error limits, indicating significant errors in precision and accuracy that would lead to misdiagnosis or inappropriate treatments (Teka & Kibatu, 2012). Thus, re-education and awareness of these basic principles are imperative to embed quality assurance protocols into laboratory environments. Quality assurance schemes must incorporate rigorous procedures to improve accuracy and precision. This could be achieved through a variety of methods, including regular equipment calibration, the use of control samples, and keeping standard testing protocols. Through the implementation of these practices, laboratories are able to minimize systematic errors and improve the quality of their results. For example, the Arkansas Water Resources Center employs a quality control report in each analysis to provide clients with useful information on the performance of testing procedures

(Austin et al., 2017). These practices not only instill greater confidence in laboratory results but also enable laboratory staff to continually improve testing procedures. Therefore, there is a need for an overarching quality assurance system with a special focus on regular audits and method validation to maintain high laboratory performance levels. Technical intervention is complemented by necessitating a culture of quality assurance among laboratory personnel as well. This involves training staff members regarding the significance of precision and accuracy in testing and instilling a feeling of responsibility and ownership for work., including laboratory technicians in the quality assurance process can enhance their vigilance during the testing process, reducing opportunities for human error that can sabotage test outcomes. Laboratories also need to check and update their quality management systems from time to time, in response to new advances in testing methodologies and technologies, so that they can continue to improve the services offered. As this Ethiopian research shows, regular surveys and assessments allow recurrent issues to be precisely identified with accuracy so that the facilities act on them in a manner that ultimately winds up adding up to patient care (Teka & Kibatu, 2012). Definitive protocols, together with a culture of quality, are the building blocks of good laboratory management.

13.2.2. Standard Operating Procedures (SOPs)

Standard Operating Procedures (SOPs) are central components of the Quality Assurance and Laboratory Management practice that ensure uniformity and reliability of laboratory procedures. Through the provision of comprehensive, crisp, and reproducible protocols, SOPs enable laboratory personnel to perform tasks consistently regardless of the individual performing them. Such consistency is particularly crucial in research environments because variations in procedures lead to incongruent outcomes and compromise the integrity of the data. The development and implementation of SOPs instill an environment in which compliance with regulatory standards becomes the norm, and ultimately, the credibility and working efficiency of the laboratory are enhanced. Moreover, SOPs facilitate training and induction of new personnel, which enables them to acquire intricate procedures quickly and easily. Incorporation of SOPs into daily activities in the laboratory also promotes continuous quality improvement measures. When procedures adhere to established standards of quality control, laboratories are in a position to objectively evaluate their performance and identify areas for improvement. Systematic revisions and reviews of SOPs take into account the dynamic process of scientific research, so methodologies remain current and aligned with present needs. This dynamic process is reflected in the revision of the ARRIVE guidelines, aimed at increasing transparency in biomedical research by instating required reporting standards in *in vivo* experiments. Implementation of updated SOPs allows laboratories to follow these standards effectively and shows a high commitment to increasing research reproducibility and reliability since the updated guidelines for hormone receptor testing in breast cancer management specify (Percie et al., 2020). Furthermore, SOPs elevate their significance above core operations by emphasizing documentation and reporting in laboratory activities. They regulate how test data, operating conditions, and quality control steps are recorded and reported. That record becomes critical in facilitating audits and inspections because it is a complete trail of compliance and performance information. The American Society of Clinical Oncology/College of American Pathologists provides a specific example with a recommendation to develop laboratory-specific SOPs specifying how results, particularly hormone receptor testing, are to be confirmed and reported. Such specificity of procedure assists laboratories in maintaining high standards in working with complicated testing regimens and promoting stakeholder confidence in the results produced (Kimberly et al., 2020). Hence, SOPs not only support operational consistency but also support the overall quality assurance system of the laboratory (Figure 13.6).

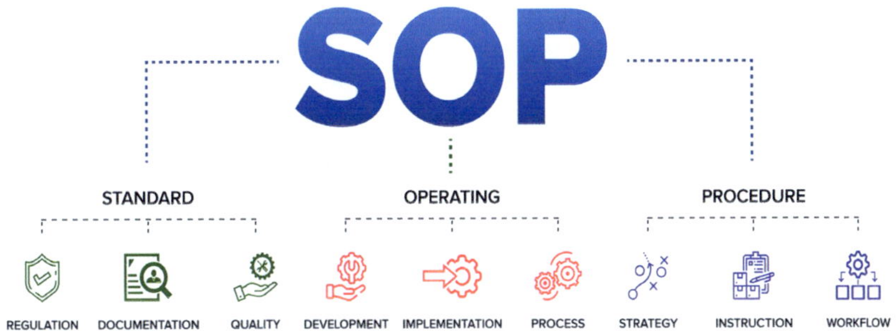

Figure 13.6. Standard operating procedures (SOPs).

Source: https://info.safelinkconsulting.com/hubfs/SOP.jpg.

13.2.3. Continuous Improvement Processes

Continuous improvement processes are of utmost importance in laboratory quality assurance and management because they provide an environment in which systematic monitoring and evaluation of laboratory processes result in better results. These processes rely on the recognition and application of quality indicators (QIs), which are measurable factors that enable laboratories to perform at high levels of care. For Point of Care Testing (POCT), these QIs are particularly important. As POCT volumes and test menus increase, formal QIs help monitor errors and ensure the quality of test results. By continuously evaluating the preanalytical, analytical, and post-analytical phases of the test, laboratories experience a spiral of ongoing quality development necessary to cope with the complexities of modern diagnostic needs (Brun et al., 2021). That which is committed to continuous improvement must adopt Total Quality Management (TQM) principles, which provide a methodical approach to quality assurance. Application of TQM relies on continuous assessment of laboratory practices against established standards and guidelines, as maintained by institutions , such as the Clinical Laboratory Standards Institute (CLSI) and the International Organization for Standardization (ISO). Through having a structured approach, laboratories ensure they comply not only with regulations but also become excellent in the delivery of quality. As noted, failure to meet regulatory requirements could result in severe outcomes like loss of accreditation and operating license. Therefore, establishing a strong TQM system that involves continuous training, auditing, and feedback mechanisms plays a vital role in keeping quality assurance activities under laboratory management (Arnold et al., 2019). Additionally, constant improvement is based on the identification of areas of strength needing enhancement. This calls for a culture that is open to receive feedback, internal audits, as well as external inspections, not just to be accepted but also to be acted upon immediately. Laboratories must track key performance indicators to identify trends, correct non-conformities and allow for corrective actions. Involving staff at all levels in these discussions ensures collective responsibility towards quality improvement and promotes mutual commitment to the laboratory's cause. Lastly, process improvement processes have a feedback loop where data analysis, staff participation, and management are in compliance to maximize laboratory performance and patient safety. Harmonizing the practice yields overall improvement that allows laboratories to properly leverage the evolving health care environment, thereby creating client trust and patient outcomes (Brun et al., 2021; Arnold et al., 2019).

13.3. Regulatory Frameworks

Regulatory frameworks are crucial for the regulation of high levels of standards in laboratory management and quality assurance across various industries. They provide structured guidelines for adherence to safety procedures and operation best practices that have been laid out. In laboratory settings, regulatory frameworks are critical for safeguarding public health by ensuring the credibility and integrity of research and testing outcomes. By adhering to guidelines , such as Good Laboratory Practice (GLP) or guidance in the format outlined in the 21 CFR Part 11, laboratories can better manage their data and process integrity. Further, regulations set expectations for equipment and human resources alike, enabling a quality management initiative across the board that minimizes risk and maximizes organizational accountability. The commitment to regulation allows for the laboratory environment to be a platform that is centered on accuracy and reliability and ultimately benefits stakeholders and end-users. Technology evolution necessitates ongoing innovation in regulatory systems, as seen in the use of informatics solutions in the laboratory. Technologies are designed not only for increasing performance but also to ensure that regulatory compliance is adequate. As pointed out by Kannan (2025), there are specific software programs like Laboratory Information Management Systems (LIMS) and Electronic Laboratory Notebooks (ELNs) that form the backbone of modern laboratory management, which encourage solid data integrity. These systems have detailed documentation mechanisms that enable laboratories to track all the parameters of their work from discovery to manufacturing.

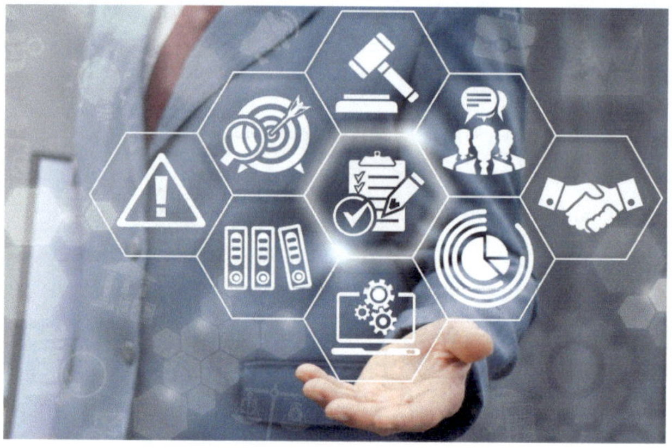

Figure 13.7. Regulatory frameworks.

Source: https://finreg-e.com/wp-content/uploads/2022/08/regulatory-framework.jpeg.

The changing nature of regulatory needs necessitates that laboratories update their practice from time to time to synchronize with new guidelines so that their quality assurance systems can hold up to scrutiny while facilitating scientific progress. Besides, the interface between regulatory frameworks and emerging technology is also changing laboratory management. By embracing Artificial Intelligence (AI) and Machine Learning (ML) technologies, laboratories can significantly enhance their quality assurance processes. With certain industries beginning to implement these technologies, the potential for increasing compliance and risk management is clearer than ever before. AI/ML makes it possible for laboratories to automate compliance testing, push data security, and ensure maximum performance testing, aligning with evolving regulatory requirements as illustrated by Pareek (2024). Not only does this forward-thinking approach render laboratory processes easy, but it also ensures a flexible environment that remains responsive to regulatory changes. Finally, by integrating these cutting-edge methodologies into their regulatory systems, laboratories can ensure their dedication to quality assurance while maintaining a high degree of flexibility in an evolving environment (Figure 13.7).

13.3.1. Overview of Relevant Regulations (e.g., ISO, GLP)

Understanding relevant regulations, the International Organization for Standardization (ISO) standards, and Good Laboratory Practice (GLP) is vital to the maintenance of quality assurance in laboratory management. ISO standards provide an approach to ensuring products and services conform to customers' requirements as well as regulations. Several ISO standards, such as ISO 9001 for quality management systems and ISO/IEC 17025 for testing and calibration laboratories, offer guidelines for quality assurance practice. Moreover, the specific conformity and accreditation procedures outlined in these standards allow laboratories to demonstrate their competence and reliability. Compliance with such guidelines not only confirms the results of a laboratory but also encourages confidence by customers in the services being provided, and this is a source of competitive edge for laboratory management. Laboratories have to adhere to rigorous practices in GLP that result in reliable and reproducible research outcomes. GLP guidelines are particularly crucial in nonclinical laboratory studies, impacting the generation, documentation, and reporting of data. GLP compliance involves satisfying set standards for qualifications of staff, equipment maintenance, and facility management, which adds to the integrity of the outcomes generated (Hukkanen et al., 2023). Adherence to these set practices helps laboratories guarantee that their research is conducted in an ethical manner and within regulatory stipulations, thus protecting public safety and health. A robust GLP system not only improves the generation of good data but also encourages regulatory filings, ensuring laboratories stay within the parameters of national and international law. Outside of the previous rules, the interplay of third-party certification and quality assurance is particularly important in laboratory settings. Third-party evaluators play a vital role in verifying that laboratories comply with the required standards, thus raising the validity of their findings. For example, in solar thermal systems, ISO certifications play a critical role in ensuring product quality as well as safeguarding consumers (Alkishriwi et al., 2021). Certification bodies, through schemes , such as ISO/IEC 17065 for product certification, conduct independent testing that helps clarify a laboratory's compliance with anticipated standards. Through the encouragement of culture in compliance and continuous improvement through third-party auditing, labs can meet the ever-evolving requirements of quality assurance and boost their market credibility.

13.3.2. Role of Regulatory Bodies in Quality Assurance

The function of regulatory institutions in ensuring quality assurance in laboratory management is central to guaranteeing that testing procedures, results, and related healthcare practices are up to the required standards. Regulatory agencies are responsible for developing frameworks and guidelines that laboratories should adhere to, which helps instill public confidence in the reliability and accuracy of laboratory findings. An example is that regulatory bodies tend to develop guidelines on performing quality inspections, dealing with compliance issues with regulations, and undertaking risk management measures. Such an initiative not only educates laboratory practice but also permits necessary audits and evaluations that ensure laboratories operate within set parameters of safety and efficacy. The involvement of regulators is crucial, as it is on their basis that laboratories are in a position to construct robust quality assurance systems that live up to domestic and international standards, placing the healthcare industry on uniformity (Devan et al., 2024). Besides this, regulatory bodies conduct regular checks and assessments to verify compliance with established standards of quality. Through these assessments, discrepancies from preferred standards could be identified, and suitable action could be quickly taken to remedy observed shortcomings. This surveillance plays an important role in ensuring that there is immense care because it aids in protecting patients against erroneous reports of diagnoses that could lead to mishandling of medical conditions. By insisting on the use of strict quality control protocols, regulatory agencies are also encouraging laboratories to adopt new technology and methodology. This fosters an environment of continuous improvement under which laboratories can optimize the efficiencies of their functions while concurrently keeping patient safety a top priority (Tauben et al., 2020). Lastly, government agencies play a decisive role in defining the education and training requirements of laboratory personnel to provide them with the qualifications and knowledge needed to ensure quality assurance standards. By defining laboratory personnel competencies and mandatory professional development, these agencies help build an effective workforce able to adapt to the evolving needs of laboratory management. Training and educational programs promoted by regulatory bodies are means of minimizing human error, which tends to be one of the primary causes of quality failures in labs. Furthermore, these kinds of programs can strengthen a culture of responsibility among lab employees, which, in the end, leads to improved patient outcomes as well as laboratory service confidence (Arnold et al., 2019) (Figure 13.8).

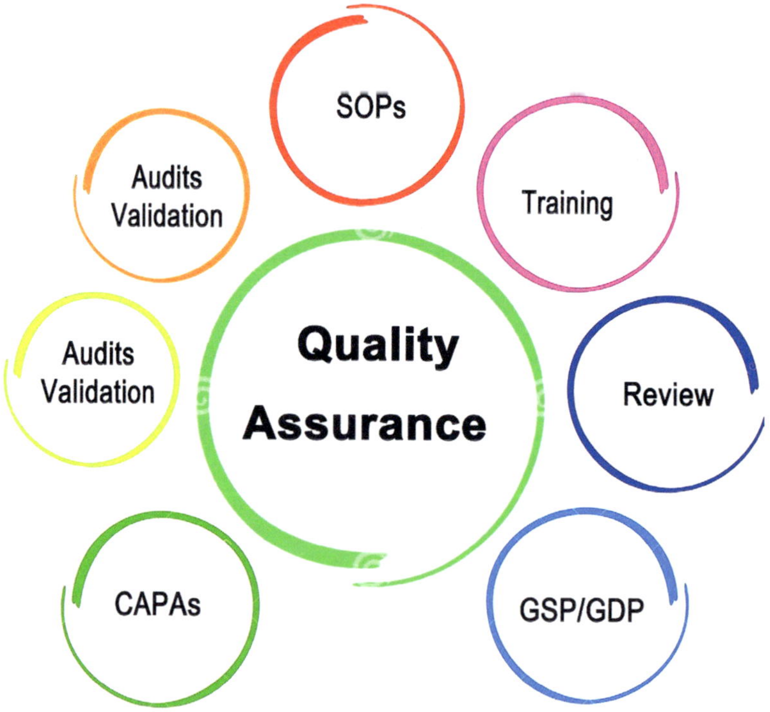

Figure 13.8. Role of regulatory bodies in quality assurance.

Source: https://1.bp.blogspot.com/-S6nr8c8-MMI/XrUUmNcc01I/AAAAAAAABBE/9JibG6tFaTohETatZ4ad44XUfkH2tzFhgCLcBGAsYHQ/s1600/quality-assurance-143478166.jpg.

13.3.3. Compliance and Its Importance in Laboratory Settings

Compliance is a required foundation for maintaining operating integrity and enhancing the quality of test results in labs. Compliance involves following standard operating procedures (SOPs), regulatory compliance, and ethical standards as prescribed by the regulating authorities. Mechanisms of compliance ensure that laboratory operations are within established limits, hence safeguarding the interests of patients, researchers, and stakeholders. For instance, when laboratories follow compliance procedures rigorously, they minimize the possibility of errors during experiments and analysis, which in turn leads to more precise outputs. The importance of this practice is well considered within institutions of learning, as observed from practices that have been adopted in health management courses that specialize in laboratory compliance (Students of Health Management 721.01, 2017). By fostering a culture of compliance, laboratories can build a valid environment that enhances the validity of their research findings. Moreover, the significance of compliance not only exceeds internal laboratory procedures but also exerts an important impact on external associations and reputations. Compliant laboratories are likely to achieve more tolerance from regulatory authorities, industry collaborators, and funding agencies. This sense of trust can lead to further collaboration opportunities and improved financing, which are essential to continued research activities. Furthermore, when laboratories demonstrate a consistent record of following regulations, they assist in advancing scientific knowledge while minimizing risks associated with legal and financial repercussions of non-compliance. For instance, the Proven Care model in healthcare emphasizes the significance of how adherence to complete standards can create better outcomes and use of resources (McCarthy et al., 2009). The same model can be transferred to laboratory environments, where adherence provides a culture of responsibility and innovation. Ultimately, the compliance culture in laboratories not only enhances quality assurance but also spurs continuous improvement in laboratory management practice. Laboratories that are actively engaged in activities of compliance are better placed to identify areas of betterment, whether methodological or technological, in application. It is through this active measure that laboratories are able to systematically apply quality management, whereby they can use data-driven information to enhance practices. Furthermore, the process of effective training programs directed at compliance guarantees that workers remain abreast of evolving standards and regulations. As scientific surroundings become increasingly sophisticated, such dedication to compliance is an invaluable asset that upholds unimpeachable standards of quality and reliability in laboratory findings. By embracing compliance as not a duty but an integral component of laboratory ethos, organizations can be confident of sustained progress in scientific research and healthcare delivery.

13.4. Quality Control Techniques

Quality control processes play a critical role in ensuring test results' accuracy and reliability in the context of quality assurance and laboratory control. These include a sequence of methodologies that are designed to oversee and improve laboratory procedures, thereby reducing errors and enhancing output quality. Among the most highly visible methods are statistical process control (SPC), analytical method validation, and proficiency testing, all contributing to an all-encompassing system of guaranteeing strict standards for laboratory work. Through the strict application of such quality control methodologies, laboratories can detect variation and inconsistency in test results, enabling a platform to identify areas of necessary improvement. Furthermore, the inclusion of quality control procedures fosters a culture of continuous learning and adaptation, which is particularly important in the dynamic world of laboratory science. An equally important aspect of laboratory quality control involves the implementation of internal quality control (IQC) and external quality assessment (EQA) schemes. IQC is defined as routines and practices used within the laboratory to ensure that each analytical run meets prescribed quality standards. This can be through the application of control materials and reagents which mimic real samples so that testing results inconsistencies can be detected before affecting patient care. Conversely, EQA schemes monitor laboratories' performance against other laboratories' results and thus provide an external measure of quality.

Participation in EQA schemes enhances laboratory results confidence and encourages laboratories to use best practice. Use of both IQC and EQA is necessary for any laboratory that wishes to achieve credibility and guarantee regulatory compliance in its quality assurance processes. The use of new technologies , such as automation and computerized data handling, has greatly enhanced the effectiveness of quality control techniques in laboratories. Automation saves time by reducing monotonous work, eliminating human error, and allowing for more precise monitoring of performance. Furthermore, electronic laboratory information management systems (LIMS) are able to facilitate real-time tracking of quality control data, hence prompt responses to deviations from the expected outcomes.

Additionally, technical advances provide laboratories with sophisticated tools to interpret quality control data more effectively and facilitate informed decision-making for continued improvement. This insertion of technology not only adds to the power of quality control measures but also aligns with the evolving needs of laboratory management, whereby the need for efficiency and precision continues to rise in tandem with the level of sophistication in testing laboratories.

13.4.1. Statistical Process Control (SPC)

Statistical Process Control (SPC) is a valuable tool in quality control, particularly in laboratory management, where precision and accuracy are paramount. By applying SPC methods, laboratories can closely monitor and control their processes such that variations in performance are identified and addressed instantly. With control charts that are part of SPC, real-time visualizations of trends and deviations of processes are enabled. Such real-time feedback is critical to laboratories striving diligently to comply with rigorous regulatory requirements and provide high-quality outputs. In addition, according to various research studies, the capacity to efficiently analyze data contributes to continuous improvement undertakings. Laboratories can thus optimize their workflow, reduce errors, and enhance the reliability of results, hence making direct contributions to enhanced health outcomes and facility operations in healthcare institutions. For healthcare interventions, the efficacy of Statistical Process Control is amply illustrated using its application in monitoring acute kidney injury (AKI). Recent analysis based on serum creatinine (SCr) data revealed the feasibility of SPC in quantifying the incidence and impact of AKI across healthcare settings. With the aid of instruments , such as Donabedian's model, SPC techniques—, such as control charts and funnel plots—can graphically illustrate AKI-related outcomes trends, facilitating the pursuit of an evidence-based quality improvement strategy. These methods also provide useful information on care interventions on patient outcomes. The ability to leverage SPC enhances not only the detection of AKI incidents but also laboratory practice culture of improvement and accountability, as it puts into perspective the worth of standardized measurement in health care quality assurance (Holmes et al., 2023). Moreover, practice applications of Statistical Process Control result in meaningful improvement in manufacturing environments from which laboratory management practices can learn. For instance, a study of machining operations of a car factory demonstrated the capability of SPC in enhancing quality indices, such as Process Capability Index (Cpk) and Process Performance Index (Ppp). Through the systematic implementation of SPC philosophy, coupled with the Plan-Do-Check-Act approach, researchers experienced notable improvement in process stability as well as a decline in defect rates. This empirical evidence resonates with the assertion that SPC can serve as a driving force to identify gaps in quality control, which ultimately means improved quality standards for laboratory work. The comparisons between manufacturing and laboratory processes demonstrate cross-domain applicability of SPC techniques to provide quality assurance, thereby spurring further development across scientific and clinical research (Devan et al., 2024) (Figure 13.9).

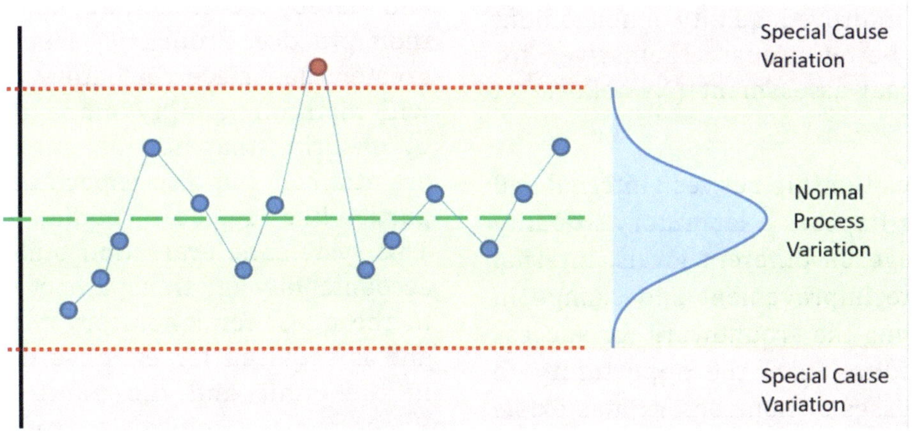

Figure 13.9. Statistical process control (SPC).

Source: https://www.zometric.com/wp-content/uploads/sites/9/2023/03/SPC-For-beginners.jpg.

13.4.2. Internal and External Audits

At the center of effective laboratory quality assurance management is the internal and external audit. Internal audits offer a key mechanism for ensuring compliance with protocols developed and identifying opportunities where improvement can be achieved. Through systematic testing, laboratories can ensure that standards of operation are concomitant with professional and regulatory standards. For instance, a systematic audit checklist for specific laboratory settings can enable proper documentation and tracking of quality controls. This move not only empowers laboratories to pass external audits but also promotes ongoing improvement. Indeed, findings of an internal audit demonstrated an overall increase in compliance by 84% over six months, illustrating the impact of rigorous internal auditing on laboratory standards (Ronny et al., 2024). Internal audits thereafter are a paramount necessity for building a quality management environment. External audits, on the other hand, are meant to verify a laboratory's compliance with external standards and regulations. These audits are typically carried out with the assistance of third-party examiners who contrast the practices, equipment, and personnel of the laboratory with pre-approved criteria. The worth of outside audits is in providing an unbiased assessment, which creates credibility and faith in lab findings and is critical for patient care, safety and outcomes. Laboratories pursuing accreditation will be required to undergo outside auditing processes not just to acquire the certification but also to enhance their working effectiveness. The application of a Quality Management System (QMS) is most beneficial here, as it provides elaborate procedures for acquiring compliance with internal and external standards. Laboratories in most parts of the world, including Nigeria, have already begun embracing QMS to address their specific issues and facilitate improved quality management practices and better prepare themselves for effective external assessment (Nwaokorie et al., 2018).

Also, the relationship between internal and external audits imposes a laboratory's quality assurance pledge on different levels. Internal audits facilitate improvement and change in operations, laying the groundwork for success in external audits. Since the opportunity to correct weaknesses or non-conformities exists through internal audits, laboratories can predict difficulties before their analysis through an external audit. This double strategy not only strengthens a laboratory's quality management capacity but also enhances the overall efficiency of health service provision. Employees' participation in internal and external audit cycles facilitates accountability and promotes professional development, leading to a culture of quality. Lastly, sound audit practices come into fruition in laboratories that not only meet but exceed quality assurance standards, therefore being in a position to deliver consistent and timely results required for patient care. The foundation of laboratory management is continual improvement, shaping not only internal audit plans and responses to external audits as key components of an integrated system of quality assurance.

13.4.3. Proficiency Testing and Benchmarking

One of the most important components of Quality Assurance and Laboratory Management is proficiency testing and benchmarking. Proficiency testing is one of the most important tools used by laboratories to gauge their analytical performance against predetermined specifications. Laboratories are provided with objective feedback through these tests on how well they can produce accurate and reliable results. This is significant feedback, for it enables laboratories to identify areas for improvement and thereby create continuous improvement in their practice. Proficiency testing has a value greater than mere regulatory requirement; it will maintain quality management systems by ensuring that not just internal standards are attained, but also expectations of external parties like regulatory bodies and customers. This systematic evaluation builds a culture of accountability and transparency that is essential in the quest for laboratory result confidence and is required for effective decision-making in the clinic and the plant (Patra, 2021). Benchmarking improves proficiency testing by providing laboratories with comparative data that can potentially lead to improved performance. Laboratories are able to compare their practice with that of peer organizations or industry-determined best practices through benchmarking. This comparative assessment helps laboratories identify their competitiveness position and informs strategy development to improve. For example, performance measurement metrics , such as turnaround time, accuracy, and cost-effectiveness can be assessed to implement certain strategies based on effective practices in other institutions. Benchmarking not only motivates laboratories to enhance operations but also fosters learning and inter-institutional collaboration. Collaborative benchmarking can lead to innovations that broaden the quality management system horizon and can ultimately find expression in improved service delivery and outcomes for patients in healthcare facilities (Nadkarni, 2005). The union of proficiency testing and benchmarking creates a solid base for quality assurance in laboratory regulation. Together, they foster a platform in which ongoing improvement is not just encouraged but also objectively recorded. Laboratories that employ these practices can achieve greater performance because they create a platform of guaranteed competency, yet are not resistant to new challenges and technology. Moreover, integrated knowledge acquired from proficiency tests and benchmarking can assist strategic decision-making so that laboratories remain ahead of their line of work. By a systemic approach to quality assurance through these measures, laboratories are able to earn the trust of clients and regulatory bodies alike, thereby enhancing their reputation and gaining a competitive edge in an aggressive market scenario (Patra, 2021) (Figure 13.10).

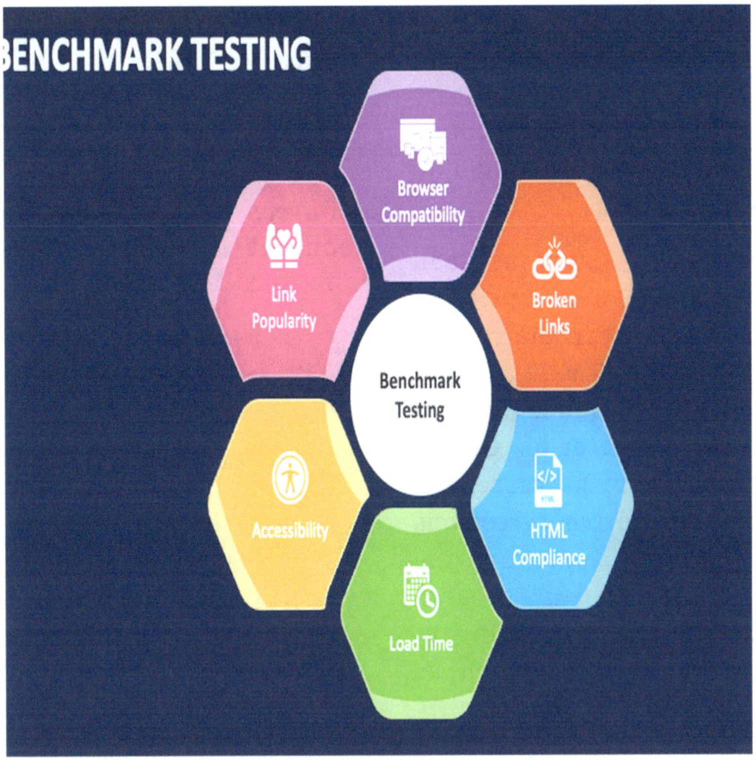

Figure 13.10. Proficiency testing and benchmarking.

Source: https://worldwidedigest.com/wp-content/uploads/2023/08/benchmark-testing-slide1.png.

13.5. Laboratory Management Practices

In today's laboratory setting, effective management practice is important in maintaining quality assurance and operational efficiency. One of the essential elements of laboratory management is building standardized operating procedures (SOPs) that govern day-to-day operation and activities. SOPs guarantee consistency and accuracy in laboratory procedures, thereby reducing errors and ensuring reliability in research outputs. In addition, ongoing training and certification programs for laboratory personnel are required to equip employees with the knowledge and capabilities to adhere to known procedures. Therefore, this emphasis on training not only improves individual performance but also collectively facilitates the laboratory's capability to produce high-quality results, demonstrating a commitment to excellence that is critical in an aggressive research setting. Moreover, the role of quality assurance programs cannot be overstated when it comes to laboratory management. Incorporation of such programs involves continuous auditing and assessment, which targets the identification of areas of improvement in laboratory operations. One of the quality assurance programs in laboratory animal facilities is to target continuous improvement through independent audits and compliance verification.

By adopting practices , such as lean management, laboratories can optimize operations, as has been evident in the case of vivarium environments where drastic changes have significantly enhanced productivity and utilization of resources (Devan et al., 2024). These practices not only simplify processes but also ensure that there are no transgressions of regulatory norms, thus complementing the laboratory's ethical stance towards research and ensuring the health and well-being of research subjects. In some cases, such as in food safety testing laboratories, quality assurance is controlled by strict regulations involving meticulous procedures for testing and monitoring. For example, in *Trichinella* spp. detection laboratories, the application of a Quality Management System (QMS) is not only effective but compulsory, considering the public health status of this parasitic infection (José et al., 2023). The QMS guarantees an organized quality assurance process by applying standard procedures, training, and inter-laboratory audits. Properly organized monitoring guarantees that laboratories maintain high standards, and in the end, public health is protected by ensuring the safety of meat products. Hence, quality assurance-based laboratory management practices play a crucial role in ensuring research integrity and public safety in the majority of scientific disciplines (Figure 13.11).

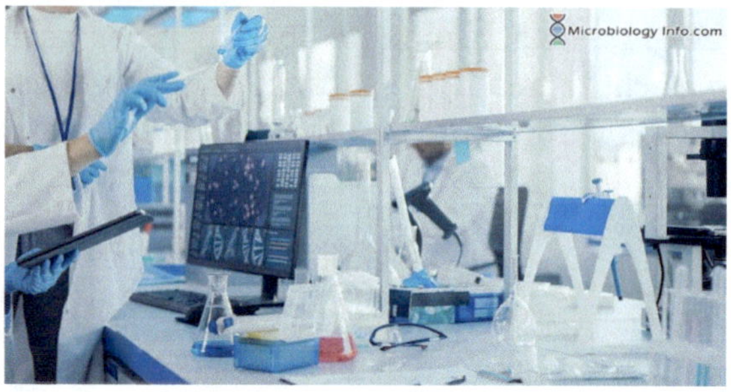

Figure 13.11. Laboratory management practices.

Source: https://microbiologyinfo.com/wp-content/uploads/featured-good-laboratory-practices-1024x538.jpg.

13.5.1. Resource Allocation and Management

Effective resource deployment is essential in laboratory management and quality assurance, as it has a direct bearing on the efficiency and capabilities of laboratory functions. With progressively complex laboratory settings occasioned by improved technology and increasingly stringent regulatory requirements, strategic deployment of human, monetary, and physical resources is increasingly important. For instance, the integration of new treatments and holistic care protocols for hemophilia emphasizes a need to furnish laboratories with not only state-of-the-art technology but also staff equipped to work utilizing new protocols (Srivastava et al., 2020). This necessitates a structured approach to the training of laboratory staff to ensure they are able to maintain high standards, thereby maximizing the use of resources and improving patient outcomes. Thus, resource allocation focuses on overall laboratory management effectiveness and the encouragement of environments in which quality assurance can gain a foothold. Resource management is rooted at the center with the coordination of open communication channels between clinical staff and laboratory teams. The two groups need to work together closely to effectively determine resource needs, prioritize, and allocate adequate funding towards equipment and human resource training requirements (Percie et al., 2020). This integration ensures that laboratory services are consistent with clinical demands, ultimately enhancing patient care quality. For example, having defined procedures for obtaining consumables and clotting factor concentrates will avoid service delivery time lags and enhance patient safety. Besides, continuous review of strategies for resource allocation allows laboratories to stay in line with evolving healthcare environments in a manner that maintains adherence to both current and future demands in quality assurance practices. Lastly, the utilization of quality assurance programs effectively is part and parcel of resource allocation activities and management within laboratories. These facilitate efficient and effective utilization of resources, leading to better overall patient outcomes. By executing evidence-based guidelines in practice, laboratories are able to enhance efficiency and minimize waste, thus being able to deliver higher standards of care (Srivastava et al., 2020). Further, regular evaluation of practices of resource allocation against known benchmarks enables laboratories to identify gaps and areas of improvement, thus promoting a culture of excellence (Percie et al., 2020). With changing demands in healthcare, continuing investment in quality assurance efforts will be critical for laboratories that intend to deliver high-quality, patient-focused care in an environment of resource shortages.

13.5.2. Staff Training and Development

Good staff development and training are integral parts of achieving quality assurance in laboratory management. Properly trained workers can use established protocols and procedures, which can reduce the level of errors significantly and render test findings more reliable. Training can be carried out using various methods, including on-the-job training, workshop training, and formal education. This multi-dimensional strategy ensures that laboratory staff are aware of the necessity of quality assurance procedures, resulting in increased accountability on their part. In settings where exact results are crucial, like clinical laboratories, continuous enhancement of staff expertise and knowledge is not only advantageous—it is necessary to achieve and sustain compliance with regulatory guidelines as well as develop a culture of excellence. In addition to higher compliance and fewer errors, robust staff development and training programs contribute to employee retention and engagement. An organization that invests in its employees' professional growth will have a more motivated and engaged workforce. Respected employees are more likely to take ownership of their work, which leads to higher productivity and organizational commitment. This upkeep of trained personnel is particularly vital in laboratory settings, in which continuity and expertise are necessary to respond to evolving complexities of scientific research. Secondly, trained individuals can better identify prospects for process improvement, enabling laboratories to be competitive and responsive to market demands and regulatory changes as identified by previous reviews of good training practices (Arnold et al., 2019). Moreover, the cost implications of accreditation and observation of quality assurance procedures in laboratories cannot be overlooked. Research has shown that organizations that prioritize personnel training as well as compliance with accreditation standards are more likely to have better business performance and innovation. Enhanced quality assurance standards can lead to a more streamlined workflow, reduced operating costs, and thereby enhanced financial performance. Aligning training initiatives with accreditation goals empowers workers with the ability to be part of contributing to the organization's reputation and success. Finally, staff training and development at length must be regarded as a strategic investment that forms an integral part of laboratory management and quality assurance, which not only promotes operational excellence but also nurtures a culture that promotes continuous improvement and professional growth (Frenz & Lambert, 2013).

13.5.3. Risk Management Strategies

Good risk management practices are a critical part of quality assurance and laboratory governance. Risk management practices allow laboratories to anticipate likely hazards and pitfalls ahead of time, enabling them to improve the reliability of experimental findings as well as overall research integrity. The use of a structured method in assessing risk facilitates the identification and assessment of risks faced in laboratory operations, such as equipment malfunctioning, human mistakes, and issues of compliance. This overall risk system forms the basis to apply targeted mitigation measures, such as regular staff safety training and robust equipment maintenance cycles. In addition, the inclusion of standard operating procedures (SOPs) not only offers workflow efficacy but also contributes to an environment of quality control and safety. Lastly, the identification and management of risks beforehand significantly lead to scientific replicability and public trust in research findings. In laboratory setups, coupling risk management and quality assurance practices sets the stage for continuous improvement. Flexibility is required since the laboratory must respond to what is attacking them, as the recent COVID-19 pandemic experience has brought about. The pandemic has led to a shift in the approach laboratories use in their work by necessitating the rapid redeployment of resources and reassessment of experimental design. Through analysis of various measures that have been taken by schools in these circumstances, based on new studies, laboratories can acquire useful lessons regarding effective risk management practices with emphasis on adaptability and prompt response (Crawford et al., 2020). These lessons not only guarantee the health of laboratory staff but also protect the integrity of research performed under extraordinary conditions, so that quality assurance is given top priority. In addition, the establishment of reporting standards, such as research ethics as provided through the ARRIVE guidelines, indicates the importance of open communication within risk management steps. The guidelines promote extensive documentation of research procedures, which is crucial for establishing the validity and replicability of scientific findings (Percie et al., 2020). Transparent reporting practices allow laboratories to identify flaws in their procedures, thus making proactive corrections to prevent future risks. Second, establishing cooperation among researchers can introduce mutual best practices and team problem-solving, enabling a more robust approach to managing risk. By promoting transparency and institution-to-institution collaboration, laboratories have the ability to build more robust quality control systems, ultimately leading to improved research findings and public confidence in scientific work.

13.6. Challenges in Quality Assurance

Within laboratory administration, ensuring quality assurance (QA) entails numerous frightening challenges that need to be resolved carefully to deliver consistent and accurate results. Application of automation technology in laboratory work has significantly enhanced diagnostic precision and accuracy in a way that rapid turnaround times for samples and results are facilitated. But such a change is not risk-free since it presents quality assurance challenges that undermine the validity of lab results. More specifically, reliance on automated systems necessitates rigorous QA measures to mitigate potential glitches or flaws that may result in sample analysis and data interpretation. Since laboratories now use more sophisticated automated technologies, it is crucial to comprehend and address the inherent issues of maintaining QA to preserve laboratory diagnosis credibility and ultimately impact patient care outcomes (Alyami et al., 2024). Moreover, diversification of laboratory tests , such as liquid chromatography-tandem mass spectrometry (LC-MS/MS), accounts for another dimension of complexity in quality assurance. While this platform enables exceptional analytical sensitivity, it also concurrently generates massive data that must be carefully monitored to ensure quality. The complexity of such data flows can overwhelm existing QA processes, creating time-consuming procedures that drain resources and decrease laboratory efficiency. Laboratories may fall into a reactive quality-control mode, addressing problems after the fact rather than being proactive about instituting safeguards. Thus, the creation of effective and automated QA systems is essential. These measures not only enhance efficiency but also reduce laboratory errors, in the end allowing for patient care and monitoring compliance to thrive (Jarrells et al., 2023). Efficient automated QA systems are used with a twofold function: enhancing laboratory efficiency and upholding results integrity. For instance, the use of web-based software for QA monitoring is an exemplary demonstration of how technology can be utilized to remedy the perennial problems of laboratories. By producing everyday QA reports showing anomalies in a readable manner, laboratories can, on a daily basis, ensure quality parameters are met. This quantum jump in QA technology allows one to monitor and audit measurements efficiently with a systematic method of correcting out-of-scope results. As laboratories become more and more inclined to embrace new technologies, the prospect of enhanced quality assurance will rise, and thus provide laboratory management practice and ultimately patient outcomes with support. Sustaining this relationship between technology and quality assurance is essential to laboratory environments' future success (Jarrells et al., 2023; Alyami et al., 2024).

13.6.1. Technological Advancements and Adaptation

The quality assurance environment in the management of laboratories has been revolutionized by technological advancements, enabling organizations to embrace better practices. Besides enabling institutions to perform detailed analysis and data handling, the technologies have also streamlined work processes. For instance, the application of open automation as well as artificial intelligence software in laboratory procedures can minimize the risk of human error and enhance reproducibility. Therefore, laboratories can attain levels of quality control higher than ever before as they provide services to the burgeoning demands of all branches of science. In addition, innovation of intelligent monitoring systems that constantly sense laboratory conditions assists in ushering in consistent results, thereby further ensuring the preservation of quality standards. While labs adopt these technological advances, the culture of built-in resilience allows them to anticipate and hurdle obstacles, ensuring resilience in a rapidly shifting science environment (Dadlani & Yadava, 2023). Parallel to the advancements of laboratory technology, the academic environment has also seen relevant debates of the implementation of Learning Management Systems (LMS) , such as Moodle. Not only do they offer learning material, but increasingly, these platforms are being utilized in support of professional training in quality assurance and laboratory management environments. Analysis suggests that although they have been quite widely adopted in STEM fields, significant research gaps continue to hamper further adoption of platforms like

Moodle in other laboratory environments (Sithara et al., 2022). By the disclosure of innovative ways of educating and creating cooperative learning communities, computer-based courses can enhance professional development. In addition, using such systems assists laboratory personnel in maintaining compliance with best practices and regulating requirements, ultimately resulting in a culture of continuous assurance of quality improvement. Furthermore, the rapid progress in technology, particularly in digital information and data integrity, necessitates ongoing adaptation from professionals in laboratory-based management. Sophisticated analytics coupled with high-end data management software facilitates smart decision-making, which allows the laboratories to efficiently address the challenges of quality assurance. Such technologies promote traceability and transparency, two of the primary components for ensuring quality levels. Besides, as reliance on digital platforms continues, addressing academic integrity and security concerns is paramount. Laboratories need to adhere to these ethics as their top priority to protect their operational systems and comply with regulatory requirements. Therefore, the interaction of technological progress and conscious adaptation in laboratory management is key to the maintenance of quality assurance and enhancing overall success in operations (Sithara et al., 2022) (Figure 13.12).

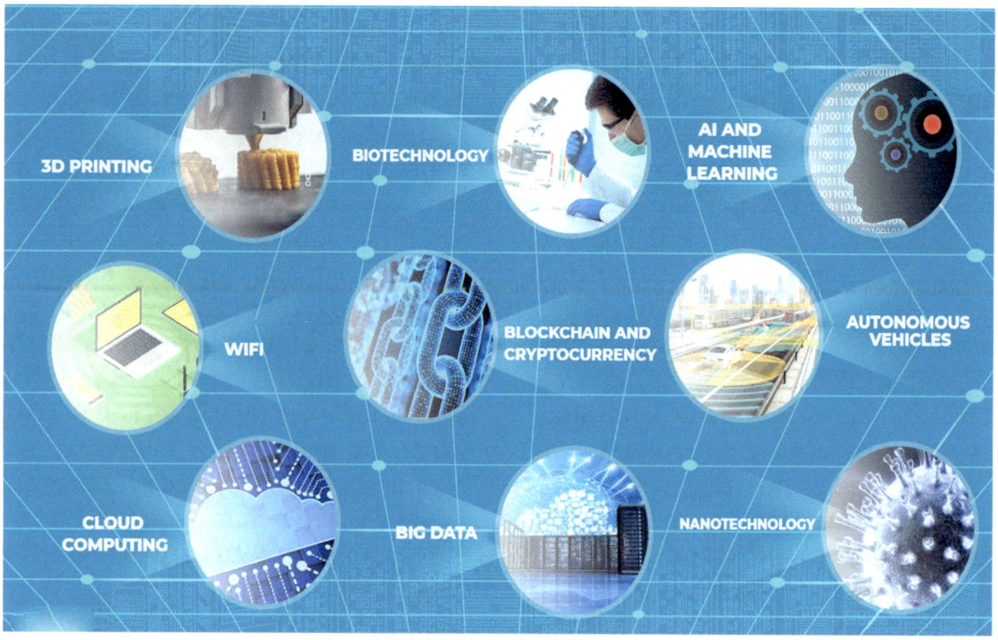

Figure 13.12. Technological advancements and adaptation.

Source: https://www.boldbusiness.com/wp-content/uploads/2018/04/In-article-Nine-TECHNOLOGIES.jpg.

13.6.2. Budget Constraints and Resource Limitations

In laboratory management, understanding of budgetary constraints and shortages of resources is critical to quality assurance. Laboratories are usually faced with having inadequate financial resources, which can have a significant impact on being capable of investing in new technology and highly skilled individuals. The limitation not only affects the efficiency of the operation but also the output quality, with likely shortcuts in research findings or diagnostic precision.

As the laboratory services market becomes increasingly competitive, laboratories need to be tactical in such financial reversals, focusing on badly needed renovations or training initiatives and deferring more aggressive reforms that could enhance their service provision. The choreography between budget constraints and the search for quality assurance thus calls for wise planning and resource allocation to keep operational standards within such cost impediments. In addition, the resource scarcity impact extends beyond capital to human resources and infrastructure. Inadequate manpower could lead to overworked technicians, resulting in increased levels of mistakes in testing and analysis, directly compromising quality assurance standards. Additionally, the presence of old or ineffectual laboratory equipment could compromise the ability to carry out certain tests appropriately, further jeopardizing the validity of results. To address such issues, laboratory directors must possess effective resource management strategies to improve productivity within budgetary limits. Adding value via innovative means, such as workflow optimization and cross-training of employees, can also alleviate some of these constraints and maintain high levels of quality. Therefore, identification and control of resource constraints effectively becomes a condition for laboratories to maintain quality assurance. The collaboration among different stakeholders can play an important role in bridging resource shortages and budget gaps. By the establishment of partnerships between government agencies, industry players, and institutions of higher learning, laboratories gain access to additional funds, shared resources, and expertise that would otherwise be unaffordable. Collaborative research work also facilitates the development of adaptable sensors and new technologies required in today's laboratory work, necessary in addressing quality assurance issues (Luo et al., 2023). Moreover, involving community-based programs, such as patient registries, facilitates more inclusive data use and collection, reinforcing evidence-based practice among laboratory management (Arnold et al., 2019). These common strategies will reduce some of the financial burdens and inspire innovation as well, with quality assurance at the center of laboratory activities under constraint. The synergistic approach to managing resources, therefore, not only increases operating efficiency but also significantly contributes towards upholding standards of quality assurance.

13.6.3. Maintaining Compliance in a Dynamic Environment

It is under the circumstances of quality assurance and laboratory management that it is an important aspect that lends credibility to scientific work and healthcare delivery to remain in line with a dynamic environment. Laboratories are usually faced with evolving regulations and standards that necessitate periodic updating of procedures and protocols. Such variability is otherwise augmented by the rapidity of developing technologies as well as the sophistication of experimental methods. Thus, organizations must establish a robust compliance system that addresses current legislation but also anticipates future changes. Through a positive compliance culture, laboratories can prevent the dangers associated with non-compliance, enhancing their credibility and protecting the integrity of their results. Ultimately, the objective is to create a learning environment where quality assurance is embedded in daily work, allowing for continuous improvement and innovation and safeguarding public health. The economic effect of remaining compliant is staggering, particularly in the way that laboratories cannot afford to implement new technologies and practices compliant with regulations. It is also exacerbated by growing antibiotic resistance within the health sector, as indicated by recent studies (Muteeb et al., 2023). Pharmaceutical and laboratory management must collaborate so that compliance actions not just meet regulatory requirements but also develop innovative solutions to combat resistant infection. This calls for spending on training staff and updating equipment to achieve best practice in quality assurance. Strategic allocation of resources to compliance functions allows laboratories to develop operational effectiveness and gain a competitive advantage in an oversaturated market. Further, this compliance vigilance ultimately leads to improved patient outcomes and reduced healthcare expenditure on antibiotic resistance and other compliance-related cases. Technological advancements, such as flexible sensors, represent a milestone achievement in laboratory management, showcasing the nature of an integrated system towards compliance despite rapid changes (Luo et al., 2023). Such sensors need to be compatible with biological processes as well as compliant with highly regulated environments, and this can complicate their implementation on a wide scale. Laboratories then have to balance compliance with innovation, and newly emerging technologies are tested and benchmarked rigorously against established standards. Furthermore, ethical as well as environmental considerations come into play in the successful roll-out of such technologies as well, and these demand a comprehensive compliance strategy that addresses all these aspects. By establishing a dynamic regulatory regime to accommodate emerging technologies, laboratories can achieve their potential and ensure the highest quality assurance. This, in turn, fosters a sustainable climate for scientific advancement and public trust in laboratory findings.

The synthesis of analysis into laboratory management and quality assurance is essential in bringing together knowledge from research and practice. The implementation of an efficient quality management system, such as ISO 9001:2008, is imperative to make the educational institution and laboratory efficient and effective. The compliance with the implementation of standard operating procedures in schools, as reflected through research in SMK Negeri 1 Purwokerto, underscores the central role of quality management in the development of curricula and teaching practices (Suprihatin, 2012). Not only does this systematic implementation guarantee adherence of academic performance to industry standards, but it also builds a foundation of tight standards that regulate operational behavior in laboratories. The ability to fit and respond to these standards shows a general mindset of quality assurance, not as a requirement for conformity but as a vehicle for ongoing enhancement in laboratory practice. In addition, the interdependency of quality assurance with laboratory operations is seen in deciding on operational processes. The research of the Texas Commission on Environmental Quality's activities in managing water quality is a classic example of the intricate interplay of technical assistance and quality assurance project planning (Montagna & Applebaum, 2006). With close observation and scrutiny, testing, and adaptability, an entire QA system comes into focus so that the laboratories are able to correctly interpret measurements and draw rational conclusions. Such systematic procedures ensure that laboratories not only meet prescribed standards but excel beyond them, exemplifying practice excellence. Thus, the conclusion drawn verifies the premise that a good quality assurance program is the master key to effective laboratory management, enabling institutions to deliver higher outputs and maintain scientific integrity. In conclusion, the recognition obtained through the study of quality assurance in laboratory management highlights its importance in fostering a culture of continuous improvement and operational excellence. Through the establishment of clear guidelines derived from standards recognized, institutions and laboratories are able to enhance their educational offerings and scientific contributions, showcasing quality-driven methodologies. The joint focus on both operational and quality aspects, as identified by the results of this research and by innovations within the field, implies an evolving future where coordination between laboratory management and quality assurance is not only desired but also mandated. As the face of laboratory practice changes, so too must quality commitment change, so that such institutions remain constantly nimble, responsive, and dedicated to excellence in all areas of their practice (Montagna & Applebaum, 2006; Suprihatin, 2012).

SUMMARY

Laboratory and quality management are the essence of ensuring credible laboratory findings and better results in clinical and research settings. Well-established quality management systems (QMS) are the requisites for obtaining consistent improvement of laboratory activities, compliance with regulations, and excellence in laboratory operations. A comprehensive QMS not only establishes quality goals but also emphasizes the importance of a culture of responsibility and cooperation at every level of the hierarchy in the laboratory environment. By establishing an organizational culture devoted to quality, laboratories are in a better position to identify and respond to sources of error and place their operations in conformity with best practice and recognized standards , such as those put forth in revised guidelines by Percie et al. (2020). This system eventually aids laboratories in increasing transparency and reproducibility of reporting, significant factors in accelerating scientific research and clinical diagnostics. Further, the regulatory environment significantly affects quality assurance practice in laboratory management, particularly within clinical settings under legal regulation , such as the Clinical Laboratory Improvement Amendments (CLIA) within the United States. Such laws impose extremely strict requirements on laboratory work that allow for standardized testing and accreditation processes that enhance the quality of laboratory results. Conversely, veterinary laboratories operate somewhat in an unregulated environment, whose variability may usher in discrepancies in the quality assurance processes. As highlighted by Arnold et al. (2019), with voluntary accreditation options for veterinary labs, the lack of requirement for regulatory compliance can increase laboratory inconsistencies. This highlight underscores the need to adopt rigid quality control measures and quality improvement programs to guard against inaccuracies that may be detrimental to patient outcomes and the validity of research findings. Overall, a solid quality assurance framework is crucial to laboratory management performance and reputation. The coupling of quality goals with clear structure and ordered processes allows laboratories to establish a culture of continuous improvement. Adopting substantive quality policies and standard operating procedures for rigid observance of established guidelines is essential to the delivery of quality products. Also crucial is ongoing monitoring of laboratory performance through internal and external audits and responsiveness to client feedback, which encourages a culture of responsibility and trust. Laboratories need to remain responsive to evolving standards and proactive towards continuous quality improvement of processes and procedures. By focusing on these key factors, laboratories are in a better position to support proper patient care and scientific advancement, ultimately achieving their overall objectives in laboratory administration and quality assurance.

A LOOK TO THE FUTURE:

CLINICAL LABORATORY IMPROVEMENT AMENDMENTS (CLIA):

The Clinical Laboratory Improvement Amendments (CLIA) of 1988 constitute a foundational framework of federal regulatory standards governing clinical laboratory testing in the United States, established to ensure that diagnostic services performed on human specimens are accurate, reliable, and timely. Prior to CLIA's enactment, laboratory testing was subject to varied state regulations and voluntary guidelines that lacked consistent national oversight. With the explosion of advanced laboratory technologies and an increasing reliance on laboratory results in medical decision-making, Congress amended the Public Health Service Act to create a unified system of quality assurance, certification, and oversight for clinical laboratories nationwide.

CLIA regulations apply to virtually all facilities conducting laboratory testing on human specimens for the purposes of diagnosing, preventing, or treating disease, as well as assessing health status. Under these standards, laboratories must obtain appropriate certification before they can legally perform testing, with the required certificate type determined by the complexity of tests they conduct. Categories range from simple waived tests (such as certain point-of-care glucose assays) to moderate and high complexity assays that demand stringent procedural controls, staff qualifications, and quality assessment practices.

The CLIA program is administered jointly by three federal agencies with defined roles: the Centers for Medicare & Medicaid Services (CMS) leads implementation and enforcement of regulatory requirements; the Food and Drug Administration (FDA) classifies test systems and assigns complexity levels; and the Centers for Disease Control and Prevention (CDC) provides scientific and technical guidance, including evaluation of proficiency testing and laboratory quality practices.

Central to CLIA is the principle that quality laboratory testing underpins effective clinical care. Ensuring the accuracy, reliability, and timeliness of laboratory results enhances diagnostic confidence for clinicians, supports appropriate treatment decisions, and protects patient safety. Compliance with CLIA involves not only certification but also participation in proficiency testing, adherence to quality control procedures, documentation of personnel qualifications and training, and oversight through periodic inspections.

Over the decades since its passage, CLIA has evolved with advances in technology and clinical practice. Amendments and regulatory updates have addressed emerging complexities, refined personnel requirements, and clarified testing categories to maintain standards that reflect contemporary laboratory science. These updates help laboratories adapt to innovations while maintaining quality assurance that supports public health.

In an era when laboratory diagnostics play a critical role in precision medicine, population health surveillance, and quality clinical care, CLIA remains a cornerstone of laboratory governance. Its emphasis on standardization, rigorous oversight, and quality performance ensures that laboratory data remain a trusted foundation for patient management and scientific discovery.

REFERENCES

1. Agresti, W., Card, D., Church, V., & McGarry, et al. (1984). *Managers Handbook for Software Development.* Document ID 19840015082 https://core.ac.uk/download/pdf/42849213.pdf (accessed on 17th July 2025).
2. Al-Fuqaha, A., Guizani, M., Mohammadi, M., Aledhari, M., & Ayyash, M. (2015). Internet of Things: A survey on enabling technologies, protocols, and applications. *IEEE Communications Surveys & Tutorials, 17*, 2347–2376. https://doi.org/10.1109/comst.2015.2444095 (accessed on 17th July 2025).
3. Alkishriwi, N., Schorn, C., & Theis, D. (2021). The International Standards for Solar Thermal Collectors and Components as a medium of quality assurance. *Volume(3)*. https://www.semanticscholar.org/paper/005b80008240c61d8e4d86840ea7c9580bf13e93 (accessed on 17th July 2025).
4. Allison, K. H., Hammond, M. E. H., Dowsett, M., McKernin, S., Carey, L. A., Fitzgibbons, P. L., Hayes, D. F., et al. (2020). Estrogen and progesterone receptor testing in breast cancer: American Society of Clinical Oncology/College of American Pathologists guideline update. *Archives of Pathology & Laboratory Medicine, 144*, 545–563. https://doi.org/10.5858/arpa.2019-0904-sa (accessed on 17th July 2025).
5. Alyami, A. A., Alaqil, N. M., Alsulayyim, A. S. M., Al Yami, R. M. K., Salem, F. J. M., Al Hatailah, A. M. H., Al Zandan, S. A., et al. (2024). Comprehensive review of laboratory automation, quality control, and workforce adaptation. *Journal of Eco Humanism*. https://www.semanticscholar.org/paper/23b9d8d1d1bb86a22de2c37049b5ac58007775bf (accessed on 17th July 2025).
6. Montagna, P. A., & Applebaum, S. (2006). *Matagorda Bay and Nearby Coastal Waters Dissolved Oxygen and pH TMDL Assessment report.* https://repositories.lib.utexas.edu/items/4eb08f76-806c-4410-adda-68cacaa62d07 https://core.ac.uk/download/211339372.pdf (accessed on 17th July 2025).
7. Arnold, J. E., Camus, M. S., Freeman, K. P., Giori, L., Hooijberg, E. H., Jeffery, U., Korchia, J., Meindel, M. J., Moore, A. R., Sisson, S. C., Vap, L. M., & Cook, J. R. (2019). ASVCP Guidelines: Principles of Quality Assurance and Standards for Veterinary Clinical Pathology (version 3.0): Developed by the American Society for Veterinary Clinical Pathology's (ASVCP) Quality Assurance and Laboratory Standards (QALS) Committee. *Veterinary clinical pathology, 48*(4), 542–618. https://doi.org/10.1111/vcp.12810accessed on 17th July 2025).
8. Aroon, A., Kavya, A., Swetha Rani, M., Harshitha, M., & Anannya, N. (2024). Evolution of quality assurance in pharmaceutical industry. *World Journal of Biology Pharmacy and Health Sciences*. https://www.semanticscholar.org/paper/c23e72a570ddcd6d170c8039e8ad7b940c04a8d9 (accessed on 17th July 2025).
9. Austin, B. J., Daniels, M., & Haggard, B. E. (2017). Laboratory Quality Control Report: Why is it Important?., 6. Retrieved from https://scholarworks.uark.edu/awrcfs/7(accessed on 17th July 2025).
10. Koenig, J. C., Billitti, J. W., & Tallon, J. M. (1979). *Photovoltaic System Criteria Documents. Volume 1: Guidelines for Evaluating the Management and Operations Planning of Photovoltaic Applications.* https://ntrs.nasa.gov/citations/19910011243. https://core.ac.uk/download/pdf/42819096.pdf (accessed on 17th July 2025).

11. Students of Health Management 721.01 (2017), University of New Hampshire and Bonica, Mark, "Healthcare Management Primer" (2017). *Open Educational Resources*. 4. https://scholars.unh.edu/oer/4(accessed on 17th July 2025).

12. Brun, M., Füzéry, A. K., Henschke, B., Rozak, K., & Venner, A. A. (2021). Identifying sources of error and selecting quality indicators for point of care testing. *Practical Laboratory Medicine, 25*, e00216–e00216. https://doi.org/10.1016/j.plabm.2021.e00216 (accessed on 17th July 2025).

13. Crawford, J., Butler-Henderson, K., Rudolph, J., Malkawi, B. H., Glowatz, M., Burton, R. L., Magni, P. A., et al. (2020). COVID-19: 20 countries' higher education intra-period digital pedagogy responses. *Journal of Applied Learning & Teaching, 3*. https://doi.org/10.37074/jalt.2020.3.1.7 (accessed on 17th July 2025).

14. Curry, N., Davenport, R., Pavord, S., Mallett, S., Kitchen, D., Klein, A. A., Maybury, H., et al. (2018). The use of viscoelastic hemostatic assays in the management of major bleeding. *British Journal of Hematology, 182*, 789–806. https://doi.org/10.1111/bjh.15524 (accessed on 17th July 2025).

15. Dadlani, M., & Yadava, D. K. (2023). *Seed Science and Technology*. https://doi.org/10.1007/978-981-19-5888-5 (accessed on 17th July 2025).

16. Devan, R. K. S., Mallikarjuna, Y., Ponraj, R., Naidu, H., & Kirana, B. (2024). Operational excellence by implementation of 5S concepts and lean management practices in vivarium. *Journal of Laboratory Animal Science*. https://www.semanticscholar.org/paper/658b4c008f8026a87acbcdad85d54b39d8b50baf (accessed on 17th July 2025).

17. Frenz, M., & Lambert, R. (2013). *The Economics of Accreditation*. https://core.ac.uk/download/20665110.pdf (accessed on 17th July 2025).

18. Gamage, S. H. P. W., Ayres, J. R., & Behrend, M. (2022). A systematic review on trends in using Moodle for teaching and learning. *International Journal of STEM Education, 9*. https://doi.org/10.1186/s40594-021-00323-x (accessed on 17th July 2025).

19. Holmes, J., Higginson, R., Geen, J., & Phillips, A. O. (2023). Utilizing routine clinical laboratory data to support quality improvement in health care: Application of a national acute kidney injury alert system as a proof of concept. *Annals of Clinical Biochemistry, 61*, 218–229. https://www.semanticscholar.org/paper/3d378c369bece46b987ce3d01d1828f4d7dc1b1f (accessed on 17th July 2025).

20. Hukkanen, R., Trapani, M., Derringer, T., Laast, V., Wojcinski, Z., Manno, R., Rinke, M., et al. (2023). Toxicologic Pathology Forum: Opinion on performing Good Laboratory Practice histopathology evaluation for nonclinical toxicity studies in a remote location. *Toxicologic Pathology, 51*, 148–152. https://www.semanticscholar.org/paper/917ee312af2f1a29b589c8c2ce76bcd56686acb4 (accessed on 17th July 2025).

21. Huq Ronny, F. H., Sherpa, T., Saquib, F. N., & Ahmad, S. (2024). Implementing laboratory internal audit to improve compliance and quality of care in the municipal public health system-based ambulatory care health clinics in New York City. *Laboratory Medicine*. https://www.semanticscholar.org/paper/8ae42ade853347a6c5a59540c0505698e029fc4f (accessed on 17th July 2025).

22. Imam, M. H., & Tasadduq, I. (2012). Evaluating the satisfaction of ABET student outcomes from course learning outcomes through a software implementation. *International Journal of Quality*

Assurance in Engineering and Technology Education, 2, 21–33. https://www.semanticscholar.org/paper/c994acbbba75d607dc5410a8c3ed0ba1ccef386c (accessed on 17th July 2025).

23. Jarrells, M., Armstrong, S., Hickey, C., Bumgardner, C., & Yu, M. (2023). B-198 Web-based application of an automated quality assurance monitoring system for a pain management panel by liquid chromatography tandem mass spectrometry (LC-MS/MS). *Clinical Chemistry*. https://www.semanticscholar.org/paper/ded513980c3f1be5d1897b2c4e8772cfaa7869fa (accessed on 17th July 2025).
24. Kannan, V. (2025). The critical role of laboratory informatics systems in ensuring public safety in pharmaceutical development. *World Journal of Advanced Research and Reviews*. https://www.semanticscholar.org/paper/ed33ea291e858168c720d24480c3f59d76ae7b18 (accessed on 17th July 2025).
25. Kharrazi, A., El Ftouh, S., El Feniche, M., Bahji, M., & Bouaiti, E. (2025). A comparative study of legislative and normative frameworks in Morocco, France and U.S.A towards progressive and evolutionary quality management in Moroccan laboratories. *Revita Romana de Medicina de Laborator, 33*, 9–20. https://www.semanticscholar.org/paper/34399af7edbd7a6b578b1d516bc15e870d2fee9e (accessed on 17th July 2025).
26. Teka, A., & Kibatu, G. (2012). Quality of Liver and Kidney Function Tests among Public Medical Laboratories in Western Region of Amhara National Regional State of Ethiopia. *Ethiopian journal of health sciences, 22*(1), 19–26.(accessed on 17th July 2025).
27. Kruk, M. E., Gage, A., Arsenault, C., Jordan, K., Leslie, H. H., Roder-DeWan, S., Adeyi, O., et al. (2018). High-quality health systems in the Sustainable Development Goals era: Time for a revolution. *The Lancet Global Health, 6*, e1196–e1252. https://doi.org/10.1016/s2214-109x(18)30386-3 (accessed on 17th July 2025).
28. Layfield, L., & Baloch, Z. (2020). Categorical systems for reporting of cytology specimens: Following the footsteps of Bethesda-like reporting systems. *Diagnostic Cytopathology, 48*. https://www.semanticscholar.org/paper/efd4169809fd2d4116b57f0d5b033c475ae3ddde (accessed on 17th July 2025).
29. Luo, Y., Abidian, M. R., Ahn, J.-H., Akinwande, D., Andrews, A. M., Antonietti, M., Bao, Z., et al. (2023). Technology roadmap for flexible sensors. *ACS Nano, 17*, 5211–5295. https://doi.org/10.1021/acsnano.2c12606 (accessed on 17th July 2025).
30. McCarthy, D., Wrenn, J., & Mueller, K. (2009). *Geisinger Health System: Achieving the Potential of System Integration Through Innovation, Leadership, Measurement, and Incentives*. https://www.commonwealthfund.org/publications/case-study/2009/jun/geisinger-health-system-achieving-potential-system-integration https://core.ac.uk/download/71351432.pdf (accessed on 17th July 2025).
31. Mishra, V., Chandra, D., & Raina, V. (2025). The evolution of quality management in laboratory services: Ensuring accuracy, safety, and efficiency. *The International Journal of Conformity Assessment*. https://www.semanticscholar.org/paper/fb5f420c9cad5fd8096f0264b2ee0dd7a21a276d (accessed on 17th July 2025).
32. Muteeb, G., Rehman, M. T., Shahwan, M., & Aatif, M. (2023). Origin of antibiotics and antibiotic resistance, and their impacts on drug development: A narrative review. *Pharmaceuticals, 16*, 1615–1615. https://doi.org/10.3390/ph16111615 (accessed on 17th July 2025).
33. Nadkarni, R. (2005). Zen and the art (or is it science) of a perfect analysis. *Journal of ASTM*

International, 2, 1–13. https://www.semanticscholar.org/paper/4d81322a56e97ed84417b3e90c8e7832d909158e (accessed on 17th July 2025).

34. Nwaokorie, F. O., & Ojo, E. A. (2018). Overview of the implementation of Quality Management System in Nigerian medical laboratories. *University of Lagos Journal of Basic Medical Sciences*. https://www.semanticscholar.org/paper/3b6e3126980908f95f46f1d00f36f59d744b1a3d (accessed on 17th July 2025).

35. Pareek, C. S. (2024). Enhancing quality assurance in annuities: A risk management approach with AI and machine learning. *International Journal of Science and Engineering Applications*. https://www.semanticscholar.org/paper/ba555d663049ceff72c0100ecd4999d70b91d5a5 (accessed on 17th July 2025).

36. Patra, N. C. (2021). Recent advances in accreditation systems in higher agricultural educational institutes (HAEI) in India: A review. *SSR Institute of International Journal of Life Sciences*. https://www.semanticscholar.org/paper/b359848dc0323c5be47919a8ffe954716fd9a28f (accessed on 17th July 2025).

37. Percie du Sert, N., Ahluwalia, A., Alam, S., Avey, M. T., Baker, M., Browne, W. J., Clark, A., et al. (2020). Reporting animal research: Explanation and elaboration for the ARRIVE guidelines 2.0. *PLoS Biology, 18*, e3000411–e3000411. https://doi.org/10.1371/journal.pbio.3000411 (accessed on 17th July 2025).

38. Pérez Vicente, H. A., Torres Bermúdez, E. G., & Morales, M. (2022). Continuous improvement using statistical process control in the Mexican automotive motor remanufacturing industry: A case study. *International Joint Conference on Industrial Engineering and Operations Management Proceedings*. https://www.semanticscholar.org/paper/d94c7c849a2b19ed38b838634aeebbaeab17cfa9 (accessed on 17th July 2025).

39. Shaikh, N. A., Sul, P. K., Shendge, A., & Sharma, K. (2024). Implementation of quality assurance and quality control in construction and management for project effectiveness. *International Research Journal of Modernization in Engineering Technology and Science*. https://www.semanticscholar.org/paper/9a284381f3a4488f9b5594a3267676c4b6c72645 (accessed on 17th July 2025).

40. Sikes, R. S. (2016). 2016 guidelines of the American Society of Mammalogists for the use of wild mammals in research and education. *Journal of Mammalogy, 97*, 663–688. https://doi.org/10.1093/jmammal/gyw078 (accessed on 17th July 2025).

41. Srivastava, A., Santagostino, E., Dougall, A., Kitchen, S., Sutherland, M. L., Pipe, S. W., Carção, M., et al. (2020). WFH guidelines for the management of hemophilia, 3rd edition. *Hemophilia, 26*, 1–158. https://doi.org/10.1111/hae.14046 (accessed on 17th July 2025).

42. Suprihatin, E. (2012). *Productive Subjects Learning Based Quality Management of ISO 9001:2008 at SMK Negeri 1 Purwokerto*. https://core.ac.uk/download/148592316.pdf (accessed on 17th July 2025).

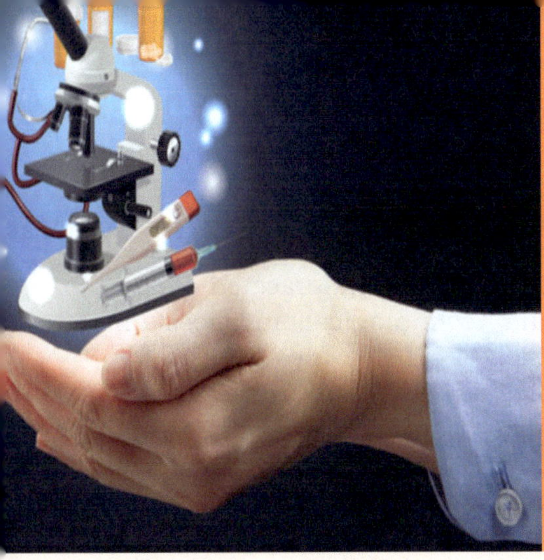

Chapter 14

ETHICAL, LEGAL, AND SOCIAL IMPLICATIONS (ELSI)

Contents

Introduction

New technologies, particularly artificial intelligence (AI) and precision medicine, have rendered it imperative to examine their ethical, legal, and social implications (ELSI). With these technologies being applied in various fields, they raise intricate issues that must be efficiently addressed by society. Concerns about the ethical use of AI, for instance, are related to ensuring equal access but not repeating existing biases that could perpetuate existing inequalities. In a similar vein, the advent of precision medicine gives rise to numerous issues of privacy, consent, and misuse of genetic information. Where these topics intersect with societal values, the need for a catch-all framework to navigate the complex map sketched by technological progress and its social implications is urgent (Lysaght, 2021). The multifaceted nature of ELSI reflects the interplay of ethical considerations, legal obligations, and societal relationships. With the development of health care and AI technologies, the uncertainty is at the center to understand the implications and the challenges spawned by these technologies. For example, in precision medicine, emergent uncertainties ironically undermine the projected benefits of individually targeted therapies, establishing a context under which patients, providers, and policymakers will have to negotiate novel complexities. The literature indicates that it is critical to grasp this uncertainty in a multilevel fashion because it is at varying levels, each possessing varying difficulties (Lohse, 2022). This degree of uncertainty requires healthy dialogue and interdisciplinarity to ensure that ethical, legal, and social frameworks are flexible and resilient. Finally, treating ELSI is not an intellectual exercise; it is essential for securing public trust and acceptability of new technology. As society increasingly relies on the innovations of precision medicine and AI, governments, technology developers, and healthcare organizations must guarantee ethical standards and legal compliance to safeguard individual rights. Merging ethical frameworks with real applications will make efforts to encourage inclusive discourse stronger, one that incorporates a variety of perspectives and values. In doing so, it will also allow informed policymaking, which diffuses the danger posed by such advances, making sure they are utilized as benefits to society at large. Thus, the topic of ELSI remains relevant, bridging the gap between capability in terms of technology and concerns of society (Lysaght, 2021) (Figure 14.1).

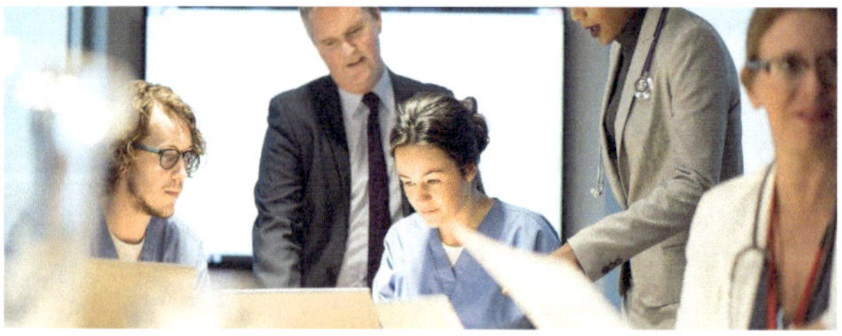

Figure 14.1. Ethical, legal, and social implications (ELSI).

Source: https://www.thehastingscenter.org/wp-content/uploads/Two-Cheers-for-Choosing-Wisely.jpg.

Definition of ELSI

The Ethical, Legal, and Social Implications (ELSI) idea has emerged to symbolize a critical basis for research regarding the multifaceted effects of scientific and technological advances on society. Essentially, ELSI provides a basis for identifying and examining the ethical issues, legal problems, and social implications that arise from innovations, particularly in fields of biotechnology and health care. With the emerging technologies being more and more integrated into the tapestry of everyday life, ELSI highlights the imperative to understand how such developments could change social relationships, access to commodities, and justice in the delivery of health care services. In this respect, ELSI is not merely a means of evaluating the benefits and burdens of scientific research but also a framework for facilitating responsible innovation in accordance with societal norms and values. A central aspect of ELSI is stakeholder engagement, with varied groups of voices that include, though are not limited to, industrial stakeholders, government departments, ethical panels, and community organizations. The broad-based strategy takes into account the opinions and interests of the people who may be affected by technological advances and ensures their rights and desires are respected. In this way, ELSI enables a participatory environment in which discussion may change, responding to the ethical and legal issues on which novel technologies are based. For instance, in debates about personalized medicine and early breast cancer detection, engaging diverse stakeholders has been critical to reconciling scientific advancement with public expectations and ethical principles, as in the project of the European Collaborative on Personalized Early Detection and Prevention of Breast Cancer (Pashayan et al., 2020). The dynamic nature of ELSI necessitates constant reconsideration and reformulation as new issues arise from technological innovation. As evident from the digitalization of rural areas and farming, there is a need to discuss the interaction between cyber, social, and physical systems within the larger context of responsible research and innovation. With that understanding of the relationships, there is a better understanding of risks and benefits provided by digital technologies, and thus policymakers and actors are guided towards meaningful responses (Rijswijk et al., 2021). Furthermore, this ongoing evaluation assures the need for accountability in managing the beneficial as well as adverse impacts of innovation. Through this, ELSI not only further enhances discussion of ethical and legal issues but also keeps social issues up front in developing new technologies and their uses, finally guiding society towards a more equal and equitable future (Figure 14.2).

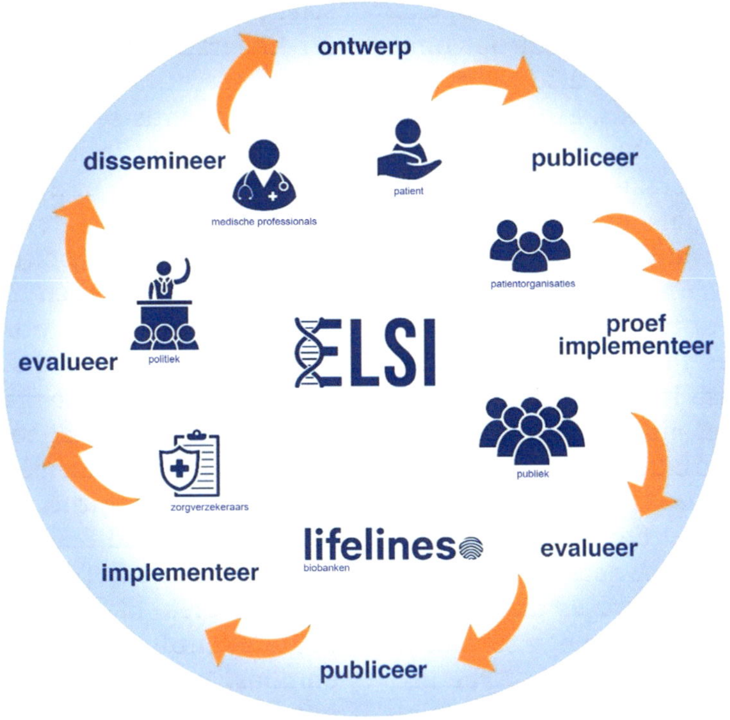

Figure 14.2. Definition of ELSI.

Source: https://www.rug.nl/research/genetics/research/elsicyclebetter.jpg.

Importance of ELSI in Contemporary Society

Today's environment of technological innovation requires more focus on the Ethical, Legal, and Social Implications (ELSI) of innovations, particularly in biotechnology and genomics. As scientists come up with tools like epigenetic clocks—procedures that measure biological aging and chronological age through DNA methylation—one cannot help but take note of the ethical concerns attached to it. For instance, the potential forensic abuse of these clocks for determining the age is problematic for privacy and consent, and for the impact on profiling individuals on the basis of their biological features (Pardede, 2025). Moreover, the moral responsibility of the creators to think about how their technologies would affect the norms and values of society is unyielding. Overlooking such ELSI can lead to social inequalities, with people who have restricted access to emerging technologies becoming increasingly discriminated against and vulnerable. Furthermore, integrating ELSI into healthcare innovation can play a key role in driving RRI. The RRI approach promotes engaging diverse stakeholders in the innovation process to make sure that health technologies are created by supporting societal values and ethical foundations (Pardede, 2025). For instance, models with transparency and public involvement can be designed to mitigate worry about abuse or misuse of complex medical technologies. This convergent strategy opens up cross-disciplinary discussion that not only addresses ethical concerns but also promotes equitable access to innovations. ELSI ideas can be incorporated into the innovation process in such a manner that stakeholders are able to create a socially responsible system that is responsive to such relevant needs of society as health equity and sustainability. Finally, what makes ELSI relevant to today's society is not only that it addresses the immediate ethical issues but also because it is able to influence future social landscapes molded by technology. While innovations continue to transform the health care industry, there is a need to analyze their long-term effects on human rights, individual autonomy, and societal welfare. An active address of ELSI encourages discussions on the trajectory of such technology so that it serves the public good rather than exacerbating inequalities. By prioritizing ethics and laws in advancing new technologies, society can develop progress that mirrors common ethical standards and contribute to social justice so that the living standards of all improve.

14.1. Historical Context of ELSI

The historical background of Ethical, Legal, and Social Implications (ELSI) dates back to the latter part of the 20th century, with the era of fast-evolving scientific breakthroughs and technologies. The era was marked by increased recognition of the necessity for ethical norms in fields like genetics, biotechnology, and information technology. Emergent technologies raised serious issues of their impact on society, which initiated appeals for mechanisms that would regulate and control their impact. The real re-establishment of the ELSI program in the early 1990s, particularly in the context of the Human Genome Project, marks a turning point in integrating ethical exploration with scientific inquiry. It brought out the necessity for integrating ethical attention into scientific advancement, and it demanded a reformation of how scientists were beginning to consider their work and its effects on society at large. As the discussion of ELSI continued, it became apparent that the ethics surrounding emerging technologies were political in nature. Based on paradigms , such as Michel Foucault's problematization of ethical conduct, it was apparent that ethics discourse existed in the sense as a prism to gauge the stability of democratic governance. The consequences of scientific advancements not only spurred debates regarding the rights of the individual but also spawned debates regarding collective social obligation. Through examining specific case studies like American and European nanotechnology programs, researchers emphasized how constitutional structures influenced the identification and prioritization of ethical issues. This helped emphasize the point that ethics are not merely abstractions; rather, they are formulated by, and formulate, political and social infrastructures and thus reveal the intricate dynamics between science, politics, and public ethics (Laurent et al., 2013). In practice, initiatives , such as the development of a Synthetic Biology Roadmap illustrate the enduring challenges and objectives of ELSI in action. By engaging Science and Technology Studies (STS) researchers in policy-making processes, advocates tried to confront the ambiguities of the emerging fields. Incorporating STS understandings was found to usually reveal drastic obstacles; however, deeply ingrained assumptions about technology as a driver of social progress were a hindrance. This mobility drew attention to tensions between scientific innovation and ethical regulation, resonating with more general resistance to challenging prevailing narratives framing technological progress as necessarily good. For this reason, the road mapping exercise illuminated not only the complexities of shaping public policy, but also the necessary challenges that scholars face in making the case for Responsible Research and Innovation (RRI) strategies when framing debates around ELSI (Dupras et al., 2019) (Figure 14.3).

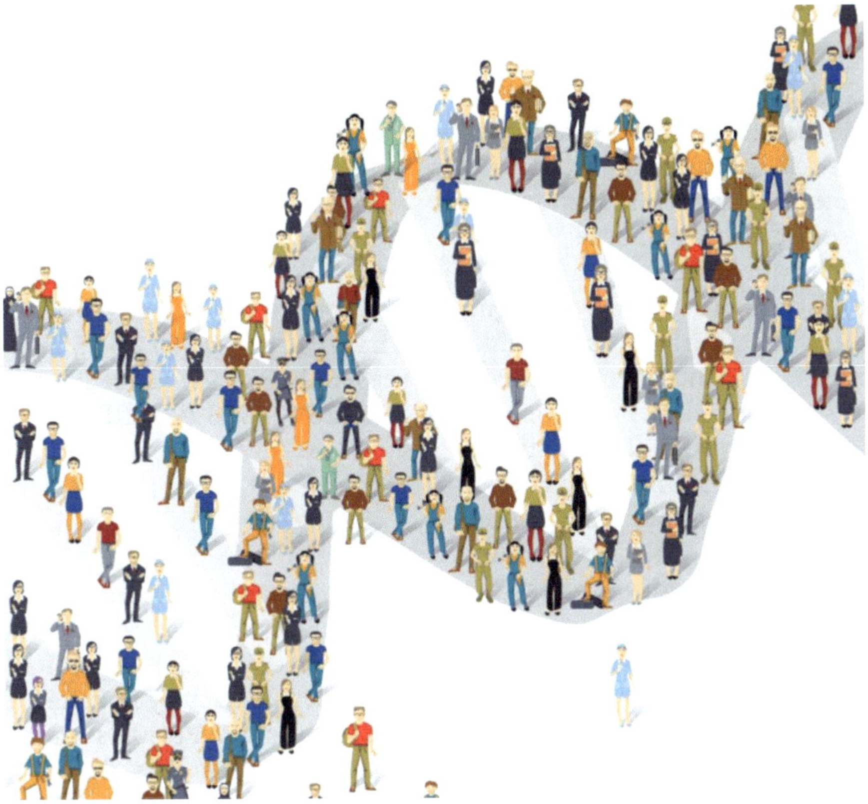

Figure 14.3. Historical context of ethical, legal, and social implications (ELSI).

Source: https://www.genome.gov/sites/default/files/media/images/2019-03/2.4.3.1_ELSI_sidebyside_CEER_0.jpeg.

14.1.1. Origins of ELSI Discussions

The discussions on the Ethical, Legal, and Social Implications (ELSI) agenda have dramatically transformed from their inception in the late 20th century. Historically, ELSI concerns initially arose as a response to advances in biotechnology and genetic research that led to the Human Genome Project. The project aimed not just to sequence human DNA but also acknowledged a fundamental imperative to address the ethical hurdles generated by genetic information. When the implications of genetic information and technology became apparent, stakeholders identified that an intersection of ethics, law, and social considerations must be explored in-depth to prevent abuse and discrimination. The first workshops, like milestone deliberations organized by the National Institute of Health and other stakeholders, aimed to formulate robust paradigms for considering these dimensions, setting groundwork principles for responding to follow-up biotechnological innovations. As concern for collateral impacts of genetic research on society as a whole grew, the ELSI topics further expanded. The developing field of gene-environment interactions (GxE) raised questions that were not explicitly covered. According to recent controversy evoked by the National Institute of Environmental Health Sciences, the complexity inherent in GxE investigation demands increased exploration of ethical, legal, and social questions, particularly if we are to understand their implications at various levels of society (Calluori et al., 2024). Through probing the intersection of genetic risk and environmental factors, researchers highlight the essential need for establishing sustainable community partnerships and incorporating social determinants of health to facilitate attention to equity and justice. As a result, the evolution of ELSI debates reflects sustained dedication to investigating scientific innovation, but to investigate it in an ethically sensitive manner. Besides, the building of ELSI frameworks attests to an essential conflict between clinical practice and theoretical discussion, more so in the case of new technologies like Preimplantation Genetic Testing (PGT). Analysis of the literature between 1999 and 2019 attests to a high rise in concern regarding the ethical aspects of PGT as a result of increased scholarly interest in aligning the debate with clinical practice (Alon et al., 2024). Despite this, there are still gaps in realizing practical applications in the real world, such that pressing concerns like funding and family concerns have not yet been fully addressed in clinical environments. This disconnect only highlights the need for intergroups consisting of ethicists, clinicians, and policymakers to establish an ELSI framework that is not merely theoretically valid but also practically feasible. From such multi-disciplinary debates, the effort done in ELSI debates may eventually lead to ethical integrity and public acceptance, paving the way for equitable access to biotechnological advancements (Figure 14.4).

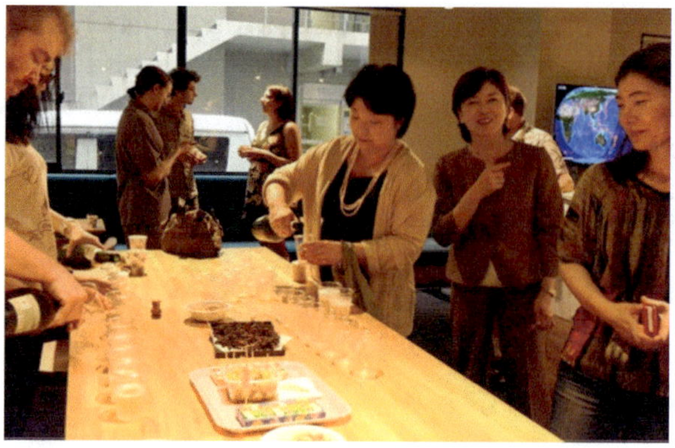

Figure 14.4. Origins of ethical, legal, and social implications (ELSI) discussions.

Source: https://wpi.elsi.jp/-/media/Project/Elsi-Tenants/Elsi-Tenant/Elsi/ELSI-blog/2015/20150820_109_PHut3.jpg%3Fh=334&w=500&la=ja-JP&hash=FD9DC836AE6941B0394DDDDAB5C258E45F18CEAE.

14.1.2. Key Milestones in ELSI Development

The history of Ethical, Legal, and Social Implications (ELSI) research has been marked by a series of historic milestones that have shaped its trajectory in genetics, biotechnology, and medicine. Perhaps the most significant early milestone was during the 1990s with the Human Genome Project (HGP), which not only sequenced the human genome but also addressed the ethical implications of genetic studies. This period saw the establishment of ELSI programs that were dedicated to infusing ethical perspectives from the very inception of scientific research. These programs emphasized the importance of diverse voices being involved in discussions about the implications of genetic advances, setting the stage for interdisciplinary ventures that are still important today. The foundation laid by this early movement continues to influence today's ELSI discourse, deeming ethical attention of paramount importance in scientific progress and policy-making. Another milestone in ELSI development emerged with the advent of personalized medicine, which served to highlight the ethical complexities of tailoring medical care to unique genetic profiles. Precision medicine advancements underscore the need for frameworks that deal with informed consent, privacy, and potential genetic discrimination. As Udegbe et al. (2024) discuss, the integration of technologies , such as bioinformatics and machine learning in the healthcare sector not only enhances the capacity to analyze large genomic data but also creates ethical concerns relating to data security and patients' rights. These discussions have resulted in the creation of guidelines and rules meant to protect people as genomics continues to evolve. Hence, the growth of personalized medicine has prompted valuable discussion on the ethical aspects of employing genetic data in clinical settings. Societal trends in general and the need to address diverse stakeholders' interests have also shaped the evolution of ELSI. Initiatives like the Breastmilk Ecology: Genesis of Infant Nutrition (BEGIN) Project are a move toward adopting translational research models combining biomedical factors and social contexts within infant nutrition. As highlighted by Nommsen-Rivers et al. (2023), developing a harmonious framework encompassing several research stages signifies the essence of interdisciplinarity and community engagement. This approach not only develops prudent research traditions but also ensures research outputs have societal and patient relevance. Overall, ELSI milestones reveal an extensive blueprint constantly adapting to address novel scientific challenges and societal needs, eventually leading to a better ethical and enlightened reaction to frontier technologies.

14.1.3. Evolution of ELSI in Response to Technological Advancements

As technology advances at breakneck pace, the ethical, legal, and social implications (ELSI) for these emerging developments have shifted dramatically. The explosion of the digital economy, i.e., software coding in technology companies, has introduced imperative ethical challenges, primarily information privacy and algorithmic fairness. Stakeholders are under increasing pressure to address these intricacies in a bid to maintain user trust while satisfying regulatory frameworks. The specter of algorithmic bias has deepened, warranting a necessary examination of the circumstances under which such algorithms operate. Work on ELSI has come to the forefront inasmuch as it seeks to handle the pressing need for ethical practice that not only strengthens the technological potential but also ensures societal well-being and justice. Without such a thesis-shifting framework, technology's benefits can inadvertently widen current social inequalities and deepen harm towards vulnerable communities, and as such may underscore the necessity for ethically motivated consideration in technological development (Ajiga et al., 2024). Moreover, with the introduction of new technologies, including virtual and augmented reality, the ELSI landscape is further complicated. The development of products like the Apple Vision Pro reflects the need for adaptable legal frameworks attuned to the speed of technological progress. As technology advances, so frequently does the law lag behind, and there appear gaps which can all too easily expose users' rights. There has been a growing debate around privacy rights and self-determination, with the need for an ongoing dialogue between technology creators, legal experts, and ethicists. The aim is to balance likely damages while encouraging democratic principles by the careful use of technology. The challenge can be addressed through an open discourse of the role of policy and law in safeguarding individual and collective rights, establishing an inclusive platform that caters to the ever-changing dynamics of technology and society (Caprioli et al., 2024). Finally, the emergence of ELSI is an ongoing response to the revolutionary impact of technology on social structure. The implications of masses embracing technology, from shifts in work to dynamics of human relationships, highlight the interdependence of ethics, law, and societal impacts. Since the process of integrating technology into human life is accelerating, it is imperative to look into the broader implications for community life and individual experience. The historical context of ELSI development draws attention to the necessity of sustained research and policy development to meet emerging ethical issues. The initiatives should focus on creating an ethical culture in technology that highlights social responsibility, justice, and fairness. Essentially, ELSI development is not merely a reaction to technological advancements but a critical framework that guides and directs responsible innovation in an ever-changing technological landscape.

14.2. Ethical Implications

The ethical implications that accompany new technologies, particularly those of artificial intelligence (AI) and genetic screening, are increasingly relevant in our ongoing discourses. With continuous advancements in AI, such frameworks not only entail technical abilities but also normative values informing their interaction with users. Such substrates of values and assumptions have the potential to lead to dumping when developers inadvertently pass on moral accountability to new users or inadequately resourced settings. This describes the necessity for robust interaction with ethical standards that are scalable to different situations to ensure responsible innovation and reduce adverse effects. As proposed in existing literature, the discussion on AI ethics has shifted from general issues to the necessity of applied frameworks that adequately integrate ethical principles into the processes of AI development and deployment, as captured in the existing investigation of how these technologies serve society overall (Jean-Christophe et al., 2024). Further, the challenges with ethically examining genetic information underscore the challenges encountered in biomedical contexts. The WISDOM trial recalls the intricate relationship between individuals and their genetic data, and most particularly regarding pathogenic variants within breast cancer-related genes. Qualitative findings from interviews showed that the majority of the participants, when provided with results on moderately penetrant breast cancer genes, perceived little difference in their own risk profile. This discrepancy poses an underlying ethical problem: the way genetic information is communicated and interpreted can be a strong influence on personal decision-making regarding health and screening. Furthermore, unwillingness to perform cascade testing is indicative of a potential shortfall in communicating the value of genetic information between relatives. Such discoveries compel moral consideration when dealing with genetic data and the release of explicit regulation in a readily accessible form, modified to suit diverse backgrounds and situations (Caprioli et al., 2024). The intersection of ethical, legal, and social considerations in AI and genetic testing calls for a multidimensional model of policymaking and regulation. The dynamic nature of these fields presents a challenge to the establishment of comprehensive guidelines confronting the specific ethical challenges they raise. Organizations tasked with implementing AI systems must evaluate the ethical considerations inherent in their application and ensure that they satisfy society's values and are sensitive to stakeholders' interests. At the same time, genetic testing programs must consider the different implications of risk information sharing by individuals and between families. Fostering transparency, user control, and engagement in ethical debate is necessary to mitigate risks potentially fueled by AI ethics dumping and subtle responses to genetic test outcomes. A shared focus on equitable ethical governance frameworks will facilitate responsibility and drive best practices in these burgeoning fields (Jean-Christophe et al., 2024) (Figure 14.5).

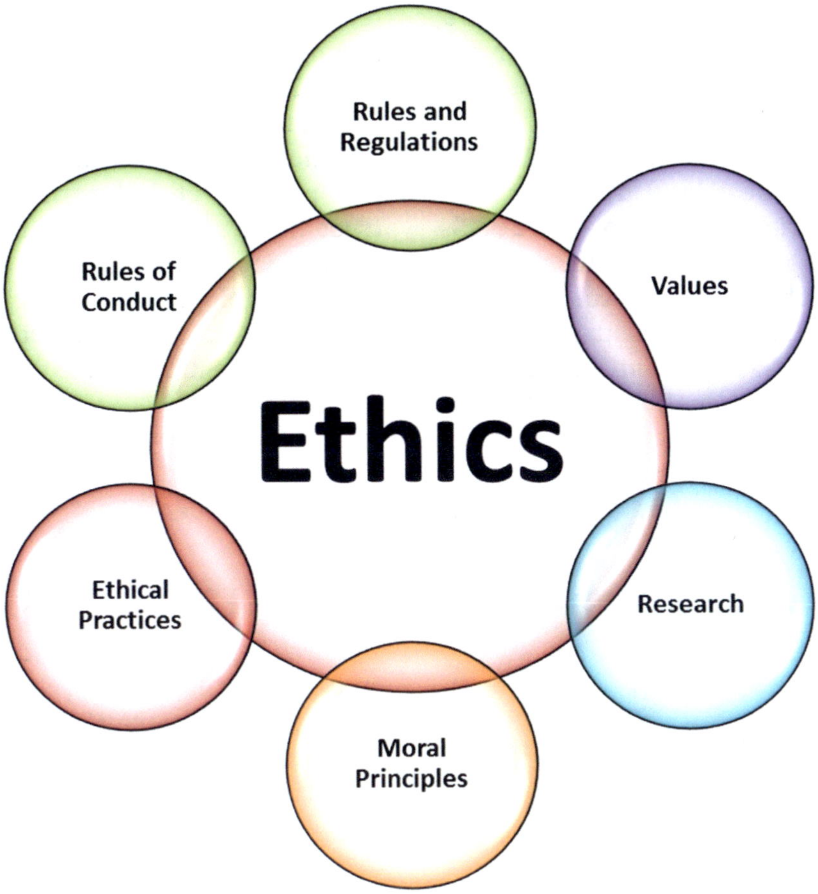

Figure 14.5. Ethical implications.

Source: https://images.saymedia-content.com/.image/t_share/MTc0MjMxNzE2NzI1NDY2NjIw/psychology-research-psychological-research-on-animals.png.

14.2.1. Moral Considerations in Research and Technology

The ethics of research and technology become increasingly pivotal with technological innovations emerging and evolving. Ethics comes to focus on the position of scientific advancement and moral responsibility to individuals and society. The applications of technologies, such as polygenic embryo screening (PES), emphasize the delicate balance in coming to make ethical choices in research. By enabling parents to select embryos based on expected genetic traits, PES raises significant ethical issues involving autonomy, the right to a future like ours for children, and the risk of creating societal disparities. As described in various media reviews, one of the common fears is that the technology might subtly steer society toward eugenics, encouraging discrimination based on genetic vulnerability (Kamenova & Haidar, 2022). Thus, the moral implications of such innovations need to be thoroughly scrutinized to help provide ethical practice at the forefront of technological uptake in reproductive medicine. Besides ethical considerations imported by new technologies, there are significant legal issues that arise, particularly under the umbrellas of patient confidentiality and informed consent. With more research conducted in fields like epigenetics, the sensitivity of the data gathered from genetic information can have severe legal and societal consequences for the individual. Issues of discrimination based on genetic information, re-identification of patients, and incidental findings management underscore the importance of robust legal frameworks to protect individuals' rights (Santal Jó et al., 2022). Unless they are properly legally protected, risks inherent in epigenetic data can create mistrust among research communities and discourage individuals' willingness to participate in studies with the potential to benefit public health. Making sure ethical standards come with legal protection will therefore be crucial to solving the complex interplay between technological advances and social implications.

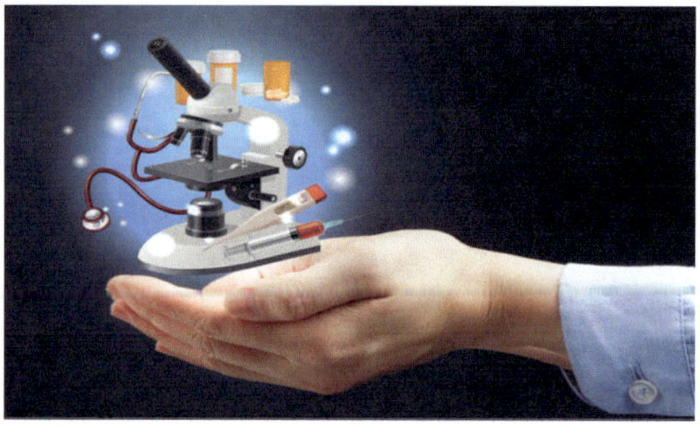

Figure 14.6. Moral considerations in research and technology.

Source: https://www.enago.com/academy/wp-content/uploads/2019/05/tinyresearchethics-1.jpg.

Moreover, the social implications of new technologies need ongoing public debate on research assumptions and resulting technologies. As society transitions toward technologies like PES and epigenetic research, not only the scientific worth but also the common cultural narratives and potential stigmas surrounding genetic information must be part of the discussion. Social equity and access issues should be a top priority in such debates to avoid exacerbating already present inequalities, especially since the benefits of genetic technologies might not be equitably distributed among different demographic groups (Santal Jó et al., 2022). Stakeholder engagement through ethicists, policymakers, and members of the community allows for an all-encompassing plan that respects ethical norms while establishing trust in scientific advancement. Last but not least, it is via this intricate discourse that the moral problems of research and technology can be dealt with correctly and leading to responsible and equitable innovations in society (Figure 14.6).

14.2.2. The Role of Informed Consent

In recent years, informed consent has emerged as the backbone of the moral universe of medical research and testing, providing genetic testing and data utilization a special significance. It safeguards individuals' autonomy by informing patients or subjects of research choices about potential risks, benefits, and results. The requirement for informed consent becomes more and more important in genetic contexts in which the information disclosed may be able to significantly influence both the individual and the familial relationships. As discussed by ELSI scholars, there has been a long-standing suspicion of genetic testing due to fear of unwelcome psychosocial consequences of becoming aware of one's genetic susceptibility. This fear is aimed at highlighting the need for strict conducted informed consent procedures that address patients' psychological and emotional needs to ensure decision-making through clarity and confidence (Parens & Appelbaum, 2019). New studies, however, suggest that initial anxieties regarding genetic information might have been exaggerated, with a re-evaluation of how to approach informed consent needed. In a few cases, negative psychosocial impacts have proven to be less frequent than initially thought, raising serious questions about the necessity of robust informed consent practices. With data indicating that the vast majority of individuals do not experience negative outcomes after learning of genetic information, some ELSI scientists advocate reducing the complexity of the informed consent process. It poses a debate regarding the ethical implications of genetic testing and data-sharing practices: whether the demand for stringent informed consent can be repealed or abandoned in light of evolving comprehension. To ensure that consent practice stays attuned to today's realities while respecting individuals' autonomy, such analysis needs to be founded on key data from various populations. Furthermore, the informed consent function extends from the medical domain to the big data research domain and its moral complexities. With neuroscience becoming more dependent on large-scale data analysis and collection, there is an urgent need to ensure that participants are informed regarding how their data will be shared, stored, and utilized. The complexity of data handling poses additional challenges to the preservation of transparent informed consent procedures, particularly in the context of international collaborations when ethical requirements are vastly different. It is ever more necessary to include informed consent procedures that bypass these complexities but continue to be in line with data protection and privacy requirements. Through this, responsible data governance becomes a core template that anticipates not just compliance with informed consent but also a dialogical approach to ethical concerns. This is critical in trust-building and guaranteeing the appropriateness of the use of data, therefore being part of the broader debate on ELSI issues (Parens & Appelbaum, 2019).

14.2.3. Balancing Benefits and Risks in Ethical Decision-Making

As far as ethical decision-making is concerned in the context of artificial intelligence and Big Data specifically, it is necessary to weigh up the subtle dynamic between anticipated gains and threats. Innovations based on data have the ability to enhance public health, augment services, and provoke economic growth, but are certain to raise significant ethical issues, primarily with regard to privacy and consent. The 'creep factor' of Big Data also points to how individual data are at risk of being lost, often unknowingly and without the consent of people, and raising issues of trust and equity. By setting down ethical standards that maximize openness and respect for people's rights, stakeholders can ensure that the benefits of Big Data technologies are harnessed without disproportionately impacting marginalized groups. This equilibrium is required not just for public acceptance but also for the development of technologies on ethical grounds in agreement with the norms and ethical values of society and hence increasing their legitimacy as well as sustainability (Da Bormida, 2021). Risk assessment in ethical decision-making frameworks must also incorporate a thought-provoking understanding of the long-term consequences of technological advancements. The automated decision-making by AI, despite being effective, can be discriminatory if not regulated properly. As seen with the increasing application of predictive models that decide life-changing implications, care must be taken to look at the accuracy and neutrality of such technologies. Moral decision-making should therefore involve ongoing evaluation of these technologies' impact on underprivileged groups and individuals' rights. There must be well-defined regulatory norms as well as mechanisms of accountability to prevent misuse and mitigate the broader societal risks associated with such innovations. Formulating a unified means of risk management not only serves to protect individual rights but also fosters an atmosphere that can be creative by ensuring the deployment of such technology to be fair and just. To this effect, ethical systems ought to cultivate discussion among stakeholders to assimilate diverse perceptions and collectively shape new technology operating norms (Maben & Bridges, 2020). Finally, the issue of reaping benefits or risks in ethical decision-making is strongly entwined in the broader narrative of social responsibility and public trust. As governments and institutions move towards leveraging data more heavily in decision-making, no greater mandate exists than to include communities themselves in meaningful ways. Openness regarding the gathering, usage of data, and implications of such contributes to building trust and facilitates public participation when discussing data ethics. This approach not only prioritizes ethical practices but also amplifies the voices of those who could be disproportionately affected by such technologies. Engaging stakeholders in the ethical dialogue of Big Data and AI operations creates a sense of responsibility and accountability, focusing attention on the public good. Placing priority on ethical issues in making decisions allows societies to truly embrace technological advancement but safeguard individual rights and ensure democratic values in an information age (Da Bormida, 2021) (Figure 14.7).

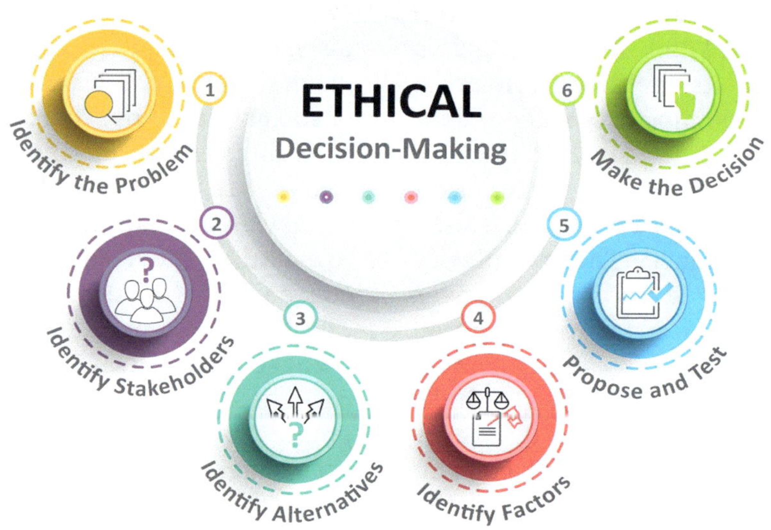

Figure 14.7. Balancing benefits and risks in ethical decision-making.

Source: https://www.islandhealth.ca/sites/default/files/2019-06/ethical_decision_making_framework.png.

14.3. Legal Implications

Legal significance of emerging scientific fields, above all in epigenetics, results in extensive debate regarding personal rights and societal obligations. The dynamics of the discipline test traditional presumptions of liability and consent, suggesting that environmental impacts on gene expression blur the line between nature and nurture. With scientists delving further into these dimensions, the scope of litigation regarding stigmatization and discrimination mounts. The legal systems can be made to adapt to meet ensuing changes in society, so that protection against discrimination is strong enough to address issues that might arise out of epigenetic research, e.g., privacy violations and misuse of genetic information. This evolving climate requires close examination of existing legislation to determine that it is well-equipped to deal with the nuances of epigenetic data and its application in public health, among other fields (Dupras et al., 2019). The implications of corporate responsibility in the context of epigenetic research also require close legal examination. In a time when the business world is globalized, it is vital to know how Corporate Social Responsibility (CSR) differs from one region to another. The comparison of CSR in the United States and Europe illustrates how legal systems govern corporate conduct and the social compact between companies and their consumers. As the legal frameworks adapt to include epigenetic considerations, companies conducting this research may be under more pressure with regard to their duties to stakeholders. This entails having openness to conduct research and utilize data that should be in line with the regulatory regimes established across jurisdictions. Hence, the legal implications extend to compliance, making it obligatory for corporations to incorporate ethical practices within their business processes all over the world (Matten & Moon, 2008). Moreover, the coincidence of genetic science and legal frameworks presents predicaments to recognize intellectual property rights. With epigenetic innovations bringing about new innovations in treatments and health technologies, problems related to patentability become more severe. Legal requirements need to address what exactly is a patentable entity when it comes to gene expression and how environmental factors affect genetics, issues of ethical concern regarding ownership and access to information. When considering the possible public health implications of epigenetic discovery, this assumes a greater significance as a means of ensuring that advances are accessible instead of being monopolized has the potential to inform future health policy. Thus, it is necessary to reconcile stimulating research with intellectual property rights while providing equitable access to progress. The ongoing argument over these legal ramifications will decide the destiny of epigenetics and how it is utilized in healthcare, policy, and society (Dupras et al., 2019).

14.3.1. Overview of Relevant Laws and Regulations

The use of large language models (LLMs) and artificial intelligence (AI) technologies in various areas , such as science research and education, has raised the question of whether existing law and regulation on their use should be reviewed in-depth. As noted at a symposium at the Walter and Eliza Hall Institute, the integration of AI tools necessitates an advanced understanding of the ethical, legal, and social implications (ELSI) surrounding such advances. The law surrounding AI technologies remains nuanced, with legislation struggling to keep pace with technological advancements. In many jurisdictions, buildings focus on privacy, intellectual property rights, and data protection, all important in the interest of safeguarding user data and ensuring ethical compliance with AI deployment (Caprioli , 2023). The major distinction between somatic and germline editing is one of the severe legal disputes in the biotechnology sector that meets with AI growth. Multiple countries have placed specific prohibitions on editing the heritable human genome, grounded in guidelines for promoting human rights and maintaining social norms. The Universal Declaration on the Human Genome and Human Rights, as approved by the United Nations, is a foundational legal instrument affecting the stance of most nations concerning the application of genetic editing tools (Andorno et al., 2020). Besides, the Oviedo Convention, which is established by the Council of Europe, imposes obligatory norms on human rights against biological advancement, supplementing the resort to responsible regulation of new technology to prevent potential malpractices. Since scientists employ AI technology for gene research, monitoring of such legal frameworks is necessary to balance the precarious interplay between innovation and conformity to the law (Caprioli et al., 2023). Moreover, the societal effects of AI technologies embrace nuances beyond the simplicity of lawfulness. Many academic bodies and organizations are now crafting policies that address the ethical concerns surrounding the employment of LLMs, particularly in education and scientific research. Those policies aim to provide a platform where academic honesty is preserved while simultaneously encouraging innovation through AI systems. The current debate within the science world reinforces the need for engagement with society and the need to create strong frameworks for responsibility in AI use (Andorno et al., 2020). As these debates unfold, stakeholders need to appreciate the worth of an interdisciplinary discourse that brings together contributions from law, ethics, and sociology to make sure that the use of AI not only meets legal requirements but also encourages fair and ethical practices in the ever-changing world of science and technology (Figure 14.8).

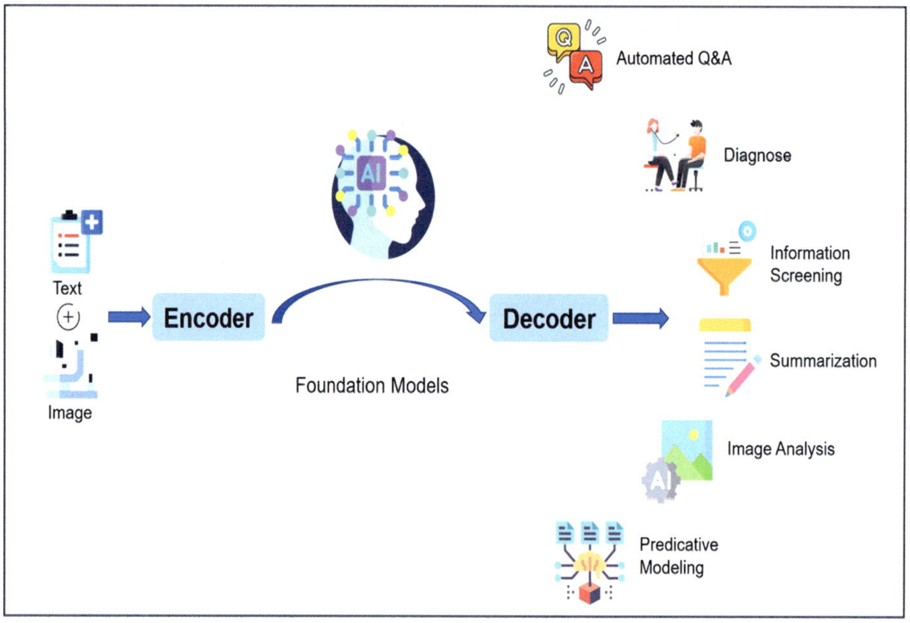

Figure 14.8. Large language models (LLMs) and artificial intelligence (AI).

Source: https://www.frontiersin.org/files/Articles/1291404/fmed-10-1291404-HTML/image_m/fmed-10-1291404-g001.jpg.

14.3.2. Intellectual Property Rights and ELSI

Intellectual property rights (IPR) are extremely significant in the new frontier of ethical, legal, and social implications (ELSI) of newer technologies, particularly artificial intelligence (AI). The more effective AI systems are at creating creative work, the more tangled the issue of ownership becomes. Authorship and copyright's similarities and traditional concepts of authorship and copyright are put to test when authors are algorithms rather than human entities. Such a revolution necessitates a rethinking of legal frameworks to respond to the unique features of AI-generated works. Current studies suggest that intellectual property implications extend way beyond authorship, and they encompass a variety of other public concerns like access to information, protection of cultural heritage, and technological fairness. Thus, policymakers need to become involved in interdisciplinary discussions that seek to balance the rights awarded to creators with the public interest in sharing knowledge and cultural creation. Incorporating AI across industries poses significant ethical concerns regarding intellectual property rights, particularly concerns of liability and responsibility. With autonomous decision-making by AI agents, it is hard not to ask who would be responsible for presumptive infringements of intellectual property rights, especially where the technology may end up plagiarizing existing works. This issue stands even more strongly in metaverse-type settings where AI avatars can interact with a degree of creativity and autonomy that renders it hard to mark boundaries of human guidance and control. The creation of AI avatars needs a responsive regulatory framework that is in a position to address these complexities appropriately. A visionary strategy of designing inclusive regulation is in a position to draw clear lines of accountability between stakeholders engaged in AI initiatives, in such a way that moral expectations and legal structures develop proportionally to technological progress (Cheong, 2024). Additionally, intellectual property rights implications in the realm of AI technologies extend to questions of data privacy and algorithmic transparency. Data collection and use for training AI call into question consent and respectful treatment of personal data. While corporations take enormous datasets to fuel AI models, it becomes increasingly vital to balance innovation with the protection of individual rights. Moreover, rendering algorithmic processes transparent enhances public trust and accountability, which neutralizes fears about the issues of bias and discrimination in AI-generated content. Initiatives like the EU's AI Act highlight the importance of constructing legal frameworks that preserve not only intellectual property rights but also community values and rights. This multilateral approach emphasizes the importance of interdisciplinarity in the process of creating effective regulatory mechanisms capable of managing the intricate interaction between intellectual property rights, ethical aspects, and social impacts (Dokumac, 2024) (Figure 14.9).

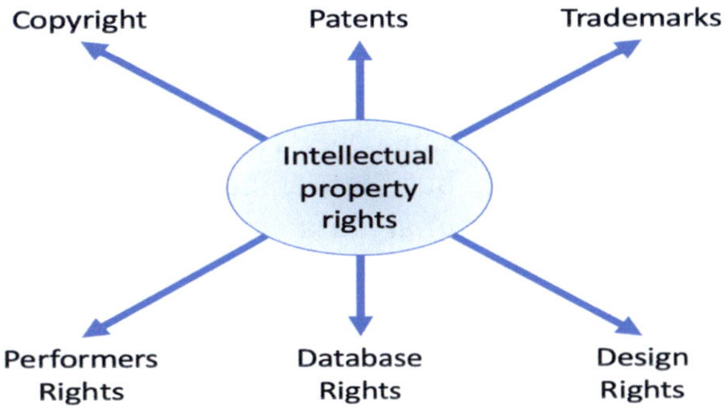

Figure 14.9. Intellectual property rights (IPR).

Source: https://pub.mdpi-res.com/algorithms/algorithms-15-00418/article_deploy/html/images/algorithms-15-00418-g001-550.jpg?1667886664.

14.3.3. Legal Challenges Arising from Technological Innovations

The rapid speed of technology advances creates a broad array of legal problems demanding immediate response in the framework of Ethical, Legal, and Social Implications (ELSI). With the diffusion of digital health technology, such as AI-based diagnostic tools and mobile health applications, in the health care setting, the legal settings are behind. Patient data privacy and informed consent issues have become increasingly pertinent, particularly in light of the fact that patients are now dealing with algorithms that analyze their health data. Such issues necessitate that existing regulatory structures be revised to make them adaptable to the evolving nature of technology. In the study, while digital health technologies enhance access, they are also likely to exacerbate already present healthcare inequities and raise ethical issues around algorithmic bias in health outcomes, and therefore, the need for uniform legal guidelines with emphasis on patient self-regulation and the protection of individual rights (McGrath et al., 2025). In addition, the convergence of augmented and virtual reality technologies, as embodied by innovations like the Apple Vision

Pro, sheds more legal complexities. In this case, privacy and autonomy rights are the dominant legal issues at stake, prompted by the immersive nature of these technologies. They not only track user interaction but also embed tremendous volumes of personal data, raising concerns of monitoring and information misuse. The challenge is in how to legislate innovation, pitted against the necessity of protecting consumers from potential overreach.

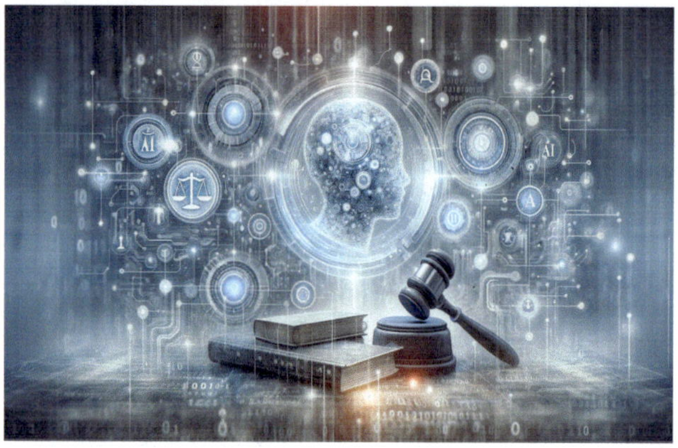

Figure 14.10. Legal challenges arising from technological innovations.

Source: https://blog.prevail.ai/content/images/size/w960/2023/12/AI-in-Law-Balancing-Legal-Tech-and-Ethics.png.

As elaborated in the relevant literature, coordination among policymakers, technologists, and lawyers is greatly needed to develop adaptable regulations that can keep up with the rapid turnover of technological innovation. This shared approach is crucial to ensure trust in technological advancements while securing individual as well as collective rights (Caprioli et al., 2024). Lastly, the legal hurdles created by technological advancements are aggravated by the digital divide, which impacts access to technology and its offerings. As society becomes increasingly reliant upon digital health technologies, the unequal access and digital literacy distribution across socio-economic groups raise equity issues in healthcare. Those who do not have the means or capability to utilize these innovations risk being left behind even further. Thus, resolving these disparities is important not only to provide equitable access but also to fortify the ethical underpinnings of technology acceptance in medicine. The debate has to move towards formulating inclusive policies considering all user communities and thereby reinforcing the ethical, legal, and social basis of new technologies in an integrated manner (McGrath et al., 2025) (Figure 14.10).

14.4. Social Implications

The advent of advanced technologies, particularly in medicine and genetics, has profound societal implications extending beyond the individual benefits to overall social dynamics. One such area of interest is how artificial intelligence , such as ChatGPT, can transform the model of health care education, research, and practice. While benefits include improved scientific communication, improved health literacy, and improved workflow efficiency, the underlying ethical issues may erode individuals' trust in medical facilities (Sallam, 2023). The excessive reliance on AI tools could lead to decreased human control, which compromises critical thinking and active participation in medical care decisions. Hence, debates regarding the transparency and accountability of such technologies are urgently needed so that the socio-cultural integrity of healthcare is ensured and marginalized groups are not further excluded from it. The risk of heritable human genome editing also raises serious issues of social justice, which cannot be neglected. Genetically modifying the coming generations carries with it the intrinsic danger of exacerbating present social inequalities and creating new forms of discrimination. Critics believe that, if commercialized, such technologies would lead to new eugenics in which genetic enhancements are reserved largely for the privileged classes and thus further solidify socioeconomic inequalities (Andorno et al., 2020). History has shown that technology has in some cases been employed to reinforce social hierarchies rather than temper them. Therefore, good public engagement is essential in negotiating these complex social landscapes. This means demanding the participation of a broad range of voices and opinions in debate about the consequences of, and the regulation of, such life-altering technologies. For these emerging social problems to be successfully addressed, there must be a strong thrust toward developing sound frameworks that prioritize ethical issues and public empowerment. This involves coming up with inclusive dialogue that offers spaces for multiplicity of viewpoints, particularly from marginalized communities whose lives are impacted by these technologies. Facilitating democratic rule in decision-making regarding artificial intelligence and genetic technologies is crucial to establishing avenues that capture society's interests and values as well as ethics (Andorno et al., 2020; Sallam, 2023). As society grapples with these social, legal, and ethical implications, an engaged public will be more capable of being involved in the thoughtful deliberations needed for responsible innovation. In the end, the goal must be to use technological advancements while creating equality and well-being in communities, so that the good extends far and wide across all levels of society.

14.4.1. Impact of ELSI on Public Perception and Trust

The Ethical, Legal, and Social Implications (ELSI) framework is a significant social measure that society employs in evaluating new technologies, particularly in biotechnology and artificial intelligence. Significant in ELSI are public attitude and trust, which play a central role in guaranteeing that the technologies are implemented successfully. A robust ELSI framework, as outlined in initiatives , such as AI4People, can engender public confidence by fostering transparency in technological progress and engaging stakeholders in meaningful discussions on ethics, legality, and societal impact. The inclusion of ethical standards formulated within such frameworks has an immediate effect on public opinion, paving the way for improved implications since social acceptance hinges on informed views on risk and advantage (Floridi et al., 2018). Acceptance of technology among the public depends to a large extent on what people believe about its ethics. The moment people realize that code writers operate under stringent ethical standards, people are likely to embrace new technologies. Dissemination of open information regarding how technologies align with societal values fosters positive attitudes and encourages engagement. For instance, collaborative consumption programs have recorded varying rates of success, which individuals' inclination to engage relies upon whether they are knowledgeable of the environmental and social benefits of engagement (Hamari et al., 2015). The above trend captures how public opinion interacts with ethical systems so as to matter since participation and trust in technology can be scaled up, that is, increased collective action for societal purposes. In addition, the impact of ELSI extends beyond public acceptance to shape the direction of policy and regulatory practice, too. Policymakers who are led by the principles of ELSI can impose regulations that ensure ethical conduct, thereby maintaining public trust. By involving the public directly in ELSI discussions, e.g., public forums and advisory groups, policymakers are in a position to address increasing demands on privacy, data protection, and discrimination. This citizen participation not only creates a sense of ownership but also brings credibility to the governance of new technology. When citizens believe that their voices are being heard and that ethical concerns are being prioritized, then they are more likely to facilitate a cooperative environment, which is required to deal with the sophistication of modern technological advancements (Floridi et al., 2018) (Figure 14.11).

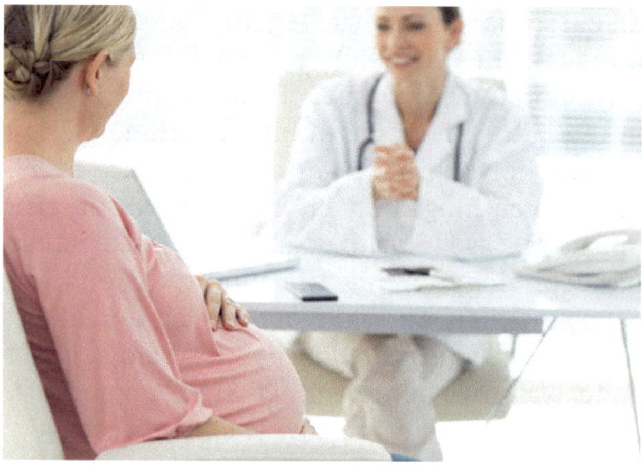

Figure 14.11. Impact of ELSI on public perception and trust.

Source: https://www.lecre.umontreal.ca/wp-content/uploads/2023/08/capture-decran-le-2023-08-22-a-081713.png.

14.4.2. Social Justice and Equity Considerations

Social justice and equity values play a critical role in informing policy and practice in ethical, legal, and social implications (ELSI). Demand for equity in biotechnology regulation extends beyond access to new therapeutic solutions; it has a broader societal consequence, including the potential to exacerbate disparities. The benefits of progress made in biotechnology, such as genetic testing and treatment, should be fairly shared so that marginalized groups are not left behind.

Most times, this can involve reconstructing what policies already are so that vulnerable groups are prioritized, thus guaranteeing a more equitable response to health equity. Policy-makers must engage with vulnerable groups to listen to their stories and learn about their particular experiences and challenges so that efforts become responsive to their needs rather than passing down measures that could further deepen injustice and inequality (McGrath et al., 2025). Informed consent and autonomy are key elements of social justice in the situation of ELSI. Forced paternity testing, for example, raises important questions regarding individual rights and individual autonomy in family matters, towards the balance of creating just systems in child support and protecting parental autonomy. While benefits , such as combating paternity fraud would function to enhance fairness in monetary commitments within the family, the moral implications of compulsory testing cannot be ignored. This conversation invokes the need for reviewing consent procedures so that individuals are given complete disclosure and the autonomy to make uninfluenced decisions without coercion. Ethical theories must be used to evaluate how legal conditions impact familial and communal social relationships with the objective of eventually balancing disclosure with individual freedoms in ways that enhance social justice (mcGrath et al., 2025). Besides, social consequences of ELSI need to be managed sensitively in matters of public awareness and trust in supervised technologies. Effective communication among the public, policymakers, and scientists is essential in building trust, especially when handling such sensitive issues as biotechnology. Misinformation and cultural discord may heavily contribute to shaping the ways communities react to genetic inquiry and testing innovations, which can further sustain health disparities in access and outcomes. Therefore, educational equity and awareness work take center stage. Everyone would have to be brought into discussions that not only identify the benefits of new biotechnologies but also genuinely understand the cultural and ethical implications at play. A socio-justice strategy of a multi-disciplinary type can finally mold and shape regulatory response, to more easily support public acceptance and the moral integration of biotechnology into a regime of justice and fairness (Singh et al., 2023) (Figure 14.12).

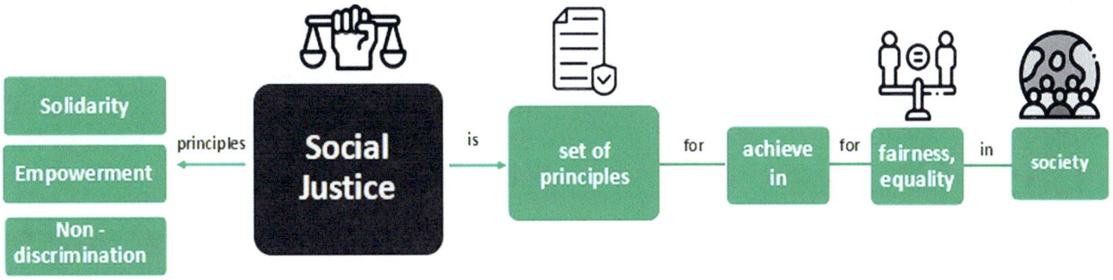

Figure 14.12. Social justice and equity considerations.

Source: https://wallstreetmojocms.recurpro.in/uploads/Social_Justice_51078484e9.png.

14.4.3. The Role of Community Engagement in ELSI

Community engagement is important in the management of the Ethical, Legal, and Social Implications (ELSI) of scientific advances, particularly those in the field of genomics and health data science. Through active interaction with members of the community, scientists can identify the intricacies of the ethical concerns and cultural sensitivities that may be raised. If communities are respected and their voices are heard, trust is established, leading to increased collaboration and participation in research studies. Such initiatives as UZIMA-DS exemplify this participatory approach by emphasizing the participation of stakeholders and creating sustainable frameworks for the release of health-related information to local populations. Focusing on such a community ensures researchers are able to form methods that are more attuned to the values and expectations of the affected, thus enhancing the overall worth of findings from the research and providing equitable access to benefits accruing from new technologies and data practices (Waljee et al., 2022). Further, the incorporation of community participation strategies provides a platform for the voice of excluded peoples, particularly Indigenous peoples, who are often excluded from decision-making around their data or biological material. The recent instances of the Biocultural Labels and Notices demonstrate the importance of the recognition and integration of Indigenous rights in the cycle of data. These funds allow Indigenous people to exert control over their cultural and biological data and allow researchers to navigate the complex landscape of consent and collaboration. Through the incorporation of ethical considerations right at the center of research in the form of interactions with communities, the ELSI approach increases the accountability of researchers and institutions to include the concerns and interests of communities into the development and realization of novel scientific technologies (Anderson & Hudson, 2020). The added stress on community engagement within the ELSI process further highlights the importance of interdisciplinary discussion between broad constituencies of stakeholders, including policymakers, ethicists, and civil society in general. The establishment of a conversation among these various perspectives leads to a more nuanced understanding of the long-term implications of scientific advancement. Community engagement not only promotes openness but also provokes the co-construction of knowledge in a value-responsive and priority-sensitive way. With evolving ethical issues, particularly the sharing of health data and privacy concerns, active participation by communities can direct researchers to engage cultural norms and promote equitable data utilization. Ultimately, by establishing a platform for collaboration, the ELSI framework can evolve to respond to emerging issues, thus promoting an ethical and social responsibility-oriented approach to scientific research and its application (Waljee et al., 2022).

14.5. Case Studies in ELSI

The increasingly visible presence of genetic technologies, particularly Next Generation Sequencing (NGS), demands scrutiny of the associated Ethical, Legal, and Social Implications (ELSI). As the capacity to recognize disease-causing variants increases, health professionals face questions about how to integrate systematic reanalysis of this data into routine diagnostics. Most importantly, studies show that while many articles cite the technological advancement in genetic diagnosis, such articles frequently neglect addressing the core ELSI concerns. For instance, the scoping review highlighted essential factors , such as consent, cost-effectiveness, and the involvement of Genetic Health Professionals (GHPs) in handling these complex circumstances. This gap in discourse underscores the importance of GHPs' active engagement with issues around ELSI, balancing the limits of the lab with the need to provide accurate diagnoses for patients with diverse needs. Such ethical input is essential to the effective use of genomic technologies in the clinical setting (Weng & Francesconi, 2023). Even in robotics, the development of social robots presents difficult ELSI issues. The case of the "LOVOT" humanoid companion robot identifies the need for consent in human-robot interaction. As robots are entering more and more private and social spheres, privacy becomes the most significant question to address. Traditional legal codes struggle to react adequately to the specific needs that originate from the rapidly evolving artificial intelligence technologies, often finding themselves behind inventions creating fuzzy ethical issues. Design-focused proponents suggest "Ethical Design" processes with user consent and privacy taking priority on the development side. While these considerations not only make valuable human-robot interactions feasible, but they also ensure that ELSI ramifications follow ethical best practices on par with technological advancements.

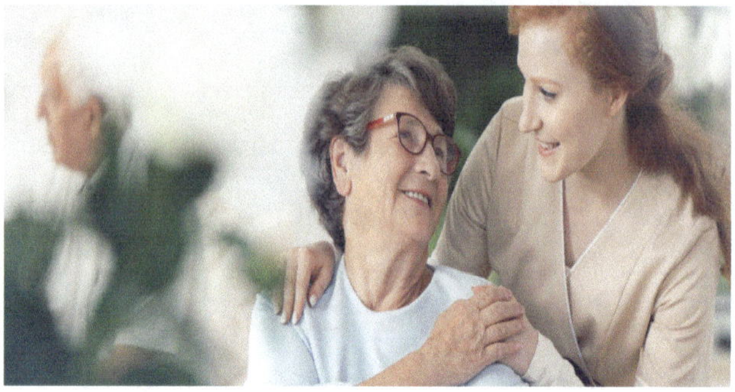

Figure 14.13. Case studies in legal, and social implications (ELSI).

Source: https://regenerage.org.uk/wp-content/uploads/2023/01/Untitled-design-21-1-1024x383.png.

The regulation of social robots, therefore, depends on in-depth knowledge about their ELSI implications (Weng & Francesconi, 2023). The exploration of ELSI through several case studies captures the intricacy of ethical issues in contemporary technology. Whether genetic diagnosis or social robots, these cases pin down one thread in common: the necessity for inclusive frameworks with ethical, legal, and social considerations. The diverging opportunities of NGS and humanoid robots challenge practitioners as well as policymakers to adopt new paradigms that not only meet the needs of today but also anticipate what is coming next. Encouraging an enabling environment among stakeholders like researchers, ethicists, and technologists allows society to navigate the complexities surrounding technological innovations. This comprehensive focus on ELSI is not only essential for the advancement of technology but for the development of a society founded on the principles of ethical integrity and social responsibility as integral values in progress. Case studies in ELSI are then imperative landmarks in our understanding of technology's interactions with ethical and social frameworks (Weng & Francesconi, 2023) (Figure 14.13).

14.5.1. Genetic Research and Its Ethical Dilemmas

The gene research landscape is rapidly evolving, with attendant possibilities for medical and health advances. The advance is accompanied by enormous ethical issues that warrant critical scrutiny. A majority of scientists are in favor of gene editing and genetic testing as pathways to enhanced disease prevention and precision medicine. However, the implication of such technology extends beyond the medical intervention, and it has raised alarms regarding enhanced inequality and the code of ethics in action. For instance, access to genetic technologies like polygenic embryo screening (PES) is privileged for the wealthy, and healthcare social justice and equity are compromised. In light of researchers' calls for inclusive regulatory frameworks to govern these technologies, public policy, informed consent, and equitable access to genetic innovation have to be tackled by interdisciplinary conversation through the rich tapestry of ethical concerns harbored within (Silva, 2023). Among the most pressing ethical concerns is the risk of genetic discrimination and the re-evolution of eugenics-type activity. Polygenic embryo screening raised worries about the normalization of designer babies, with selecting embryos based on intelligence or physical attributes potentially redefining social norms and expectations. PRC critics argue that reliance on polygenic risk scores (PRS) for embryo screening may induce unrealistic hopes in prospective parents and amplify social inequalities. Moreover, the inaccuracy of making exact predictions of an individual's outcome from such genetic analysis gives rise to significant ethical issues surrounding parents' duty and children's rights to an open future. The moral argument always asks stakeholders to consider the long-term consequences of these technologies, not only for the science but also for broader societal considerations interlaced with human genetics (Kamenova & Haidar, 2022). Keeping these complex moral challenges in mind, the argument for genetic studies asks for a robust model of regulation and control. Scholars and bioethicists advocate for inclusive rules that steer through the opaque terrain of genetic interventions, emphasizing community involvement. Initiatives must involve a diversity of perspectives, particularly from marginalized communities who may bear the disproportionate risk of these innovations. Equally important is maintaining transparency in the design and use of genetic technologies. This increased focus demands ongoing education of healthcare professionals as well as the population for informed decision-making about genetic interventions. Finally, encouraging an interdisciplinary response to genetic research and its ethical implications is critical to safeguarding the future of human genetic technologies under the principles of equality, justice, and dignity (Silva, 2023).

14.5.2. Artificial Intelligence and Legal Ramifications

The emergence of artificial intelligence (AI) throughout sectors has totally altered the dominant paradigms of operation, but at the same time, generated an abundance of legal implications. With the development of AI technologies, they present complex challenges to the widespread paradigms of law, which are apt to fall behind lawmakers' ability to adopt adequate regulations. This paradox raises pressing questions regarding the accountability of AI systems, particularly in cases where consequences arising from actions by these systems amount to harm or are immoral. Where there is no good legal system in place, it becomes more difficult to assign responsibility in cases of AI malfunction or abuse. Furthermore, the responsibility also changes depending on whether the AI is considered an agent in its own right or merely a means by which human actors act. Therefore, the relationship between law and AI requires urgent consideration to make legal expectations align with moral standards in this rapidly evolving field. The intersection of AI and legal ethics only contributes to the richness of dialogue regarding its use, especially when ethical considerations are pushed to the side by competency. Bringing AI into fields , such as social work is an ideal example, where the potential gains of increased efficiency will have to be weighed against compromising the client relationship and trust. As per current debates about AI's role in social work, teachers need to provide students with the appropriate skills for working through these ethical considerations wisely and responsibly (Reimer, 2024). The challenge is not merely in grasping the technical nuances of AI but in developing an awareness of how it affects equity, privacy, and informed consent. Students should be prepared to analyze AI outputs critically and align them with ethical standards implicit in professional activity. Ultimately, the creation of a legally attentive ethical framework is most imperative to avoid danger and errors in incorporating AI in sensitive situations. Scholars and experts in law have also been deeply troubled by the moral aspects that lie at the source of AI usage, such as discrimination, privacy violation, and transparency concerns (Ayub & Banday, 2023). Such issues demand strict regulatory frameworks capable of coping with the fluidity that characterizes technological development. The absence of a comprehensive ethical framework has resulted in a fragmented way of addressing these issues, exposing organizations across the board to public scandal and litigation. The potential for unfair algorithms to perpetuate social injustice, for instance, underscores the need for adequate regulation and the adoption of accountability measures. As AI continues to evolve, the legal community has a responsibility to engage in a proactive dialogue that involves technologists, ethicists, and policymakers. By so doing, we can endeavor to develop a harmonized legal environment focusing on ethical factors while being able to contain the risks presented by artificial intelligence (Figure 14.14).

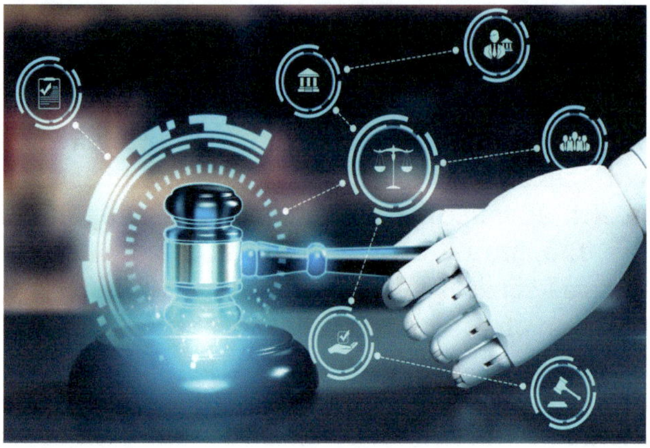

Figure 14.14. Artificial intelligence and legal ramifications.

Source: https://commonlegalquestions.com/wp-content/uploads/2023/07/ai-generated-content-copyright-law-scaled.jpeg.

14.5.3. Public Health Initiatives and Social Implications

Public health programs are necessary to counter the numerous health issues besetting populations, especially those in at-risk communities. They are designed to enhance overall health conditions via prevention, education, and the provision of vital services. Yet, program implementation is usually fraught with profound ethical, legal, and social concerns. With the goals of public health evolving to meet emerging needs of society, dilemmas like non-discriminatory access to care, respect for autonomy, and informed consent must be confronted with prudence. Engaging multiple stakeholders , such as policymakers, healthcare professionals, and community members, is critical to establishing trust and ensuring that health programs are grounded in the values and priorities of the populations of interest. Neglecting these ethical aspects could lead to public health interventions that, instead of lessening the inequities, further perpetuate them, thus undermining the very foundations of public health's purpose. The legal framework of public health activities also deserves scrutiny, especially in regard to individual rights versus collective welfare. Public health laws can serve to improve the effectiveness of interventions, imposing sanctions upon measures that safeguard the public against threats to health. But these regulations can also infringe on individual liberties, causing ethical debates about the equilibrium of rights. This tension occurs in debates concerning immunization mandates or quarantine during disease outbreaks. As indicated in debates concerning ethical norms underlying the development of health policies, the legislators should consider the overall social effect of their measures. Hasty choices without sufficient consideration of the rights of the populations can lead to social unrest and lost confidence in healthcare systems, making it crucial to adopt an integrative strategy respecting the autonomy of individuals while asserting priority on public health outcomes (Floridi et al., 2018). Moreover, social impacts of public health interventions extend beyond short-term benefits on health to restructuring community dynamics as well as social relationships. Efforts for health improvement can promote social cohesion and decrease stigmatization of some health conditions, thus promoting community solidarity. However, public health interventions are likely to become divisive if they are conceived as top-down or dissonant with local values. Most notably, the success of such interventions relies on their capacity to connect and empower local populations. As per the definitions in existing health system reviews, guaranteeing high-quality care is a population-based approach that focuses on equity, access, and responsiveness to emerging health needs (Silva, 2023). By optimizing collaborative arrangements that include the local voice and those targeting systemic inequities, public health programs can catalyze sustained social change, ultimately yielding healthier communities (Figure 14.15).

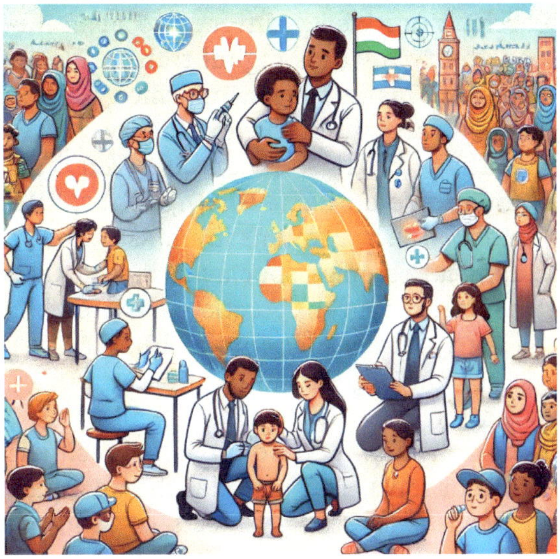

Figure 14.15. Public health initiatives and social implications.

Source: https://5minuteenglish.com/wp-content/uploads/2024/06/Global-Health-Initiatives-2.webp.

14.6. Future Directions in ELSI

As society keeps embracing technological developments, particularly in biomedicine and digital, the Ethical, Legal, and Social Implications (ELSI) infrastructure must evolve alongside the dynamism such advancements introduce. The new fronts for ELSI involve a critical analysis of how socio-cyber-physical systems influence areas like healthcare and agriculture. With the increasing interconnection of the world through digital technology, patterns that fully assess the interlinkages between social, cyber, and physical dimensions will be required. For instance, a responsible research and innovation approach demands increased sensitization to the normally unforeseen effects of the integration of technology, necessitating stakeholders to approach system complexities responsibly. In analyzing such interdependency on several levels, researchers are well positioned to push moral responsibility towards digital transformations, and thereby make proper, informed decisions regarding accountability for positive as well as negative impacts, as emphasized in the fresh literature on ELSI (Rijswijk et al., 2021). Personalized interventions are most in need in the healthcare sphere, specifically within areas , such as breast cancer detection and prevention at an early stage. All future ELSI research needs to converge around priority areas for intervention in health, which will allow for the development of varied population-specific risk assessment tools. This includes the elimination of the ethical and legal aspects of using such methods to make them accessible and equitable. Stakeholder engagement is crucial here as it allows for varied social norms and values to be embedded in health systems. By creating a collaborative environment, health interventions can address diverse community needs while simultaneously addressing ethical concerns that arise from discrimination or prejudice in medical technology. Interwoven research frontiers of effectiveness and implementation are thus able to remake ELSI discourse, unveiling opportunities for potent public health policies (Pashayan et al., 2020). Additionally, with additional developments in digital technologies that reshape human organization and individual experience, interdisciplinary approaches are increasingly necessary in ELSI research. Researchers, policymakers, and practitioners must collaborate to address the ethical and legal concerns introduced by such new technologies as artificial intelligence and gene editing. It will ensure the multidisciplinary nature of ELSI to facilitate the identification of new solutions sensitive to the social nuances and legal framework. *Responsibilisation* will underpin the discussion of responsibility for the ethical burden of decision-making for technology adoption. It will also ensure participation in the design of policies that govern the use of these technologies. By emphasizing group responsibility and accountability, ELSI research can substantially impact how society meets the challenges of the future of innovation and ethical governance, thereby validating its continued relevance in the evolving technological environment.

14.6.1. Emerging Technologies and Their ELSI Challenges

The rapid development of emerging technologies is accompanied by problematic ethical, legal, and social implications (ELSI) that must be addressed systemically to enable the responsible innovation. Emerging technologies , such as artificial intelligence, gene editing, and biotechnology are accompanied by issues that cannot be addressed in terms of traditional regulatory frameworks. For instance, the use of epigenetic clocks in criminal forensic contexts raises serious ethical concerns regarding privacy, consent, and misusing biological age as a metric of culpability or behavior. As can be observed in research for such clocks, there is a significant need to examine drivers and regulators of aging changes to understand their implications in detail, especially when applied to sensitive fields , such as criminal justice and medicine (Pardede, 2025). Such challenges need to be tackled using a multi-faceted approach that considers not just the technology's immediate benefits but also its broader implications for society. Furthermore, the discussion of responsible innovation (RI) increasingly focuses on the significance of integrating ELSI concerns in the process of technological development. Both in Europe and the United States, the concept of RI stresses transparency, stakeholder involvement, and responsibility in science and technology management. Though still incipient in countries like China, the roots of RI are gaining footing because policymakers and researchers are more and more conscious of the need for models that guarantee ethical considerations as well as technological advancement (Zhao & Liao, 2019). The participation is necessary because it provides a participatory model that incorporates diverse voices, therefore guaranteeing harmonization of new technologies with ethics and values within society.

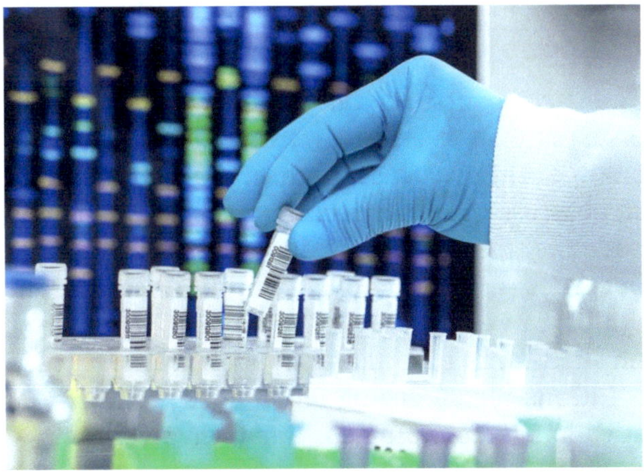

Figure 14.16. Emerging technologies and their ELSI challenges.

Source: https://www.thehastingscenter.org/wp-content/uploads/shutterstock_genetics-research-CERA-2025910559.jpg.

The evolution of RI practices can help mitigate the potential harmful effects stemming from technology misuse or misconception and hence guarantee more harmonized outcomes. Finally, addressing the ELSI challenges posed by emerging technologies requires proactive and active engagement by various actors. These involve policymakers, technologists, ethicists, and the general populace, whose joint expertise is essential in developing ethical paradigms that are compatible with innovation. Of particular importance, however, is that ELSI discussion must be transformed so that it can address the realities of increasingly interlinked global environments, where technologies might have disproportionately damaging effects on specific groups. Through cross-sector coordination, we can establish policies that not merely react to risks but also anticipate them, addressing dangers ahead of when they might become issues. Engaging stakeholders can ground technological advancement in ethical concerns, building trust among innovators and citizens. Attaining that balance is crucial to creating a context of appropriate technology usage that advances societal welfare and prevents unwanted repercussions (Figure 14.16).

14.6.2. The Importance of Interdisciplinary Collaboration

The complexity of ethical, legal, and social implications (ELSI) demands interdisciplinarity from various fields, particularly in environments like healthcare and technology. With advancing artificial intelligence (AI) transforming healthcare practices, the integration of knowledge from ethicists, lawyers, and medical professionals is inevitable. This cross-disciplinary approach deepens the richness of knowledge on AI's potential contribution to care and outcomes for patients and confronts the ethical dilemma of decision-making algorithms. The collaboration of multiple experts makes possible the comprehensive exploration of the potential benefits and limitations of AI, finally leading healthcare organizations to effective implementation. Through interdisciplinary work, stakeholders can better manage the intricacies of marrying technology and human well-being, ensuring that ethical norms keep up with technological advancements (Alowais et al., 2023). The new environment of new technologies, for instance, the metaverse, also highlights the need for interdisciplinary work in managing its extensive ELSI. With the intersection of physical and virtual borders, experts from different fields like sociology, psychology, and law are forced to research the sociocultural effects of such innovations collaboratively. A common framework supports these experts in interpreting issues of privacy, trust, and bias alongside observing social consequences of technology adoption. The case of how virtual reality worlds affect human relationships necessitates technical expert knowledge inputs alongside social scientist inputs. Through syncretizing various disciplinary perceptions, researchers can build an integrated narrative that informs policy-making and anticipates the ethical challenges introduced by the metaverse (Alowais et al., 2023). Hence, interdisciplinarity is a crucial tool for creating multi-dimensional observations that ultimately inform ethical technological assimilation. Finally, encouraging interdisciplinary culture fuels innovation in addressing ELSI, particularly in developing learning programs and policies.

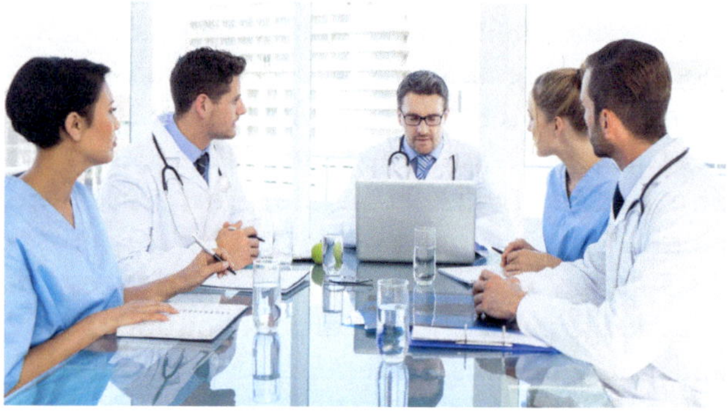

Figure 14.17. Importance of interdisciplinary collaboration.

Source: https://www.sermo.com/wp-content/uploads/2023/02/effective-communication-img6-min.jpg.

The inclusion of scholars and professionals across various fields calls for the offering of multiple methodologies and paradigms that finally lead to the formation of multidimensional strategies for increasing stakeholders' awareness of ethical matters. For example, crafting workshops and curricula that synthesize concepts from law, ethics, and technology can support intellectual examination and empower professionals to manage ELSI appropriately. Thus, interdisciplinary collaboration not only supports immediate solutions for ethical dilemmas but also allows future generations to address complex issues with an equilibrium perspective. As technology evolves, an interdisciplinary education setup will allow professionals to prepare themselves to address the complexity of ethical, legal, and social factors and ultimately create a more just and responsible technological future (Alowais et al., 2023) (Figure 14.17).

14.6.3. Anticipating Societal Changes and Ethical Frameworks

The terrain of societally changing landscapes is usually marked with sudden technological change that is faster than current ethical structures. With new technologies unfolding, the necessity for responsive governing mechanisms becomes all the more compelling. Current ethics have to not just respond to current implications but also have to frame future solutions for emerging challenges arising from advancing technologies. Early involvement by a wide range of stakeholders in the research and innovation process can ensure that all societal needs and values are understood thoroughly. This proactive approach allows the development of technologies that are not only scientifically reliable but also ethically justifiable. Scholars have recognized the place of compliance programs and Environmental, Social, and Governance (ESG) practices, emphasizing how these can assist organizations in mitigating risks while promoting ethical behavior as a reflection of evolving societal norms and support for Sustainable Development Goals (SDGs) (Silva, 2023). Anticipatory governance systems are necessary in the case of challenging the emergent complexity presented by new scientific fields, such as reprogramming technologies and the implications of human embryoid research. Traditional precautionary approaches fail to consider the dynamism of scientific development, and consequent law can actually serve to discourage progress rather than encourage it. New scholarly writing has proposed competing systems, such as Responsible Research and Innovation (RRI), placing stress on reflexivity and deliberation. By encouraging dialogue between policymakers, researchers, and the broader public, anticipatory strategies can be capable of anticipating ethical dilemmas while guiding socially equitable trajectories for technology. This kind of dialogue is particularly crucial in fields that are very uncertain, where emerging scientific advancements' ontological status and potential remain uncertain (Lysaght, 2021). Finally, the secret to forecasting change in society is to establish ethical standards that are robust as well as flexible during times of rapid change. The importance of foresight cannot be overstated; it is a guiding concept in designing policies that are adaptive and not reactive. Through the integration of ethical reflection into the early phases of technological innovation, societies can aim towards morally desirable objectives based on common human values. The integration of ethics in the governance of technology stimulates a culture of responsibility required to balance innovation with welfare. By actively taking these steps, policymakers and scientists can virtually ensure that progress builds flourishing, just futures and does not worsen current ethical challenges (Lysaght, 2021; Silva, 2023).

SUMMARY

In bringing to a conclusion an examination of the Ethical, Legal, and Social Implications (ELSI) of the issues of today, it is increasingly evident that the intersection of ethics, law, and social forces requires tact. Among the most important factors in these discussions is the capacity of marginal points of view to lead to change. The narrative of Zelophehads daughters, as it appears in Numbers 27:1–11, is a strong reminder that ethical consequences have a way of emanating from those who have been historically disenfranchised in models of decision-making. Their rebellious demand for equitable rights of inheritance creates the necessity of inclusiveness in legal frameworks. This basic realignment not only permitted legislative reform but also showed the possibility of the coexistence of divine and human laws peacefully, altering the ethical requirements produced by the excluded. Thus, reformative initiatives by citizens can shape normative legal habits, widening the scope of justice. Over the passage of time, transhumanism emerges and introduces difficult philosophical and ethical concerns that complicate conventional legal patterns. The consequences of using advanced technologies for the development of human potential raise fundamental questions about matters of autonomy and human freedom, as well as the limits of legal responsibility. Quoted in diverse academic literature, such debates affect a broader framework of understanding individual liberty and human rights and necessitate a rethinking of what it means to be human when immersed in a technology-heavy world. Critics argue that transhumanism is capable of creating new inequalities, with access to the technologies of enhancement stratified along socio-economic lines. It is therefore essential that stakeholders like legislators and ethicists accept the implications of such developments. These new realities necessitate a rethinking of ethical regimes, and of the legal regimes upon which they are based, to better protect people and communities from exploitation. Finally, the common exploration of ELSI needs to determine the interdependence of ethical theory, legal code, and social justice movements. Continued deliberation on tales of empowerment, such as that of the daughters of Zelophehads, and the challenge of transhumanism, reminds us of the necessity for an integrated response to the ethical issues of today. Listening to the voices of the oppressed and responding well to technological advancement, society can build a more just world. As the pursuit of justice evolves over time, it is more essential to maintain the values of human dignity and equality at the focal point of legal and ethical discourse. This holistic approach is not merely a way of developing further knowledge about justice but is also a foundation for incorporating future ethics, law, and societal thoughts.

The ethical, legal, and social implications (ELSI) of new technologies are a complex system that requires thorough scrutiny. In the middle of the controversy are concerns regarding governance and public involvement, particularly in the context of synthetic biology. Experts argue that initiatives like the UK's Synthetic Biology Roadmap demonstrate challenges to integrating Science and Technology Studies (STS) perspectives into policymaking processes. These academics describe the difficulty of changing policies that have a tendency to refer to deeply ingrained beliefs over what causes and affects the technological innovation-economic growth connection. Furthermore, the tendency to perceive public skepticism as an obstacle rather than as a critical voice in the rhetoric of scientific advancement denotes a failure to foster responsible research and innovation (RRI) (Dupras et al., 2019). Thus, ELSI controversy highlights the importance of reframing stakeholders' roles and understanding a range of societal values framing technological adoption. Another essential aspect of ELSI is legitimation of technological advancement through employing narratives that do not necessarily align with public interests. The controversy surrounding agricultural innovation, particularly regarding genetically modified organisms (GMOs), illustrates this dynamic. While technologies of modernity are generally hailed as precursors of the future, the examination above reveals a more nuanced interdependence under which the empowerment of oppressed groups and climate protection are given priority over the glorification of technology. This is a viewpoint that advocates for a utilitarian approach to technology where ethical concerns are not bypassed but woven into the fabric of technological advancement (van der Weele & Keulartz, 2009). The ethical lesson underlying this is that by placing the welfare of humans and the environment over technological advancement for its own sake, society can steer innovations toward more socially responsible purposes and thus improve the ELSI debate. In addition, interlinking ethical, legal, and social concerns in the technology-oriented world necessitates self-reflection about the ramifications of neglecting public discussion in this context. As also reflected in debates over synthetic biology and agricultural biotechnology, failure to engage with societal values can create huge resistance to scientific work. Public distrust that results from a lack of engagement and understanding highlights the need for open communication and participative policy-making. ELSI models encourage the instruments that guarantee communication between scientists, decision makers, and the public, and thus guarantee a scenario in which everyone contributes to building the future of technology. Not only should one guarantee that the legitimacy of innovation is enhanced, but also that it is designed specifically to meet the requirements of society and thus pave the way towards responsible and inclusive scientific progress (Bélisle-Pipon & Victor, 2024).

A LOOK TO THE FUTURE:

HEALTH DATA SCIENCE:

Health data science has rapidly emerged as a transformative interdisciplinary field at the nexus of data analytics, computer science, and healthcare. It encompasses the collection, processing, and interpretation of vast and complex datasets generated throughout the healthcare ecosystem—from electronic health records and medical imaging to wearable devices and genomic profiles—to derive actionable insights that improve health outcomes, optimize clinical workflows, and support evidence-based decision-making. By applying advanced techniques such as machine learning, predictive modelling, and statistical inference, health data science enables researchers and clinicians to turn raw health data into meaningful information that drives innovation, enhances patient care, and strengthens health systems.

The importance of health data science stems from the exponential growth of digital health information and the increasing complexity of modern healthcare delivery. With electronic health records now widely adopted, and diverse sources such as sensor data from mobile health devices complementing traditional clinical results, there is unprecedented potential to analyse and integrate multifaceted data types to predict disease risk, tailor personalized treatments, and monitor population health trends. Predictive analytics, for example, can identify patients at high risk for chronic conditions or hospital readmission, thereby enabling proactive intervention strategies that improve outcomes while reducing costs.

In addition to patient-level benefits, health data science strengthens healthcare systems by supporting operational efficiencies and resource planning. Analyses of admissions, bed occupancy, and clinical workflows help health organizations allocate resources more effectively and anticipate demand. At the population level, data science can reveal patterns in disease outbreaks and health disparities, informing public health policies and preventive strategies. Such capabilities are particularly valuable in responding to public health emergencies and managing long-term challenges like aging populations.

Beyond clinical care and public health, health data science has profound implications for medical research and innovation. Large, well-curated datasets facilitate drug discovery, biomarker identification, and the validation of clinical decision support tools. When combined with secure, ethical data sharing practices, these insights can accelerate scientific discovery and expand the frontiers of precision medicine.

Nevertheless, the application of data science in health also raises important challenges. Ensuring data privacy, maintaining the security of sensitive information, and addressing algorithmic bias are critical to sustaining trust and equity in health data practices. As the field continues to mature, interdisciplinary collaboration between data scientists, clinicians, ethicists, and policymakers will be essential to realise the full potential of health data science in improving global health.

In summary, health data science represents a critical and dynamic domain that leverages computational power and analytical ingenuity to transform data into insights that benefit individuals and populations alike. Its growth reflects a broader shift toward data-driven healthcare—where evidence, prediction, and personalized strategies guide the future of medicine.

REFERENCES

1. Silva, A. de O. (2023). Academic Literature on Compliance Programs, ESG, Corporate Governance, Fraud Prevention, Human Rights, Corruption, Data Protection, and SDGs. *Journal of Sustainable Institutional Management, 10*(gc), e0138. https://doi.org/10.21434/IberoamericanJCG.v10igc.138(accessed on 17th July 2025).
2. Ajiga, D., Okeleke, P. A., Folorunsho, S. O., & Ezeigweneme, C. (2024). Navigating ethical considerations in software development and deployment in technological giants. *International Journal of Engineering Research Updates*. https://www.semanticscholar.org/paper/6b0b76136d4c32d113cb88ab7f953ae271f335d4 (accessed on 17th July 2025).
3. Alon, I., Bussod, I., & Ravitsky, V. (2024). Mapping ethical, legal, and social implications (ELSI) of preimplantation genetic testing (PGT). *Journal of Assisted Reproduction and Genetics, 41*, 1153–1171. https://www.semanticscholar.org/paper/236efb6461f4bfc62adf8102594168dcd64cb073 (accessed on 17th July 2025).
4. Alowais, S. A., Alghamdi, S. S., Alsuhebany, N., Alqahtani, T., Alshaya, A., Almohareb, S. N., Aldairem, A., et al. (2023). Revolutionizing healthcare: The role of artificial intelligence in clinical practice. *BMC Medical Education, 23.* https://doi.org/10.1186/s12909-023-04698-z (accessed on 17th July 2025).
5. Anderson, J., & Hudson, M. (2020). The Biocultural Labels Initiative: Supporting Indigenous rights in data derived from genetic resources. *Biodiversity Information Science and Standards*. https://www.semanticscholar.org/paper/3b17f54b8cf00b290516dffbcf7814781c26141c (accessed on 17th July 2025).
6. Andorno, R., Baylis, F., Darnovsky, M., Dickenson, D., Haker, H., Hasson, K., Lowthorp, L., et al. (2020). Geneva statement on heritable human genome editing: The need for course correction. *Trends in Biotechnology, 38*, 351–354. https://doi.org/10.1016/j.tibtech.2019.12.022 (accessed on 17th July 2025).
7. Ayub, Z., & Banday, M. T. (2023). Ethics in artificial intelligence: An analysis of ethical issues and possible solutions. https://doi.org/10.1109/stcr59085.2023.10396966 (accessed on 17th July 2025).
8. Bélisle-Pipon, J.-C., & Victor, G. (2024). Ethics dumping in artificial intelligence. *Frontiers in Artificial Intelligence, 7.* https://doi.org/10.3389/frai.2024.1426761 (accessed on 17th July 2025).
9. Bell, C. G., Lowe, R., Adams, P. D., Baccarelli, A., Beck, S., Bell, J. T., Christensen, B. C., et al. (2019). DNA methylation aging clocks: Challenges and recommendations. *Genome Biology, 20.* https://doi.org/10.1186/s13059-019-1824-y (accessed on 17th July 2025).
10. Borger, J. G., Ng, A. P., Anderton, H., Ashdown, G. W., Auld, M., Blewitt, M. E., Brown, D. V., et al. (2023). Artificial intelligence takes center stage: Exploring the capabilities and implications of ChatGPT and other AI-assisted technologies in scientific research and education. *Immunology and Cell Biology, 101*, 923–935. https://doi.org/10.1111/imcb.12689 (accessed on 17th July 2025).
11. Calluori, S., Heimke, K. K., Caga-Anan, C. F., Kaufman, D., Mechanic, L. E., & McAllister, K. A. (2024). Ethical, legal, and social implications of gene-environment interaction research. *Genetic Epidemiology, 49.* https://www.semanticscholar.org/paper/fd44033be51122f0f609118478c412c1ece5c42e (accessed on 17th July 2025).

12. Caprioli, E., de Barros Vitta, J., Nieddermeyer, H. L., & Pardo, P. (2024). Ethical challenges of technological advance: Apple Vision Pro. *Caderno Pedagógico*. https://www.semanticscholar.org/paper/c65df43d2e8aef9b0c0f078e8b1a53a76f5b0f95 (accessed on 17th July 2025).

13. Cheong, B. C. (2024). The rise of AI avatars: Legal personhood, rights and liabilities in an evolving metaverse. *SSRN Electronic Journal*. https://www.semanticscholar.org/paper/902df8034c087e415ee91cef7f536ffe710c61cf (accessed on 17th July 2025).

14. Chibugo Udegbe, F., Ebulue, O. R., Ebulue, C. C., & Ekesiobi, C. S. (2024). Precision medicine and genomics: A comprehensive review of IT-enabled approaches. *International Medical Science Research Journal, 4*, 509–520. https://doi.org/10.51594/imsrj.v4i4.1053 (accessed on 17th July 2025).

15. Da Bormida, M. (2021). The big data world: Benefits, threats and ethical challenges. *Advances in Research Ethics and Integrity*. https://doi.org/10.1108/s2398-601820210000008007 (accessed on 17th July 2025).

16. Dokumacı, M. (2024). Legal frameworks for AI regulations. *Human Computer Interaction*. https://www.semanticscholar.org/paper/09d9bae5bc69d20df47ad8a3fd1d54a4d7344787 (accessed on 17th July 2025).

17. Dupras, C., Saulnier, K. M., & Joly, Y. (2019). Epigenetics, ethics, law and society: A multidisciplinary review of descriptive, instrumental, dialectical and reflexive analyses. *Social Studies of Science, 49*, 785–810. https://doi.org/10.1177/0306312719866007 (accessed on 17th July 2025).

18. Dwivedi, Y. K., Hughes, L., Baabdullah, A. M., Ribeiro-Navarrete, S., Giannakis, M., Al-Debei, M. M., Dennehy, D., et al. (2022). Metaverse beyond the hype: Multidisciplinary perspectives on emerging challenges, opportunities, and agenda for research, practice and policy. *International Journal of Information Management, 66*, 102542–102542. https://doi.org/10.1016/j.ijinfomgt.2022.102542 (accessed on 17th July 2025).

19. Floridi, L., Cowls, J., Beltrametti, M., Chatila, R., Chazerand, P., Dignum, V., Luetge, C., et al. (2018). AI4People—An ethical framework for a good AI society: Opportunities, risks, principles, and recommendations. *Minds and Machines, 28*, 689–707. https://doi.org/10.1007/s11023-018-9482-5 (accessed on 17th July 2025).

20. Fothergill, B. T., Knight, W., Stahl, B. C., & Ulnicane, I. (2019). Responsible data governance of neuroscience big data. *Frontiers in Neuroinformatics, 13*. https://doi.org/10.3389/fninf.2019.00028 (accessed on 17th July 2025).

21. Fridmanskyy, R. M., Badyda, A., Pifko, O. O., & Dir, I. Y. (2024). Human rights in the context of transhumanist medicine: Ethical and legal aspects. *Wiadomosci Lekarskie, 77*(10), 2077–2082. https://www.semanticscholar.org/paper/550635442a9567b659de7d61a7359fce22849bb5 (accessed on 17th July 2025).

22. Hamari, J., Sjöklint, M., & Ukkonen, A. (2015). The sharing economy: Why people participate in collaborative consumption. *Journal of the Association for Information Science and Technology, 67*, 2047–2059. https://doi.org/10.1002/asi.23552 (accessed on 17th July 2025).

23. James, J. E., Riddle, L., Caruncho, M., Koenig, B. A., & Joseph, G. (2022). A qualitative study of unaffected *ATM* and *CHEK2* carriers: How participants make meaning of 'moderate risk' genetic results in a population breast cancer screening trial. *Journal of Genetic Counseling, 31*, 1421–1433. https://doi.org/10.1002/jgc4.1617 (accessed on 17th July 2025).

24. Kamenova, K., & Haidar, H. (2022). The first baby born after polygenic embryo screening. *Voices in Bioethics, 8*. https://doi.org/10.52214/vib.v8i.9467 (accessed on 17th July 2025).

25. van der Weele, C., & Keulartz, F. W. J. (2009). *Heroes of Agricultural Innovation*. Genomics, Society and Policy 5 (3):1-15 (2009) https://core.ac.uk/download/pdf/29246888.pdf (accessed on 17th July 2025).

26. Kruk, M. E., Gage, A., Arsenault, C., Jordan, K., Leslie, H. H., Roder-DeWan, S., Adeyi, O., et al. (2018). High-quality health systems in the Sustainable Development Goals era: Time for a revolution. *The Lancet Global Health, 6*, e1196–e1252. https://doi.org/10.1016/s2214-109x(18)30386-3 (accessed on 17th July 2025).

27. Laurent, B. (2013). *The Constitutional Effect of The Ethics of Emerging Technologies*. https://core.ac.uk/download/576796379.pdf (accessed on 17th July 2025).

28. Lohse, S. (2022). Mapping uncertainty in precision medicine: A systematic scoping review. *Journal of Evaluation in Clinical Practice, 29*, 554–564. https://doi.org/10.1111/jep.13789 (accessed on 17th July 2025).

29. Lysaght, T. (2021). Anticipatory governance and foresight in regulating for uncertainty. *The American Journal of Bioethics, 22*, 51–53. https://www.semanticscholar.org/paper/4492788bde28fc4e1a14d01a325ead215b9c14f5 (accessed on 17th July 2025).

30. Maben, J., & Bridges, J. (2020). Covid-19: Supporting nurses' psychological and mental health. *Journal of Clinical Nursing, 29*, 2742–2750. https://doi.org/10.1111/jocn.15307 (accessed on 17th July 2025).

31. Matten, D., & Moon, J. (2008). "Implicit" and "explicit" CSR: A conceptual framework for a comparative understanding of corporate social responsibility. *Academy of Management Review, 33*, 404–424. https://doi.org/10.5465/amr.2008.31193458 (accessed on 17th July 2025).

32. McGrath, C., Chau, C. W. R., & Molina, G. (2025). Monitoring oral health remotely: Ethical considerations when using AI among vulnerable populations. *Frontiers in Oral Health, 6*. https://www.semanticscholar.org/paper/41c620944a85e5b2f734c4fa07e3ae09cd889eec (accessed on 17th July 2025).

33. Nommsen-Rivers, L., Black, M. M., Christian, P., Groh-Wargo, S., Heinig, M. J., Israel-Ballard, K., Obbagy, J., et al. (2023). An equitable, community-engaged translational framework for science in human lactation and infant feeding—a report from "Breastmilk Ecology: Genesis of Infant Nutrition (BEGIN)" Working Group 5. *American Journal of Clinical Nutrition, 117*, S87–S105. https://doi.org/10.1016/j.ajcnut.2023.01.020 (accessed on 17th July 2025).

34. Pardede, N. (2025). Perempuan sebagai pembaru: Telaah teologis-naratif kisah anak-anak Zelafehad. *EPIGRAPHE: Jurnal Teologi dan Pelayanan Kristiani*. https://www.semanticscholar.org/paper/aafc2b129b260c145284a3272b63da068c6457c4 (accessed on 17th July 2025).

35. Parens, E., & Appelbaum, P. S. (2019). On what we have learned and still need to learn about the psychosocial impacts of genetic testing. *The Hastings Center Report, 49*. https://doi.org/10.1002/hast.1011 (accessed on 17th July 2025).

36. Pashayan, N., Antoniou, A. C., Ivanuš, U., Esserman, L. J., Easton, D. F., French, D., Sroczynski, G., et al. (2020). Personalized early detection and prevention of breast cancer: ENVISION consensus statement. *Nature Reviews Clinical Oncology, 17*, 687–705. https://doi.org/10.1038/s41571-020-0388-9 (accessed on 17th July 2025).

37. Reimer, E. (2024). Examining the role of generative AI in enhancing social work education: An analysis of curriculum and assessment design. *Social Sciences, 13*, 648–648. https://doi.org/10.3390/socsci13120648 (accessed on 17th July 2025).
38. Rijswijk, K., Klerkx, L., Bacco, M., Bartolini, F., Bulten, E., Debruyne, L., Dessein, J., et al. (2021). Digital transformation of agriculture and rural areas: A socio-cyber-physical system framework to support responsibilities. *Journal of Rural Studies, 85*, 79–90. https://doi.org/10.1016/j.jrurstud.2021.05.003 (accessed on 17th July 2025).
39. Sallam, M. (2023). ChatGPT utility in healthcare education, research, and practice: Systematic review on the promising perspectives and valid concerns. *Healthcare, 11*, 887–887. https://doi.org/10.3390/healthcare11060887 (accessed on 17th July 2025).
40. Santaló, J., & Berdasco, M. (2022). Ethical implications of epigenetics in the era of personalized medicine. *Clinical Epigenetics, 14*. https://doi.org/10.1186/s13148-022-01263-1 (accessed on 17th July 2025).
41. Sheikh, H. I., Prins, J. E. J., & Schrijvers, E. (2023). *Mission AI. Research for Policy*. https://doi.org/10.1007/978-3-031-21448-6 (accessed on 17th July 2025).
42. Silva, H. P. da, Lehoux, P., Miller, F. A., & Denis, J. L. (2018). Introducing responsible innovation in health: A policy-oriented framework. *Health Research Policy and Systems, 16*. https://doi.org/10.1186/s12961-018-0362-5 (accessed on 17th July 2025).
43. Singh, K., Zeeshan, Z., & Karna, S. (2023). The regulation of biotechnology: Ethical, legal, and social implications. *Interdisciplinary Studies in Society, Law, and Politics.* https://www.semanticscholar.org/paper/5bc242ff775e1512373ea6e67a757771f3c3e4f6 (accessed on 17th July 2025).
44. van der Geest, M. A., Maeckelberghe, E. L. M., van Gijn, M. V., Lucassen, A. M., Swertz, M., van Langen, I. V., & Plantinga, M. (2024). Systematic reanalysis of genomic data by diagnostic laboratories: A scoping review of ethical, economic, legal and (psycho)social implications. *European Journal of Human Genetics, 32*, 489–497. https://www.semanticscholar.org/paper/495af02717947fb1d652d8d113f215e83dc69a6e (accessed on 17th July 2025).
45. Waljee, A., Weinheimer-Haus, E. M., Abubakar, A., Ngugi, A., Siwo, G. H., Kwakye, G., Singal, A., et al. (2022). Artificial intelligence and machine learning for early detection and diagnosis of colorectal cancer in sub-Saharan Africa. *Gut, 71*, 1259–1265. https://www.semanticscholar.org/paper/440492a4d6b7faf05e0302a0a2401d7109dc403c (accessed on 17th July 2025).
46. Y. -H. Weng and E. Francesconi, "Ethical Design for Privacy-related Communication in Human-Robot Interaction," *2023 32nd IEEE International Conference on Robot and Human Interactive Communication (RO-MAN)*, Busan, Korea, Republic of, 2023, pp. 2427-2432, doi: 10.1109/RO-MAN57019.2023.10309553.(accessed on 17th July 2025).
47. Zhao, Y., & Liao, M. (2019). Chinese perspectives on responsible innovation. *Edward Elgar Publishing eBooks.* https://doi.org/10.4337/9781784718862.00039 (accessed on 17th July 2025).

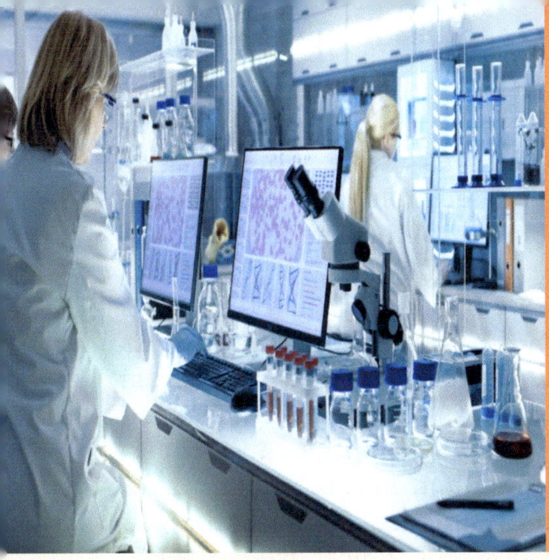

Chapter 15

EMERGING TECHNOLOGIES AND FUTURE DIRECTIONS

Contents

Introduction

With the rapidly evolving 21st-century world, emerging technologies are simply revolutionizing various sectors, with unprecedented opportunities as well as complex challenges. With technologies , such as artificial intelligence, blockchain, and machine learning, traditional operating procedures in sectors have been recharted, resulting in a critical reassessment of their impact on economic growth as well as social life. These technologies promise to contribute to operational efficiency, improve decision-making, and give birth to new business models. But along with rising complexity and interconnectivity of these technological advancements comes a monumental agenda of problems related to ethical aspects, regulatory aspects, and the requirements of acquiring skills. While organizations are grappling with such changing dynamics, charting the trajectory of emerging technologies becomes vital to realizing their full potential as much as withstanding attendant risks and liabilities. The debate regarding up-and-coming technologies is not one-sided in their favor; it also encompasses the necessity for robust frameworks and regulatory measures that can facilitate their growth and address the challenges that ensue. For instance, efficient adoption of blockchain and artificial intelligence technologies into accounting processes, as discussed in Bangladesh national research, brings the government's role and development of specific standards of regulation to light (Islam et al., 2024). Such measures can facilitate safe adoption of these technologies and resolve problems of data security, technology architecture, and the need for industry-specific training modules.

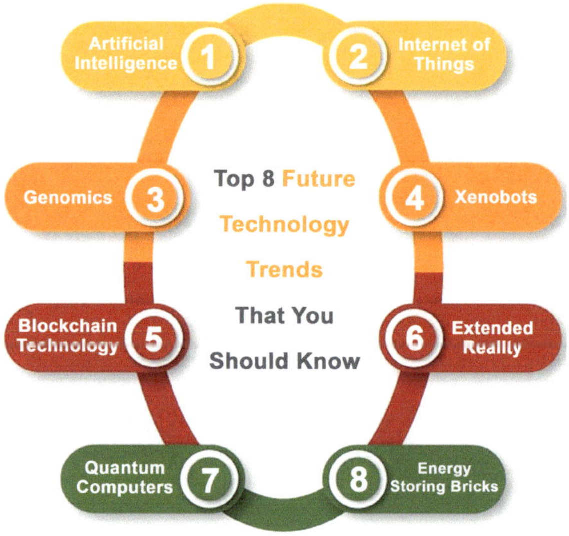

Figure 15.1. Emerging technologies and future directions.

Source: https://www.conurets.com/wp-content/uploads/2022/10/Technology-Trends-That-You-Should-Know-2-01.jpg.

Moreover, the role of learning facilities takes a central position in developing the workforce with the desired skills for future jobs affected by such transformation. Alignment of the education curriculum to suit the demands of future technologies is critical to preparation in a changing labor market. In addition to education and regulation concerns, the promise of innovative diagnostic technologies and capabilities reminds us of the transformative potential of new technology in healthcare. Access to genomic profiling, next-generation sequencing, and artificial intelligence has the possibility of improving early diagnosis and treatment of advanced tumors, such as neuroendocrine neoplasms (NENs) (Massironi et al., 2024). Despite phenomenal advances, challenges , such as limited awareness, budget constraints, and seeking noninvasive alternatives still dominate. Bridging the gap between innovation and clinical use is the key to maximizing patient benefit. Future emphasis here likely lies in leveraging future technologies to establish precision medicine tailored to the specific requirements of individual patients, optimizing the efficiency of diagnosis, and revolutionizing treatment paradigms amidst rapid technological progress (Figure 15.1).

Definition of Emerging Technologies

New technologies are often characterized as new innovations that bring about fundamental changes in existing systems, processes, and paradigms. They vary from general advances in numerous areas, including artificial intelligence, robotics, biotechnology, and information and communication technology (ICT). Besides rendering efforts more productive and efficient, these technologies alter the character of human interactions in business and life contexts. For instance, the advent of cyborgian technologies presents a new type of service interaction wherein human capabilities are augmented by highly sophisticated technological assistance, leading to more empathetic and intuitive solutions when faced with highly complicated situations in the management of services. This kind of paradigm necessitates a redefinition of current roles, particularly frontline service employees (FLEs), who now, most likely, will coexist with such new-fangled technologies and completely revolutionize customers' experiences and expectations (Garry & Harwood, 2019). In addition, the definition of emerging technologies includes their potential to change industries, such as architecture, engineering, and construction (AEC). The integration of ICTs in these industries reflects a strategic direction that views technology as a vital resource to achieve competitive advantage. Previously, the AEC industry's strategy towards ICT investment has been dispersed, primarily devoid of any strategic purpose. However, studies find a growing recognition of ICT as a value-creating resource, and thus it is becoming imperative for business change drivers and operational capacity improvement. Such transformation caters to the requirement of putting ICT at the focal point of organizational strategies, whereby corporations utilize such emerging technologies to tap innovation and expansion (Isikdag et al., 2009).

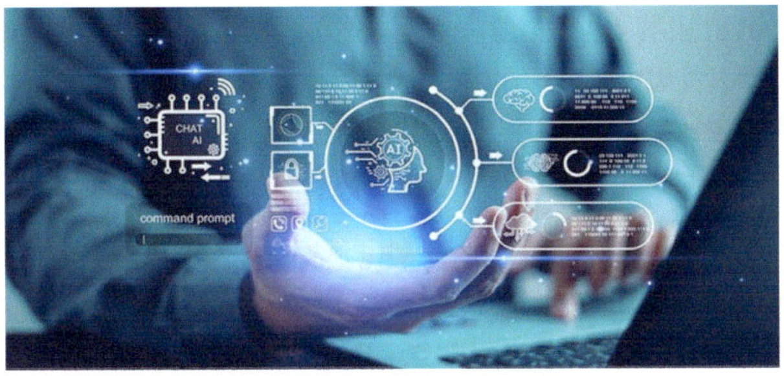

Figure 15.2. Emerging technologies.

Source: https://img-s-msn-com.akamaized.net/tenant/amp/entityid/AA1HNLiM.img?w=768&h=576&m=6.

As new technologies expand, so do they present complex ethical challenges to be confronted in an enlightened way. The overlap of human and technological abilities brings questions of privacy, consent, and the socio-economic implications of such unions into focus. For example, applications of cyborgian technology require proper scrutiny of ethical principles embracing human enhancement in work settings. It is noteworthy that researchers and practitioners enter these unexplored waters carefully, trying to balance the benefits of technological advancement with the potential risks they might impose on personal liberty and cultural norms. On our path towards a more technologically dominated future, sober discussion around their definition, ramifications, and ethical implications is necessary for ensuring their balanced and sustainable inclusion in all aspects of life (Figure 15.2).

Importance of Studying Future Directions

The importance of research on future trends within the arena of new technologies cannot be overstated, considering the profound implications that these technologies have on disease and health control. Understanding the interaction of more than one organ system, as presented in ongoing research, is vital in solving difficult health issues. For instance, advances in mechanistic explanation of interorgan signaling have provided insight into the intricate relationship between metabolic processes and cardiovascular health. Such advances not only provide opportunities for improved and earlier diagnosis but also make targeted and effective therapy for conditions like cardiovascular disease possible, and therefore emphasize the need for forward-looking research to plug gaps in current medicine. In this regard, proactive strategies allow researchers and practitioners to anticipate and address oncoming health emergencies according to our rapidly evolving biological and technological contexts (Bae et al., 2025). In addition to advances in medicine, research on forthcoming trends in technology, particularly in the Metaverse, is a vital area of study worthy of focused attention. With blockchain, artificial intelligence, and immersive technologies like virtual and augmented reality, economic transactions and social paradigms are totally revamped. As the Metaverse opens up, it becomes imperative to have a grasp of how digital payment systems work and how they impact economic inclusiveness. Patterns of research reveal growing recognition of the need to address regulative issues and technological constraints associated with such systems, requiring ongoing dialogue between researchers and technology developers. Through critical analysis of such advances, we can create contexts supportive of security and sustainability of digital transactions, thus vindicating the need for forward thinking in navigating the new digital economy (Mariana et al., 2025). In addition, the study of future trends equips scholars and policy analysts with the toolset of competencies to deal with the constraints inherent in high-speed technical development. As technologies emerge, dominant paradigms must evolve alongside the complexities of such technologies. This is particularly essential in scenarios where the ethical implications and policy paradigms lag behind technical development. A thorough analysis of trends and patterns, such as the case of the integration of blockchain technology and internet payment platforms, can create a road map to effective policy-making that is sensitive to technological potential and social effects. Addressing such problems provides room for new technologies to be harnessed for the common good while addressing possible harms, underscoring the urgent need for continued investigation of the future of technology and its impact on society (Bae et al., 2025; Mariana et al., 2025).

15.1. Artificial Intelligence (AI)

While Artificial Intelligence (AI) is growing its reach, it is paving the path towards future Web 3.0 development, which is a revolutionary shift toward a decentralized internet. This shift is characterized by developments , such as blockchain, which is inherently designed to accomplish transparency and security. AIs purpose here is crucial, as it can digest and interpret huge volumes of information with ease, thus ensuring viable information that facilitates intelligent decision-making. The use of AI in Web 3.0 not only enhances the user experience but also enhances systems across various industries—healthcare, finance, and education, to name a few, by harnessing analytics to attain revolutionary outcomes. However, with these challenging opportunities lie several essential challenges to be addressed, particularly on issues of data privacy and ethics. This delicate dance between opportunity and risk is most important as society embraces this future wave of digital innovation (Kansal, 2024). Furthermore, the union of AI and blockchain technology promises even more avenues for innovation, as each serves to complement the use and stability of the other. AI's computational power complements blockchain's decentralized structure, creating systems that are more autonomous and intelligent. Areas , such as supply chain management are already seeing the potential of this synergy, where AI can predict trends and automate procedures and blockchain maintains transactions transparent and safe. This combined strategy can potentially make operations smoother, less expensive, and more responsible. However, the actual application of converging such technologies in the real world is not a problem-free process. There are the technical challenges, the issues of regulation and policy, and the ethical question of applying AI technologies that must be met to maximize the societal benefits and minimize risks from these emerging technologies (Kapoor et al., 2024). Artificial Intelligence is, in short, an overarching force in determining and directing the future of emerging technologies. As businesses move towards the Web 3.0 principles and explore the intersection of AI with blockchain, the larger social implications entail that fundamental issues must be raised about trust, bias, and data safeguarding. The potential of AI to act as a driver for revolutionary changes across industries must be balanced with an appropriate examination of ethical standards and user-initiated policy. In the future, our research must address these challenges and unlock the full potential of AIs for the good in society. Through partnerships between policymakers, technologists, and ethicists, we can unravel the complexities of these emerging technologies and work towards a future where innovation is balanced with wise stewardship (Kansal, 2024; Kapoor et al., 2024).

15.1.1. Current Applications in Various Industries

New technologies have found extensive application across various industries in ways that completely transformed traditional practice and enhanced efficiency. In shipping, for example, the integration of intelligent design and operation methods becomes increasingly vital to the promotion of energy efficiency. Ship operators and builders now apply Industry 4.0 thinking, which advocates for the full rethinking of ship design, manufacture, and operation processes. With smart ship design and the integration of computational intelligence into cyber-physical systems, the industry is moving in the direction of sustainable practice that will be able to reduce operational costs as well as environmental impacts.

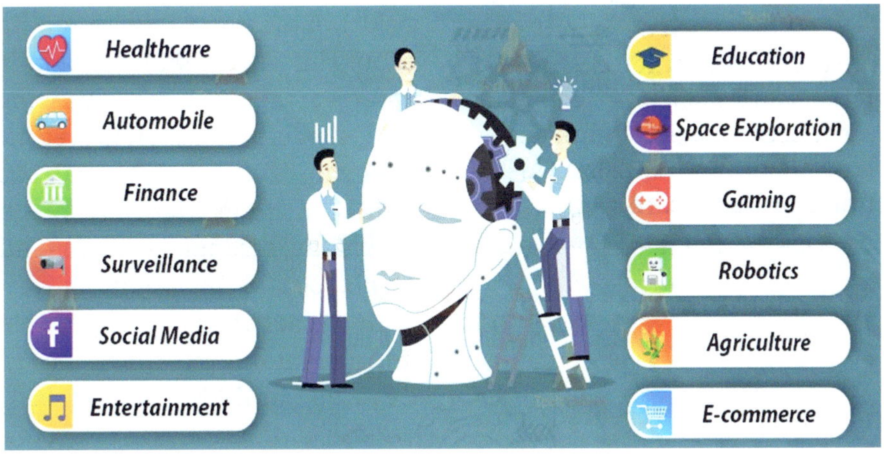

Figure 15.3. Current applications in various industries.

Source: https://techvidvan.com/tutorials/wp-content/uploads/sites/2/2020/04/applications-of-AI.jpg.

Aside from presenting a response to the pressing concerns of global competition, these innovations provide a vision for energy-efficient ships and guide the way to a more sustainable maritime industry (Ang et al., 2017). The Internet of Things (IoT) is another innovative idea, revolutionizing how companies operate. By bringing physical items and the internet together, IoT enables real-time data collection and analysis, significantly enhancing operational efficiency and decision-making. IoT is being used by agriculture, manufacturing, and the healthcare industry to monitor systems, predict machinery failure, and improve resource use. Also, the convergence of IoT and big data analytics introduces new possibilities for businesses to enhance their market strategies and operational models. Through real-time processing of sensor data, organizations can gain valuable insights into their operations, thereby making well-informed decisions that deliver growth and innovation. While companies are attempting to get their heads around using such technology, there has always existed a sense of distrust regarding the statements made by IoT advertisements, indicative of the necessity for more research and verification in this sector (Alansari et al., 2018). In the healthcare sector, emerging technologies are changing patient treatment, diagnosis, and treatment patterns. Telemedicine is becoming more and more an essential component of healthcare delivery, particularly in rural areas, to make medical care previously limited more accessible. Health apps and wearable devices empower individuals with the ability to monitor their health data and communicate with healthcare workers in real time, thus enabling self-management of health. Artificial intelligence and machine learning algorithms are also utilized to break down large volumes of data to use predictive analytics and personalized medicine approaches. Such advancements are maximizing organizational functions and improving patient outcomes, positioning healthcare to revolutionize rapidly due to technological advancements. The constant intersection of such technologies emphasizes the importance of flexibility and vision in navigating the future of healthcare (Ang et al., 2017; Alansari et al., 2018) (Figure 15.3).

15.1.2. Ethical Considerations and Challenges

With new technology being created and disseminated, the ethics of using it are only getting more complex. A major concern centers on data privacy and security, particularly with how much personal information these technologies collect and utilize.

As has been debated in recent scholarship, advances in artificial intelligence (AI) have underscored new issues regarding the use of data in innovation management processes, and it has now become a matter of consent and data exploitation implications.

The stakeholders must navigate through the thin line of using data to yield more effective operations and ensuring the rights of people are preserved privately, necessitating a firm framework that corrects these ethical dilemmas while promoting effective innovation (Saur-Amaral et al., 2024). The integration of several future-generation technologies also brings along other ethical challenges, especially in healthcare and caregiving. The deployment of technology-based interventions is intended to empower and support individuals, yet inadvertently raises questions regarding access and equity. The barriers to technology adoption can serve as a source of disparities among different socioeconomic groups and hence marginalize the poor with access to assets or information to benefit from such innovation. Recent studies have highlighted the need for human-centered and inclusive design approaches in technology solution design, recommending that equity should inform the building of technology-enabled care systems. Not merely being equitable but also capable of resolving ethical concerns by ensuring that all potential users have equal access to innovation advantages, the practice would be strongly recommended (Lindeman et al., 2020). In resolving such multifaceted ethical challenges, policymakers, researchers, and technologists need to join hands and develop holistic strategies that promote ethical conduct in every sector of technology. Well-defined regulatory environments can aid ethical compliance, particularly in areas where technology is constantly evolving. There is always the possibility of abuse when regulatory mechanisms lag behind technological advancements, and this necessitates an active mode of governance that will be capable of adapting to future challenges. In addition, encouraging ongoing discussion of ethical issues among the technology community can increase awareness and sensitivity to issues as they arise. Finally, by putting ethical issues front and center and integrating them into the innovation process, stakeholders can use emerging technology to achieve positive social change while mitigating potential harms (Saur-Amaral et al., 2024) (Figure 15.4).

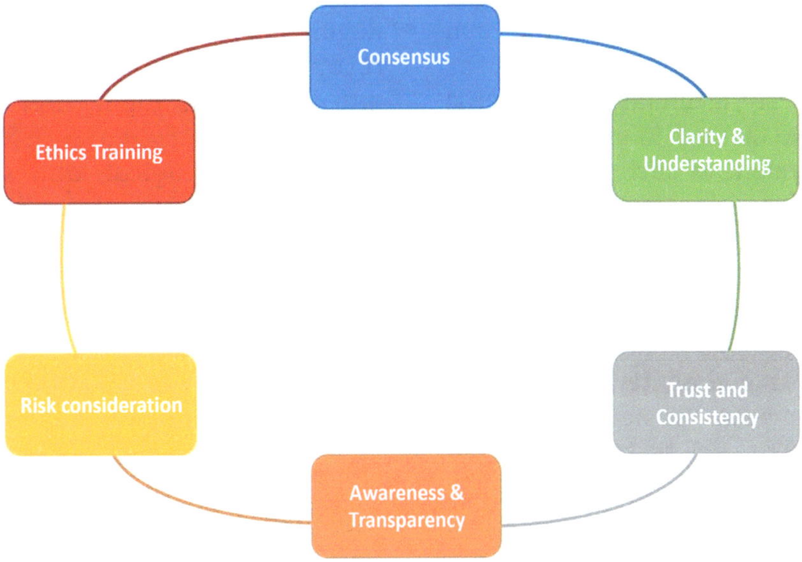

Figure 15.4. Ethical considerations and challenges.

Source: https://research.aimultiple.com/wp-content/uploads/2022/09/best-practices-for-data-collection-ethics.jpg.

15.1.3. Future Potential and Advancements

Stepping into a new era dominated by emerging technologies, the anticipated developments in artificial intelligence (AI) serve as a critical juncture in the direction of future developments. Science fiction stories, particularly in games like Cyberpunk 2077, reveal possible directions in the development of AI and its integration into everyday life. This game illustrates AI not only as a machine but as a living entity with the capability to engage in advanced interaction and anthropomorphic qualities, calling attention to ethical concerns and societal reception of such technologies. By looking at the possible future of AI through models created in fictional representations, we are in a better position to see the thin line between innovation and human values and understand the significance of responsible design approaches that prioritize user experience and ethically based technology uptake (L'opez & Casado, 2023). Alongside AI, the development of cyborgian technologies presents promising ways for enhancing human capabilities in various service contexts. Research outlines the formation of melded frontline service employees (FLEs) where advanced technologies are integrated into human actors, thereby transforming the interaction dynamics of customer services. These innovations have the potential to improve the delivery of services through the enhanced cognitive and emotional capacities implanted into cyborg technologies. The integration of neural interfaces, for instance, would enable FLEs to react instinctively to the needs of customers, improving the empathetic and effective experience of the service. However, such advancement also poses ethical questions that warrant due consideration, prompting scientists to ponder what it means to bring human intelligence together with artificial augmentation (Garry & Harwood, 2019). As technology horizons are extended, the merging of high-end augmented reality (AR), virtual reality (VR), and biotechnology presents groundbreaking opportunities for revolutionary breakthroughs across disciplines. Such technologies can transform industries as wide-ranging as education and healthcare, facilitating experiential learning and creative therapy in mental health. Through the deployment of such instruments, professionals are able to gain access to simulated environments that enhance knowledge retention and functional skills. However, the extensive adoption of such technologies also necessitates research on how these impact human interaction and integrity over the long term. Research and development investment needs to factor in possible changes to society to ensure that technological advancements can be aligned with human values. This will be imperative in utilizing emergent technologies to enhance life while not sacrificing the essence of the common human experience (L'opez & Casado, 2023).

15.2. Biotechnology

Biotechnology is a critical field of emerging technologies that offers novel and innovative solutions outside traditional laboratory parameters in medicine, agriculture, and the environment. With the world faced with severe global challenges, including food security and health crises, the application of biotechnological innovation holds the potential to create a new wave of sustainable development. The combination of genetic engineering with advanced molecular biology techniques allows the enhancement of crop resilience and yield and consequently the relief of food shortages in a growing population. Furthermore, researchers are now more often creating organisms with specific purposes in mind using synthetic biology, exposing biotechnology's potential for the revolutions in production processes as well as the utilization of resources. The sustained research and development in this area are crucial in framing a sustainable future, necessitating robust frameworks to ensure the ethical application of biotechnological advances and their prolonged social implications. Regulation of biotechnology holds significant resonance with its successful integration into society. As highlighted in China's rising biotech industry analysis, the meeting of policy, technological, and societal forces is paramount to the long-term sustainability of biotechnological innovation. The putting in place of successful governance arrangements will require stakeholder collaboration among government, business, and civil society to establish frameworks for producing responsible innovation while managing risks. The dynamics of the biotechnological innovations bring about challenges that demand a new approach that encompasses multifaceted thinking to guarantee access to the accrued benefits on equitable terms. In China, where biotechnology is a strategic necessity for economic development, governance models emerging will also shape global practice and emphasize the importance of balancing social responsibility with innovation (Chen et al., 2011). The emerging biosimilar market is the revolutionary footprint of biotechnology in the field of healthcare. As biologic products approach patent expiration, the emergence of biosimilars, particularly from emerging markets like India and China, is a paradigm shift in the pharmaceutical sector. This market disruption not only destabilizes the monopoly of traditional pharma players but also facilitates the democratization of access to breakthrough therapeutics, enhancing patient care across segments. The capacity of emerging market firms to produce biosimilars at low costs makes it easier for there to be enhanced access to healthcare, research, and innovation, especially where there has been historically limited access to biologics (Huzair et al., 2011). The ongoing growth in the sector draws attention to the requirement for monitoring regulatory regimes and market trends because they will, in turn, dictate the pace at which biosimilars will revolutionize global health outcomes (Figure 15.5).

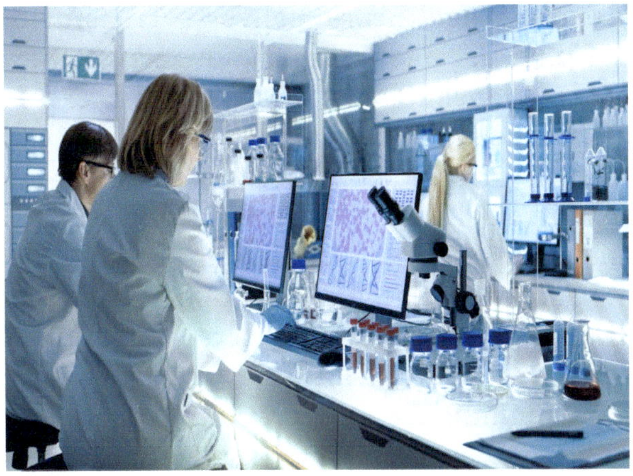

Figure 15.5. Biotechnology represents a critical facet of emerging technologies.

Source: https://www.process-insights.com/wp-content/uploads/2021/05/shutterstock_1073659406_2560x1707-min.jpg.

15.2.1. Innovations in Genetic Engineering

The technological breakthroughs in genetic engineering are a milestone in the history of biotechnology, providing revolutionary methods to each industry ranging from agriculture to medicine and the environment. CRISPR-Cas9 technology demonstrates the precision and effectiveness with which modern genetic engineering technology can provide, as scientists can directly cut and edit DNA with great accuracy. This technology is already revolutionizing how scientists are dealing with genetic disease, which could possibly cure it by directly modifying faulty genes. In addition, gene manipulation for cultivating crop varieties that are tolerant to climatic stresses not only maximizes food security but also sustains it. Institutions and policymaking institutions must harmonize the ethical implications of such powerful technology to ensure that these advancements benefit the greater good of society without posing risks around genetic manipulation, a point that has started intense debates in scientific and ethical arenas (Dwivedi et al., 2023). Surprisingly, the use of lignocellulosic biomass in genetic engineering presents a groundbreaking way of resolving global energy issues. By altering the biochemical processes of plants, researchers can optimize the production of biofuels, thus developing a sustainable source of fuel to supplement fossil fuels. Genetic modification that lowers the content of lignin in biomass allows for better conversion of plant matter to sugars that can be fermented into biofuels. This transition is particularly pertinent in light of the increasing need to stem climate change, as a successful bioeconomy based on renewable biomass can make a significant contribution to mitigating greenhouse gas emissions. The promise of such innovations is underpinned by recent advances that not only enhance productivity effectiveness but also generate high-value co-products, which suggest a diversified approach towards the utilization of agricultural resources that benefits both the economy and the environment (Alowais et al., 2023). Moreover, the convergence of genetic engineering and public health intervention has increasingly gained significance in the last few years, particularly because of the obstacle created by emergent infectious diseases. The development of recombinant vaccines, such as those based on tobacco plants that generate strong antibodies against Ebola viruses, shows the therapeutic potential of genetic engineering for countering urgent health crises. The vaccines take advantage of the inherent capability of plants to produce complex biomolecules, offering a cost-effective solution to vaccine production that is both rapid and scalable. In the face of shifting global health issues, the role of genetic engineering in the development of therapeutic treatments is increasing its pace. There must be ongoing research to reveal the extent of this technology while following safe procedures, thus establishing grounds for new-age health treatments that have the ability to develop with the pace of future challenges (Dwivediet al., 2023) (Figure 15.6).

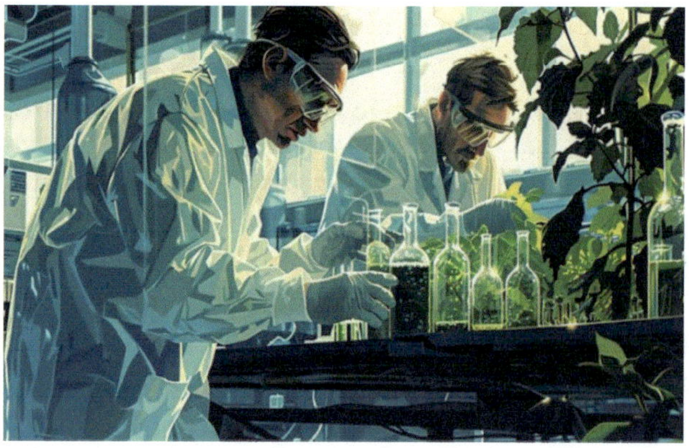

Figure 15.6. Innovations in genetic engineering.

Source: https://img.freepik.com/premium-photo/innovations-genetic-engineering-diseaseresistant-crops-path-sustainable-agriculture_49047-5148.jpg.

15.2.2. Impact on Healthcare and Medicine

The intersection of new technologies is reshaping the healthcare and medical sector, revolutionizing patient care and medical practice efficiency. The application of machine learning algorithms ranks as one of the most important of these innovations as a tool for predictive analytics and personalized medicine. The algorithms utilize enormous amounts of patient information to calculate potential health threats and prescribe tailored treatment protocols. Apart from that, remote patient monitoring technology is also an important tool whereby practitioners can track the status of patients in real time, improving outcomes and reducing face-to-face consultations.

Their implementation not only optimizes the consumption of resources but also empowers patients to have active roles in their own care, thereby leading the healthcare system towards more patient-centered practice. With advancements in healthcare, the congruence between clinical practice and technology will only continue to grow, with far-reaching effects on future healthcare delivery. Transfusion medicine is one such major area where emerging technologies are playing a crucial role, particularly in securing blood safety and enhancing transfusion effectiveness. Emerging trends are headed towards blood storage innovation and the transfusion process, with the impetus coming from omics technology advancements as well as personalization of therapies. Research identifies trends towards rising dominance of particular transfusion modes, such as plasma and platelet transfusions, and proper management of the same to attain optimal patient results. Secondly, blood safety is a distinguishable realm of interest, and persistent inquiry and technological progress need to be addressed to counteract risks associated with transfusion-related complications. The resilience of transfusion medicine in remaining committed to its core structure, yet developing alongside these advances, bears testament to the adaptive principle of the field. The strategic application of cutting-edge technologies will assist in enhancing the quality of treatment for the transfusion patients and related therapies (Lin et al., 2025).

The second important advancement in the health industry is the use of big data analytics that allows for better decision-making and better allocation of resources. This is especially evident in urban health systems, where the combination of data-driven strategies enhances patient outcomes via evidence-based interventions and streamlined healthcare resource management. Data privacy and scalability issues await resolution, but the possible payoffs are significant. For instance, combining Internet of Things devices with big data may facilitate real-time surveillance of health and disease management in the urban population. By leveraging these technologies, health workers are able to formulate more predictive and preventive models of care. As we move into a world increasingly characterized by interconnected digital spaces, the seamless evolution of such technologies provides the platform for game-changing healthcare and systems management—enabling maximum potential for personalized and effective healthcare interventions (Pasupuleti et al., 2024) (Figure 15.7).

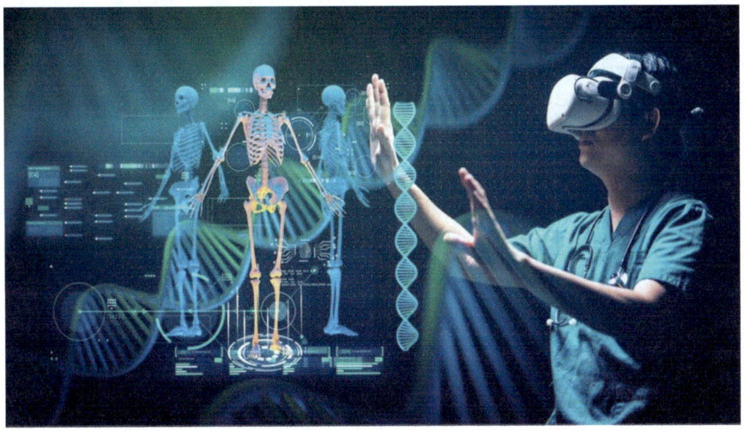

Figure 15.7. Impact of emerging technologies on healthcare and medicine.

Source: https://inventixlabs.com/wp-content/uploads/2023/12/Smart-Medicine-AIs-Trailblazing-Impact-on-Healthcare.jpg.

15.2.3. Regulatory and Ethical Implications

The development of new technology, particularly nanotechnology, calls for close examination of regulatory and ethical matters. The European Commissions approach illustrates a living and developing framework that simultaneously involves new forms of governance tools and more traditional regulation tools. This form of hybrid model tries to address the complexity involved in nanotechnologies through coupling consultations and self-regulation with traditional regulations and directives. But the case-by-case approach is coherence-challenged because it can lead to incoherent applications when faced with dynamic threats. Overreliance on data collection and lack of proactive engagement with ethical standards, i.e., human rights, may restrict monitoring and mechanisms of ethical good governance in new tech sectors (Ruggiu et al., 2015). Moreover, as new technologies are brought into caregiving procedures on every level, privacy and access ethics become issue points that emerge. More applications of mobile, cloud, and robotics technologies have great benefits for family caregivers, but at the same time introduce risks that must be cleverly contained. Equity and access concerns specifically become very acute as some groups can be put in harm's way by not being able to utilize these technologies. These difficulties must be addressed with a regulatory framework that promotes interoperability while, at the same time, being mindful of the ethical aspects of the implementation of technology. A lack of standardized standards will heighten inequalities, ultimately undermining the good intentions of empowering caregivers in their profession. A harmonized equilibrium between ethics and regulation will be required to enable that technological innovation impacts all stakeholders proportionately (Lindeman et al., 2020). As such technologies develop, continued discussion between stakeholders—policy-makers, developers, and citizens—ensues to foster ethical practices and optimal regulations. Innovation-regulation interaction needs to address priority ethical concerns in devising and using new technologies so that solutions meet practical requirements as well as consider larger societal implications.

This involves adherence to human-centered design ethics that include empathy and ethical anticipation. Through the development of an intellectual framework to address the numerous challenges posed by emerging technologies, actors will be better positioned to navigate the complex legal landscape and promote responsible innovation. The quest for such frameworks will work to bring technological potential together with ethical oversight and ultimately influence future directions in technology development and application (Lindeman et al., 2020).

15.3. Renewable Energy Technologies

With the world being confronted with the urgent task of a sustainable supply of energy, renewable energy technologies took center stage in the transition from fossil to clean fuels. One such technology is wind energy, which stands out with its rate of growth and economic potential. The United States wind turbine industry, for example, has brought enormous employment, with an estimated 30,000 Americans working directly and indirectly in the industry in 2011, an impressive increase from just 2500 in 2004. Such a rise not only increases cleaner energy production but also improves the welfare of local economies through jobs and infrastructure investment. Thus, the history of wind power reveals how an acceptance of renewable technology can contribute to environmental as well as economic benefits, and help achieve a more sustainable future while addressing pressing climate challenges (Platzer, 2011). Another revolutionary shift in the field of renewable energy is the development of Smart Grids (SGs). Traditional power grids are increasingly lacking in managing the complexities of integrating renewable energy due to their dependence on unidirectional flow and limited ability to manage real-time data. SGs bypass such limitations by enabling service providers and consumers to share information and energy in bi-directional terms. Powered by the Internet of Things (IoT), these grids enable comprehensive monitoring, analysis, and control over generation, transmission, and distribution systems. The deployment of IoT devices, such as smart sensors and smart meters, enhances grid reliability, security, and efficiency. With expanding Smart Grids, there is an opportunity for a more agile, resilient energy system that can enable higher penetration of the renewable sources (Saleem et al., 2019). Besides, the integration of renewable energy technologies is needed to realize their maximum potential. Non-traditional sources , such as solar, wind, and hydroelectric power, mean that holistic solutions , including energy storage media and grid management, are needed. Emerging technologies , such as battery storage and demand response programs, play significant roles in controlling the intermittency of renewable resources. Through their buffering of excess energy produced during hours of peak generation, such solutions ensure that power is available during peak demand or low generation periods. Not only does this capacity to balance supply and demand make grids more stable, but it also stimulates further investment in renewable energy technologies. With further innovations emerging all the time in this burgeoning field, the possibility of a sustainable and economically viable future is ever more imminent.

15.3.1. Types of Renewable Energy Sources

Studies on the utilization of renewable energy are key to addressing the pressing issues of climate change and environmental degradation. Solar, wind, hydroelectric, geothermal, and biomass energy are just some of the large types, each with specific advantages and potential for sustainability. Solar energy harnesses sunlight to energize photovoltaic cells that transform light into electricity. Wind energy harnesses kinetic energy by using it through turbines that generate energy clean and efficiently. Hydroelectric power plants take advantage of the gravitational force of water in motion and are therefore a key contributor to supplying power to the grid across most regions, especially where water is plentiful. It is imperative to make the transition to these renewables because they not only reduce reliance on fossil fuels but also assist in reducing carbon footprints—an important consideration in evaluating newer technologies and their effects on the environment. Biomass and geothermal energy are other channels of sustainable energy production. Geothermal energy uses the heat trapped under the Earth's surface, with the advantage of a steady and consistent source of energy capable of generating electricity as well as direct heating. Geothermal energy is most suited in tectonically active areas where there are reservoirs beneath the ground. Biomass energy derived from organic waste, such as residues from agriculture, and forest by-products, provides a twofold advantage by providing waste disposal solutions while providing a renewable energy alternative. As technology improves, innovations in the conversion processing of biomass and the geothermal reservoirs can provide more efficient power harvesting. As research has established, this pattern among countries to invest in renewable forms of energy demonstrates their ability to minimize environmental footprint and ensure energy sustainability, as illustrated by Scandurra & Romano (2011). The integration of renewable sources of power into existing power grids is an operation that addresses both technological innovation and efficiency in resources through a multi-dimensional approach. Emerging technologies are central to the realization of these goals, particularly in the control of the smart grid and energy storage.

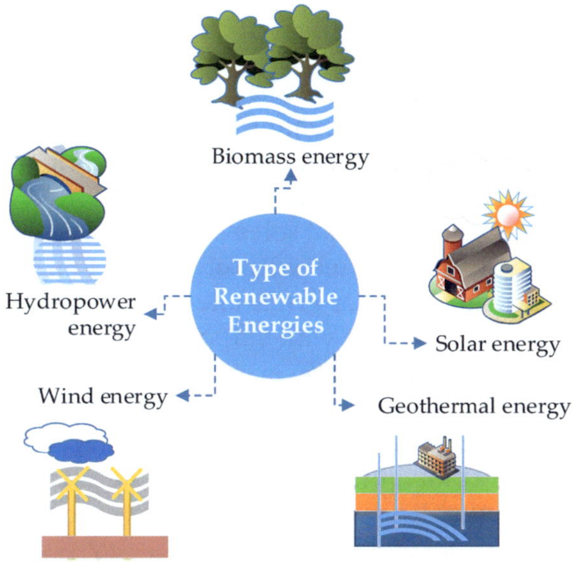

Figure 15.8. Types of renewable energy sources.

Source: https://pub.mdpi-res.com/resources/resources-08-00149/article_deploy/html/images/resources-08-00149-g001.png?1571741481.

Smart sensors and high-grade forecasting systems make efficient energy distribution and usage possible, utilizing renewable energy to its optimum level. Also, breakthroughs in efficient energy storage technologies, like batteries and pumped hydro storage, play a critical role in offsetting the intermittent nature of certain renewables, solar and wind electricity being prominent cases. Herein, as discussed by Fagas et al. (2017), there is a need for multidisciplinarity that transcends different techno-sectors to enhance energy sustainability. The complementarity of information and communications technology (ICT) with renewable energy technologies can optimize the overall efficiency of energy systems as well as encourage even greater investments in renewable resources, thus directing the world's energy consumption path towards sustainability (Figure 15.8).

15.3.2. Technological Advancements in Energy Efficiency

The increasing need to fight climate change has driven radical technological innovation in the efficiency of energy generally. Technologies , such as smart grids and energy-efficient appliances play crucial roles in reducing overall energy consumption without compromising performance. Smart grids allow for real-time data analysis that will empower utilities to more efficiently manage electricity distribution, hence reducing waste. All these developments not only facilitate improved energy management but also contribute to the enhanced utilization of renewable energy sources in national networks. An efficient energy efficiency system is imperative to the realization of sustainability targets, particularly as patterns of energy consumption keep evolving. As America focuses on cutting down carbon emissions, research into energy-efficient technologies will be at the forefront. This need is brought into focus through scenarios that examine the way U.S. energy security would have to adapt in the case of aggressive emissions reduction policies (Staley et al., 2009). The use of artificial intelligence (AI) for energy efficiency is an emerging influence on becoming a revolutionary force for shaping how energy systems are built and operated. AI-driven analytics enable precise monitoring and predictive maintenance of energy-consuming equipment, thereby saving significant amounts of energy. For instance, machine learning software can automate HVAC systems in offices to optimize usage rates and adjust operations. AI also facilitates demand and supply trend forecasting in renewable energy production so that utilities respond quickly to changes. With organizations employing such technologies, there is a greater scope for optimized performance at operations, leading to the possibility of carbon footprint reduction. These developments are characteristic of a general tendency wherein intelligent systems are being increasingly integrated into energy systems, thereby remodeling the consumption and preservation patterns of energy within living and industrial spaces (Garry & Harwood, 2019). Furthermore, analysis of cyborgian technologies in service environments promises bright future avenues for energy efficiency. The planned integration of melded frontline service employees (FLEs) utilizing the latest technologies has the potential to maximize functions and reduce energy consumption in the service industry. By embedding technologies , such as neural interfaces and AI directly into human capabilities, business organizations can maximize service delivery while also maximizing their sustainability profiles in the process. Such fusion of humans and technology maximizes not only efficiency but also overcomes multidimensional challenges in customer interaction and service management. The ethical implications of cyborg integration also warrant consideration, as it raises questions regarding the very nature of work and human roles in energy-efficient activities. The establishment of these cyborgian applications represents a critical shift of technology and human labor into an intriguing future where energy efficiency becomes an omnipresent aspect of our economic framework (Staley et al., 2009).

15.3.3. Future Trends in Energy Consumption

The energy consumption of the future is poised for transformation, led primarily by innovation in leading-edge technologies and calls for sustainability. With growing energy demands worldwide while climate change anxieties heighten, emerging solutions , such as artificial intelligence (AI) and smart grid technology can potentially recast the generation, transmission, and usage of energy. AI, in particular, has a vital role to play in optimizing the performance of renewable energy sources like solar and wind power. AI can reduce the cost of operations and improve grid reliability through energy forecasting, fault detection, and real-time analysis and thereby make a sustainable, low-carbon future a reality. The symbiotic potential of renewable energy and AI is a turning point in overcoming the challenges of the current environment and marks the beginning of an effective energy age, as highlighted in recent case studies and emerging trends (Khaleel & Abdulkareem, 2025). Further, increasing levels of integration of renewable energy sources into the energy mix necessitate a reinterpretation of traditional patterns of energy use. Water treatment plants (WTPs), for example, are significant consumers of energy but absolutely essential to enable access to safe and clean water. The energy efficiency status of WTPs identifies the need to introduce high-tech treatment technologies and operation strategies to minimize their footprints. Through a study of alternatives to install advanced monitoring systems and new treatment technologies, such as forward osmosis and electrochemical treatment, energy consumption can be greatly reduced. Not only are these reforms likely to save operational costs by making WTPs more energy-efficient, but they also conform to broader sustainability goals, underscoring the interconnectedness of energy efficiency and water quality management (Skoczko, 2025). In addition to the technological revolution behind transforming energy consumption, shifting consumers' behavior and policy development will also shape the future. Increased awareness regarding the environment and the economic benefits of energy conservation is making individuals and businesses more environmentally friendly. The advent of electric cars and energy-efficient appliances, for instance, indicates a large-scale move towards reducing energy consumption in everyday life. Policymakers are also responding with the creation of incentives for the use of renewable energy and stricter controls over carbon emissions. Together, these reforms constitute a progressive energy use strategy balancing growth and sustainability. As technology advances further, the dynamic relationship between consumer choice, policy frameworks, and technological progress will be critical to building an even more sustainable energy future (Figure 15.9).

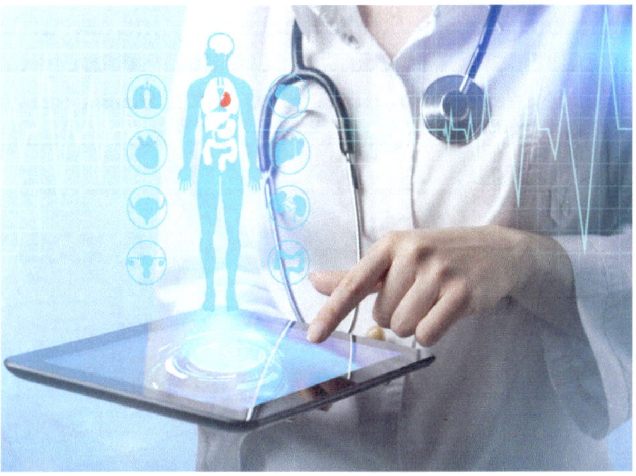

Figure 15.9. Future trends in energy consumption and artificial intelligence (AI).

Source: https://healthwire.pk/wp-content/uploads/2022/06/Future-Technology-Trends-in-Healthcare.jpg.

15.4. Internet of Things (IoT)

Internet of Things (IoT) is an underlying shift in the manner by which devices communicate and interact with one another, opening up new opportunities for data integration and application development. This network of connected devices from consumer products to industrial machinery offers the platform to collect and transfer massive amounts of data in real-time. By incorporating IoT technologies, organizations can maximize their operational efficiency, optimize decision-making, and create new ways of addressing the needs of an increasingly digital future. As mentioned in future frameworks, such as those that consolidate Industry 4.0 technologies, IoT is tasked with sustainable supply chain management, shaping the circular economy strategy that seeks to reduce waste and increase the use of resources (Liu et al., 2023). This networked world of things is more than a technological breakthrough; it is an across-the-board move toward an even more interconnected and intelligent future. The rate of exponential growth of IoT is primarily set by the progress in wireless communication technologies, particularly in 5G networks. These new technologies provide the necessary infrastructure to support the high-density connectivity required by billions of devices to share data securely and feasibly in near real-time. Through this area, the interconnection of devices to a combined network enhances not only efficiency but even the scope for analytics of data that can transform industries like healthcare, transport, and smart cities.

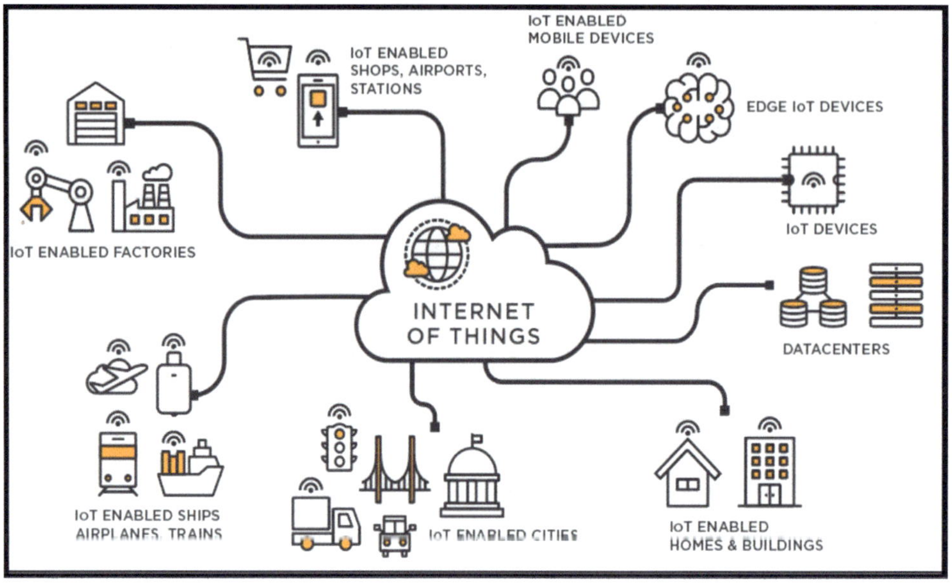

Figure 15.10. Internet of Things (IoT).

Source: https://businesstech.bus.umich.edu/wp-content/uploads/2023/01/iot2.png.

The purpose behind IoT is not only connectivity; it is to extract insights from data collected, which enables a better quality of life and promotes economic growth. The presence of smart algorithms in IoT spaces also reflects a move towards more sophisticated applications with the use of machine learning and data smarts, thus spurring innovation in various industries (Vaezi et al., 2022). When talking about the future of IoT, the necessity to end challenges , such as security, interoperability, and data management cannot be overstated. As more devices are interconnecting, the scope for vulnerabilities is higher, and robust cybersecurity must be established to protect critical information and instill user trust. Additionally, the development of universal protocols for IoT devices would be necessary to enable smooth operation across different platforms, enhancing the effectiveness of IoT systems. Additional research activities must focus on increasing energy efficiency and scalability to manage more devices without compromising performance. As the capabilities of IoT expand, the integration of emerging technologies , such as artificial intelligence and edge computing, will enhance the versatility and robustness of IoT applications, leading to a smarter and connected global ecosystem that will respond to current issues (Liu et al., 2023; Vaezi et al., 2022) (Figure 15.10).

15.4.1. Definition and Scope of IoT

The Internet of Things (IoT) is increasingly becoming a central paradigm in technology advancement, defined by the interconnection of devices through the internet. The technological advancement enables ordinary items to communicate and exchange information with one another without the intervention of human beings, thereby enhancing efficiency in operation and decision-making in many industries. With embedded system technologies, the interconnectivity of these elements forms what are termed federated embedded systems. The scope of IoT is far beyond automation; it's an ecosystem of devices, networks, and data coming together to create meaningful insights. The IoT ecosystem presents issues that it must overcome, like delivering secure data transmission and protecting sensitive data from cyber-attack, which is important in establishing user trust and increasing adoption of the technology (Bouzidi et al., 2022). Also, the infrastructure of IoT systems is structured by default in layers that define their scope of work. The perception layer, for example, is responsible for data acquisition through devices and sensors, while the middleware layer is responsible for processing data as well as device communication. The structured format allows for the convergence of various enabling technologies, like hardware platforms, as well as software solutions that facilitate the overall IoT ecosystem. The intersection of new technologies, such as IQRF, enhances the performance and security of IoT applications. With innovative protocols and architectures, IoT systems are becoming increasingly robust, opening up to more sophisticated functionalities and a broader color box of applications in smart cities, healthcare, and agriculture (Kobetski & Axelsson, 2012). In addition to facilitating automation and efficiency, IoT provides unrivaled opportunities for creating interconnected systems that dissolve conventional boundaries. These types of systems, also called systems of systems, bring together cyber-physical components with advanced analytics to expand functional capability. The intersection of IoT with philosophies like ubiquitous computing and multi-agent systems is an indicator of its multi-faceted nature, suggesting that it's not a fleeting technological trend but a paradigm shift in the design and functioning of systems. As researchers and developers delve into IoT complexities, more focus is directed towards filling security gaps and determining avenues of future research that can provide secure and sustainable IoT infrastructures. Such ever-increasing pursuit underscores IoT's instrumental role in determining the world's leading-edge technology and the world's future of connected spaces (Bouzidi et al., 2022).

15.4.2. Applications in Smart Homes and Cities

The application of Internet of Things (IoT) to the infrastructure of smart cities and homes is a technology that significantly enhances the quality of city life. IoT technology is applied in smart homes to make routine tasks automatic, allowing for personalized experiences that simplify and enhance comfort. For example, smart thermostats, lighting, and security cameras can be controlled remotely, adjusting to the residents' preferences and work patterns. The ubiquity of networked devices in urban areas also leads to effective utilization of energy, which is the signature of sustainability. As more smart city projects take flight, they allow planners to manage and monitor resources more effectively, thereby establishing a framework that is congenial to economic growth and environmental conservation. The incorporation of smart technology within urban infrastructure makes way for the potential of a future where inhabitants get to live better as their environments respond in a dynamic manner to their behavior and needs. For smart cities, V2X technology is an important advance that can revolutionize transportation infrastructure.

V2X utilizes a communication system that connects cars, to traffic lights, and even pedestrians to share information in real-time. This interaction is used to enhance road safety and optimization of traffic, which can lead to reduced congestion and lower emissions. Additionally, through the processing of data gathered from vehicles and infrastructure, city planners can calculate trends and make informed decisions regarding the use of roads and public transport. The potential of V2X systems is beyond mere convenience; it assists in the development of intelligent transportation systems capable of adapting to changing circumstances. Solving security problems concerning V2X communications can help urban cities develop a safe and trustworthy transportation system that goes beyond the concept of smart cities.

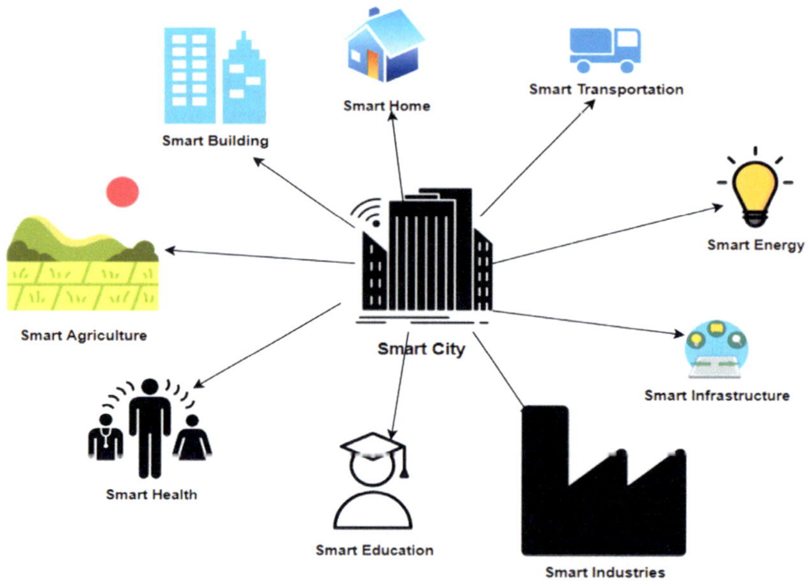

Figure 15.11. Applications in smart homes and smart cities.

Source: https://www.mdpi.com/smartcities/smartcities-04-00064/article_deploy/html/images/smartcities-04-00064-g003.png.

The implications of IoT are more than mere convenience; they are the potential for far-reaching change to society in terms of enhanced standards of living. Smart cities that get IoT technologies right benefit from enhanced data analysis, enabling real-time management and control of municipal services like garbage collection, water provision, and public safety. Real-time management translates to cities being able to act proactively on newly emerging issues, directing resources to where they are most needed. In addition, smart cities and homes create new challenges, particularly concerning data security and consumer privacy. As more individuals use smart technologies, robust security protocols become even more critical. Addressing these challenges not only protects the integrity of the information being communicated between smart systems but also lays the groundwork for broader public acceptance and confidence in the technology. As the cities themselves evolve, the path of IoT and its applications will shape a great deal of the urban future, showcasing a commitment to sustainability, efficiency, and security in a more interlinked world (Figure 15.11).

15.4.3. Security and Privacy Concerns

In today's discourse on emerging technologies, security and privacy have emerged as priorities that need to be carefully examined. With the prevalence of cloud computing in various sectors, particularly in banking institutions, storage and processing of data pose dangers that become front-page news. Such technologies are employed by businesses for increased agility and cost reduction but unleash a series of security threats that endanger confidential information. Mukherjee (2025) outlines the necessity of robust regulatory compliance in the wake of these evolving challenges, emphasizing the critical intersection of cybersecurity and regulatory policy. This can include the application of advanced encryption standards and continuous risk analysis, both of which are essential in sustaining consumer trust and protecting data integrity throughout its life cycle. The Internet of Things (IoT) is another sector that has been at the center of debates when it comes to security and privacy concerns. With organizations increasingly applying networked devices to streamline the efficiency of operations, threats to the systems increase exponentially. Threats on IoT networks can lead to intrusion and data leakage that expose both organizational and customer data to risks. AlQahtani et al. (2025) identify these problems, addressing the fundamental necessity of data privacy for IoT fire security systems and the broader effect of our reliance on network technologies. Businesses subsequently have the responsibility to attach great importance to the implementation of strong cybersecurity solutions, including real-time surveillance systems and end-to-end incident response planning, to remediate these problems. The complexity of the IoT environment necessitates an interdisciplinarity of focus not only on technological measures but also on the socio-economic undertones of information loss. The future prospects include the antagonism between emerging technologies and security risks, pointing to an imperative necessity for unrelenting innovation in cybersecurity mechanisms. With artificial intelligence and machine learning becoming the very fabric of data protection design, organizations are likely to shift their approaches in synchronization. Evolving threat landscapes demand proactive measures, including AI-based threat detection technologies with the capability to move swiftly in the event of imminent breaches and strengthen data privacy legislation. Furthermore, enhancing multi-stakeholder collaborations, as suggested by Mukherjee (2025), will enhance the resilience of the digital infrastructure, particularly in regions most susceptible to cyber-attacks. While companies face this rapidly evolving environment, an emphasis on cutting-edge cybersecurity best practices will be key to leveraging the potential of emerging technologies while securing vital data for the long term.

15.5. Virtual and Augmented Reality

Virtual and Augmented Reality (VR and AR) development is a pioneering frontier in the area of emerging technologies, where unprecedented opportunities for application lie in varied fields, notably education and cultural heritage. As immersive technologies, VR and AR are engaging platforms for experiential learning, which trigger very high retention of knowledge and user interaction. For instance, the use of VR in learning environments facilitates simulated real-life experiences that are capable of putting the learners in places that are otherwise inaccessible. Such engagement is particularly critical for adult education, where personalized learning experiences are capable of adapting in accordance with specific requirements, thereby facilitating better understanding and applicability. With the inclusion of technologies , such as Large Language Models (LLMs), students can now benefit from content that addresses their unique learning pathways, and the vast possibilities for VR and AR in shaping future pedagogical approaches (Storey & Wagner, 2024). Furthermore, the intersection of VR and AR with cultural heritage is a demonstration of the cutting-edge paths on which these technologies can travel to preserve and experience history. By utilizing augmented-reality applications, teachers and museums are able to offer rich narratives that complement traditional learning resources. Such technology not only improves access to cultural heritage artifacts but also the depth of learning experience through facilitating users' engagement interactively with digital replicas of heritage settings or artifacts. Such an interactive experience calls forth a deeper appreciation of cultural heritage, especially where physical access is limited. Moreover, the ability to deliver cultural heritage in a digitally shareable format reflects growing expectations for interactive and user-centered experiences, increasingly regarded as central components of effective educational approaches (Bekele et al., 2018). The ethical implications regarding the application of VR and AR technology must not be overlooked. With greater integration of these technologies into learning environments and cultural heritage sites, concerns with respect to data privacy, bias in algorithms, and academic honesty also emerge. For instance, as helpful as personalization of the learning experience is, it creates concerns around how the data is collected and used and potential bias in algorithm-driven content recommendations. Solving these ethical problems is crucial to establishing trust among users and ensuring equitable access to technological innovation. Moreover, the direction should be marked for VR and AR through ongoing debate of policy implications for establishing frameworks that not only guide ethical usage but also optimize the educational and cultural benefits of these technologies (Bekele et al., 2018; Storey & Wagner, 2024) (Figure 15.12).

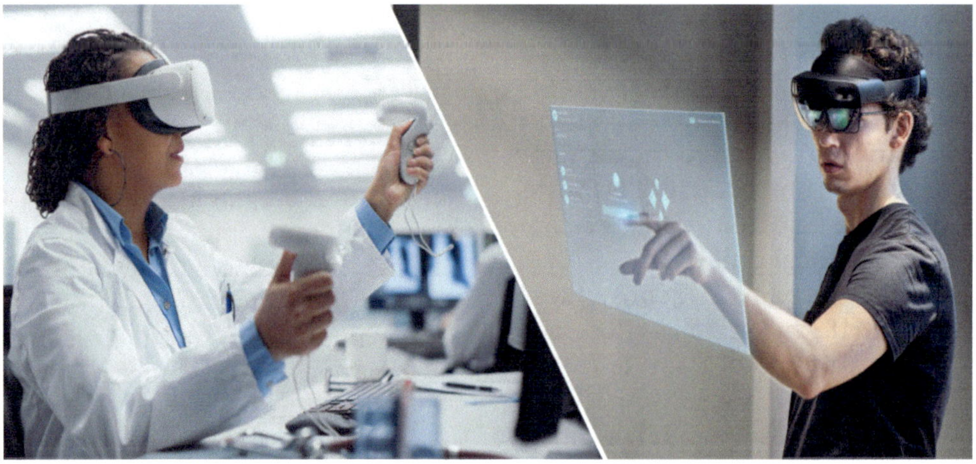

Figure 15.12. Virtual reality (VR) and augmented reality (AR).

Source: https://www.xmreality.com/hubfs/AR%20vs%20VR%20mindre-2.png.

15.5.1. Current Uses in Entertainment and Education

The use of new technologies in entertainment has changed the way people consume media, and the front-runners are VR and AR. These new technologies produce experiences that engage users and have them interact with the surroundings in ways traditional media hasn't been able to. In the entertainment sector, for instance, VR technology allows users become part of the story and have them navigate virtual worlds or read narration interactively. Further, the use of AR in mobile provides more immersive experiences for users by overlaying virtual information on the real world and therefore enhancing gaming and live event experiences. However, with the development of such technology comes concerns regarding the ethical impacts as well as misinformation, particularly with the development of deepfake technology. Solving these issues is crucial to maintaining trust and integrity in entertainment as it adapts to keep pace with technological advancements (Ansar & Kumar, 2025). In education, the incorporation of new technologies , such as AI and digital twins, has introduced new pedagogy and learning approaches. AI-based platforms can allow learning to be tailored, and students can learn at their own pace while getting personalized coaching. Digital twins, or copies of actual systems and processes in virtual form, have also found application in educational institutions, where they can simulate innovative concepts and complement the learners' perspective through learn-by-doing. For example, architecture and engineering students can work with virtual replicas of buildings to comprehend structural principles better. As schools incorporate these technologies more and more, so too must they address implications of data privacy and security, particularly as highlighted in analyses of cybersecurity threats to cyber systems (Alhamam et al., 2025). The convergence of technology in entertainment and education foresees a future with both sectors contributing more and more directly to inform and support one another. For example, edutainment games employ entertainment principles for user engagement and better learning outcomes, bridging the divide between learning and play. Similarly, employing entertainment storytelling techniques, educators can present information in a more interactive and credible form with higher retention and understanding. Such a convergence, however, creates fundamentally important questions about the quantity of educational material and the risk of diversion. As industries shift to more integrated approaches, ongoing research in the efficacy and morality of such technologies will be crucial in deciding their future applications (Alhamam et al., 2025; Ansar & Kumar, 2025).

15.5.2. Potential for Training and Simulation

The future for training and simulation through emerging technologies has actually been transforming educational paradigms in various sectors, particularly the Architecture/Engineering/Construction (AEC) sector. While organizations increasingly recognize information and communication technologies (ICT) as strategically important, integrating training schemes based on such technologies is increasingly essential. Specifically, the AEC sector begins to think of ICT as not only an accessory, but also as a strategic asset that supports competitive advantage. According to research, ICT training priority is emerging as an important factor to achieve sustainable improvements and to facilitate innovation in organizations (Isikdag et al., 2009). The shift of emphasis reinforces the assumption that high-quality training has the potential to yield more informed stakeholders, effective projects, and ultimately improved outcomes in operational and financial terms. Further, the integration of computational science and engineering (CSE) with training and simulation methods outlines a promising avenue to the development of an informed workforce able to tackle complex issues. CSE's accelerated growth has revolutionized conventional problem-solving practices to provide a more enhanced learning experience through experiential simulations and computational experiments that mimic actual situations. Using advanced computing methods, instructors can develop interactive simulation settings that encourage critical thinking and decision-making among trainees. This forward-thinking strategy challenges learners to experiment with various outcomes within a simulated framework, thereby enhancing their capacity for negotiating complex systems and innovating within fields (Biros et al., 2016).

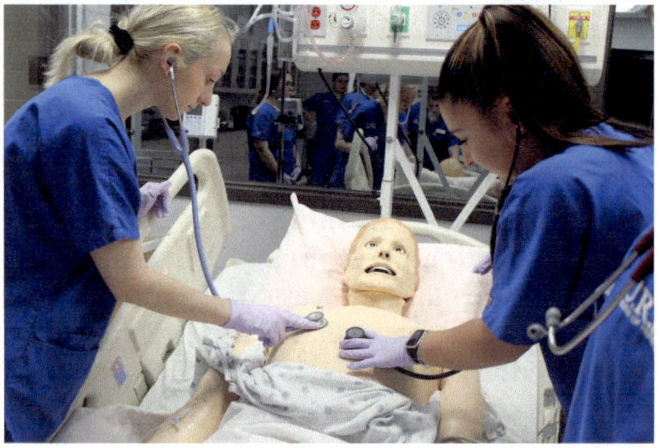

Figure 15.13. Potential for training and simulation.

Source: https://web.uri.edu/nursing/wp-content/uploads/sites/963/IMG_6552-2.jpg.

Thus, the use of simulation-based training in CSE holds immense potential towards creating a workforce that is not just knowledgeable but also skilled in adaptability in methods and approaches. Lastly, the advancement of training and simulation technologies crosses disciplinary boundaries, affecting more and more fields. This interdisciplinarity highlights the importance of adaptive training models that can leverage cutting-edge technological advancements, framing a new workforce learning paradigm. The effective use of interactive simulations drives collaboration, knowledge sharing, and real-time decision-making between cross-functional teams. Hence, organizations can cultivate innovation and responsiveness among their staff members and prepare them to effectively meet the challenges that lie ahead. As markets evolve and face unforeseen setbacks, the activity of tailored training and simulation experience will definitely set the pace for their development and sustenance. The need for ongoing learning and skill acquisition highlights the importance of integrating such technologies in educational institutions and professional programs, making them indispensable in the pursuit of achievement (Figure 15.13).

15.5.3. Future Developments and Market Growth

In line with the changing digital landscape, technological growth in the future promises to revolutionize market growth in unprecedented ways. One of the central driving forces of this revolution is artificial intelligence (AI), which is revolutionizing businesses by enabling data-driven decision-making as well as maximizing operational effectiveness. Companies are increasingly turning to AI to unlock insights from vast amounts of data to enable greater customer customization, predictive analytics, and improved resource allocation. This transformation not only optimizes existing operations but also creates new avenues of revenue as firms use AI for product innovation and improving services. Moreover, the advent of blockchain technology is driving market growth through secure and transparent transactions that are building customer trust industry-wide. Organizations adopting these new technologies will be capable of gaining a competitive edge in the marketplace, as seen in recent research, making the need for disruptive approaches to tackling complexities in a rapidly evolving business environment (Prerna, 2025). Green business practice is also a critical element of future innovations that affect market growth. With increasingly environmentally conscious consumers, firms are compelled to adopt more responsible practices that align with the aspirations of individuals. This is leading to the emergence of sustainable technologies that address environmental issues and create economic opportunities as well. For instance, progress in renewable energy, waste reduction, and sustainable supply chain management is becoming a critical component of corporate strategy. Such action is not only beneficial to the planet but also assists in creating brand reputation and attracting environmentally conscious consumers, which in turn results in market growth. Moreover, organizations concentrating on ethical aspects in their functions are certain to attain massive returns on investment as they develop customer loyalty and better community relationships. This revolutionary wave signifies a turning point towards the integration of sustainability into business models, confirming the interdependence of economics and ethics (Arinze, 2024). Lastly, the interplay between exponential growth drivers and emerging technologies presents unique opportunities for business expansion. As illustrated in ongoing studies, the convergence of AI, biotechnology, and digitalization allows for rapid innovation across multiple industries. This exponential growth can lead to unbounded innovation, where companies that successfully leverage these developments can gain enormous market shares and control. Yet this potential does come with ethical and regulatory issues that have to be managed wisely. For instance, facing public health issues and ethical questions surrounding technological advancements requires visionary leadership and stakeholder cooperation. A fine-grained comprehension of these dynamics thus becomes imperative for organizations that want to thrive in the midst of high-speed change. By embracing a multidisciplinary approach and sustainable development, organizations can not only innovate but promote the well-being of society so that technological innovation serves future generations and existing ones alike (Arinze, 2024).

15.6. Quantum Computing

Quantum computing is a groundbreaking leap in computational power that draws on quantum mechanics laws to perform tasks that are not possible for ordinary computers. A bit is used in normal computing as the smallest unit of data, 0 or 1. Quantum computing employs qubits that can exist in many states simultaneously due to superposition. This special feature makes quantum computers capable of handling huge amounts of data at unprecedented rates, which can potentially transform areas like cryptography, materials science, and modeling of complex systems. As they advance, we can see the emergence of a different paradigm in not just the resolution of problems but in the concept of computation itself, with the promise of an era where quantum algorithms might be orders of magnitude faster than their classical counterparts. In addition, the applications of quantum computing reach far into the realm of information security. As quantum technologies develop, classical cryptography, relying in large part on the computational hardness of some mathematical problems, is confronted with a daunting challenge. Quantum computers can crack commonly used encryption systems, prompting the establishment of new cryptographic methods that are resistant to these developments. Therefore, there should be a robust quantum-resistant cryptography platform; researchers now develop hybrid systems that integrate the use of both the classical and quantum methods to enable data privacy and security. Post-quantum cryptography, derived from mathematical problems that are still secure against quantum attacks, is a critical research area as society increasingly depends on digital communications and data storage technology (Kabanov et al., 2018). Computational science and engineering (CSE) is also facing a parallel revolution, embracing quantum computing within its scope to achieve its computational strength. CSE has emerged as the center of discovery in many fields of science, discovering solutions to the complexities of current data with advanced computational techniques.

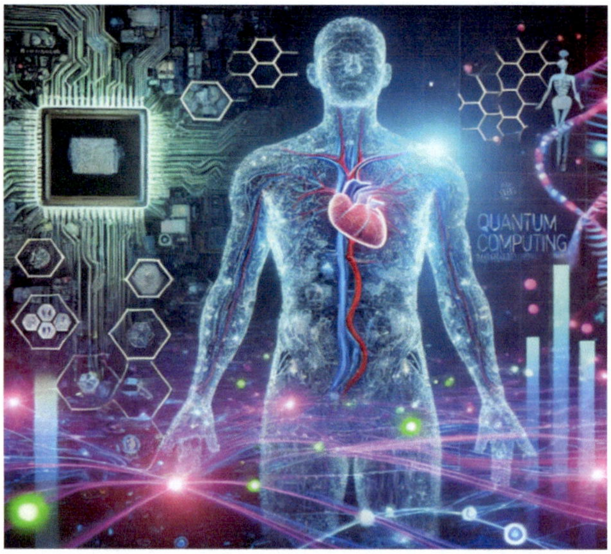

Figure 15.14. Quantum computing represents a transformative advancement in biomedical science.

Source: https://external-content.duckduckgo.com/iu/?u=https%3A%2F%2Fuplink.weforum.org%2Fuplink%2Fsfc%2Fservlet.shepherd%2Fdocument%2Fdownload%2F069TE000009wEDWYA2&f=1&nofb=1&ipt=25d037e0358a04bf9b87581521c6c27dde01ceb9ac11a548ae1923d996911c6f.

With quantum technology maturing, it will refurbish CSE by providing methods of resolving problems that require very high computational strength. The integration of quantum algorithms into practice in CSE potentially could enable new avenues for simulating complex systems, optimizing resource allocation, and designing innovative materials. But this convergence is not without challenges, such as coping with architectural complexities inherent to extreme-scale computing, as well as the explosive growth of data-driven science. Welcoming such challenges and cultivating such a workforce proficient in both quantum and classical computations will be the key to maintaining progress in CSE and its applications (Biros et al., 2016) (Figure 15.14).

15.6.1. Basics of Quantum Computing Technology

Quantum computing is a computer paradigm change that utilizes the principles of quantum mechanics to calculate. Unlike classical computers, which employ bits as the most basic unit of data, quantum computers employ quantum bits or qubits, which can be in numerous states simultaneously due to the superposition effect. This property allows quantum computers to carry out an incredible number of computations in parallel, significantly enhancing their processing power for specific tasks over classical computing. Qubits are also entangleable, producing correlations that enable these systems to execute complex algorithms more efficiently. Therefore, this technology opens new avenues in various industries, like cryptography, drug discovery, and optimization issues, thereby marking its importance to redefine computational problem-solving in the coming future. An interesting innovation in the field of quantum computing technology is the emergence of quantum cloud computing, in which customers can rent quantum computers remotely via the cloud. This model makes quantum resources accessible to the public, enabling developers and scientists to experiment with quantum algorithms without needing to invest significant resources into proprietary hardware. Quantum cloud platforms provide a variety of services , including being able to run quantum simulations and develop quantum applications to address real-world problems. The latest advancements in the area have further solidified the infrastructure required to make quantum cloud computing effective in managing resource management, quantum serverless computing, and addressing issues of privacy and security, which are most critical in safeguarding secret information. The advancements put focus on the position of quantum cloud computing as a building block of quantum technologies of the future, transforming the way applications are deployed and executed (Nguyen et al., 2024). With the continuous progress of quantum computing, it is also necessary to consider its intersection with other revolutionary technologies, in this scenario, particularly security orchestration in networking.

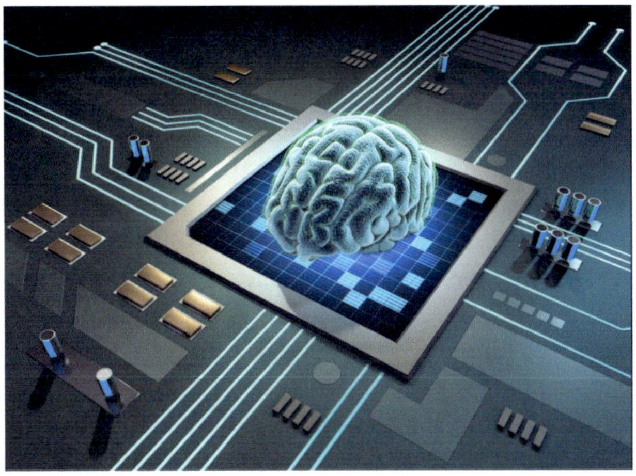

Figure 15.15. Basics of quantum computing technology.

Source: https://www.amsterdamsciencepark.nl/wp-content/uploads/2022/10/Digitale-hersenen-1920x1440.jpg.

Quantum computing can potentially enhance next-generation network security capabilities, such as those in 5G and beyond 5G (B5G) networks. Based on quantum principles, researchers are exploring new ways of encrypting information and protecting data that may have an advantage over existing ones. For instance, quantum key distribution (QKD) offers a never-before-seen level of security by utilizing the fundamental principles of quantum physics to offer secure channels for communication. This association of quantum computing with other technologies helps to highlight the necessity of continuous research and development in both fields to address the challenge of increasing complexity in security management. Thus, the mastery of the basics of quantum computing technology is a requirement for comprehending the future world in communication and information security (Batewela et al., 2025) (Figure 15.15).

15.6.2. Comparison with Classical Computing

With newer technologies pushing against conventional boundaries, the analogy with classical computing becomes ever more important, especially in areas of computational efficiency and resource allocation. Classical computing uses a centralized framework, solving resource allocation problems (RAPs) through structured algorithms that tend to be very time-consuming and computationally intensive. However, greater information and communication technology (ICT) has initiated proposals of market-based solutions that offer dynamic frameworks for RAPs to achieve maximum efficiency and flexibility for application purposes. Comparative analyses of the performance of such methods have appeared in the literature, particularly in settings with uncertainty, e.g., the mobile task allocation problem (MTAP). This indicates a revolutionary shift in which classic computational methodologies are complemented, or even supplanted, by more agile methods better suited to the intrinsic complexities of today's challenges, indicating a groundbreaking transformation in computing paradigms. Aside from efficiency, resource management of the networking aspect is an example of pointing out the drastic divergence in classic computing and emerging technologies. Network slicing is an emerging path of departure from traditional networking that allows operators to create customized virtual networks according to precise requirements. Network slicing facilitates differentiated provisioning of service and thus operators have the option to sell differentiated slices at varying prices. Traditional networks, by default, are not capable of such flexibility, and thus, network slicing invokes sophisticated resource handling to make these slices offer optimum performance. Deep reinforcement learning (DRL) is brought to the fore here as an effective instrument, sharpening resource allocation processes by directly learning from real-time experiences in the network environment. The comparative analysis of the traditional and modern approaches to network management highlights a shift towards intelligent systems, which can much more easily adapt to users' demands, a characteristic that traditional computing is less able to simulate. The consequences of this shift to advanced computational methods go beyond efficiency; they redefine the landscape of technology innovation. By integrating intelligent systems , such as DRL for resource management for network slicing, businesses are able to optimize operating efficiencies and cost reductions to create a more adaptive environment for digital services. This trend is particularly relevant in the context of increased complexity and demand for services, which require systems that respond quickly to change. Future research directions seek to unveil the full potential of combining classical fundamentals and emerging technologies to enable innovations in areas , such as mobile task allocation and dynamic resource management. As these technologies become realities, the constant juxtaposition of traditional computing models with new approaches will be instrumental in the determination of the viability and trajectory of future computational models, requiring ongoing review and adjustment.

15.6.3. Future Implications for Data Processing and Security

The shifting data processing and security environment poses huge implications for numerous sectors, particularly now that companies are increasingly embracing the use of advanced technologies , such as artificial intelligence (AI) and big data analytics. These facilitate better decision-making and operational efficiency, allowing companies the capacity to spur growth and innovation. However, the use of such technology is fraught with threats, most significantly in terms of cybersecurity threats. As organizations use real-time data analytics for more productivity, they must also be prepared for the weaknesses associated with greater access to data. Further, the rapid development of these technologies necessitates ongoing research to bridge gaps in compliance and training in all industries to prepare organizations adequately to manage the threats associated with digital transformation. As emphasized under the heading on financial risk management, the two-edged aspect of such tools needs to be comprehended along with each other to leverage opportunities and mitigate threats (Sunaryo et al., 2025). In the retail business, the implementation of real-time analysis of data profoundly reengineers order management systems as well as supply chain potential. Greater emphasis on sophisticated analytics programs makes for a business culture concerned with customers' happiness and operational bliss. Nonetheless, such growth calls for intense concentration on the technical aspect of data processing, like system integration, scalability, and security controls. Companies must be confident that their environment of analytics is not just effective in handling bulk data but also robust enough to safeguard against expected security vulnerabilities. The implications of these technologies can provide enhanced market competitiveness, but they are accompanied by data integrity and customer sensitivity stewardship implications. Toggling between robust security measures and maximizing analytics potential will be critical to retail businesses that want to operate in this technology landscape (Raketla, 2025). In the future, the confluence of upcoming technologies , such as blockchain and edge computing, continues to shape future implications on data processing and security. Blockchain offers unmatched transparency and security in data transactions that prove to be of essential importance in sectors like finance and supply chain. Blockchain offers integrity and accountability with reduced threats associated with data fraud and breaches. Edge computing, on the contrary, allows organizations to process data closer to its source, cutting down latency and response time for analytics. This shift also necessitates reassessing traditional cybersecurity controls because data proliferation at the edge introduces more probable points of exposure. To successfully realize the promise of these emerging technologies, organizations must pursue an integrated strategy that combines innovative processing power with robust security systems to develop a secure and effective operating platform for the future (Raketla, 2025; Sunaryo et al., 2025) (Figure 15.16).

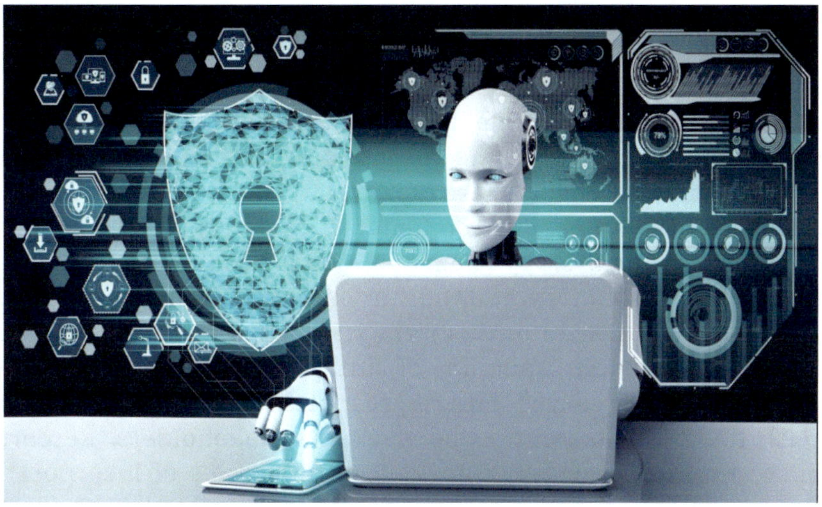

Figure 15.16. Future implications for data processing and security.

Source: https://nohack.net/wp-content/uploads/2023/11/ai-robot-using-cyber-security-protect-information-privacy-scaled.jpg.

SUMMARY

As one observes the trajectory of emergent technologies, it is clear that the intersection between innovation and applied uses is profoundly transforming various industries. As illustrated throughout this essay, technology in the future is not merely about creating tools and systems but also about constructing human capability and addressing social wants. Non-contact sleep monitoring analysis illustrates how the new advances can be utilized for disease control, emphasizing the importance of interdisciplinary studies. As Shi et al. (2025) put it, monitoring systems are set to integrate developing technologies for improved patient care as well as prevention in healthcare. These developments are evidence of a broader trend under which technology is not merely an enabler but a change agent in addressing complex health-related issues. The impact of embracing future technologies in traditional areas, such as medicine and accounting, also supports the necessity for facilitative frameworks and infrastructure. The analysis of AI and blockchain applications illustrates that while countries like India and Thailand are making advances, there are still significant barriers that must be overcome across various environments, such as regulatory issues and the need for certain education programs. An analysis by Islam et al. (2024) shows the importance of government support systems to promote technology adoption in emerging economies. As the transformation takes place, companies are committed to also driving training and development that fills the skills gap. Without such support, the full capability of future technology can be left untapped, with significant opportunities going unrealized. Future prospects for emerging technologies are positive, but they need a push toward collaboration between the stakeholders. Researchers, companies, and policymakers have to work together to tackle the intricacies of incorporating technology in a manner that addresses ethical questions and security concerns beforehand. The future of non-contact sleep tracking and blockchain technologies is indicative of innovation strands capable of revolutionizing dominant paradigms when dealt with in an integrated fashion. Future directions in this space, as indicated by ongoing research, need to be directed towards not just pushing technology but sustainable systems that foster trust and openness. With the environment shifting, these complexities will have to be embraced to craft a future where upcoming technologies realize their full potential for the benefit of society.

In researching new technologies, the intersection of digital payment platforms and the Metaverse is a key economic paradigm shift. Amongst the focus areas delivered is blockchain technology use, which has become an imperative to introduce depth in security and transparency in financial transactions in virtual worlds. As the Metaverse expands, adopting such technologies as virtual reality (VR) and augmented reality (AR) becomes increasingly important. These technologies support immersive experiences that enhance user interaction, thus maximizing the potential for economic exchange. In spite of increased growth in blockchain and decentralized finance (DeFi), issues continue to discourage inclusivity and sustainability within the Metaverse economy. Thus, future work should try to improve these electronic payment systems for greater access and efficiency and overcome recurring problems clarified in the study (Mariana et al., 2025). Secondly, energy consumption sustainability in water treatment plants (WTPs) becomes a major issue for emerging technologies. WTPs are likely to use large amounts of energy, which contributes to greenhouse gas emissions and is a primary operating cost. The research reveals that conventional treatment technologies are ineffective, an aspect that underscores the need for revolutionary solutions towards enhancing energy efficiency. The prime reasons for such a scenario are not only outdated infrastructure but also energy-intensive characteristics of processes , such as reverse osmosis and

UV disinfection. As the literature suggests, the use of renewable energy sources , such as solar and wind power, combined with intelligent monitoring systems evolved from IoT and AI, can potentially reduce energy consumption and operation costs in WTPs significantly. Such new approaches are significant avenues for future research committed to water management activities' sustainability (Skoczko, 2025). Finally, constructing a consensual space among stakeholders remains essential as new technologies redefine traditional frameworks in various industries. The interaction between researchers, policymakers, and technology developers is essential in the development of technologies that are technologically effective and socially aware. The understanding of the cooperative networks made public in recent studies illuminates how such interactions can translate into mutual knowledge and means, eventually resulting in better implementation of sustainable practices. Future strategic plans should be centered on implementing such collective frameworks to facilitate the development of technologies that address critical societal needs and reduce environmental impacts. While science practitioners and researchers chart these complex linkages, continued dialogue on future technologies will be vital to determine future-proof and participatory infrastructures (Mariana et al., 2025; Skoczko, 2025).

A LOOK TO THE FUTURE:

PATIENT TREATMENT:

Patient treatment is a foundational concept in healthcare, reflecting the comprehensive set of actions and interactions that clinicians undertake to diagnose, manage, and improve the health status of individuals receiving care. At its most basic level, treatment refers to the provision and coordination of medical services aimed at alleviating illness, restoring function, and enhancing quality of life through therapeutic interventions that are tailored to a patient's needs. These interventions can range from preventive measures and diagnostic evaluations to pharmacologic therapy, surgical procedures, rehabilitation, and long-term care strategies. Patient treatment begins with accurate assessment and diagnosis, which form the basis for developing a treatment plan that responds effectively to the underlying health condition. This plan often integrates contributions from multidisciplinary teams—including physicians, nurses, therapists, pharmacists, and other healthcare professionals—who work collaboratively to ensure that care is evidence-based and patient-centered. Effective treatment not only addresses the physical aspects of disease but also considers psychological, social, and emotional factors that influence healing and recovery.

Central to modern patient treatment is the concept of shared decision-making, which respects the patient as an active participant in their care journey. Rather than simply following provider directives, patients are informed about treatment options, potential benefits, risks, and alternatives so they can help decide the course that aligns with their values and preferences. This approach fosters trust, improves adherence to treatment regimens, and enhances overall satisfaction with care.

The goals of patient treatment extend beyond symptom relief to encompass prevention, stabilization, and long-term well-being. For chronic conditions such as diabetes, cardiovascular disease, or cancer, effective treatment involves not only addressing current health problems but also implementing strategies that minimize progression, prevent complications, and optimize quality of life over time. This requires continuous monitoring, follow-up care, and adjustment of treatment plans to reflect changes in the patient's condition or response to therapy.

In recent years, the delivery of patient treatment has also embraced broader dimensions of care, including patient education, counseling, and resource coordination, which support individuals in understanding their conditions, participating actively in their care, and managing their health outside clinical settings. These aspects have become increasingly important as healthcare systems strive to enhance patient engagement, reduce unnecessary readmissions, and promote sustainable health outcomes.

In essence, patient treatment is not a single intervention but a dynamic and patient-centered process that integrates clinical expertise, compassionate care, and active patient involvement to achieve the best possible health outcomes.

REFERENCES

1. Isikdag, U., Underwood, J., Kuruoglu, M., Goulding, J.S., & Acikalin, U. (2009). Construction informatics in Turkey: strategic role of ICT and future research directions. *J. Inf. Technol. Constr., 14*, 412-428. (accessed on 17th July 2025).
2. Alhamam, N., Rahman, M. M. H., & Aljughaiman, A. (2025). A comprehensive review on cybersecurity of digital twins: Issues, challenges, and future research directions. *IEEE Access, 13*, 45106–45124. https://www.semanticscholar.org/paper/91215532cc187425008307c2ee324d20f29cd49e (accessed on 17th July 2025).
3. AlQahtani, A. A. S., Sulaiman, M., Alshayeb, T., & Alamleh, H. (2025). From Inception to Innovation: A Comprehensive Review and Bibliometric Analysis of IoT-Enabled Fire Safety Systems. *Safety, 11*(2), 41. https://doi.org/10.3390/safety11020041(accessed on 17th July 2025).
4. Alowais, S. A., Alghamdi, S. S., Alsuhebany, N., Alqahtani, T., Alshaya, A., Almohareb, S. N., Aldairem, A., et al. (2023). Revolutionizing healthcare: The role of artificial intelligence in clinical practice. *BMC Medical Education, 23.* https://doi.org/10.1186/s12909-023-04698-z (accessed on 17th July 2025).
5. Andorno, R., Baylis, F., Darnovsky, M., Dickenson, D., Haker, H., Hasson, K., Lowthorp, L., et al. (2020). Geneva statement on heritable human genome editing: The need for course correction. *Trends in Biotechnology, 38*, 351–354. https://doi.org/10.1016/j.tibtech.2019.12.022 (accessed on 17th July 2025).
6. Ang, J. H., Goh, C., Saldivar, A. A. F., & Li, Y. (2017). Energy-Efficient Through-Life Smart Design, Manufacturing and Operation of Ships in an Industry 4.0 Environment. *Energies, 10*(5), 610. https://doi.org/10.3390/en10050610(accessed on 17th July 2025).
7. Ansar, H., & Kumar, M. S. (2025). Video deepfake detection: Current trends, methodologies, and future directions. *2025 International Conference on Machine Learning and Autonomous Systems (ICMLAS).* https://www.semanticscholar.org/paper/1906ef59210cb2e3fe20afe9757047432dc17cf1 (accessed on 17th July 2025).
8. Lindeman, D. A., Kim, K. K., Gladstone, C., & Apesoa-Varano, E. C. (2020). Technology and Caregiving: Emerging Interventions and Directions for Research. *The Gerontologist, 60*(Suppl 1), S41–S49. https://doi.org/10.1093/geront/gnz178(accessed on 17th July 2025).
9. Saur-Amaral, I., Aragonez, T., & Lopes, J. M. (2024). Artificial intelligence for innovation in business & engineering. https://core.ac.uk/download/629226572.pdf (accessed on 17th July 2025).
10. Arinze, E. (2024). Unravelling exponential growth dynamics: A comprehensive review. *IAA Journal of Scientific Research.* https://www.semanticscholar.org/paper/c0ba85fbc6fbac427c1aca0e84da7adbab990917 (accessed on 17th July 2025).
11. Kobetski, A., & Axelsson, J. (2012). Federated embedded systems–A review of the literature in related fields. Software and Systems Engineering Laboratory Swedish Institute of Computer Science https://core.ac.uk/download/11434985.pdf (accessed on 17th July 2025).
12. Bae, H., Nguyen, C. M., Ruiz-Orera, J., Mills, N., Snyder, M., Jang, C., Shah, S. H., et al. (2025). Emerging technologies and future directions in interorgan crosstalk cardiometabolic research. *Circulation Research, 136*, 1494–1506. https://www.semanticscholar.org/paper/9edabc684a07db38b4ca86ae28785fdeb2882f51 (accessed on 17th July 2025).

13. S. Batewela, P. Ranaweera, M. Liyanage, E. Zeydan and M. Ylianttila, "Addressing Security Orchestration Challenges in Next-Generation Networks: A Comprehensive Overview," in *IEEE Open Journal of the Computer Society*, vol. 6, pp. 669-687, 2025, doi: 10.1109/OJCS.2025.3564788.(accessed on 17th July 2025).

14. Mafkereseb Kassahun Bekele, Roberto Pierdicca, Emanuele Frontoni, Eva Savina Malinverni, and James Gain. 2018. A Survey of Augmented, Virtual, and Mixed Reality for Cultural Heritage. J. Comput. Cult. Herit. 11, 2, Article 7 (June 2018), 36 pages. https://doi.org/10.1145/3145534(accessed on 17th July 2025).

15. Biros, G., Bungartz, H., Corones, J., et al. (2016). Research and education in computational science and engineering. Report from a workshop sponsored by the Society for Industrial and Applied Mathematics (SIAM) and the European Exascale Software Initiative (EESI-2), August 4-6, 2014, Breckenridge, Colorado https://core.ac.uk/download/148025463.pdf (accessed on 17th July 2025).

16. M. Bouzidi, N. Gupta, F. A. Cheikh, A. Shalaginov and M. Derawi, "A Novel Architectural Framework on IoT Ecosystem, Security Aspects and Mechanisms: A Comprehensive Survey," in *IEEE Access*, vol. 10, pp. 101362-101384, 2022, doi: 10.1109/ACCESS.2022.3207472. (accessed on 17th July 2025).

17. Nguyen, H.T., Krishnan, P., Krishnaswamy, D., Usman, M., & Buyya, R. (2024). Quantum Cloud Computing: A Review, Open Problems, and Future Directions. *ArXiv, abs/2404.11420.*(accessed on 17th July 2025).

18. L'opez, M.B., & Casado, C.Á. (2023). A Cyberpunk 2077 perspective on the prediction and understanding of future technology. *Entertain. Comput., 54*, 100952.(accessed on 17th July 2025).

19. Chen, X., I, C. L., Li, R., et al. (2018). Deep reinforcement learning for resource management in network slicing. http://arxiv.org/abs/1805.06591 (accessed on 17th July 2025).

20. Chen, Y., & Ely, A. (2011). Health biotechnology innovation for social sustainability – A perspective from China. https://core.ac.uk/download/2731317.pdf (accessed on 17th July 2025).

21. Childs Staley, B., Goodward, J., Zyla, K., & Ladislaw, S. (2009). Evaluating the energy security implications of a carbon-constrained U.S. economy. https://core.ac.uk/download/71351146.pdf (accessed on 17th July 2025).

22. Saleem, Y., Crespi, N., Rehmani, M.H., & Copeland, R. (2017). Internet of Things-Aided Smart Grid: Technologies, Architectures, Applications, Prototypes, and Future Research Directions. *IEEE Access, 7*, 62962-63003.(accessed on 17th July 2025).

23. Dr. Prerna. (2025). Emerging trends and innovative strategies in commerce: Navigating the future of business practices. *International Journal of Business and Management Invention.* https://www.semanticscholar.org/paper/3ec51b9b2dde2df3017ec8358e498969347d40df (accessed on 17th July 2025).

24. Dwivedi, Y. K., Kshetri, N., Hughes, L., Slade, E., Jeyaraj, A., Kar, A. K., Baabdullah, A. M., et al. (2023). Opinion paper: "So what if ChatGPT wrote it?" Multidisciplinary perspectives on opportunities, challenges and implications of generative conversational AI for research, practice and policy. *International Journal of Information Management, 71*, 102642–102642. https://doi.org/10.1016/j.ijinfomgt.2023.102642 (accessed on 17th July 2025).

25. Iwona Skoczko, 2025. "**Energy Efficiency Analysis of Water Treatment Plants: Current Status and Future Trends**," Energies, MDPI, vol. 18(5), pages 1-35, February.(accessed on 17th July 2025).

26. Fagas, G., Gallagher, J. P., Gammaitoni, L., et al. (2017). "Energy challenges for ICT." In *ICT - Energy Concepts for Energy Efficiency and Sustainability*, IntechOpen, pp. 1-36, DOI: 10.5772/66678. (accessed on 17th July 2025).

27. I. S. Kabanov, R. R. Yunusov, Y. V. Kurochkin, A. K. Fedorov; Practical cryptographic strategies in the post-quantum era. *AIP Conf. Proc.* 28 February 2018; 1936 (1): 020021. https://doi.org/10.1063/1.5025459(accessed on 17th July 2025).

28. Garry, T., & Harwood, T. (2019). Cyborgs as frontline service employees: a research agenda. *Journal of Service Theory and Practice, 29*, 415-437.(accessed on 17th July 2025).

29. Islam, R., Islam, M. H., & Islam, S. (2024). Blockchain and AI: Integrating emerging technologies into Bangladesh's accounting practices. *International Journal of Science and Business.* https://www.semanticscholar.org/paper/9791aa8c464f6a3c2aae9c2b6c2b6596d4446df9 (accessed on 17th July 2025).

30. Kansal, K. (2024). Exploring the prospects and challenges of artificial intelligence in shaping the future of Web 3.0. *International Journal for Research in Applied Science and Engineering Technology.* https://www.semanticscholar.org/paper/38b4849e6fccdb455f343005790ee75a867d3a72 (accessed on 17th July 2025).

31. Kapoor, D., Gupta, D., Uppal, M., Mapari, S., & Saini, S. (2024). Unveiling the dimensions of Internet of Things: A comprehensive bibliometric analysis. *2024 First International Conference on Data, Computation and Communication (ICDCC).* https://www.semanticscholar.org/paper/3e92c5acfb5620716a6cee2298ffabb1d23fc207 (accessed on 17th July 2025).

32. Mahdi Fadil Khaleel, & Zainab Mohammed Abdulkareem. (2025). A study on the role of artificial intelligence and renewable energy technologies in building a sustainable future. *Journal of Artificial Intelligence,Machine Learning and Neural Network* , *5*(1), 14–27. https://doi.org/10.55529/jaimlnn.51.14.27(accessed on 17th July 2025).

33. Liu, L., Song, W., & Liu, Y. (2023). Leveraging digital capabilities toward a circular economy: Reinforcing sustainable supply chain management with Industry 4.0 technologies. *Computers & Industrial Engineering, 178*, 109113–109113. https://doi.org/10.1016/j.cie.2023.109113 (accessed on 17th July 2025).

34. Mane, S. S., & Jadhav, S. S. (2024). Artificial intelligence in blockchain technology. *International Journal for Research in Applied Science and Engineering Technology.* https://www.semanticscholar.org/paper/bfddd6a5bcac6cdc04f7dbfd89b6292721456ab4 (accessed on 17th July 2025).

35. Mariana, C. D., Husodo, Z., Ekaputra, I. A., & Fahlevi, M. (2025). The digital payment revolution in the metaverse: A systematic review of emerging technologies, challenges, and future directions. *Strategic Change.* https://www.semanticscholar.org/paper/aaf918819f0d0f05edad485a872922867e48544e (accessed on 17th July 2025).

36. Massironi, S., Franchina, M., Ippolito, D., Elisei, F., Falco, O., Maino, C., Pagni, F., et al. (2024). Improvements and future perspective in diagnostic tools for neuroendocrine neoplasms. *Expert Review of Endocrinology & Metabolism, 19*, 349–366. https://www.semanticscholar.org/paper/3f10150420340ad6993172c5de5552bfedea3ba8 (accessed on 17th July 2025).

37. Mukherjee, D. (2025). Cloud security and privacy in financial institutions: Challenges, frameworks, and future directions. *International Journal of Research in Science, Commerce, Arts, Management and Technology.* https://www.semanticscholar.org/paper/04f0b923dfe9f22b261421b11705aa9ea8141f83 (accessed on 17th July 2025).

38. Pasupuleti, V., Thuraka, B., & Kodete, C. S. (2024). Machine learning and big data analytics in smart cities and healthcare: Applications, challenges, and future directions. *2024 International Conference on Computer and Applications (ICCA).* https://www.semanticscholar.org/paper/098b962710e8ff89a449039a75281c85d9484a4f (accessed on 17th July 2025).

39. Alansari, Z. *et al.* (2018). Challenges of Internet of Things and Big Data Integration. In: Miraz, M., Excell, P., Ware, A., Soomro, S., Ali, M. (eds) Emerging Technologies in Computing. iCETiC 2018. Lecture Notes of the Institute for Computer Sciences, Social Informatics and Telecommunications Engineering, vol 200. Springer, Cham. https://doi.org/10.1007/978-3-319-95450-9_4c(accessed on 17th July 2025).

40. Platzer, M. D. (2011). U.S. wind turbine manufacturing: Federal support for an emerging industry. https://core.ac.uk/download/19958933.pdf (accessed on 17th July 2025).

41. Raketla, R. G. (2025). Real-time analytics revolutionizing retail order management. *International Journal of Science and Research Archive.* https://www.semanticscholar.org/paper/d92c67f68852e89134dd2717d5e213f4a9211ef9 (accessed on 17th July 2025).

42. Rishiwal, V., Agarwal, U., Alotaibi, A., Tanwar, S., Yadav, P., & Yadav, M. (2024). Exploring secure V2X communication networks for human-centric security and privacy in smart cities. *IEEE Access, 12*, 138763–138788. https://www.semanticscholar.org/paper/2e21d4a48515073ad495362f197ec5a833857278 (accessed on 17th July 2025).

43. Scandurra, Giuseppe & Romano, Antonio Angelo, 2011. "**The investments in renewable energy sources: do low carbon economies better invest in green technologies?**," MPRA Paper 34216, University Library of Munich, Germany.(accessed on 17th July 2025).

44. Ruggiu, D. (2015). The consolidation process of the EU regulatory framework on nanotechnologies: Within and beyond the EU case-by-case approach. https://core.ac.uk/download/53525097.pdf (accessed on 17th July 2025).

45. Shi, H., Qian, J., Kang, J., Cui, Y., Shao, Y., Bao, K., Fang, L., et al. (2025). Bibliometric analysis of research hotspots and trends in non-contact sleep monitoring. *Journal of Computational Methods in Engineering Applications.* https://www.semanticscholar.org/paper/7f81c4f9b6d6a0bb983cf90d5cfffd739ed8a44f (accessed on 17th July 2025).

46. Storey, V. A., & Wagner, A. (2024). Integrating artificial intelligence (AI) into adult education: Opportunities, challenges, and future directions. https://core.ac.uk/download/618236236.pdf (accessed on 17th July 2025).

47. Sunaryo, D., Hamdan, H., Pramesylia, D. A., Oktariani, W., & Imelda, E. (2025). Digital transformation in financial risk management: Opportunities, challenges, and future trends. *Management Dynamics: International Journal of Management and Digital Sciences.* https://www.semanticscholar.org/paper/86fb0b543be987ed8f0612d54ab101efb0bc94b7 (accessed on 17th July 2025).

INDEX

D

E

N

O

P

U

V

W

X

Z